Policy and Governance of Artificial Intelligence

Principles and Practices

Azamat Ali
Associate Professor, Lovely Professional University
Punjab, India

CRC Press
Taylor & Francis Group
Boca Raton London New York

CRC Press is an imprint of the
Taylor & Francis Group, an **informa** business
A SCIENCE PUBLISHERS BOOK

First edition published 2027
by CRC Press
2385 NW Executive Center Drive, Suite 320, Boca Raton FL 33431

and by CRC Press
4 Park Square, Milton Park, Abingdon, Oxon, OX14 4RN

CRC Press is an imprint of Taylor & Francis Group, LLC

Library of Congress Cataloging-in-Publication Data (applied for)

ISBN: 978-1-041-30896-6 (hbk)
ISBN: 978-1-041-30901-7 (pbk)
ISBN: 978-1-003-77665-9 (ebk)

DOI: 10.1201/9781003776659

Typeset in Times New Roman
by Prime Publishing Services

Preface

The concept of artificial intelligence (AI) has become a common characteristic of modern society. AI systems have begun to be applied in government, business, education, health care, finance, and public administration. They affect the decision-making process, the service delivery process, and the allocation of resources. The issue of responsibility, accountability, and control is also brought to the fore by AI technologies as they grow in size and influence. The concerns have resulted in the development of AI governance as an important field of scholarly research and policy.

AI governance can be described as the guidelines, rules, regulations, and organisation, which govern the design, development, deployment, and management of AI. It aims at making sure that AI systems are run in a manner that is legal, ethical, transparent, and socially valuable. The use of AI requires AI governance since it is not a neutral technology. Human options, information, and institutional settings define AI systems. Through this, they are able to strengthen pre-existing inequalities, bring about new hazards, and redistribute power in manners that are not foreseeable or challenging to challenge.

This book is aimed at creating a layered, simple introduction to AI governance. The book treats AI governance as an interdisciplinary subject, which relates technology, ethics, law, and the general public policy. It will assist the reader in grasping not only the way AI systems work, but also the way they may be managed. The chapters are organised such that they establish a knowledge base incrementally starting with fundamental principles and proceeding to policies of application and future pathways of governance challenges.

In Chapter 1, the fundamental notions of AI governance, its scope, and importance are outlined. It justifies why governance has been critical in the face of the rapid technological change. This chapter sets the structure used in analysis in the rest of the book. Chapter 2 dwells on AI system architecture. It describes the primary technological characteristics that are applicable to governance, data, algorithms, and automated decision-making. The chapter is composed in a way that it is accessible to any reader with no technical background and focuses on relevance to policy making than the engineering specifics.

In Chapter 3, issues of ethical principles in AI are discussed and focused especially on fairness, accountability, and transparency. The role of ethical guidelines in present day governance is also significant in areas where there is no formal regulation (or a regulation is undergoing development). The chapter also discusses the merits of the use of ethics-based AI governance as well as its restrictions. Chapter 4 examines the legal and regulatory cases of AI globally in a comparative manner. It shows the response of various jurisdictions to the opportunities and risks of AI in the form of law and regulation.

Chapter 5 is dedicated to the national strategies of AI and policy implementation. Most governments have come up with national policies to enhance innovation in reducing social and economic risks. The chapter looks at the design of such strategies and their manifestations in the governance practices. Chapter 6 deals with the application of AI in the government. It talks about the possibilities to enhance efficiency and service delivery as well as issues of accountability, transparency, and trust by the population.

In Chapter 7, the authors focus on algorithmic bias and discrimination. It also describes how bias can arise in AI systems, based on data, design decision-making and institutional applications. The chapter also talks of policy instruments and decision-making mechanisms in an attempt to diminish discriminating results. Chapter 8 is about privacy and data governance. Since AI depends on data existing in large quantities, data protection, consent, and surveillance are the key concerns associated with AI governance.

In Chapter 9, the authors examine the issue of the connection of AI and human rights. Automated systems have the potential to violate equality, privacy, expression of freedom, and due process rights. This chapter looks at the ways in which AI governance can be implemented through human rights frameworks. Chapter 10 discusses AI and the future of work. It takes into consideration the impact of automation and algorithmic management on employment, labour conditions, and workforce policy.

Chapter 11 studies how AI has been managed by critical industries such as healthcare, education, and finance. These are areas that have high risks of making decisions and vulnerable groups and should be properly monitored. Chapter 12 is devoted to AI and democracy, and such issues as disinformation, political manipulation, and electoral integrity. Chapter 13 tells the purpose of international organisations and global cooperation in controlling AI.

Chapter 14 highlights the approaches of inclusive/participatory governance. It claims that the proper management of AI cannot be done without the participation of different stakeholders such as civil society and the communities being impacted. The last chapter of Chapter 15 explores the further perspectives of AI policy and governance.

The book is targeted at students, researchers, policymakers, and practitioners. It employs clear and straightforward sentences and an academic tone to render clarity and understanding. Its major thesis is that AI governance is necessary to make sure that AI helps to achieve social well-being, equity, and sustainable development.

Contents

1 Introduction to AI Governance

Concepts, Scope, and Significance

Artificial Intelligence (AI) has turned out to be one of the leading trends determining contemporary society, economies, and regimes. Due to the proliferation of AI technologies in industries, the necessity to establish proper governance has become remarkably important. AI governance offers the systems, concepts, and procedures necessary to make AI systems safe, ethical, and in accordance with human values. This chapter presents the main ideas, the scope, and the relevance of AI governance in an understandable and well-organised way. It describes the principles, the key areas of governance, and functions of key actors, and institutions. Another problem that has emerged, and is mentioned throughout the chapter, is bias, privacy concerns, and transparency, and explains how these challenges can be addressed to advance responsible and human-centred AI development. All in all, it offers a general insight into why AI governance is crucial in the digital era.

1.1 Introduction

Artificial intelligence (AI) has already become one of the most powerful technologies of the 21st century that influences the development of the economy, science, and life in general. In the current state, AI systems are involved in automated decision-making, language processing, prediction, and pattern recognition. These applications have wide use in the fields of healthcare, finance, education, and governance, transport, and communication. The promotion of big data, cloud computing, and machine learning has also increased the use of AI (Abbas Khan et al., 2024). With increased dependence on digital systems by societies, AI is steadily becoming a central element of digital transformation. The possibility to process a great amount of information and generate real-time insights has transformed AI into a vital instrument that can be used to address difficult problems, enhance productivity, and facilitate innovation. Nevertheless, the fast development of AI also contributes to the significant questions of the way these systems are to be designed, monitored, and controlled to be beneficial to society (Brandao, 2025).

The growing use of AI in society, both in government and business, demonstrates the significance of issues of AI governance in AI societies. Facing uncontrolled supervision, AI systems may contribute to unintended harms, such as biased results, intrusion of privacy, misinformation, and unequal resource accessibility. There needs to be governance to make sure that AI technologies are utilised in a responsible, open, and in accordance with societal values (Taeihagh, 2021). Good governance assists in establishing checks and balances to ensure

DOI: 10.1201/9781003776659-1

that individuals and communities are not exposed to any form of danger. It also aids in accountability through the establishment of roles and responsibilities of the developers, organisations, as well as policymakers. Moreover, effective governance systems can help to build goodwill among the population by making AI systems just, secure, and trustworthy. The necessity of adequate governance is even more urgent as AI gains additional penetration in such important areas of life as healthcare, policing, and state administration. The need to govern is thus not just a technical need but also social and ethical necessity (Camilleri, 2024).

The development of AI governance is a sign of the increased awareness of these issues. Back in the early years, AI was discussed primarily in terms of ethical concerns, which include fairness, transparency, and respect of human rights. Numerous international organizations, universities, and technology firms unveiled ethical standards, which were supposed to foster responsible AI practices (Whittlestone & Clarke, 2022). These guidelines focused on values-based strategies; however, these strategies did not usually have formal enforcement mechanisms. With the proliferation of the use of AI applications into sensitive and high-risk regions, policymakers started noticing the fact that ethical recommendations could not be implemented on their own. This transition resulted in the emergence of regulatory frameworks which brought about legal requirements, compliance requirements, and risk-based appraisals (Walter, 2024).

Examples are the AI Act in the European Union, the AI Principles of the OECD, the recommendations on AI ethics of the UNESCO, and new national legislations in countries like the United States and Singapore. Such laws are intended to establish formal mechanisms of assessing AI risks, establishing norms of data utilisation, and providing human control. Formal regulation is a significant step of AI governance maturity, as it implies the transition of ethical discourse to formal regulation. It demonstrates the ways in which the international community is shifting to more complex, binding, and unified frameworks that inform the safe and positive application of AI in contemporary communities (Corrêa et al., 2023).

1.2 Conceptual Foundations of AI Governance

1.2.1 Defining AI Governance: Meaning, Components, and Objectives

AI governance is a term that denotes rules, procedures, and frameworks that inform the development and utilisation of AI. It offers an effective framework of the safe, ethical, and responsible management of AI technologies. AI governance entails technical controls, legal requirements, and organisational policies. It also takes into account social and ethical implications of AI on people and society. AI governance is primarily aimed at ensuring that AI systems do not harm people but benefit them (Ghosh et al., 2025). The elements of AI governance are varied. These are policies that direct developers, and standards assuring quality and control mechanisms that watch the behaviour of AI systems. The other elements involve the risk assessment tools, reporting systems, and independent audits. These are the factors that aid organisations to identify their issues at an early stage and rectify them before they can lead to damages. They also assist in enforcing the fact that AI systems act according to the principles and carry out their functions as planned. These structures of governance involve a number of actors, such as governments, companies, universities, and civil society organisations (Mäntymäki et al., 2022).

AI governance objectives are viable and justifiable. Achieving one of the goals is to decrease the risks that could be produced by the AI systems in terms of unfair decisions or unsafe outcomes. The other goal is to facilitate innovation through establishment of a stable and reliable environment to encourage technological development. The purpose of AI governance is also to make people more trustful, as individuals tend to be more ready to use AI systems, which they think are transparent, fair, and reliable. Another target is to make sure that there is accountability. This involves determining who is to make decisions on AI technologies. Such goals make the system of AI balanced due to the ability to improve it without posing a threat to safety, fairness, and human rights (De Almeida et al., 2021).

1.2.2 Core Principles: Transparency, Accountability, Fairness, Safety, Privacy

AI governance is based on core principles. These principles are used in making decisions at any level of the AI lifecycle. The first principle is transparency. It implies that AI systems also must be comprehensible to people, regulators, and auditors. Transparency can clarify the process of making a decision, the data utilised, and the constraints that can be in place. It builds confidence and assists in finding mistakes and prejudices. Another important principle is accountability. It implies that a person has to be accountable for AI decision consequences. Effective chains of command are used to ensure that issues are solved promptly. Redress and corrective measures in the case of harm are also supported by accountability. Fairness will focus on ensuring that AI systems will not discriminate against particular people or groups of people. AI models are trained on large data and this data can have historical biases. Unless there is a proper government of AI systems, it can repeat or augment these biases. The principles of fairness are intended so that organisations are supposed to test models, find bias, and enhance data quality (Radanliev, 2025).

One of the major principles of AI governance is safety. The AI systems should be dependable and secure particularly in such a risky setting as a hospital, airliners, banks, or authorities. Such safety measures are testing, validation, monitoring, and continuous improvement. The measures can be used to avoid accidents and unintended consequences. AI governance is also focused on privacy. Many AI systems usually need people to operate. The governance should make sure that this information is legally gathered, stored, and utilized. The privacy safeguards can be used to curb the abuse of sensitive data and guard on individual rights.

They also enhance the confidence between users and the AI developers (Hosseini Tabaghdehi & Ayaz, 2025). These are fundamental values that collaborate with the aim of ensuring responsible and trustful AI development.

1.2.3 Distinguishing AI Ethics, AI Regulation, and AI Governance

AI ethics, AI regulation, and AI governance are different concepts related to each other. Their differences can be used to explain why they are involved in the management of AI. The term AI ethics describes moral principles and values in how AI is to be utilised. Fairness, respect, safety, autonomy, and human dignity are some of the ethical principles. Ethical rules will help developers and organisations to consider the social implications of their systems. They are however voluntary and not legally binding. They guide and do not dictate behaviour (Huang et al., 2022). AI regulation is defined as rules which are legally enforceable and which are made by governments or other bodies that regulate. Laws establish the actions to be performed by the organisations in the development or implementation of AI systems. These are transparency, risk assessment requirements, record keeping, and data protection requirements. The regulation also provides punishments against offences. It tries to safeguard the citizens, minimise harm, and establish responsibility (Schuett, 2023). Ethics and regulation are narrower in their scope than AI governance. It comprises ethical values, regulations, institutional policies, and technical controls. Governance offers an integrated structure through which the efforts of the developers, regulators, and institutions are synchronised. It holds AI systems responsible for designing, testing, deploying, and monitoring. As long as ethics gives moral guidance and regulation offers legal action, governance offers long-term organisation, coordination, and control throughout the entire AI ecosystem (Radu, 2021).

1.2.4 Theoretical Perspectives and Governance Models

A number of theoretical views can be used to explain how AI governance can be organised.

The risk based model aims at determining the degree of risk of an AI system. Very critical systems like ones employed in medical diagnosis or law enforcement are to be under tight control, thoroughly documented, and monitored. Less protection is necessary on low risk systems. The model will make governance proportional to harm that may arise (Novelli et al., 2024). The anthropocentric model involves the development of AI around human values. It makes sure AI assists people in decision-making and promoting human welfare. The model aims at the concept of human rights, dignity, inclusivity, and accessibility. It promotes the designs that ensure that man is in command and is not abused (Koval et al., 2025). The Multi-stakeholder governance model focuses on collaboration between governments, companies, academic institutions, civil society organisations, as well as users. AI touches numerous industries, so none of the actors can handle it independently. This model encourages group responsibility and action (Capasso & Umbrello, 2023).

The Adaptive governance model promotes flexibility in the making of policies. AI technologies are changing rapidly, and the policies should keep up with the changes. Adaptive governance promotes frequent changes, constant education, and early detection of emerging concerns. It helps to avoid the out-datedness of the rules (Taeihagh, 2021). The Principles-based model does not have specific but general guidelines. It enables the organisations to make sense of principles like fairness and transparency in a manner that fits the context. The model is flexible and has strong ethical bases (Durante & Floridi, 2022).

1.3 Scope and Domains of AI Governance

1.3.1 Technical Dimensions: Algorithms, Data Quality, Safety, and Security

The technical aspect is concerned with the process of AI system creation, training, testing, and maintenance. This dimension is concerned with algorithms, the data that is being modeled, the safety of AI operations, and the security of systems. It gives the basis to the implementation of ensuring that AI is reliable and does not create unintended damage. AI systems consist of algorithms. The governance demands that the algorithms should be transparent and the user and auditor should be able to comprehend the way of decision-making. This does not necessarily imply the disclosure of source code, but it includes the description of the rationale, inputs, and potential constraints of the model. Using algorithmic transparency allows identifying any unfair tendencies and minimises the possibility of concealed bias. It also facilitates outside audit as well as enhanced decision-making (Jauhiainen & Lehner, 2022). Another factor of technical governance is data quality. AI systems are trained on data, and bad data results in bad outputs. Any incomplete, biased, or inaccurate data may lead to unfair outcomes. Governance demands that organisations should gather quality information that is reflective of the population. It additionally requests the records of data sources and data processing techniques. The responsible use of data can avoid discrimination and enhance the accuracy of the AI forecast (Cheong, 2024).

AI systems require safety and particularly where risks are high. The AI models should be tested in various conditions to make sure that they should work properly. Safety procedures involve checking of models, stress testing, and monitoring after implementation. Such processes aid in detecting failures, unforeseen behaviour, and weaknesses of the system. The sensitivity of the application particularly to healthcare diagnosis, transportation, financial-decision systems, and public administration makes safety measures critical (Gyevnar & Kasirzadeh, 2025). The issue of security is a significant one since AI systems can be hacked or spoilt. Data poisoning, model tampering, or unauthorised access are examples of cyber attacks that can alter the behaviour of the AI models or reveal personal information. AI governance demands high standards of security measures such as encryption, access control, secure storage, and frequent vulnerability testing. Security guarantees that AI systems are reputable and not subjected to any technical or human attacks (Oseni et al., 2021). The technical aspect encompasses the entire AI lifecycle, including the gathering of data to the implementation of a model. It can make sure that systems are safe, fair, transparent, and secure at all levels.

1.3.2 Organisational and Institutional Dimensions: Policies, Standards, and Compliance

The organizational and institutional aspect is concerned with the management of AI in the internal organisation of organisations. It consists of policies, norms, mechanisms of compliance, and responsible management practices, which are used to guide AI development and use. The policies of organisations dictate the responsible use of AI. These policies outline the methods of data collection, testing of AI models, and means of risk management. They also define internal review procedures, duties, and obligations. Policies make employees know what is acceptable and it assists organisations to realise uniformity in the operations of the various departments (Mikalef et al., 2022). The value of standards lies in the fact that they establish similar regulations in the development of AI. A variety of organisations adhere to the international standards that have been introduced by the organisations like the International Organization of Standardization (ISO) or the Institute of Electrical and Electronics Engineers (IEEE). The standards offer the guidelines in the data handling, documentation, model testing and system evaluation. Standards also contribute to the assurance that AI systems created in various organisations should be able to collaborate and reach global standards to be considered as of high quality and safety (De Almeida et al., 2021).

Another significant aspect of institutional governance is compliance. It makes sure that organisations comply with the law, ethics, and internal regulations. Compliance systems encompass periodic audits, risk assessment, documentation, and reporting. These systems assist companies in proving that they are within the regulatory systems. Legal risk is also minimised through compliance since AI systems should comply with data protection legislation, transparency regulations, and accountability (Wirtz et al., 2022). Organizations also need training and capacity building. The developers, managers, and employees should be aware of the AI governance principles. They should be trained about data management, equity, privacy, and risk evaluation. The organisations should also establish means of reporting issues, reporting errors, and handling complaints. Responsible behaviour can be promoted with the help of strong institutional governance, and confidence in AI systems grows among the population. The organisational aspect also makes sure that AI is not just technically healthy but in line with ethical and legal requirements in institutions (Birkstedt et al., 2023).

1.3.3 Societal and Global Dimensions: Human Rights, Public Trust, and International Cooperation

The social and international aspect is concerned with the impact of AI on people, society, and states. It is a matter of guarding human rights, ensuring national trust, as well as fostering international collaboration. One of the key elements of governance in society is human rights. The AI systems should not violate human dignity, autonomy, and equality. The governance structures demand that AI must not discriminate or harm the vulnerable populations. They also help people to make sure that they are in control of personal information and can appeal against unjust rulings. Human rights approach guards human beings against technology abuse and misuse (Randazzo & Hill, 2024). AI technologies are only accepted by the population when they trust them. Individuals will be more willing to embrace AI in case they are sure that systems are just, open, and responsible. Trust construction is possible through unambiguous communication on how AI systems operate, information they use and decision-making. Social engagement, consultations, and feedback systems assist organisations with social issues and enhance AI design (Choung et al., 2023).

Cooperation between countries is required since AI is a universal technology. Data is transferred across the borders and the AI tools created in one country can find their application in a different one. Nations need to collaborate in order to establish similar principles, practices of risk management, and uniform standards. The OECD, UNESCO, and European Union are some of the organisations that help in global governance by proposing some principles of responsible AI. Collaboration assists in minimising regulatory disputes, fosters innovation, and ethical conduct on an international level (Ala-Pietilä & Smuha, 2021). Access and inequality are also societal and global aspects. AI can be beneficial to not all groups equally. There are communities with no digital infrastructure and those characterised by a greater risk of being surveilled or discriminated against. Governance should be able to make AI contribute to social inclusion and not to increase the existing inequalities. This involves policies that expand digital access, provide digital literacy, and cushion marginalised groups against being disadvantaged (Imran, 2023).

1.4 Key Actors, Institutions, and Governance Frameworks

1.4.1 Governmental and Regulatory Authorities

The key players in AI governance are the government and regulatory bodies. They develop laws, regulations, and policy frameworks which dictate the way AI systems should be developed and utilised. The governments also control the working of these rules in order to safeguard the population against any possible damage. Regulators establish legal requirements of those organisations dealing with AI. Such requirements can be those of transparency, risk assessment, data protection, and accountability. Governments also create agencies or committees that are in charge of monitoring AI applications, evaluating risks, and compliance. Indicatively, a few nations have established national AI councils, data protection authorities, or digital regulatory commissions (Taeihagh, 2021). The guidelines on ethical and responsible AI are provided by governments. Such codes promote equity and privacy values and safety. Research and innovation is also aided by the government in terms of funding, national strategies, and capacity-building programmes. They encourage the use of AI and strike a balance between economic objectives and the well-being of the population (Camilleri, 2024). Complaints can also be researched by the regulatory authorities and the violation can be dealt with as well as penalties may be administered when the organisations do not comply with regulations. They play a significant role in ensuring that there is trust and no abuse. The role of governments is to act as the guardians of the common good, and AI is expected to promote the social, economic, and developmental interests safely and responsibly (Züger & Asghari, 2023).

1.4.2 Industry Stakeholders and Standard Setting Bodies

Technology companies are key players in the field of AI governance since they create and implement the majority of AI. These corporations develop algorithms, gather information, develop AI tools, and provide online services. Their choices are directly related to the way AI impacts society (Mäntymäki et al., 2022). Numerous organisations come up with their own internal governance systems. These are moral provisions, risk evaluation instruments, and review procedures. Responsible AI teams and audit systems are also investments made by companies to determine fairness, privacy, and safety. Players in the industry can add technical skills and practical knowledge which can provide a better governance practice. Standard setting authorities are significant in the regulation of industry behaviour. The standards of AI development are offered by organisations like the International Organization of Standards (ISO) and the Institute of Electrical and Electronics Engineers (IEEE). Such standards include data management, algorithmic transparency, system testing, systems documentation, and safety (Oviedo et al., 2024). These standards can be followed to make sure the quality, reliability, and consistency of various AI systems are guaranteed. There are also industry associations and professional associations that help in governance. These organisations facilitate the best practices, exchange knowledge, and come up with common principles of responsible AI. They contribute to increasing awareness about such issues like the bias of the algorithms, threats to privacy, and vulnerabilities of the systems. Other collaborators of technology firms are governments, research institutions, and civil society. They are needed to participate since they possess means, information, and technical abilities to deploy massive AI solutions. Their contribution to governance is hence technical and ethical, which influences the development of AI and its impact on daily life (Kamila & Jasrotia, 2025).

1.4.3 Academia, Civil Society, and Multi-Stakeholder Partnerships

Academia can be a significant part of AI governance because it conducts research, educates, and critiques. Universities generate evidence and theories, as well as technical innovations that facilitate responsible AI. The social, ethical, and legal implications of AI are studied by researchers. They also come up with audit, transparency, and fairness tools. Future professionals who will design and operate AI systems in industry and government are trained in academic institutions (Chan, 2023). The civil society organisations come in with the role of voicing the interests of the people. They ensure that AI is tracked on its impact on communities, promote fairness, human rights, and social inclusions. Civil societies have issues with discrimination, surveillance, breach of privacy, and transparency. They also inform the citizens on risks and enable them to be part of policy deliberations (Moon, 2023).

Multi-stakeholder partnerships involve governments, companies, researchers, and the civil society actors. Such coalitions provide forums of mutual communication and decision-making. These collaborations are essential to AI governance since one actor cannot handle the intricacy of AI independently. The partnership is useful to create a balance among various points of view, avoid conflict, and work out ethical solutions. Multi-stakeholder initiatives can be examples of a national AI task force, international working groups, and ethical advisory boards. These platforms facilitate sharing of knowledge and building coordinated action. They assist in making sure that AI governance possesses a variety of opinions and tries to meet the requirements of various social groups (Dreier et al., 2022). Academia and civil society also assist in keeping the strong institutions in check. Their own research and advocacy efforts help create transparency and oversight and democratic involvement in AI governance.

1.4.4 Global Frameworks: OECD Principles, UNESCO Guidelines, and Risk-Based AI Regulatory Models

AI is technology that is global and regulation would need global collaboration. There are a number of international laws which help to regulate responsible AI practices nationally. OECD AI Principles are common knowledge. The values they advance include fairness, transparency, accountability, human-based design, and sustainable development. The principles make countries create policies that promote innovation without causing harm. Another significant point they make is the significance of international co-operation and adaptive governance (Schmager et al., 2025). UNESCO has come up with international principles on AI ethics. These principles are human rights, dignity, and social justice. They demand transparency, accountability, and good data governance. The methodology of UNESCO aims at safeguarding cultural diversity, limiting inequality, and ensuring that AI is beneficial to every society, even the developing countries (Bean et al., 2025). The EU AI Act has brought about one of the most detailed regulatory frameworks by the European Union. This legislation has a risk based approach with the following categories: unacceptable risk, high risk, limited risk, and minimal risk. Risky systems need to be well documented, tested, manned by human beings, and transparent. The EU AI act provides powerful guidelines on the quality, safety, and accountability of data. It is among the initial significant efforts to control AI on a large scale (Cancela-Outeda, 2024).

Germany is working on its AI regulatory system in a blend of European Union laws and national policy projects. The privacy of personal data and the rights of individuals is regulated by the main law the General Data Protection Regulation (GDPR), which determines the formed data processing and automated decision-making patterns in the field of AI in Germany. Moreover, EU Artificial Intelligence Act (Regulation (EU) 2024/1689) creates a risk-based, harmonised regulatory framework of AI systems in Member States directly affecting the regulatory environment in Germany (Justo-Hanani, 2022). The new national AI strategy of Germany focuses on responsible innovation, human-centric AI, and enhancing research and industrial competitiveness. The system of governance entails coordination between the federal ministries, research agencies, players in the industry, and standardisation of organisations. Germany implements its policies at the international level in line with international frameworks like the OECD AI Principles to establish regulatory coherence and ethical AI development on a global level (Liebig et al., 2024). All these measures are designed to meet the objective of stabilising technological innovation and the preservation of basic rights, legal certainty, and trust of the population.

1.5 Emerging Challenges and Opportunities in AI Governance

1.5.1 Key Risks: Bias, Inequality, Privacy Issues, and Systemic Failures

AI systems also have several risks since they are based on information and algorithms that might not be fair during social realities. Bias is a critical challenge. The AI models are trained on historical data, and in case the information in the historical data is biased, the model generates an unjust decision. This may result in discrimination during hiring, lending, healthcare, policing, and education. Marginalised groups are usually subject to prejudice and thus, governance is required to promote fairness (Nishant et al., 2024). Another significant threat is inequality. The AI technologies can be helpful to the more digitally privileged individuals. The rural population, the poor, and the underserved may not get the same benefits. Consequently, the social inequalities that are already there could increase. There should be inclusiveness and equal access in AI governance (Imran, 2023). The dangers to privacy are considerable since AI systems can be based on huge amounts of data. Such data sets might be personal and sensitive. Bad data management may result in abuse, unauthorised access, profiling, or tracking. These practices force the person into suspicion and contravene the rights of individuals.

Privacy needs to be ensured to ensure that the users are not compromised (Martin & Zimmermann, 2024). Systemic failures are the situations where AI systems act erratically or fail in cases of conditions they have not encountered before. Such failures may result in the damage to some very sensitive fields like healthcare or transport. Certain system failures may propagate to adjacent systems causing massive outages. Such failures should be minimised by making governance demand testing, validation, and constant monitoring (Macrae, 2022). Table 1.1 summarises how each risk arises and what governance actions are required to mitigate harm.

Table 1.1 Key Risks in AI Governance and Their Implications.

Risk Type	*Description*	*Possible Harm*	*Governance Need*
Bias	Model outcomes influenced by unfair data patterns	Discrimination, unequal treatment	Fairness testing, data audits
Inequality	Unequal access to AI technologies	Wider digital divide, social exclusion	Inclusion policies, digital access programmes
Privacy Issues	Misuse or leakage of sensitive personal data	Surveillance, identity theft, loss of autonomy	Strong data protection and consent rules
Systemic Failures	Errors or breakdowns in AI performance	Safety risks, financial losses, system instability	Continuous monitoring and safety checks

1.5.2 *Ethical and Societal Dilemmas: Labour Impact, Surveillance, and Trust*

Ethical dilemmas and social problems that the AI systems introduce are complicated and should be governed carefully. The fact that labour is changing is one of the biggest dilemmas. Automation using AI can substitute human labour during the production process, transportation, customer services, and administration. Although AI provides new employment opportunities in the sphere of data science, robotics, and analytics, it decreases the number of low skilled workers. This generates destabilisation of the economy. The ability to govern should facilitate the armed forces to acquire skills, job transition schemes, and equitable labour regulations (Camilleri, 2024). Another ethical issue is surveillance. People can be monitored with the help of AI tools, like facial recognition, tracking their behaviour, and predictive analytics. They are tools that can be used to aid the cause of public safety, but breach the privacy and civil liberties. In the absence of an appropriate governance system, surveillance technologies can be employed to control or discriminate against politics. There should be clear regulations on what surveillance should be permitted, who will own the data, and the duration of storage (Fontes et al., 2022).

One of the key problems of AI acceptance is trust. The reluctance to use AI systems by many people is caused by their lack of understanding of how the decisions are made. The absence of transparency decreases trust. There are also previous examples of discriminatory or unsafe AI, which influence perception. To achieve trust, one has to explain things clearly, communicate honestly and be accountable. The users should have the ability to challenge AI decisions and obtain corrections when needed (Choung et al., 2023). Ethical dilemmas are not usually simple to solve. They also demand respectful communication, inclusive policy making, as well as the involvement of various players such as societies that are impacted by AI systems.

1.5.3 Opportunities: Enhancing Innovation, Safety, and Responsible Digital Transformation

Challenges are not the only issues that AI governance deals with. It also provides significant opportunities. The first opportunity is safe and sustainable innovation promotion. Well-formed governance frameworks give business enterprises a sense of direction in the way they should create ethical and trustworthy AI. This stability promotes investment, research, and technological expansion. Once people have confidence in an AI system, that adoption will rise, resulting in significant innovation (Alhosani & Alhashmi, 2024). Safety also is enhanced in AI applications by governance. AI has the potential to assist in medical diagnostics, climate change, disaster management, and transport systems. The robust safety protocols will make AI tools work in such high impact industries. Periodic checks and balances enhance the quality of a system and eliminate malicious errors (Ali, 2025). The other opportunity is accountable digital transformation. Through its appropriate governance, AI can assist governments to deliver better services to the people, control urban infrastructure, support learning, and promote agriculture. Digital transformation is led with ethical considerations in place, so that AI does not serve the privileged groups but everyone. AI is also capable of helping to achieve accessibility by speech recognition, automatic translation, and assistive technologies (Yigitcanlar et al., 2024).

Another valuable opportunity is international cooperation. Nations are able to exchange best practices and come up with unified principles. The international collaboration limits the conflict among various regulatory systems and enhances the formation of equitable international standards. International collaboration is achieved by institutions like the OECD and UN agencies, UNESCO, and others (von Ingersleben-Seip, 2023). Governance is also useful in assisting organisations to enhance internal operations. It promotes ethical design, responsible use of data, and human supervision. The practices mitigate against risks and enhance organisational credibility. AI governance thus promotes safety and invention, which forms a balanced technological landscape (Ghosh et al., 2025).

1.6 Conclusion

The concept of AI has become an integral part of society in many respects. This change opens up new opportunities which can be utilised in innovation, efficiency and better decision-making. Nevertheless, it presents the risks of fairness, privacy, human rights, and the trust of the people. The necessity of effective and responsible leadership is evident, with AI still determining the economic system, public services, and life. The principles of governance including transparency, accountability, safety, and fairness should be understood well to make sure that AI can be used to benefit people without harming them. Governance should also be concerned with technical considerations, institutional tasks, and social effects. It needs intergovernmental, inter-industry, inter-research, and inter-civil society collaboration to establish common standards and safeguard the good of the people. The spread of AI governance systems on the global stage is an indication of a greater realisation of challenges and opportunities. The major risks include prejudice, discrimination, and breach of privacy that should be strictly controlled. Simultaneously, governance may promote innovation that contributes to social and economic development. Overall, AI development will be responsible and human-centred to govern to achieve results that would ensure equality, security, and long-term sustainability.

References

Abbas Khan, M., Khan, H., Omer, M.F., Ullah, I. and Yasir, M. (2024). Impact of artificial intelligence on the global economy and technology advancements. In: *Artificial General Intelligence (AGI) Security: Smart Applications and Sustainable Technologies* (pp. 147– 180). Singapore: Springer Nature Singapore. https://doi.org/10.1007/978-981-97-3222-7_7.

Ala-Pietilä, P. and Smuha, N.A. (2021). A framework for global cooperation on artificial intelligence and its governance. In: *Reflections on Artificial Intelligence for Humanity* (pp. 237–265). Cham: Springer International Publishing. https://doi.org/10.1007/978-3-030-69128-8_15.

Alhosani, K. and Alhashmi, S.M. (2024). Opportunities, challenges, and benefits of AI innovation in government services: A review. *Discover Artificial Intelligence*, *4*(1), 18. https://doi.org/10.1007/s44163-024-00111-w.

Ali, A. (2025). Ethical Implications of Artificial Intelligence: Ensuring Patient Data Security. In: *Transforming Healthcare Sector Through Artificial Intelligence and Environmental Sustainability* (pp. 149–164). Singapore: Springer Nature Singapore. https://doi.org/10.1007/978-981-97-9555-0_8.

Bean, E., Burleigh, C., Haskell, C., Burris-Melville, T., Payne, J. and Pathak, B. (2025). Eavesdropping on UNESCO AI Policy, Leadership, and Ethics. *Journal of Leadership Studies*, *18*(4), 98–110. https://doi.org/10.1002/jls.70007.

Birkstedt, T., Minkkinen, M., Tandon, A. and Mäntymäki, M. (2023). AI governance: Themes, knowledge gaps, and future agendas. *Internet Research*, *33*(7), 133–167. https://doi.org/10.1108/INTR-01-2022-0042.

Brandao, P.R. (2025). The impact of artificial intelligence on modern society. *AI*, *6*(8), 190. https://doi.org/10.3390/ai6080190.

Camilleri, M.A. (2024). Artificial intelligence governance: Ethical considerations and implications for social responsibility. *Expert Systems*, *41*(7), e13406. https://doi.org/10.1111/exsy.13406.

Cancela-Outeda, C. (2024). The EU's AI act: A framework for collaborative governance. *Internet of Things*, *27*, 101291. https://doi.org/10.1016/j.iot.2024.101291.

Capasso, M. and Umbrello, S. (2023). Big tech corporations and AI: A social license to operate and multi-stakeholder partnerships in the digital age. In: *The Ethics of Artificial Intelligence for the Sustainable Development Goals* (pp. 231–249). Cham: Springer International Publishing. https://doi.org/10.1007/978-3-031-21147-8_13.

Chan, C.K.Y. (2023). A comprehensive AI policy education framework for university teaching and learning. *International Journal of Educational Technology in Higher Education*, *20*(1), 38. https://doi.org/10.1186/s41239-023-00408-3.

Cheong, B.C. (2024). Transparency and accountability in AI systems: Safeguarding well-being in the age of algorithmic decision-making. *Frontiers in Human Dynamics*, *6*, 1421273. https://doi.org/10.3389/fhumd.2024.1421273.

Choung, H., David, P. and Ross, A. (2023). Trust in AI and its role in the acceptance of AI technologies. *International Journal of Human–Computer Interaction*, *39*(9), 1727–1739. https://doi.org/10.1080/10447318.2022.2050543.

Corrêa, N.K., Galvão, C., Santos, J.W., Del Pino, C., Pinto, E.P., Barbosa, C., ... & de Oliveira, N. (2023). Worldwide AI ethics: A review of 200 guidelines and recommendations for AI governance. *Patterns*, *4*(10). 100857.

De Almeida, P.G.R., Dos Santos, C.D. and Farias, J.S. (2021). Artificial intelligence regulation: A framework for governance. *Ethics and Information Technology*, *23*(3), 505–525. https://doi.org/10.1007/s10676-021-09593-z.

Dreier, V., Gelissen, T., Oliveira, M., Riezebos, S., Saxena, R., Sibal, P. and Yang, S.Y. (2022). *Multi-stakeholder AI development: 10 Building Blocks for Inclusive Policy Design*. UNESCO Publishing.

Durante, M. and Floridi, L. (2022). A legal principles-based framework for AI liability regulation. In: *The 2021 Yearbook of the Digital Ethics Lab* (pp. 93–112). Cham: Springer International Publishing. https://doi.org/10.1007/978-3-031-09846-8_7.

Fontes, C., Hohma, E., Corrigan, C.C. and Lütge, C. (2022). AI-powered public surveillance systems: why we (might) need them and how we want them. *Technology in Society*, *71*, 102137. https://doi.org/10.1016/j.techsoc.2022.102137.

Ghosh, A., Saini, A. and Barad, H. (2025). Artificial intelligence in governance: Recent trends, risks, challenges, innovative frameworks, and future directions. *AI & Society*, 1–23. https://doi.org/10.1007/s00146-025-02312-y.

Gyevnar, B. and Kasirzadeh, A. (2025). AI safety for everyone. *Nature Machine Intelligence*, 1–12. https://doi.org/10.1038/s42256-025-01020-y.

Hosseini Tabaghdehi, S.A. and Ayaz, Ö. (2025). AI ethics in action: A circular model for transparency, accountability, and inclusivity. *Journal of Managerial Psychology*. https://doi.org/10.1108/JMP-03-2024-0177.

Huang, C., Zhang, Z., Mao, B. and Yao, X. (2022). An overview of artificial intelligence ethics. *IEEE Transactions on Artificial Intelligence*, *4*(4), 799–819. https://doi.org/10.1109/TAI.2022.3194503.

Imran, A. (2023). Why addressing digital inequality should be a priority. *The Electronic Journal of Information Systems in Developing Countries*, *89*(3), e12255. https://doi.org/10.1002/isd2.12255.

Jauhiainen, T. and Lehner, O.M. (2022). Good governance of AI and big data processes in accounting and auditing. In: *Artificial Intelligence in Accounting* (pp. 119–181). Routledge.

Justo-Hanani, R. (2022). The politics of Artificial Intelligence regulation and governance reform in the European Union. *Policy Sciences*, *55*(1), 137–159. https://doi.org/10.1007/s11077-022-09452-8.

Kamila, M.K. and Jasrotia, S. S. (2025). Ethical issues in the development of artificial intelligence: Recognizing the risks. *International Journal of Ethics and Systems*, *41*(1), 45–63. https://doi.org/10.1108/IJOES-05-2023-0107.

Koval, E., Zhadunova, N. and Martynova, M. (2025, May). Artificial Intelligence Ethics: Anthropocentric Approach. In: *2025 IEEE Ural-Siberian Conference on Biomedical*

Engineering, Radioelectronics, and Information Technology (*USBEREIT*) (pp. 45–48). IEEE. https://doi.org/10.1109/USBEREIT65494.2025.11054203.

Liebig, L., Güttel, L., Jobin, A. and Katzenbach, C. (2024). Subnational AI policy: Shaping AI in a multi-level governance system. *AI & Society*, *39*(3), 1477–1490. https://doi.org/10.1007/s00146-022-01561-5.

Macrae, C. (2022). Learning from the failure of autonomous and intelligent systems: Accidents, safety, and sociotechnical sources of risk. *Risk Analysis*, *42*(9), 1999–2025. https://doi.org/10.1111/risa.13850.

Mäntymäki, M., Minkkinen, M., Birkstedt, T. and Viljanen, M. (2022). Defining organizational AI governance. *AI and Ethics*, *2*(4), 603–609. https://doi.org/10.1007/s43681-022-00143-x.

Martin, K.D. and Zimmermann, J. (2024). Artificial intelligence and its implications for data privacy. *Current Opinion in Psychology*, *58*, 101829. https://doi.org/10.1016/j.copsyc.2024.101829.

Mikalef, P., Conboy, K., Lundström, J.E. and Popovič, A. (2022). Thinking responsibly about responsible AI and 'the dark side' of AI. *European Journal of Information Systems*, *31*(3), 257–268. https://doi.org/10.1080/0960085X.2022.2026621.

Moon, M.J. (2023). Searching for inclusive artificial intelligence for social good: Participatory governance and policy recommendations for making AI more inclusive and benign for society. *Public Administration Review*, *83*(6), 1496–1505. https://doi.org/10.1111/puar.13648.

Nishant, R., Schneckenberg, D. and Ravishankar, M.N. (2024). The formal rationality of artificial intelligence-based algorithms and the problem of bias. *Journal of Information Technology*, *39*(1), 19–40. https://doi.org/10.1177/02683962231176842.

Novelli, C., Casolari, F., Rotolo, A., Taddeo, M. and Floridi, L. (2024). AI risk assessment: A scenario-based, proportional methodology for the AI act. *Digital Society*, *3*(1), 13. https://doi.org/10.1007/s44206-024-00095-1.

Oseni, A., Moustafa, N., Janicke, H., Liu, P., Tari, Z. and Vasilakos, A. (2021). Security and privacy for artificial intelligence: Opportunities and challenges. *arXiv preprint arXiv:2102.04661*. https://doi.org/10.48550/arXiv.2102.04661.

Oviedo, J., Rodriguez, M., Trenta, A., Cannas, D., Natale, D. and Piattini, M. (2024). ISO/IEC quality standards for AI engineering. *Computer Science Review*, *54*, 100681. https://doi.org/10.1016/j.cosrev.2024.100681.

Radanliev, P. (2025). AI ethics: Integrating transparency, fairness, and privacy in AI development. *Applied Artificial Intelligence*, *39*(1), 2463722. https://doi.org/10.1080/08839514.2025.2463722.

Radu, R. (2021). Steering the governance of artificial intelligence: National strategies in perspective. *Policy and Society*, *40*(2), 178–193. https://doi.org/10.1080/14494035.2021.1929728.

Randazzo, M.S. and Hill, G. (2024). Human dignity in the age of Artificial Intelligence: An overview of legal issues and regulatory regimes. *Australian Journal of Human Rights*, *30*(3), 386–408. https://doi.org/10.1080/1323238X.2025.2483822.

Schmager, S., Pappas, I.O. and Vassilakopoulou, P. (2025). Understanding Human-Centred AI: A review of its defining elements and a research agenda. *Behaviour & Information Technology*, 1–40. https://doi.org/10.1080/0144929X.2024.2448719.

Schuett, J. (2023). Defining the scope of AI regulations. *Law, Innovation, and Technology*, *15*(1), 60–82. https://doi.org/10.1080/17579961.2023.2184135.

Taeihagh, A. (2021). Governance of artificial intelligence. *Policy and Society*, *40*(2), 137-157. https://doi.org/10.1080/14494035.2021.1928377.

von Ingersleben-Seip, N. (2023). Competition and cooperation in artificial intelligence standard setting: Explaining emergent patterns. *Review of Policy Research*, *40*(5), 781–810. https://doi.org/10.1111/ropr.12538.

Walter, Y. (2024). Managing the race to the moon: Global policy and governance in Artificial Intelligence regulation: A contemporary overview and an analysis of socioeconomic consequences. *Discover Artificial Intelligence*, *4*(1), 14. https://doi.org/10.1007/s44163-024-00109-.4

Whittlestone, J. and Clarke, S. (2022). AI challenges for society and ethics. In: *The Oxford Handbook of AI Governance* (pp. 45–64). New York, NY: Oxford University Press.

Wirtz, B.W., Weyerer, J.C. and Kehl, I. (2022). Governance of artificial intelligence: A risk and guideline-based integrative framework. *Government Information Quarterly*, *39*(4), 101685. https://doi.org/10.1016/j.giq.2022.101685.

Yigitcanlar, T., David, A., Li, W., Fookes, C., Bibri, S.E. and Ye, X. (2024). Unlocking artificial intelligence adoption in local governments: Best practice lessons from real-world implementations. *Smart Cities*, *7*(4), 1576–1625. https://doi.org/10.3390/smartcities7040064.

Züger, T. and Asghari, H. (2023). AI for the public. How public interest theory shifts the discourse on AI. *AI & Society*, *38*(2), 815–828. https://doi.org/10.1007/s00146-022-01480-5.

2 The Architecture of AI
Understanding the Technology behind the Policy

The chapter provides the technological foundations to consider how AI architecture supports policy and governance discussion. The components that define intelligent behaviour include key aspects of AI systems, namely, algorithms, data, computational models, and infrastructure. The chapter underscores the importance of machine learning, deep learning, and natural language processing, as the basis of modern AI applications. It highlights the role of data quality, training, and computational resources in defining system performance and reliability. This chapter illustrates the reasoning behind the necessity of comprehending AI design to regulate and govern AI ethically and responsibly by connecting technical structures to social policy and policy outcomes. Technical decisions in areas like healthcare, teaching, and finance are examples of how the decisions can be positively impactful. Altogether, the discussion paints a clearer picture of how technology is a driver of policy needs and why governance structures should be enlightened by technical realities.

2.1 Introduction

Artificial intelligence (AI) currently ranks among the strongest technologies of the 21st century. It is applied in many areas such as healthcare, education, finance, transportation, and governance. To comprehend the functioning of AI and how it can be controlled, it is vital to pay attention to its inner structures. AI architecture is the design of AI systems, including algorithms, data, computation models, and infrastructure that together generate intelligent behaviour (Serrano, 2022). As the architecture of a building dictates how you use that building, so will the architecture of AI dictate how you use it and the risks and benefits thereof. Accordingly, the task of defining AI architecture is not simply a technical problem, but also a starting point in policy and governance debates.

The applicability of AI architecture to governance is easily justified: policies strive to govern outcomes that are tightly linked to system design. Here are a few examples of how fairness in automated decision-making can be ensured based on training data and algorithm design. Transparency needs systems that can be interpreted or explained, a decision that was made during the development of these systems (Camilleri, 2024). The key to accountability depends on the capability to trace and audit AI decision paths, which can only occur when the system has been designed to permit it. Policymakers lack the awareness of the architectural properties that shape system behaviour, hence they are unable to develop efficient rules to govern fairness, privacy, and accountability (Novelli et al., 2024).

DOI: 10.1201/9781003776659-2

The policy/technology design relationship can also be observed when it comes to the topic of bias and discrimination. Biased data can be used to train AI systems that can generate or even exacerbate inequalities in society. Technical solutions can be closely related to policy solutions, like training data diversification or adding fairness constraints to algorithms. In the same manner, AI systems should process, store, and collect data on the basis of informed data protection and privacy policies (Villegas-Ch & Garcia-Ortiz, 2023). The quality of privacy regulations depends on technical decisions, such as data anonymisation, encryption, and secure storage. Therefore, the governance constructions are intimately connected with the technology design options of AI architecture (Neuwirth, 2024).

Scalability and deployment of AI systems is another connection between policy and architecture. Large-scale computing, facilitated by cloud computing and edge devices, and the high performance computational resources is often needed by AI applications. The exploitation of these infrastructures creates concerns of energy use, digital divide, and cross national data flows. Policies around sustainability, equity, and international cooperation should be informed by technical realities of AI infrastructure, unless regulation will be overly responsive or fail to control underlying risks (Bolte & Van Wynsberghe, 2025).

Lastly, by gaining insight into AI architecture, one can look at AI prospects and opportunities equally. On the one hand, recent progress in deep learning and natural language processing (NLP) is facilitating innovation never seen before. Conversely, these innovations bring with them complexity, opaqueness, and vulnerability to abuse. The principles of governance must be anchored on a good understanding of how AI systems are constructed. Connecting technical foundations to policy agendas may help policymakers construct structures that are pragmatic and can keep up with the fast pace of technological advancements (Nordström, 2022). It is this view that allows this chapter to proceed: there is no way to think of AI policy without the architecture that constitutes it.

2.2 Core Components of AI Systems

AI systems are composed of several key components that dictate their functionality, their output, and their controllability. These basic building blocks are algorithms, data, computing infrastructure, and feedback loops. All these components contribute to the behaviour of AI systems and affect the risks and opportunities posed by the system. These constituents need to be understood in order to create governance structures that will tackle technical and social challenges.

2.2.1 Algorithms

The core of any AI system is algorithms, which are sets of rules or instructions that a system follows to process input and generate output. The initial AIs used were based on rule-based algorithms where human experts coded logical rules to determine actions. These systems were simple and predictable, but they were not well equipped to deal with complex or changing environments. Systems of rules could be used only within the domain of human coded knowledge, which restricted their application in dynamic scenarios (Rao et al., 2024).

The next step in AI evolution was machine learning algorithms, which allow the systems to learn patterns based on the data and not just rely on a set of rules. Machine learning involves training algorithms to identify patterns or relationships and make predictions on data sets.

This is a more versatile and robust method, because the system can infer the new information based on other rules outside the fixed rules. These are decision trees, support vector machines, and clustering algorithms (Sarker, 2021). Deep learning is another development that makes use of multi layered artificial neural networks. The use of deep learning algorithms has provided advances in NLP, computer vision, and speech recognition. They are very good at unstructured data (images, text, and audio). However, deep learning systems are regarded as black boxes since understanding the rationale behind its decision is not readily accessible, which makes them an area of concern regarding accountability and governance (Montesinos Lopez et al., 2022). Overall, although algorithms underpin AI systems, their nature and design have a direct impact on questions of interpretability, fairness, and reliability.

2.2.2 Data

Data is the second key element of AI systems. Depending on the information fed to it, AI systems learn, develop, and generate valuable output. Information may be structured or unstructured. Data are grouped into predetermined sequences (e.g., in rows and columns) like financial reports or demographics, and are therefore simpler to store and manipulate. Unstructured data, such as text files, photos, videos, or social media posts, do not have this prearranged structure and are more difficult to process; however, they may have more profound insights needed in advanced AI use. The quality of data is essential to the performance of an AI system. Poor quality data: Data that is not complete, biased, or accurate results in poor models and incorrect results. Hiring or lending algorithm training data can be biased, and missing medical records may provide erroneous healthcare predictions. Thus, an essential element of AI governance consists of strong data quality management (Ali, 2025a; Whang et al., 2023). The next important detail is the data pipeline: the mechanism of gathering, cleaning, storing, and providing the data to AI models. Good data pipelines guarantee a continuous, high quality, secure information flow between source and system. Governance should focus on all stages of this process to maintain privacy, equity, and compliance with the law (Aldoseri et al., 2023).

2.2.3 Computational Infrastructure

AI systems require powerful computational infrastructure to operate. This comprises hardware elements, such as processors, memory, and storage devices that enable algorithms to process a large amount of data. Modern deep learning models and models with higher complexity may surpass the power of traditional CPUs (central processing units). Consequently, dedicated hardware, such as graphics processing units (GPUs), and tensor processing units (TPUs), optimised to perform parallel tasks, have become widespread in AI development. Besides hardware, the cloud computing platforms become a fundamental component in AI development and deployment. Cloud computing offers scalable infrastructure that enables companies to train and deploy AI models without having to maintain costly physical infrastructure. Another potential application of cloud platforms in collaboration is access to data and tools through shared accessibility (Prangon & Wu, 2024).

Another emerging infrastructure paradigm is edge computing, wherein AI processing is done on local devices (e.g., smartphones, sensors, or autonomous vehicles) and not on centralised servers in the cloud. By making data more accessible to its source, edge computing can bring down latency, better efficiency, and privacy. But it does cause difficulties with standardisation, security, and interoperability (Singh et al., 2022). The performance and scalability of AI systems is therefore supported by computational infrastructure. Algorithms and data are not the only aspects of governance to be considered, but resources and infrastructure enabling massive AI should also be taken into account.

2.2.4 Feedback Loops and System Adaptability

AI systems are not fixed but developed through a feedback process. The feedback loop is a situation in which the output of a system affects other future inputs or the behaviour of the system. Supervised learning uses feedback through comparison of assumptions to real performance and makes changes to the model to meet the goal. In reinforcement learning, the agent trains through trial and error, where the agent is rewarded or punished to inform them on how to act next. AI systems can adjust to changing conditions due to feedback loops, though there are dangers to this. When feedback relies on poor or skewed data, an AI system may solidify malicious behaviour in the long run. An illustrative case is that a predictive policing algorithm that was taught discriminatory crime data can over-police some communities and perpetuate a cycle of discrimination. Likewise, the existence of recommendation systems can lead to the formation of so-called echo chambers, which strengthen the preconceived notions of a user, which in turn may strengthen misinformation or extremist beliefs (Arriagada-Bruneau et al., 2025). Flexibility is strength but it is also a weakness: it allows AI systems to become better and better, but this also makes their actions less predictable and more difficult to control. Therefore, the governance should incorporate all the monitoring, auditing, and correcting loops, and ensure that they do not generate any unintended effects.

2.3 Machine Learning and Deep Learning Foundations

Current AI systems are mostly developed using machine learning and deep learning algorithms to achieve difficult tasks. These techniques allow machines to identify a pattern in the data and reach a prediction or decision even without being coded to handle all cases. It is important to understand these foundations in order to identify the opportunities they bring with them as well as the issue of governance they present.

2.3.1 *Supervised, Unsupervised, and Reinforcement Learning Models*

There are three general types of machine learning models: supervised learning, unsupervised learning, and reinforcement learning (Morales & Escalante, 2022). In supervised learning, the model is trained on data that is labelled and, in other words, all inputs have a correct output. An example would be to train a medical diagnosis system on X-ray images classified as either diseased or healthy. Through these examples, the algorithm is able to make predictions about labels of new and previously unknown data. Supervised learning is also popular in spam detection, credit scoring, and image classification tasks. No labelled outputs are given in unsupervised learning. The model itself has to discover patterns or groupings in the data that were not evident. As an example, without labels, customers can be grouped based on purchasing behaviour by clustering algorithms. Unsupervised learning can apply to market segmentation, anomaly identification, and exploratory data analysis. Nevertheless, since ground truth cannot be evaluated, it may be difficult to assess unsupervised methods results. Reinforcement learning works based on trial and error. An agent acts on an environment and learns through feedback in terms of rewards or penalties to its behaviour. An illustrative example is a robot controlling a maze, where it can learn what actions result in successful behaviour by positive or negative feedback. There have been significant successes in applying reinforcement learning to game playing (e.g., AlphaGo), and it is used in robotics, autonomous driving, and resource optimisation (Souchleris et al., 2023).

2.3.2 *Neural Networks: Architecture, Layers, and Training Processes*

Deep learning is a branch of machine learning that relies on artificial neural networks that are based on the structure of the human brain. A neural network is a system of networked layers of computing nodes (neurons). In most cases, an input layer receives raw data (e.g., pixel values of an image or words of a text). The data is then transformed by a series of multiple less obvious layers, using mathematical functions to extract progressively more abstract features. Lastly, the result of prediction or classification appears as an output layer. The process of training a neural network consists in balancing the connection weights among neurons with the goal of reducing errors. It does this by a process termed back propagation wherein the prediction of the model is checked against the actual result and the difference is propagated backward to the network to adjust weights.

By repeating this process a number of times, the network becomes increasingly accurate. Deep learning has many hidden layers, making them able to represent patterns that are much more complex in data, but also more computationally costly and less interpretable (Montesinos Lopez et al., 2022).

2.3.3 Advances in Deep Learning: CNNs, RNNs, and Transformers

Current advances in deep learning have given rise to neural network architectures that perform well on some data types. CNNs are created to process images and videos. They apply convolutional layers which serve as filters to identify visual patterns of various complexity including edges, shapes and textures. Applications such as facial recognition and medical image analysis use CNNs, and even the vision of self-driving vehicles (Krichen, 2023). RNNs are constructed to process sequential data, including speech or text. They retain some kind of memory of past inputs, hence they can encode context across sequences (e.g., sentences or time series). However, classical RNNs do not work with very long sequences because it is difficult to maintain long term dependencies (Das et al., 2023).

In 2017, NLP was transformed by the introduction of the Transformer architecture. Transformers, in contrast to RNNs, simultaneously process input sequences and weigh the relevance of various aspects of the input, including attention (Myers et al., 2024). This breakthrough facilitated massive language models like BERT and GPT that perform impressively on various tasks including translation, summarisation, and conversational AI (Annepaka and Pakray, 2025). All these architectures promise enormous potentials, yet bring with them new governance challenges. (convolutional neural networks) (CNN)-enabled surveillance systems are privacy threatening, and giant Transformer-based models require massive computing power, creating problems in both environmental and equity practices.

2.3.4 Implications for Scalability, Interpretability, and Trustworthiness

Although machine learning and deep learning are potent tools, governance problems also arise and must be faced (Li et al., 2022).

- **Scalability:** The current AI models have the potential to use large amounts of data and scale globally, driving innovation but also creating concerns about resource concentration, energy usage, and expanding the digital divide.
- **Interpretability:** It is a property of many designed models, especially deep neural networks, to be black boxes. Their inner processes are sophisticated and difficult to comprehend, making it hard to hold them to account in sensitive areas such as health care or law enforcement.
- **Reliability:** Public confidence in AI requires performance and transparency. Even the most precise models cannot be relied upon when they make their decisions behind closed doors. Things that are explainable, assessable, and safeguarded against abuse are needed to create trust.

The policymakers need to look at what such complicated models can do and how their technical features meet ethical and social values. Governance options like a mandate to be interpretable, evaluate energy consumption, or make AI technology accessible equitably are critical as AI systems grow. Table 2.1 summarises the major types of machine learning approaches, their definitions, common applications, and key governance challenges linked to fairness, accountability, and transparency.

Table 2.1 Machine Learning Paradigms: Definitions, Examples, and Governance Implications.

Type	*Definition*	*Examples*	*Governance Implications*
Supervised Learning	Learns from labelled input output pairs.	Spam filters, medical diagnosis, credit scoring.	Bias in training data may lead to unfair outcomes.
Unsupervised Learning	Finds hidden patterns in unlabeled data.	Market segmentation, anomaly detection.	Lack of ground truth makes evaluation difficult, potentially leading to unreliable use.
Reinforcement Learning	Learns through trial and error with feedback.	Robotics, self-driving cars, game AI.	Decisions may be unpredictable or unsafe in real world scenarios without proper constraints.
Deep Learning (CNNs, RNNs, Transformers)	Learns complex patterns using multi layer neural networks.	Image recognition, language models, translation.	High complexity leads to opaqueness and heavy resource demands, raising issues of transparency, privacy, and fairness.

2.4 Natural Language Processing and Computer Vision

AI has gone a long way to allow machines to process human words and images. NLP and computer vision are two prominent fields, driving AI to the level of human communication and perception. NLP is concerned with making machines interpret, understand, and generate human language, whereas computer vision allows machines to interpret and extract meaning out of images and video. Applications based on these technologies include machine translation, medical image analysis, surveillance systems, and generative text modelling, among others. NLP and computer vision are everywhere in governance, business, healthcare, education, and in everyday life, no longer limited to research laboratories. Yet, they also introduce additional challenges in governance, such as bias, transparency, privacy, and accountability.

2.4.1 Overview of Natural Language Processing

NLP is designed to help computers understand and produce human language. The initial NLP systems were programmed rule-driven systems with manually crafted dictionaries and grammar rules. Although these systems may have been able to process simple tasks such as part of speech tagging, they had difficulty with ambiguity, slang, and context. Machine learning techniques brought progress to the field as systems learned language patterns based on the data they had received instead of being limited to a fixed set of rules. The focus of modern NLP is language models. Conventionally, short sequences of word probabilities based on n-grams have been used to capture long-range dependencies or complex contexts, which were not as effective. Later, recurrent neural networks (RNNs) enabled sequential patterns to be learned, but they continued to suffer long-term dependencies. The breakthrough was the Transformer architecture (circa 2017), which relies on attention mechanisms to establish the importance of words in context. Powerful models were developed based on transformers, including BERT, GPT, and T5, which are highly accurate and fluent at solving complex language problems (Myers et al., 2024; Annepaka & Pakray, 2025).

Semantic analysis is another important component of NLP. It attempts to go beyond a superficial level of word recognition to meaning, intent, and relationships. Semantic analysis can allow machines to derive sentiment in a social media post, discover themes in policy documents, or detect relationships in legal texts, which give more contextual and accurate results (Qian et al., 2022). Generative AI has also revolutionised NLP. Big language models can generate human-like text that is coherent. They are able to write essays, summarize long papers, answer questions, and even create original material such as poetry or stories. These capabilities hold potential uses in education, journalism, business communication, and policy formulation. The risks associated with generative AI also include the spread of false data, creation of harmful or biased content, and the threat to conventional ideas of who is an author and the ownership of intellectual assets (Golec & Hachaj, 2025).

2.4.2 Applications of NLP

NLP methods find their applications in multiple fields and are now some of the most common AI technologies (Shrivastava et al., 2025). Key applications include:

- **Text Mining:** NLP systems have the ability to compute large amounts of unstructured text (e.g., research articles, news stories, social media posts) to extract patterns, trends, or new problems. As an example, in case of a general health crisis, text mining can assist governments with identifying issues of interest to citizens and tracking the evolution of discussions on the topic.
- **Machine Translation:** Machine translators such as Google Translate and DeepL translate dozens of languages in real-time using powerful language models (transformers). A better machine translation eases international trade, diplomacy, and cross cultural communication.
- **Chatbots and Virtual Assistants:** Voice or text-based assistants (e.g., Siri, Alexa, customer service chatbots) use NLP to interpret user requests and answer in a natural way. Chatbots can be used in governance to provide public

services, address the questions of citizens (such as taxes or administrative procedures), and lead people in bureaucracy.

- **Policy Analysis:** NLP tools are used by policy makers to examine legal documents or legislative records or comments by people. An example of how NLP can be used is to divide citizen responses and generalise their opinions during public consultations using NLP to guide decision-makers on which issues or interests are most common among citizens.

Such applications show that NLP could significantly enhance efficiency, access, and decision making. Meanwhile, they expose threats that should be carefully monitored. The consequences of misunderstanding by NLPs, biased reactions, or cloudy decision-making in crucial areas (legal, political, healthcare) can be severe.

2.4.3 Computer Vision Basics

The area of AI known as computer vision deals with allowing machines to analyse what they see. Essentially, computer vision algorithms are used to process digital pictures or video just as the human visual system processes information with the eyes and the brain. CNNs are fundamental to modern computer vision, where visual features are detected on a progressively more complex level by using a series of filters (Krichen, 2023).

Critical activities in computer vision are:

- **Image Recognition:** Determining the existence of certain objects (e.g., a person, animal, and landmark) in an image. This is the basis of applications such as photo tagging, product recognition, and forensics.
- **Object Detection:** The identification and classification of multiple objects in an image or a video. Autonomous vehicles, as an example, detect objects to identify and follow pedestrians, other vehicles, and road signs in real-time.
- **Medical Imaging Analysis:** Diagnostic image (X-rays, CT scans, MRIs) with AI, suspicious areas can be pointed out and the model can help doctors identify ailments like cancers or retinal illnesses.

These crude tasks are building blocks to more sophisticated computer vision tasks in fields like surveillance, robotics, and augmented reality.

2.4.4 Applications of Computer Vision

Applications of computer vision in industry are on the rise:

- **Healthcare:** The uses of vision systems include radiology, ophthalmology, and pathology. Diagnostic devices based on AI could assist doctors in recognising diseases faster and more accurately (Alowais et al., 2023).
- **Security and Surveillance:** Airports, stadiums, and cities utilise facial recognition and other vision-based surveillance to deter crime or to improve security. These systems can enhance safety but at a significant cost to civil liberty and privacy because they can be used to conduct mass surveillance.

- **Transportation:** Autopilot vehicles and computer-controlled driver aids rely on computer vision to identify road signs, traffic lights, pedestrians, and other cars. It is very imperative that these systems are really precise and dependable to ensure that individuals are secure.
- **Retail and Agriculture:** In retail, computer vision can be used to check out in self-service lanes, check inventory, and quality in warehouses and stores. Drones and smart sensors in agriculture monitor crops, detect diseases or pests, and optimise irrigation and harvesting based on vision.

These are efficient and innovative applications that are prone to misfortune due to errors or abuse. To illustrate, a facial recognition system may identify an individual as the wrong person leading to false arrests and missed diagnosis in a patient, which can be detrimental.

2.4.5 Governance Challenges in NLP and Computer Vision

The emergence of NLP and computer vision has brought AI governance challenges to the fore (Mueller, 2025). Key challenges include:

- **Bias and Discrimination:** AI models tend to have biases that are reflected in their training data. NLP models could give discriminatory results or support stereotypes when trained on biased text, and facial recognition technology has been found to be more error prone with some ethnic backgrounds. Discrimination must be addressed using different data sets, bias reduction algorithms, and accountability.
- **Privacy:** Generative language models can produce fake news or impersonate individuals, putting information integrity and personal reputation at risk. Meanwhile, AI-based surveillance may spy on people without their written consent, undermining the right to privacy and democratic liberties.
- **Transparency:** There are a lot of NLP and vision models that are complicated and obscure. Stakeholders should be mindful of decision-making processes when it comes to sensitive areas like criminal justice or health care when such systems are implemented. Without transparency, accountability and trust is compromised.
- **Responsibility:** NLP or computer vision errors pose challenging responsibilities. Who is to blame when a chatbot provides life threatening medical information or a self-driving car does not see a pedestrian, the developer, the user, or the system? It requires well-designed accountability arrangements in order to allocate responsibility.
- **Resource Inequality:** NLP and vision models of the state-of-the-art require both big data and massive computational resources. Only a few large corporations or well-funded countries can access these assets, which results in the concentration of power. This disparity influences the ownership and the beneficiaries of AI technologies.

The challenges explain why governance structures should not be limited to technical standards. Policies must be fair, protect citizens and encourage transparency. The moral and legal contexts within which AI can be used also define the level of public trust in AI rather than the technical functionality.

2.5 Data, Infrastructure, and System Performance

The key elements of AI systems are data, computational capacity, and deployment infrastructure. Quality of these elements is directly associated with the accuracy, efficiency, and reliability of AI models. Also, policymakers and regulators should know the effect that data and infrastructure have on the functioning of a system to develop effective regulations. Here, the importance of big data, the importance of computational resources, the value of cloud versus edge computing to deploy AI, and the relevance of performance metrics and benchmarks are discussed.

2.5.1 Importance of Big Data and Data Governance Frameworks

Today, modern AI, especially machine learning and deep learning models, is based on big data, which is a huge volume, variety, velocity, and veracity dataset large data. The increase in digital information, such as social media, sensors, healthcare records, and government databases, has led to the use of AI growing rapidly. Nevertheless, big data comes with massive risks. Data of bad quality yields bad results. Prejudiced or incomplete data can lead to unfair or inaccurate predictions. To use a medical example, the failure of diagnostic systems in some population groups is a possibility if the data used to train the system does not represent the entire population. These problems highlight the necessity of effective data governance models (Ali, 2025b; Batko & Ślęzak, 2022). The term data governance refers to policies, procedures, and standards that guide ethical, legal, and responsible data use. Good governance systems address every facet of data management in collecting, storing, sharing, anonymising, and accessing it. They also feature protection of privacy and adherence to laws such as the General Data Protection Regulation (GDPR) in Europe or the Health Insurance Portability and Accountability Act (HIPAA) in the United States. AI systems can pose a danger of violating rights, disseminating false information, or reinforcing social injustices without effective governance (Moon, 2023).

2.5.2 The Role of Computational Resources

State-of-the-art AI systems demand huge computations to build and implement. Whereas early AI programs could be implemented using a regular CPU, more recent applications often need dedicated hardware (Mishra et al., 2023). Key resources include:

- **Graphics Processing Units (GPUs):** GPU is designed to handle parallel processing, and thus it is best suited to train deep learning models with millions of parameters. They are now the standard hardware used in research and development over AI.

- **Tensor Processing Unit (TPUs):** TPU is a special chip (developed by Google) which is optimised to perform machine learning. They are also more effective when it comes to deep learning on a large scale.
- **Distributed Systems:** AI tasks can be projected on many machines or clusters when dealing with large datasets and complex models. This similarity enables workloads to be executed and scaled more quickly.

The availability of computational resources is making the difference as to who can develop state-of-the-art AI systems. The ability to have many GPUs, TPUs, and distributed computing power advantages organisations whereas smaller institutions can be disadvantaged. Governance issues include the unfairness of this and the concentration of power in a select few corporations or nations that own the vital AI infrastructure.

2.5.3 Cloud Computing and Edge Computing in AI Deployment

AI systems need platforms where they can execute and provide their services. These two are cloud computing and edge computing. Cloud computing provides a centralised structure in which companies can use the services of powerful computing systems without the hardware. Cloud services such as Amazon Web Services (AWS), Microsoft Azure, and Google Cloud offer data storage, training, and deployment services. Cloud computing is scalable and flexible; it is also cost-effective and can be used in research and in commerce. It, however, introduces governance issues associated with cross-border data flows, lock in with the vendor, and dependence on a small number of big providers (Misra et al., 2022).

Edge computing is a decentralised data processing approach where computation is done nearer to the data source, or on a smartphone, an IoT device or an autonomous car. Instead of transporting all information to the cloud, edge computing enables local processing, which results in lower latency and privacy improvement, because sensitive data is on premise. An example is wearable health sensors, which could process patient data on the sensor without necessary transmission to the server. Edge computing is also used in real-time applications such as autonomous driving or industrial automation. At the same time, edge computing has challenges with interoperability, standardisation, and device-level security (Prangon & Wu, 2024). Both edge and cloud computing are essential to the implementation of AI, but each presents different policy concerns. Cloud systems mandate the international treaties on data security and sovereignty, and edge systems robust local measures and standards to avoid abuse and guarantee the security.

2.5.4 Performance Metrics and Benchmarks for Policy Relevant Systems

Evaluation of AI performance is a key factor when making systems trustworthy. Regulators, policymakers, and developers require indicators and standards with which to measure whether a system is precise, just, and credible (Nastoska et al., 2025). Typical performance measurements are:

- **Accuracy:** How many predictions the system makes are correct, which is the success rate of the system.
- **Precision and Recall:** Precision is the number of items identified by the system that were relevant, whereas Recall is the number of relevant items identified. These are commonly added together in an F1 score, the harmonic mean of precision and recall.
- **Latency:** This is the responsiveness of the system, which is very important in real-time systems such as health monitoring or automated driving.
- **Energy efficiency:** Model execution energy consumption, which is vital in sustainable AI, particularly large models and deployments.
- **Robustness and Fairness:** Measures of system performance in diverse circumstances or among diverse population groups, in terms of model reliability and equity.

Commonly used tests or datasets are called benchmarks. Similar to language understanding performance in NLP, benchmarks like GLUE or SuperGLUE exist, and in vision, there is the ImageNet challenge which has led to advancements in image recognition. Considering the governance aspect, it is important that evaluation is not merely technically accurate but must also meet fairness, interpretability, and ethics standards. In the absence of these, a system may be technically marvellous, but harmful when implemented in society. Table 2.2 identifies the key technical elements that enable AI systems, including data structures to computer infrastructure, and the associated governance implications of fairness, equity, privacy, and accountability.

Table 2.2 Key components of AI infrastructure and their governance implications.

Component	*Description*	*Governance Implications*
Big Data	Large scale datasets characterised by high volume, variety, velocity (and variable quality).	Raises risks of bias and privacy violations; necessitates regulations for responsible data collection and sharing.
Data Governance	Policies and standards for managing data ethically and legally.	Ensures compliance with laws, protects individual rights, and demands transparency in data use.
GPUs and TPUs	Specialised processors for machine learning computations.	Concentration of these resources in wealthy organisations raises equity concerns and can widen the AI innovation gap.
Distributed Systems	AI computation spread across multiple machines or clusters.	Introduces questions of equitable access and scalability; requires international collaboration to share resources.

Contd.

Table 2.2 *Contd.*

Component	*Description*	*Governance Implications*
Cloud Computing	Centralized, scalable computing resources provided over the internet.	Involves cross border data flows and dependency on a few big providers, highlighting the need for international agreements and data sovereignty protections.
Edge Computing	Localized processing on devices at the edge of the network.	Improves latency and privacy, but demands strong device level security and standardisation to ensure interoperability.
Performance Metrics	Evaluation criteria (accuracy, precision, recall, latency, fairness, etc.).	Governance must ensure metrics capture ethical and social aspects, not just technical performance.

2.6 Linking Architecture to Policy and Governance

AI is a technological system and a topic of social and policy interest. Construction and design of AI has a direct influence on whether this can be practised fairly, transparently, and with accountability. User experiences and impacts on society are defined by technical factors: algorithms, data, and model architectures. It is because technology and governance are not two separate things. Understanding the connection between AI architecture and governance is essential to the creation of responsible, trustworthy, and ethical AI systems.

2.6.1 How Technical Features Affect Fairness, Accountability, and Transparency

The architecture of an AI system is an important factor affecting its fairness. Whether the system is fair to different groups depends on the selection of the training data, the algorithms to apply, and the way the results are handled. When the training data reflect the pre-existing inequalities within the community, the algorithm is likely to reproduce them. In that case, a system of hiring with a high degree of training on male resume may tend to give advantage to the male candidates. In this regard, AI fairness depends on both design responsibility and continuous supervision (Camilleri, 2024).

Accountability is another important governance concern. To ensure that an AI system or its operators are accountable, there should be a clear method of tracking the decision-making process. This can be achieved by the use of technical mechanisms which record the activities of the document systems and allow the process to be audited. However, when AI systems are used as black boxes, it might not be obvious who to blame, when something goes wrong. Without a clearly explained system design, it can lose its accountability to the technology instead of being distributed to organisations and individuals, which is both unlawful and unethical (Novelli et al., 2024).

Interpretability relates closely with transparency. Basic algorithms such as linear regressions or decision trees are very easy to understand, and deep neural networks are much more complicated and not explainable. This is a difficulty in the minds of the user, regulators as well as developers because it clouds judgements. Transparency is not so much a technical problem but a governance necessity, as citizens and regulators otherwise have to speculate on how decisions are made (Mittelstadt, 2021).

2.6.2 Risks from Biased Datasets, Black-Box Algorithms, and Limited Interpretability

Some of these risks are inherent in the technical implementation of AI systems (Şahin et al., 2025):

- **Partisan Datasets:** No objective data. Data are indicative of the state, circumstances, and worth of the community where they are gathered. Algorithms can therefore detect and even boost the presence of historical discriminatory patterns in the data. Therefore, lending, hiring, or policing AI systems may skew against some groups in a disproportionate way, perpetuating the cycle of inequality by introducing past biases into current judgements.
- **Black-Box Algorithms:** Black-box algorithms represent many of the most powerful models of AI that provide results without justifications explainable to a human. This is a government issue since actions that touch the lives of individuals (loans, medical procedures, admission to school) can be questioned. When a system refuses a loan or a medical treatment recommendation without justification, the affected cannot be given a clear explanation. AI makes black-box systems less credible and responsible.
- **Limited Interpretability:** Although developers may try to describe their models, the description may be overly technical and not comprehensible to non-experts. Opaqueness in technical reasoning does not permit easy assessment by policy makers, judges or the citizens. Low interpretability introduces a disconnection between technology and governance in which systems may formally comply with the rules but are not practically controllable by those charged with this responsibility.

These dangers support the rationale that the technical design must be aligned with the principles of governance. They highlight the necessity of laws demanding fairness testing, explainability, and bias auditing.

2.6.3 Case Examples in Healthcare, Finance, and Education

The influence of AI structure on governance can be well demonstrated in particular areas:

- **Healthcare:** AI is becoming more common in the field of medical diagnosis (diagnosing diseases based on X-rays, predicting patient risk scores, and so on). When training datasets are restricted to specific populations, other populations can have worse health outcomes as the model is not specifically designed to support them. In fact, a diagnostic AI that has been trained on mostly Western data may not be able to generalise to other patients. The management of healthcare must thus require various training data, equity audit, and the imposition of error accountability. Notably, the utilisation of AI does not hold physicians or hospitals accountable for error (Zhang & Zhang, 2023).

- **Finance:** Banks and financial services use AI to score credit and detect fraud. These systems are dependent on data quality and representativeness. Distorted financial information may lead to the injustice of refusing loans to minorities or low income earners. Furthermore, when the credit scoring model is a black box, customers cannot understand why they were turned down. Many countries now require explainable AI in their financial decisions to safeguard consumer rights and maintain anti-discrimination laws (Akhtar et al., 2024).
- **Education:** AI is applied in the education field in the areas of student admissions, grading, and personal learning. A predictive model could identify students as high-risk or low-potential based on biased or a small amount of data, which creates inequalities. The automated grading systems may focus on a specific writing style or dialect making the results unfair. Governance on AI systems should require that they are transparent, accountable, and protect student privacy. It also requires policies to prevent excessive automation where human judgement is paramount (Nguyen et al., 2023).

These illustrations demonstrate that the impact of technical design decisions has a long-term scope. They show that good governance cannot afford to be oblivious to AI architectural decisions and their practical consequences.

2.6.4 Importance of Technical Literacy for Policymakers

Policymakers must have some fundamentals of technical literacy regarding AI to effectively address the challenge posed by AI. It is hard to create effective and fair regulations without knowing how AI systems are developed and how they work. Technical literacy does not mean that policymakers need to turn into engineers or data scientists. Instead, it implies that they need to understand the fundamentals of algorithm training, what types of data bias could happen, and what is the significance of explainability (Chiu, 2025). Such knowledge will help them pose some very important questions like:

- What data was used to train such a system?
- Does the model work equally well with diverse population groups?
- Does the process of decision-making make sense to non-experts?
- What responsibility measures are available in case the system does harm?

The improvement of technical literacy can be achieved by way of training, special advisory committees, and increased cooperation between government, academia, and technological institutions. Such attempts guarantee that policy makers may provide a critical evaluation of AI technologies and make a reasonable judgement. Essentially, enhancing the technical knowledge of policymakers can reduce the gap between the complexity of AI and the governance requirements.

2.7 Conclusion

AI systems are designed to behave in a particular manner and influence society based on those designs. Algorithms, data, computational infrastructure, and feedback loops are core components that determine the performance, flexibility, and reliability of an AI system. Machine learning and deep learning models, NLP, computer vision, are all examples of technical design opportunities and risks. These aspects are not neutral; they dictate results in the areas of healthcare, finance, and education. This discussion has shown that there is a close relationship between technology and governance. The impartiality, responsibility, and transparency of the AI systems depend on technical decisions: what model is designed, what data is used, how to provide explanations. Regimes of governance that fail to recognise these realities are likely to be ineffective or unfair. To prevent it, policymakers need to be technically literate enough to understand the consequences of AI architecture and create regulations that are well-balanced, flexible, and inclusive. Moving forward, the correlation between AI architecture and governance will be expanded into the larger questions of ethics, law, and international regulation. The problems will be addressed in further chapters, touching upon how societies can safeguard human rights, promote responsible innovation, and build global structures of AI governance. Building a robust connection between policy and technical architecture of AI is a core initial step to achieve the goal of creating reliable and long lasting AI systems.

References

Akhtar, M.A., Kumar, M. and Nayyar, A. (2024). *Towards Ethical and Socially Responsible Explainable AI*. Springer. https://doi.org/10.1007/978-3-031-66489-2.

Aldoseri, A., Al-Khalifa, K.N. and Hamouda, A.M. (2023). Re-thinking data strategy and integration for artificial intelligence: Concepts, opportunities, and challenges. *Applied Sciences, 13*(12), 7082. https://doi.org/10.3390/app13127082.

Ali, A. (2025a). Ethical Considerations and Bias in AI Applications in Healthcare. In: *Artificial Intelligence in Healthcare Information Systems: Security and Privacy Challenges* (pp. 129–146). Cham: Springer Nature Switzerland. https://doi.org/10.1007/978-3-031-84404-1_7.

Ali, A. (2025b). Ethical Implications of Artificial Intelligence: Ensuring Patient Data Security. In: *Transforming Healthcare Sector through Artificial Intelligence and Environmental Sustainability* (pp. 149–164). Singapore: Springer Nature Singapore. https://doi.org/10.1007/978-981-97-9555-0_8.

Alowais, S.A., Alghamdi, S.S., Alsuhebany, N., Alqahtani, T., Alshaya, A.I., Almohareb, S.N., ... & Albekairy, A. M. (2023). Revolutionizing healthcare: The role of artificial intelligence in clinical practice. *BMC Medical Education, 23*(1), 689. https://doi.org/10.1186/s12909-023-04698-z.

Annepaka, Y. and Pakray, P. (2025). Large language models: A survey of their development, capabilities, and applications. *Knowledge and Information Systems, 67*(3), 2967–3022. https://doi.org/10.1007/s10115-024-02310-4.

Arriagada-Bruneau, G., López, C. and Mendoza, M. (2025). *Ethics in Artificial Intelligence and Information Technologies*. CRC Press.

Batko, K. and Ślęzak, A. (2022). The use of big data analytics in healthcare. *Journal of Big Data, 9*(1), 3. https://doi.org/10.1186/s40537-021-00553-4.

Bolte, L. and Van Wynsberghe, A. (2025). Sustainable AI and the third wave of AI ethics: A structural turn. *AI and Ethics, 5*(2), 1733–1742. https://doi.org/10.1007/s43681-024-00522-6.

Camilleri, M.A. (2024). Artificial intelligence governance: Ethical considerations and implications for social responsibility. *Expert Systems, 41*(7), e13406. https://doi.org/10.1111/exsy.13406.

Chiu, T.K. (2025). AI literacy and competency: Definitions, frameworks, development, and future research directions. *Interactive Learning Environments, 33*(5), 3225–3229. https://doi.org/10.1080/10494820.2025.2514372.

Das, S., Tariq, A., Santos, T., Kantareddy, S.S. and Banerjee, I. (2023). Recurrent neural networks (RNNs): Architectures, training tricks, and introduction to influential research. In: *Machine Learning for Brain Disorders* (pp. 117–138). https://doi.org/10.1007/978-1-0716-3195-9_4.

Golec, J. and Hachaj, T. (2025). Ten natural language processing tasks with generative artificial intelligence. *Applied Sciences, 15*(16), 9057. https://doi.org/10.3390/app15169057.

Krichen, M. (2023). Convolutional neural networks: A survey. *Computers, 12*(8), 151. https://doi.org/10.3390/computers12080151.

Li, X., Xiong, H., Li, X., Wu, X., Zhang, X., Liu, J., ... & Dou, D. (2022). Interpretable deep learning: interpretation, interpretability, trustworthiness, and beyond. *Knowledge and Information Systems, 64*(12), 3197–3234. https://doi.org/10.1007/s10115-022-01756-8.

Mishra, A., Cha, J., Park, H. and Kim, S. (Eds.). (2023). *Artificial Intelligence and Hardware Accelerators*. Springer. https://doi.org/10.1007/978-3-031-22170-5.

Misra, S., Tyagi, A.K., Piuri, V. and Garg, L. (Eds.). (2022). *Artificial Intelligence for Cloud and Edge Computing*. Springer.

Mittelstadt, B. (2021). Interpretability and transparency in artificial intelligence. In: *The Oxford Handbook of Digital Ethics* (pp. 378–410). Oxford University Press.

Montesinos López, O.A., Montesinos López, A. and Crossa, J. (2022). Fundamentals of artificial neural networks and deep learning. In: *Multivariate Statistical Machine Learning Methods for Genomic Prediction* (pp. 379–425). Springer. https://doi.org/10.1007/978-3-030-89010-0_10.

Moon, M.J. (2023). Searching for inclusive artificial intelligence for social good: Participatory governance and policy recommendations for making AI more inclusive and benign for society. *Public Administration Review, 83*(6), 1496–1505. https://doi.org/10.1111/puar.13648.

Morales, E.F. and Escalante, H.J. (2022). A brief introduction to supervised, unsupervised, and reinforcement learning. In: *Biosignal Processing and Classification Using Computational Learning and Intelligence* (pp. 111–129). Academic Press. https://doi.org/10.1016/B978-0-12-820125-1.00017-8.

Mueller, M.L. (2025). It's just distributed computing: Rethinking AI governance. *Telecommunications Policy, 49*(3), 102917. https://doi.org/10.1016/j.telpol.2025.102917.

Myers, D., Mohawesh, R., Chellaboina, V.I., Sathvik, A.L., Venkatesh, P., Ho, Y.H., ... & Jararweh, Y. (2024). Foundation and large language models: Fundamentals, challenges, opportunities, and social impacts. *Cluster Computing, 27*(1), 1–26. https://doi.org/10.1007/s10586-023-04203-7.

Nastoska, A., Jancheska, B., Rizinski, M. and Trajanov, D. (2025). Evaluating trustworthiness in AI: Risks, metrics, and applications across industries. *Electronics, 14*(13), 2717. https://doi.org/10.3390/electronics14132717.

Neuwirth, R.J. (2024). The global institutional governance of AI: A four-dimensional perspective. *International Journal of Digital Law and Governance, 1*(1), 113–153. https://doi.org/10.1515/ijdlg-2024-0004.

Nguyen, A., Ngo, H.N., Hong, Y., Dang, B. and Nguyen, B.P.T. (2023). Ethical principles for artificial intelligence in education. *Education and Information Technologies, 28*(4), 4221–4241. https://doi.org/10.1007/s10639-022-11316-w.

Nordström, M. (2022). AI under great uncertainty: Implications and decision strategies for public policy. *AI & Society, 37*(4), 1703–1714. https://doi.org/10.1007/s00146-021-01263-4.

Novelli, C., Taddeo, M. and Floridi, L. (2024). Accountability in artificial intelligence: What it is and how it works. *AI & Society, 39*(4), 1871–1882. https://doi.org/10.1007/s00146-023-01635-y.

Prangon, N.F. and Wu, J. (2024). AI and computing horizons: Cloud and edge in the modern era. *Journal of Sensor and Actuator Networks, 13*(4), 44. https://doi.org/10.3390/jsan13040044.

Qian, C., Mathur, N., Zakaria, N.H., Arora, R., Gupta, V. and Ali, M. (2022). Understanding public opinions on social media for financial sentiment analysis using AI-based techniques. *Information Processing & Management, 59*(6), 103098. https://doi.org/10.1016/j.ipm.2022.103098.

Rao, V.S., Satish, M.A. and Prasad, M.B. (2024). *Artificial Intelligence: Principles and Applications.* Leilani Katie Publication.

Şahin, E., Arslan, N.N. and Özdemir, D. (2025). Unlocking the black box: An in-depth review on interpretability, explainability, and reliability in deep learning. *Neural Computing and Applications, 37*(2), 859–965. https://doi.org/10.1007/s12559-023-10179-8.

Sarker, I.H. (2021). Machine learning: Algorithms, real-world applications, and research directions. *SN Computer Science, 2*(3), 160. https://doi.org/10.1007/s42979-021-00592-x.

Serrano, W. (2022). iBuilding: Artificial intelligence in intelligent buildings. *Neural Computing and Applications, 34*(2), 875–897. https://doi.org/10.1007/s00521-021-05967-y.

Shrivastava, N., Tewari, P., Sujatha, S., Bogireddy, S.R., Varshney, N. and Sharma, V. (2025, March). Natural language processing for conversational AI: Chatbots and virtual assistants. In: *2025 IEEE International Conference on Interdisciplinary Approaches in Technology and Management for Social Innovation* (*IATMSI*) (Vol. 3, pp. 1–6). IEEE. https://doi.org/10.1109/IATMSI64286.2025.10984818.

Singh, A., Satapathy, S.C., Roy, A. and Gutub, A. (2022). AI-based mobile edge computing for IoT: Applications, challenges, and future scope. *Arabian Journal for Science and Engineering, 47*(8), 9801–9831. https://doi.org/10.1007/s13369-021-06348-2.

Souchleris, K., Sidiropoulos, G.K. and Papakostas, G.A. (2023). Reinforcement learning in game industry: Review, prospects, and challenges. *Applied Sciences, 13*(4), 2443. https://doi.org/10.3390/app13042443.

Villegas-Ch, W. and García-Ortiz, J. (2023). Toward a comprehensive framework for ensuring security and privacy in artificial intelligence. *Electronics, 12*(18), 3786. https://doi.org/10.3390/electronics12183786.

Whang, S.E., Roh, Y., Song, H. and Lee, J.G. (2023). Data collection and quality challenges in deep learning: A data-centric AI perspective. *VLDB Journal, 32*(4), 791–813. https://doi.org/10.1007/s00778-022-00775-9.

Zhang, J. and Zhang, Z.M. (2023). Ethics and governance of trustworthy medical artificial intelligence. *BMC Medical Informatics and Decision Making, 23*(1), 7. https://doi.org/10.1186/s12911-023-02103-9.

3 Ethical Principles in AI
Fairness, Accountability, and Transparency

To achieve healthy results for people, and society, AI systems should be designed and implemented using the best ethical standards. In this chapter, fairness, accountability, and transparency are explored as key components of ethical AI. Justice demands that AI decisions be fair and cannot be influenced by unreasonable prejudices; responsibility demands that human stakeholders own AI consequences and results, and transparency demands that AI behaviours and conclusions be comprehensible. We talk about practical issues in areas like health, money, and education, how infringements of these principles can be detrimental to stakeholders. We also discuss measures and best practices to incorporate these principles into AI governance. Fairness, accountability, and transparency are the three components of trustworthy and human-centred AI.

3.1 Introduction

Artificial intelligence (AI) has become one of the most popular and fast improving forms of technology, attracting significant ethical concerns. Healthcare, financial, educational governance, and daily decision-making have all implemented AI systems (BaniHani et al., 2024). These systems affect the distribution of resources, development of opportunities, and safeguarding of rights. Consequently, AI ethics is not a hypothetical consideration but an essential part of AI, and it influences the influence of AI on humans and society. In the absence of clear ethical basis, AI systems may reproduce bias, harm people, and undermine trust (Bleher & Braun, 2023).

Ethics in AI defines a series of concepts, sometimes encapsulated as the FAT framework (Fairness, Accountability, and Transparency) which informs responsible AI use. These values have been identified as fundamental aspects of responsible and trustworthy AI, which guides developers, policymakers, and organisations implementing AI. Essentially, fairness suggests that AI must not discriminate against people or strengthen social inequalities, accountability implies that there are recognisable humans or organisations behind AI choices (particularly when the outcomes of these choices are serious), and transparency implies that AI systems are accessible and comprehensible to stakeholders. All of these principles promote a culture of trust, safety, and legitimacy regarding AI usage (Radanliev, 2025).

The key concept of fairness in AI is the absence of prejudice and discrimination. AI models are conditioned using statistics that often indicate historical and social disparities. Unmitigated, these biases may become integrated in AI models and

DOI: 10.1201/9781003776659-3

influence decisions in fields such as hiring, lending, or policing. Equity requires critical management of training information, algorithm testing to yield biased results, and result analysis to encourage equal treatment. This is particularly important when AI decisions affect vulnerable populations or access to necessary services (Varona & Suarez, 2022).

AI accountability deals with the question of responsibility. The high level of autonomy allowed in AI systems makes it difficult to clearly identify who one should hold responsible when something goes awry: the programmer, the user, or the machine. In the absence of explicit responsibility, victims of AI decisions will have no remedy, and society will lose confidence in the technology. An ethical AI thus involves clearly defined lines of accountability in terms of control, company rules, and human interventions. Finally, AIs are supposed to be controlled by humans, and the final decision must be able to be traced back to human behaviours (Novelli et al., 2024).

Transparency is a fair solution to the black box behaviour of a lot of modern algorithms. There are numerous examples of high performing AI systems, particularly deep learning systems, that are opaque and complex, and their operation cannot be easily understood by users or regulators. Transparency implies that organisations disclose data regarding the design of AI systems, the data they work with, and the way they operate. The mechanisms of documentation and explainability allow stakeholders to diligently monitor AI decisions, challenge them when needed, and have confidence in the integrity of the system. Transparency also facilitates fairness and accountability as biases or errors can be identified and corrected (Von Eschenbach, 2021).

To conclude, ethics provide a framework of rules to make sure that AI development and deployment address human values and the common good. Transparency, accountability, and fairness are effective responses to the threat of discrimination, irresponsibility, and obscurity in AI systems (Jain et al., 2025). Through its technical design and governance, society can create an innovative AI that is trustworthy and has useful social value. This chapter explores each of these principles separately and justifies why they are crucial to responsible AI and how they guide policy and governance.

3.2 Fairness in AI

3.2.1 Meaning of Fairness in Algorithmic Decision-Making

Fairness in AI denotes the belief that AI-based systems should produce a decision that is fair, just, and not injuriously discriminatory. When individuals are seeking a loan, a job, or university admission, they want to be judged based on relevant qualifications, and not on irrelevant factors such as race, gender, and age. The purpose of fairness in AI is to support these values, meaning that the decisions by the algorithm are made based on legitimate factors (Casillas, 2024). But the notion of fairness is not a one-size-fits-all concept; it may have various interpretations in different settings and societies. In employment, equity could apply to give the most skilled candidates an equal chance whether they are born in America or not. In lending, it may imply that borrowers with comparable creditworthiness will be given comparable loan judgements. Fairness in healthcare is understood as equal access to proper diagnostic and treatment procedures across demographic lines. Due to these subtleties, fairness is a relative concept that should be operationalised and moralised to fit each use. Technically, fairness can be defined through the outcomes and error rates of groups. An AI system would be considered unfair when it generates greatly different error rates or success rates across demographic groups. If a facial recognition system is found to have a much greater error rate with women versus men, then it would be deemed to be unfair. Precisely, fairness in AI entails not focusing on biased outcomes and trying to achieve similar performance across groups (Afreen et al., 2025).

3.2.2 *Types of Bias in AI*

One of the biggest challenges towards fairness is the existence of bias within AI systems. Bias is a systematic deviation of outcomes or groups towards some groups or outcomes, rather than others. It can be added during different levels of AI system design, training, or implementation. Data bias, algorithmic bias and societal bias are the main types of bias in AI. Table 3.1 describes these types of bias, their most common causes, and some of their effects.

Table 3.1 Major types of bias affecting fairness in AI, with descriptions and examples.

Type of Bias	*Description and Example*
Data Bias	Bias due to incomplete, unrepresentative, or biased training information. As an illustration, when a medical AI system develops on Data containing primarily middle-aged men, it might not effectively identify conditions in women or older patients. The under or over representation of specific groups in the data results in a poor performance of said groups (Hanna et al., 2025).
Algorithmic Bias	Discrimination caused by the design of the algorithm or the objective form, even in balanced data. An example of this is a predictive hiring algorithm that may prefer people who have attended specific universities due to previous hiring record that shows that such hire has worked well. The design may have an unfairly negative impact on minority candidates with equal qualifications (Casillas, 2024).
Societal Bias	Bias based on the prejudices or historical disparities that exist in a society and are enshrined in AI behavior. As an example, a predictive policing system that is trained with historical crime data could send additional police to areas with a higher rate of past arrests. In many cases, such rates involve previous over-policing of a particular group, instead of the real crime rates, leading the AI to continue disproportionately tracking a particular group (Pulivarthy & Whig, 2025).

3.2.3 Real World Examples

To see the physical effect of AI bias and injustice, we take several high-profile examples in various spheres:

- **Hiring:** AI systems are already being used in the hiring process of big companies. In a single instance, an AI trained on resumes of a male majority workforce was trained to prefer male candidates. It rated resumes with signs of female gender (such as mention of participation in a women chess club) down. The gender discrepancy in the historical training data caused the AI to discriminate against female candidates in a systematic manner. This caused the imbalance in the employment of qualified women because it led to unfair hiring results (Albaroudi et al., 2024).
- **Credit Scoring:** Banks are applying AI to help them evaluate loan applications and estimate credit risk. When the training data is based on past lending differences, the AI may end up refusing loans to creditworthy members of minority groups. As an example, a potential applicant in a disadvantaged neighbourhood could be classified as high risk just due to the address and not due to their individual credit history. These consequences reproduce structural inequalities and deprive some groups of equal access to financial services (Raji et al., 2024).
- **Predictive Policing:** Certain police forces have implemented AI technologies to predict crime hotspots and distribute law enforcement resources. Such systems are trained using historical crime and policing data, which are often biased (e.g., one neighbourhood recorded more police crimes in the past because it was over policed). The AI can declare those places as risky, and the police focus patrol on those places, and create more arrests in a vicious circle. This feedback loop implies that marginalised communities will be disproportionately monitored and implicated in enforcement, which will perpetuate stereotypes and undermine trust in police officers (Almasoud & Idowu, 2025).

These illustrations demonstrate that AI fairness concerns are not abstractions but they have a direct impact on people, their lives, possibilities, and rights. Without mitigation, unfair AI systems have the potential to enhance discrimination and inequality.

3.2.4 Approaches to Achieve Fairness

AI fairness is not a self-sustaining process; it needs technical and organisational initiatives. Principles of encouraging equity are the following:

- **Diverse and Representative Datasets:** One of the most successful methods of reducing bias is to use training data that is both diverse and representative of all pertinent user groups. This includes the inclusion of data on different genders, ethnicities, age brackets and geographical localities. As an example, a medical AI system must have patient data of a variety of populations (not just one group) to avoid diagnostic performance bias. This type of dataset expansion and balancing enhances the usability and fairness of AI systems to every user (Kurapati et al., 2025).

- **Fairness Metrics:** Scholars have developed explicit methods of assessing AI system fairness. These measures of fairness are used to verify whether algorithms treat certain groups equally, are biased, or commit unfair errors. They transform fairness into quantifiable and easy to measure values that drive model design, testing, and refinement (Palumbo et al., 2024).
- **Demographic Parity:** This principle of fairness means that there should be equal distribution of positive outcomes, like through job offers, approvals, or loans, across various demographic groups. It implies that race, gender, or background should not determine an individual probability of being favoured.
- **Equal Opportunity:** The concept ensures that persons possessing the same qualifications or creditworthiness are given an equal opportunity to produce positive results irrespective of their group identity. It addresses the equal treatment of similar qualified individuals along demographic lines to eliminate systemic discrimination.
- **Predictive Parity:** Making sure that the model works equally well on different groups (e.g., the percentage of correct loan approvals is the same across groups). These metrics are used to assess the developer's models; when they quantify the differences in error rates or results, they are able to identify unfair trends and affect the model or data.
- **Bias Audits:** A proactive approach to fairness is to perform a periodic audit of AI systems to detect biased results. Bias audits (either internal or conducted by third parties) assess whether the decisions made by an AI system impact any population differently, and whether it adheres to non-discrimination laws and ethical guidelines. As an example, an AI credit rating system can be audited periodically to confirm that applicants of other races or genders are being treated fairly. Periodic audits bring a sense of responsibility and allow organisations to identify and rectify bias in its initial stages (Murikah et al., 2024).
- **Human Oversight:** Even highly automated AI systems require human oversight and intervention. Humans are expected to examine algorithm decisions and allow exceptions in situations of possible injustice. As an example, a loan officer is expected to read through hand loan applications that an AI is warning about should there be reason to suspect that a qualified applicant might be unfairly rejected by the algorithm. The maintenance of a human in the loop will provide fairness not just in the design of the model but also through moral decision-making and common sense (Holzinger et al., 2025).
- **Legal and Ethical Systems:** Governments and entities are putting in place regulations and guidelines to enforce fairness in AI. In particular, proposed AI Act in the European Union would entail stringent testing to ensure fairness and non-discrimination in high-risk AI systems. Ethical guidelines issued by

professional bodies and industry groups also lay fairness as a core value. These regulations and standards will make sure that fairness is not a voluntary and a post factum issue, but an obligatory part of AI implementation (Fessenko & Jasperse, 2025).

3.3 Accountability in AI Systems

3.3.1 Defining Accountability in the AI Context

Regarding AI, accountability implies that a person, company, or institution is responsible for the result of the AI-powered processes. It also includes the accountability concerning the correctness, impartiality, and security of algorithmic choices. Notably, accountability is not merely a question of having someone to blame when something bad occurs; rather it is a matter of establishing systems and procedures to avoid harm, prior to its occurrence (Hosseini Tabaghdehi & Ayaz, 2025). People participate in every life cycle phase of an AI system, whether it is writing algorithms, training data, deploying models, or policy rules regarding their use. This implies that AI systems are influenced by developers, data scientists, companies, and policymakers alike. Responsibility in AI involves ensuring that these stakeholders recognise, and take responsibility for the results of the systems that they develop or run. As an example, when an AI medical device results in a false diagnosis, accountability would require determining whether it was the developers of the model who should be held responsible, the doctors who operated the device without due diligence, or the hospital that implemented it. The high autonomy and complexity of AI systems in comparison to conventional tools make it difficult to hold AI systems accountable. However, AI cannot be left to work in empty space outside the control of humans. The principle of accountability is what makes technology fall under human judgement and under human values, making AI a human tool instead of an uncontrollable force (Rezaei et al., 2024).

3.3.2 The Challenge of Responsibility in Automated Decision-Making

There are multiple reasons why assigning responsibility to automated decisions may be hard (Jedličková, 2025):

- **Complexity of AI Systems:** Current AI systems (and in particular deep learning networks) are black boxes with millions of parameters. Even the developers may not understand why a given input led to a given output. This obfuscation contributes to the inability to identify the source of a mistake or damage and place the blame or responsibility.
- **Shared Accountability:** AI systems are often used by more than one party. A single organisation can gather and read the data, another creates the algorithm, and others implement the system in various settings. An illustration is of a bank buying a credit scoring AI vendor and the decisions taken apply to the

bank customers. Developers, vendors, and users share responsibility and it is difficult to know who is ultimately in charge of what the AI does.

- **Decision-making Independence:** There are AI systems that require a small amount of human input, such as autonomous cars or high speed trading algorithms. These systems autonomously arrive at rapid decisions. In case an autonomous car leads to an accident, it is not known if it is because of the fault of the car programme, its producer, or the human occupant who may have not intervened. The independent decision-making capacity of the AI confuses the conventional concept of liability.
- **Legal and Ethical Uncertainties:** AI capabilities have not been completely reflected by laws and regulations. The question of the allocation of liability in cases where an AI system inflicts harm remains unclear in most jurisdictions. Such ambiguity indicates that accountability gaps can exist: victims do not know who is to be responsible, and organisations are not explicitly required to pay damages related to AI.

3.3.3 Case Examples

In order to demonstrate the problems related to accountability in practice, we take into consideration the situation in various sectors:

- **Medical Diagnosis:** AI is finding more applications in medical diagnosis (such as cancer detection in radiography images). These are tools that can enhance efficiency and accuracy, though not fool proof. Assume an AI system has not identified a tumour in the scan of a patient, resulting in late diagnosis. Should the supervision cause injury then who is responsible? One might say that the developers trained a flawed model, the hospital implemented it without proper validation, or the doctor was too much of an AI recommendation adherent. The lack of clear accountability can make the patient unable to pursue justice, and these cases may undermine the confidence in medical AI (Ali, 2025a; Zhang & Zhang, 2023).
- **Financial Services:** Banks have used AI in activities such as credit scoring and fraud detection. An example is an AI turning down a loan to a qualified applicant due to a bias in the training data. In cases where the applicant appeals the decision, the bank may accuse the software vendor, and the vendor may accuse the bank of abusing the system. In the eyes of the customer, there must be a well-defined responsible side to give an answer and correct the situation. This case highlights why accountability must be clearly defined: customers should be able to get clear explanations and recourse to unfair automated decisions (Leal, 2022).
- **Self-driving Cars:** one of the most advanced uses of AI is self-driving cars, which use sensors and complicated algorithms to navigate. Questions of responsibility arise urgently in case an autonomous vehicle is the victim of an accident. Did the vehicle object detection algorithm (the task of a developer) have a flaw? Does the car manufacturer not conduct proper safety tests? Or

had the human passenger not intervened in time? These cases frequently cannot comfortably fall into law, demonstrating the necessity of novel forms of accountability towards AI-directed autonomous systems (Siegel & Pappas, 2023).

Such instances prove that accountability is not a matter of theory only, but there are practical implications of accountability in various sectors. In both cases, the absence of a clear sense of accountability may negatively impact the affected population and reduce trust in AI solutions.

3.3.4 Mechanisms to Enforce Accountability

To enhance AI system accountability, a combination of technical, organisational, and regulatory approaches is possible using several mechanisms:

- **Regulation and Legal Frameworks:** Governments and international organisations are starting to develop laws that would hold AI systems to account. To illustrate, the European Union proposed AI Act would require companies to perform risk assessments and ensure transparency of high risk AI applications. With these regulations, the responsibilities of the AI developers, deployers, and operators are defined, so no one can avoid liability. Legal regulations also have a solution to not following the rules, which introduces the motivation of making organisations accountable (Huang et al., 2024).
- **Human Oversight:** The major step toward accountability is ensuring human oversight of AI decisions. Humans should be either in the loop (where they have to approve AI decisions before they become effective), or on the loop (observing decisions as they happen and capable of interfering). As an example, physicians must go over AI-generated diagnoses with their doctors before they settle on treatment plans, and loan officers need to question AI-generated credit refusals. The level of human control is that the final decision-making authority lies with humans as opposed to machines (Holzinger et al., 2025).
- **Audit Trails and Documentation:** AI systems are expected to be traceable. This implies maintaining records (audit trails) of how they make decisions in terms of the data they input, the calculations they perform and the results. Other important issues in developing a model, like the origin of data, training technique, and performance measurement, are to be properly documented as well. These documentation and audit trails allow the investigation to reverse engineer the decision-making process and find areas of failure or bias and responsibility in an error. They also enable the regulators and auditors to ensure the system meets the standard of fairness and transparency (Mökander et al., 2021).
- **External Review and Independent Audits:** Organisations can enhance accountability by having external professionals audit their AI systems. Third party audits, which are conducted by independent agencies or auditors, evaluate the compliance of AI models with specific fairness, accuracy, and

safety standards. An external audit of a credit scoring algorithm could, as an example, ensure that it does not unfairly target any ethnic group. These audits are objective as well as give confidence to the people. Publicising the results of audits (or even the presence of audits) allows companies to demonstrate that these companies are ready to be responsible, not only to themselves but also to the regulator and society (Falco et al., 2021).

- **Ethical Guidelines and Industry Standards:** Professional bodies and industry consortia have been setting codes of ethics and best practice guidelines on AI that focus on accountability. As an example, in most responsible AI models, companies will have defined roles and protocols to follow in case of AI system failures or harm. Although these guidelines are not a legal obligation, it is important to set them as it provides important standards. Firms that comply with these norms will determine who in the organisation is responsible regarding AI results and how concerns will be managed (e.g., internal review boards or incident response plans). These best practices may eventually become norms which the populace and regulators expect organisations to adhere to (Sarkar & Paul, 2025).

3.4 Transparency and Explainability

3.4.1 Transparency vs. Explainability: Key Differences

Explainability and Transparency are somewhat different terms in AI ethics. Transparency is a matter of openness: it means that organisations disclose information regarding the development and functioning of an AI system. For example, transparency could mean publishing information about the training data, releasing information about the algorithm methods, or describing the limitations known to the system. Transparency gives easy access to regulators, auditors, or even users to investigate the components and development process of the system.

On the other hand is explainability, which is concerned with interpretation: it is about allowing people (in particular users and persons that are impacted by the AI) to know the reason behind certain decisions or outputs. As an example, when an AI system denies a loan application, explainability implies that the system can give the loan applicant agreeable explanations of how and why it made the loan decision to reject the loan, say because of inadequate income to support the debt. Explainability is also relevant to end users as well as regulators and developers who must check that the system is operating appropriately and fairly.

Transparency and explainability are in essence complementary, with the former offering sufficient information to judge an AI system and the latter offering insight in a format understandable by humans. A system may be transparent (the code and data can be viewed) but not be explainable by a layperson when the technical aspects are too complicated. A system, on the other hand, may give you easy answers to why it does what it does with little information about how it does it. Both of these are essential: transparency allows informed stakeholders to audit and verify the AI, and explainability allows non-experts to understand the reasons behind a decision. Stakeholders do not know what they do not know about AI decisions without transparency, and without explainability, even a transparent system may seem a black box to a non-technical audience (Speith & Xu, 2024).

3.4.2 The Problem of Black Box Algorithms

Most of the most sophisticated AI systems of today can be said to be black boxes since it is not straightforward to see what is going on inside the box. This non-interpretability raises some governance challenges:

- **Lack of Accountability:** When an AI system gives a negative or biased result and no one can answer why an event occurred, it becomes extremely hard to charge anybody. In situations in which the decision-making process is not adherable, accountability (as addressed above) fails.
- **Mistrust:** When people do not understand how the system works, they are likely to mistrust it. When users, or the general population, do not know how AI decisions are made, particularly in serious cases such as medical diagnoses or criminal justice, they will have less trust in such decisions.
- **Legal Compliance:** In most legal systems, people are entitled to an explanation of any decision that carries significant consequences (like being denied credit or parole). Black box algorithms are not very good at providing the rationalisations that laws or regulations may demand, so organisations can hardly rely on such algorithms without violating the right to explanation provisions or other laws.
- **Ethical Risks:** It is difficult to uncover any latent biases or errors within an AI model without explainability. These may cause systematic unfair or inaccurate results that are not corrected due to the ignorance of the occurrence by anyone. Making ethical oversight transparent and explainable is therefore crucial; otherwise there will be no control over unfair practices.

The performance and interpretability of a model are often traded off. In general, highly complex models (such as deep neural networks with billions of parameters) are more accurate but less interpretable, whereas simpler models (such as decision trees or linear regressions) may be easier to understand but not as accurate on complex problems. One key problem with AI governance is how to strike this trade off, such that we neither lose too much interpretability in the name of performance nor the reverse. Continued AI research aims to create a system that is not only highly performing but also more transparent.

3.4.3 Case Examples

Absence of transparency and explainability may cause practical problems in other areas:

- **Medical AI:** AI can now be used to read X-rays or determine health risks. Although these devices may be as effective as human beings are at times, they are not always able to reason why. When an AI diagnostic system recommends a specific treatment or can diagnose (or fails to diagnose) a condition without a clear explanation, doctors may be unwilling to rely on it, and patients may be unwilling to follow its advice. Further, when an AI errs (e.g., does not see a tumour on a scan), the absence of an explanation makes it harder to hold the AI accountable and learn about the mistake. Thus, interpreting the medical AI output is paramount to patient safety and confidence between patients and caregivers (Shastry & Sanjay, 2022).

- **Credit Scoring:** AI models allow banks and other lenders to determine whether to give out loans or not. Consumer protection laws in most locations, including the USA, require that the lender explain why the applicant was denied credit. Black box credit scoring models may produce a bare approve or deny result, with no explanation, which in consumer rights terms is unacceptable. Beyond legality, when specific groups are repeatedly declined credit without a reason why, it causes suspicion of discrimination. Some regulators in turn are now asking credit scoring algorithms to be auditable, with key influencing factors to be recorded. This is why explainability is an important aspect of financial services: it ensures consumer safety and can be used to detect potential biases in lending (Leal, 2022).
- **Automated Hiring:** AI is also employed to sift through resumes and category job applicants. In a couple of salient situations, the training data used to train these systems was based on previous hiring bias and as such, was biased towards certain groups (e.g., male candidates or individuals attending particular schools). When an AI system rejects an applicant without feedback, the applicant is not able to determine whether the decision made was fair or, what improvements could be made. In the case of organisations, , lack of explainability in hiring AI implies that organisations may be unwittingly reproducing biases and may not easily be able to demonstrate to auditors or the general public that they are fair. It is also essential to ensure that automated hiring systems are transparent about their requirements (and that the candidates are told why they were not hired) because this is the way to hold the company accountable to its hiring processes (Hunkenschroer & Luetge, 2022).

These case studies demonstrate that AI systems can be genuinely harmful and lead to public backlash when they are used in black box mode, when they are not transparent or explainable. The more people learn about how AI decisions are made and understand that the decisions are based on reason and evidence, the more they will trust and accept them.

3.4.4 Tools for Transparency and Explainability

Diverse tools and methods can contribute to making AI systems more understandable and transparent:

- **Explainable AI (XAI):** XAI is a set of methods and models that help to humanise the outputs of AI. Certain AI models (as decision trees or linear regression) are explainable in nature as their decision-making process can be followed in a simple manner. In more complex models (such as deep neural networks), further methods are employed to derive explanations. These can be used to indicate which attributes had the greatest effect on a decision (feature importance), demonstrate the internal model behaviour (such as heat maps of what part of an image affected a classification), or provide counterfactual explanations (e.g., if the applicant had made $5,000 more money, the loan would have been approved). The tools assist users of the model and regulators in knowing why a model arrived at a particular decision. XAI specifically plays a crucial role in stakes-intensive areas (healthcare, finance, law enforcement) where the rationale supporting an AI-based choice is crucial (Chamola et al., 2023).

- **Algorithmic Audits:** The standard approach to auditing AI systems is through systematic assessment of AI systems based on whether they are biased or whether they meet ethical or legal norms. Such audits may be performed both in-house by the preparing organisation and by external auditors (the latter may prove to be more convincing). To give one example, an audit of a hiring algorithm could look at whether there is a significant difference between how the system suggests applicants of different gender or ethnicity, with the same qualifications. Through these checks, algorithmic audits can help shed light on the inner workings of AI and give an assurance that the system is being held to standards of fairness and accuracy (Mökander, 2023).
- **Model Documentation:** Detailed documentation of AI models and datasets is a viable resource to improve transparency. The documentation must contain information regarding the model construction and training: descriptions of the training data (where it came from, demographics, any other pre processing done on the data), the model architecture used, the training process, and performance measures on many groups. Researchers proposed common documentation formats like model cards to report the properties of an AI model and data sheets to report the composition and biases of a dataset. These practices help developers explain to others the design and limitations of AI systems. It can then be possible to regulate, audit, and even use AI to learn the context that it will be utilised in and whether it is suitable to address a specific usage (Königstorfer & Thalmann, 2022).
- **Open Source Practices:** Open source (or at least partially open source) AI systems can also enhance transparency. The source code, model weights, or sample datasets can be published to allow external experts to check and test the AI by themselves. Open source AI allows the general research community to detect bugs, biases, or security vulnerabilities that could have been overlooked by the original developers. Nonetheless, it is not always practical and wise to open source everything and enterprises might have certain intellectual property issues, and there is a chance that strong AI models will be abused when they are open source. Practically, other organisations prefer to take an intermediate position: to provide models and data to researchers with some

license or confidentiality agreement. The point is that increased transparency is likely to result in increased oversight and eventually more reliable AI systems (Mora-Cantallops et al., 2021).

It is always good to recapitulate the relation of these different aspects before proceeding with the next section. Table 3.2 summarises the most important ethical AI principles (fairness, accountability, transparency) and the concepts based on them (explainability and trust), their definitions, the challenges they solve, and some of the methods to implement them.

Table 3.2 Key aspects of ethical AI (fairness, transparency, explainability, accountability, and trust).

Aspect	*Definition*	*Challenge*	*Approach*
Fairness	Equitable, non-discriminatory outcomes	Biased data or algorithms; embedded inequalities	Diverse datasets; fairness metrics
Transparency	Openness about AI design, data, and processes	Organisational secrecy; lack of disclosure	Model documentation; open source sharing
Explainability	Ability to interpret and understand AI decisions	Black box model complexity; technical opacity	XAI techniques (feature importance, counterfactuals)
Accountability	Linking outcomes to responsible actors	Diffused responsibility among developers/users	Clear audit trails; regulatory requirements
Trust	Public confidence in AI decisions	Errors, unfair outcomes; unclear reasoning	Transparent communication; ethical guidelines

3.5 Interconnections and Practical Applications

3.5.1 Overlap and Mutual Reinforcement of FAT Principles

The FAT principles are closely interrelated and mutually reinforcing concepts. One principle can be used to help the other. As an illustrative example, transparency can help create fairness by exposing biases within datasets or algorithms, lacking which some discriminatory trends may not be visible. Likewise, accountability requires a certain level of transparency: it is impossible to hold a person or organisation accountable to an AI decision when the decision-making process remains completely hidden. Fairness also increases accountability, since accountability is not valuable when its consequences are also unfair (it is of little value to hold actors accountable who cause unfair or harmful outcomes). As a matter of fact, these principles must cooperate. Technical fairness without transparency will not be credible to the masses of people and a transparent system that always brings unfair results will not be seen as legitimate. Accountability would be empty without fairness, unfortunately, actors may be accused or penalised, yet suffering by detrimental decisions will be experienced by vulnerable populations. To the point, the FAT principles offer a holistic framework to guarantee the social acceptability of AI systems and their technical soundness (Panarese et al., 2025).

3.5.2 Ethical Dilemmas and Trade offs

In the practical use of the FAT principles in AI systems, they are frequently balanced with other factors such as efficiency, privacy, or accuracy. Common dilemmas include (Wu, 2024):

- **Fairness vs. Efficiency:** It is sometimes observed that the faster an AI system is, the more work can be done to make it fairer (e.g., adding constraints or other processing to even out the final results among groups). The processing of more data or more complex calculations may be essential to achieve fairness in an algorithm, and can slow down decision-making or be costly. Companies that are pressurised to maximise performance and reduce costs are confronted with the ethical dilemma of how far they are prepared to sacrifice efficiency in order to attain more fair results.
- **Transparency vs. Privacy:** Transparency with regard to data and processes may be in conflict with privacy issues and confidentiality. When a dataset is published to allow it to be audited by others, e.g., by not taking care, sensitive personal data may be disclosed. Likewise, to determine the functioning of a credit scoring model, the disclosure of proprietary information or personal data about individuals may be necessary. Engineers and policymakers should find a balance between transparency and privacy of personal data (and intellectual property) to prevent infringement of privacy, yet allow oversight.
- **Accountability vs. Innovation:** AI failure and high oversight requirements can be a major barrier to innovation since strong accountability mechanisms may be necessary. When companies/developers are worried about legal responsibility in case of any errors that an AI could commit, they could be reluctant to test AI applications or implement AI at scale. Although accountability is essential to trust, it must be adjusted to ensure it does not inordinately suppress technological innovation. This trade off can be balanced by creating so-called safe sandboxes in which experiments can be performed or tiered accountability on the basis of risk.
- **Fairness vs. Accuracy:** In certain situations, increasing fairness can cause a small decrease in the predictive accuracy of a model. An example of this is when trying to make a model equal between groups of people (such as by trying to make sure that an algorithm used in hiring gets a certain proportion of people of various backgrounds to come out top) it may result in not necessarily picking the best-ranked candidate if it disturbs the balance. The moral dilemma is whether we ought to tolerate a slight decrease in the total accuracy to obtain a fairer outcome. Governance systems might have to offer prescriptions as to

how to navigate such trade offs, e.g., by establishing tolerances of acceptable accuracy loss in the name of fairness.

These paradoxes show that the FAT principles cannot be implemented in vacuum or using simple checklists. They should be implemented with close attention to values and context and to dialogue between stakeholders. The one-size-fits-all solution is quite a rare case; rather, all the competing values have to be evaluated and reasonable trade offs have to be made in each situation. Finally, these trade offs are specific to the context in which they are resolved. As an example, in a life critical system such as healthcare, fairness, and transparency may reasonably outweigh concern about efficiency or even a modest loss of accuracy, but in other contexts a higher degree of accuracy may be reasonable as long as minimum fairness thresholds are not violated. The trick here is to think these decisions over in a very inclusive way that includes moral deliberation as opposed to handling them purely on technical or market grounds.

3.5.3 Sector Specific Applications

Fairness, accountability, and transparency may hold varied significance in different sectors. Here are some of the areas that we emphasise in practice:

- **Healthcare:** Fairness in healthcare AI: Fairness refers to the accuracy of the diagnostic or treatment recommendations, regardless of the demographic subset of a patient population. A common fairness issue is that, when the training data of a medical AI biases one population (such as middle aged males), it can perform poorly on another population. The concept of accountability in healthcare means that despite the use of AI tools, patient outcomes are the responsibility of a doctor or a hospital. When AI makes a misdiagnosis, the healthcare providers are not off the hook either, they must confirm AI results and are responsible for making decisions. Explainability and transparency are important as physicians and patients should believe and comprehend AI assisted diagnoses. In the case of a cancer patient, say the AI model predicted the risk of cancer was high, the system should tell the patient why (e.g., because of a pattern in an MRI scan). Best practices associated with this area are bias audits of medical data, human control over AI suggestions (e.g., a radiologist revisiting AI marked images), and comprehensive documentation of medical AI systems to ensure transparency (Ali, 2025b; Zhang & Zhang, 2023).
- **Finance:** In the financial sector, fairness requires AI credit scoring systems, lending systems, or insurance systems to be free of discrimination on the basis of race, gender, or socioeconomic status. AI cannot continue to perpetuate historical biases in lending (including redlining). Accountability implies that financial institutions cannot seek to shirk responsibility onto an algorithm, as in the event that an automated decision has a negative impact on a customer, the financial institution has to shoulder the responsibility and offer recourse.

It also relates to explainability: denied a loan, the customer has the right to be informed why. Financial transparency means that the rules by which algorithms (at least at a high level) operate are accessible to regulators and, to a degree, to customers. Models of black box credit, such as black box credit models, have been discovered to discriminate against minorities inadvertently, making them subject to regulatory scrutiny. Financial regulators in turn are now promoting or mandating the use of explainable AI and periodic fairness audits. It is an industry best practice to test lending models with fairness measures, perform autonomous algorithm audits, and follow the frameworks of consumer protection, so that automated decisions can be clarified and appealed (Akhtar et al., 2024).

- **Education:** In education, the fairness of AI implies it should not disfavour a group of learners (such as non-native speakers, or learners at a particular school or region) when performing its task (e.g., grading tests, suggesting learners to a programme, or even proctoring tests). An A-based grading system must be tested to make sure that, e.g., it does not systematically assign low scores to essays written by a certain group of people. The responsibility of education means that educational decisions are held accountable by teachers, administrators, or institutions. In case an AI algorithm incorrectly refuses a student admission or shows that a student is behaving improperly, a human teacher has to be able to look into the situation and be answerable to the decision. Transparency is necessary to make students aware of how decisions concerning them are made. To illustrate, in the case of a student being denied by an AI-based university admissions system, transparency would involve disclosing the primary factors (academic scores, extracurricular, and so on) and may also include how these factors were combined. An illustrative case: when an AI-based writing evaluation systematically scores lower grades to essays written by students with their first language not being English, an open-ended analysis would expose this bias, and remedies (such as tweaking the algorithm or introducing human review) could have been applied. Educational best practices involve integrating AI-based assessment with human assessment (such as evaluations of AI-based assessment conducted by teachers), conducting frequent fairness reviews of educational AI systems, and disclosing information about the use of AI in assessments to students (Memarian & Doleck, 2023).

These illustrations underscore the idea that the fundamental concepts of FAT can be universal, but their application should be specific to the field. Fairness may have different specific measures in medical care compared with finance, transparency may mean posting a model card to a medical AI compared with a simple reason code about a loan decision, and accountability may involve different parties (doctors vs. loan officers vs. teachers). However, in all these areas, it is crucial to consider FAT principles in order to make AI technology complementary instead of detrimental to equity, trust, and responsibility.

3.5.4 *Best Practices for Integrating FAT Principles into Governance Frameworks*

To make sure that fairness, accountability, and transparency are not mere ideals but elements of the very fabric of AI development and deployment, organisations and policymakers are establishing several best practices. Some of the essential practices are:

- **Bias Audits and Fairness Testing:** AIs are expected to be frequently tested in terms of fairness. It entails cross demographic measurement of outcomes and ensuring for disparities through the fairness measures mentioned above. External audits (by independent parties) can be particularly beneficial, as they can be an objective evaluation of the presence of negative effects of an algorithm in specific groups and recommendations to address them. On uncovering bias via such audits, they must prescribe specific measures to mitigate that bias, which may include retraining the given model on more diverse data or changing its decision thresholds.
- **Well-defined Responsibilities:** AI systems must have clear lines of responsibility within an organisation. This implies determining who will be tasked with different phases of the AI lifecycle and who will assume the lead just in case something goes amiss. As an example, a company could require that the AI development team address the performance of the model, the compliance team address its legal and ethical compliance, and a specific AI officer addresses the incidents. Human control must be preserved particularly in dangerous applications so that at all times decisions made in areas such as healthcare or finance are ultimately made by a human decision-maker.
- **Transparency Requirements:** Internal policy and external regulations must require some level of transparency. This may involve mandates to record models and datasets (via tools such as model cards and datasheets), to publish the origin and quality of training data, and to explain to people impacted by automated decisions what those decisions are. These practices of documentation can be easily standardised so that auditors, regulators, and even locals can learn to understand AI systems. Examples include a regulator asking companies to document any consumer facing decisions made by an AI system, including its purpose, data sources, performance, and the limitations that are known.
- **Explainable AI Tools:** When forming their AI systems, organisations need to consider the elements of explainability at the design stage. Instead of attaching explanations as the system is run, it can be designed to create decision explanations as it executes. Applying XAI techniques (such as those outlined above) will increase confidence among users and regulators. To illustrate, an AI-based credit decision-making company in the fintech industry could introduce an explanation module that generates the most important factors that affect an applicant's credit related decision, operationalising transparency and fairness.

- **Balance of Trade Offs:** Governance systems (both in organisations and in public policy) must provide a way of navigating trade offs among ethics and other goals. As an example, a policy could stipulate that it is fine to slightly decrease the accuracy of a model when it treats a disadvantaged demographic much better, but that further decline in accuracy must be prevented. Decision-makers will be less likely to address such issues on a case by case basis by explicitly recognising trade offs (such as fairness vs. accuracy, or transparency vs. privacy) and restricting or defining them by explicit criteria. The idea is to ensure the ethical considerations are not an after-thought in system optimisation.
- **Public Engagement:** Involvement of the public and stakeholders during the creation of AI ethics guidelines is the best practice that will help to ensure that the ensuing policies are valued by the society. Organisations can learn what different communities view as fair, or the level of transparency desired, through public consultations, community groups workshops, and disclosure of AI use cases. Such interaction can inform more socially acceptable and culturally sensitive AI applications. It also adds civic confidence when citizens believe their voices can be heard and their issues can be addressed in the process of governance.
- **International Cooperation:** AI technology and its effects are international and cross-national. Consequently, global cooperation is necessary to develop uniform ethical codes of conduct and prevent ethics shopping (when businesses move to jurisdictions with less stringent rules and regulations). Governments, global groups, and industry are starting to collaborate to align AI principles of trust. Global collaboration (e.g., through the OECD, UNESCO, or specialized AI ethics consortia) can contribute to setting of general guidelines and best practices. This will lessen fragmentation and contribute towards meeting the expectations of AI developers around the world in terms of fairness, accountability and transparency.

When these best practices are implemented into governance structures, we will be one step closer to a world where fairness, accountability, and transparency are not requirements that an AI system has, but it is expected of all systems.

3.6 Conclusion

Three main pillars of ethical AI include fairness, accountability, and transparency. Combined, they promote the principles of justice, responsibility, and trustworthiness in the design and implementation of AI systems. Being fair implies that unfair biases should be avoided and different groups should be treated equally. To be responsible is to ensure that human actors are accountable to the outcomes of AI decisions and liabilities are explicitly defined in the event of harm or failure. To achieve transparency implies that AI decision-making processes are open and comprehensible, which, in turn, makes users trust it and can efficiently supervise it. To come up with highly innovative and reliable AI technologies, it is important to integrate the FAT principles into AI governance. This involves a set of ethical standards, regulatory policies, and technical provisions. Fairness, accountability, and transparency are not to be perceived as added features, but rather as essential characteristics of any AI system that can be implemented in society.

Much work needs to be done to put these principles into practice. We need to strike a wise balance between fairness and efficiency, transparency and privacy, accountability, and innovation. These are the trade offs that are too complicated to solve with technologists only. They will have to be addressed through interdisciplinary teamwork, a team of computer scientists, policy makers, ethics, legal, and civil society representatives. Through collaborative efforts, the stakeholders can make AI more responsible so that its development ensures maximum benefits and preservation of core rights and values. Finally, pursuing fairness, accountability, and transparency in AI is necessary to maximise the potential of AI to benefit society and reduce its risks. By assembling more and more conversation, building strong governance systems, and dedicating ourselves to ethical standards, we can put AI on a course that earns the confidence of the public and functions in the service of humanity.

References

Afreen, J., Mohaghegh, M. and Doborjeh, M. (2025). Systematic literature review on bias mitigation in generative AI. *AI and Ethics*, 1–53. https://doi.org/10.1007/s43681-025-00721-9.

Akhtar, M.A.K., Kumar, M. and Nayyar, A. (2024). Transparency and accountability in explainable AI: Best practices. In: *Towards Ethical and Socially Responsible Explainable AI: Challenges and Opportunities* (pp. 127–164). Cham: Springer Nature Switzerland. https://doi.org/10.1007/978-3-031-66489-2_5.

Albaroudi, E., Mansouri, T. and Alameer, A. (2024). A comprehensive review of AI techniques for addressing algorithmic bias in job hiring. *AI*, *5*(1), 383–404. https://doi.org/10.3390/ai5010019.

Ali, A. (2025a). Ethical Implications of Artificial Intelligence: Ensuring Patient Data Security. In: *Transforming Healthcare Sector through Artificial Intelligence and Environmental Sustainability* (pp. 149–164). Singapore: Springer Nature Singapore. https://doi.org/10.1007/978-981-97-9555-0_8.

Ali, A. (2025b). Ethical Considerations and Bias in AI Applications in Healthcare. In: *Artificial Intelligence in Healthcare Information Systems: Security and Privacy Challenges* (pp. 129–146). Cham: Springer Nature Switzerland. https://doi.org/10.1007/978-3-031-84404-1_7.

Almasoud, A.S. and Idowu, J.A. (2025). Algorithmic fairness in predictive policing. *AI and Ethics*, *5*(3), 2323–2337. https://doi.org/10.1007/s43681-024-00541-3.

BaniHani, I., Alawadi, S. and Elmrayyan, N. (2024). AI and the decision-making process: A literature review in healthcare, financial, and technology sectors. *Journal of Decision Systems*, *33*(sup1), 389–399. https://doi.org/10.1080/12460125.2024.2349425.

Bleher, H. and Braun, M. (2023). Reflections on putting AI ethics into practice: How three AI ethics approaches conceptualize theory and practice. *Science and Engineering Ethics*, *29*(3), 21. https://doi.org/10.1007/s11948-023-00443-3.

Casillas, J. (2024). Bias and discrimination in machine decision-making systems. *Ethics of Artificial Intelligence*, 13–38. https://doi.org/10.1007/978-3-031-48135-2_2.

Chamola, V., Hassija, V., Sulthana, A.R., Ghosh, D., Dhingra, D. and Sikdar, B. (2023). A review of trustworthy and explainable artificial intelligence (XAI). *IEEE Access*, *11*, 78994–79015. https://doi.org/10.1109/ACCESS.2023.3294569.

Falco, G., Shneiderman, B., Badger, J., Carrier, R., Dahbura, A., Danks, D., ... & Yeong, Z.K. (2021). Governing AI safety through independent audits. *Nature Machine Intelligence*, *3*(7), 566–571. https://doi.org/10.1038/s42256-021-00370-7.

Fessenko, D.S. and Jasperse, A. (2025). Ethics at the heart of AI regulation. *AI and Ethics*, *5*(3), 3387-3398. https://doi.org/10.1007/s43681-024-00562-y.

Hanna, M.G., Pantanowitz, L., Jackson, B., Palmer, O., Visweswaran, S., Pantanowitz, J., ... & Rashidi, H.H. (2025). Ethical and bias considerations in artificial intelligence/machine learning. *Modern Pathology*, *38*(3), 100686. https://doi.org/10.1016/j.modpat.2024.100686.

Holzinger, A., Zatloukal, K. and Müller, H. (2025). Is human oversight to AI systems still possible? *New Biotechnology*, *85*, 59–62. https://doi.org/10.1016/j.nbt.2024.12.003.

Hosseini Tabaghdehi, S.A. and Ayaz, Ö. (2025). AI ethics in action: A circular model for transparency, accountability, and inclusivity. *Journal of Managerial Psychology*. https://doi.org/10.1108/JMP-03-2024-0177.

Huang, K., Joshi, A., Dun, S. and Hamilton, N. (2024). AI regulations. In: *Generative AI Security: Theories and Practices* (pp. 61–98). Cham: Springer Nature Switzerland. https://doi.org/10.1007/978-3-031-54252-7_3.

Hunkenschroer, A.L. and Luetge, C. (2022). Ethics of AI-enabled recruiting and selection: A review and research agenda. *Journal of Business Ethics*, *178*(4), 977–1007. https://doi.org/10.1007/s10551-022-05049-6.

Jain, D.K., Bhatele, K.R., Garg, D. and Dhiman, G. (Eds.). (2025). *A Compendium of Responsible Artificial Intelligence*. CRC Press.

Jedličková, A. (2025). Ethical approaches in designing autonomous and intelligent systems: A comprehensive survey towards responsible development. *AI & Society*, *40*(4), 2703–2716. https://doi.org/10.1007/s00146-024-02040-9.

Königstorfer, F. and Thalmann, S. (2022). AI documentation: a path to accountability. *Journal of Responsible Technology*, *11*, 100043. https://doi.org/10.1016/j.jrt.2022.100043.

Kurapati, S.S., Yaghy, A. and Shukla, A.G. (2025). Data bias: Ethical considerations for understanding diversity in medical artificial intelligence. *AI and Ethics*, *5*(3), 3399–3405. https://doi.org/10.1007/s43681-024-00589-1.

Leal, A.A. (2022, April). Algorithms, creditworthiness, and lending decisions. In: *International Conference on Autonomous Systems and the Law* (pp. 321–353). Cham: Springer International Publishing. https://doi.org/10.1007/978-3-031-47946-5_17.

Memarian, B. and Doleck, T. (2023). Fairness, accountability, transparency, and ethics (FATE) in Artificial Intelligence (AI) and higher education: A systematic review. *Computers and Education: Artificial Intelligence*, *5*, 100152. https://doi.org/10.1016/j.caeai.2023.100152.

Mökander, J. (2023). Auditing of AI: Legal, ethical, and technical approaches. *Digital Society*, *2*(3), 49. https://doi.org/10.1007/s44206-023-00074-y.

Mökander, J., Morley, J., Taddeo, M. and Floridi, L. (2021). Ethics-based auditing of automated decision-making systems: Nature, scope, and limitations. *Science and Engineering Ethics*, *27*(4), 44. https://doi.org/10.1007/s11948-021-00319-4.

Mora-Cantallops, M., Sánchez-Alonso, S., García-Barriocanal, E. and Sicilia, M.A. (2021). Traceability for trustworthy AI: A review of models and tools. *Big Data and Cognitive Computing*, *5*(2), 20. https://doi.org/10.3390/bdcc5020020.

Murikah, W., Nthenge, J.K. and Musyoka, F.M. (2024). Bias and ethics of AI systems applied in auditing: A systematic review. *Scientific African*, *25*, e02281. https://doi.org/10.1016/j.sciaf.2024.e02281.

Novelli, C., Taddeo, M. and Floridi, L. (2024). Accountability in artificial intelligence: what it is and how it works. *AI & Society*, *39*(4), 1871-1882. https://doi.org/10.1007/s00146-023-01635-y.

Palumbo, G., Carneiro, D. and Alves, V. (2024). Objective metrics for ethical AI: A systematic literature review. *International Journal of Data Science and Analytics*, 1–21. https://doi.org/10.1371/journal.pdig.0000864.

Panarese, P., Grasso, M.M. and Solinas, C. (2025). Algorithmic bias, fairness, and inclusivity: A multilevel framework for justice-oriented AI. *AI & Society*, 1–23. https://doi.org/10.1007/s00146-025-02451-2.

Pulivarthy, P. and Whig, P. (2025). Bias and fairness addressing discrimination in AI systems. In: *Ethical Dimensions of AI Development* (pp. 103–126). IGI Global. https://doi.org/10.4018/979-8-3693-4147-6.ch005.

Radanliev, P. (2025). AI ethics: Integrating transparency, fairness, and privacy in AI development. *Applied Artificial Intelligence*, *39*(1), 2463722. https://doi.org/10.1080/08839514.2025.2463722.

Raji, A.A. H., Alabdoon, A.H.F. and Almagtome, A. (2024, April). AI in credit scoring and risk assessment: Enhancing lending practices and financial inclusion. In: *2024 International Conference on Knowledge Engineering and Communication Systems* (*ICKECS*) (Vol. 1, pp. 1–7). IEEE. https://doi.org/10.1109/ICKECS61492.2024.10616493.

Rezaei, M., Pironti, M. and Quaglia, R. (2024). AI in knowledge sharing: Which ethical challenges are raised in decision-making processes for organisations? *Management Decision*. https://doi.org/10.1108/MD-10-2023-2023.

Sarkar, B. and Paul, R.K. (2025). AI safety and ethical considerations. In: *AI for Advanced Manufacturing and Industrial Applications* (pp. 141–154). Cham: Springer Nature Switzerland. https://doi.org/10.1007/978-3-031-86091-1_6.

Shastry, K.A. and Sanjay, H.A. (2022). Cancer diagnosis using artificial intelligence: A review. *Artificial Intelligence Review*, *55*(4), 2641–2673. https://doi.org/10.1007/s10462-021-10074-4.

Siegel, J. and Pappas, G. (2023). Morals, ethics, and the technology capabilities and limitations of automated and self-driving vehicles. *AI & Society*, *38*(1), 213–226. https://doi.org/10.1007/s00146-021-01277-y.

Speith, T. and Xu, J. (2024, September). Explainability and transparency in practice: A comparison between corporate and national AI ethics guidelines in Germany and China. In: *Explainable and Transparent AI and Multi-Agent Systems: 6th International Workshop, EXTRAAMAS 2024,* Auckland, New Zealand, May 6–10, 2024, *Revised Selected Papers* (Vol. 14847, pp. 205–223). Cham: Springer Nature Switzerland.

Varona, D. and Suárez, J.L. (2022). Discrimination, bias, fairness, and trustworthy AI. *Applied Sciences*, *12*(12), 5826. https://doi.org/10.3390/app12125826.

Von Eschenbach, W.J. (2021). Transparency and the black box problem: Why we do not trust AI. *Philosophy & Technology*, *34*(4), 1607–1622. https://doi.org/10.1007/s13347-021-00477-0.

Wu, C. (2024). Data privacy: From transparency to fairness. *Technology in Society*, *76*, 102457. https://doi.org/10.1016/j.techsoc.2024.102457.

Zhang, J. and Zhang, Z.M. (2023). Ethics and governance of trustworthy medical artificial intelligence. *BMC Medical Informatics and Decision Making*, *23*(1), 7. https://doi.org/10.1186/s12911-023-02103-9.

4 Legal and Regulatory Frameworks for AI
Comparative Global Perspectives

Artificial Intelligence (AI) is swiftly altering governance and business systems, and governmental service systems in the globe. With the growth of AI application, there is a strong necessity to establish legal and regulatory frameworks that are clear, safe, fair, and accountable. This chapter offers a global comparison of the regulation of AI and looks at the way various countries and regions are coping with emerging risks. It also examines the key regulatory paradigms such as the risk-based framework of the European Union, sector-based regulation of the United States, the state-centric governance framework of China, and the evolving regime of data protection and AI regulation in Germany. The chapter shows both similarities and differences of the legal priorities, enforcement mechanisms, and human rights protections. It also addresses issues of balancing worldwide standards and being innovative. The results highlight the significance of regulatory systems of adaptive and inclusive development of responsible AI.

4.1 Introduction

Artificial Intelligence (AI) is a disruptive technology that is swiftly changing social, economic, and administrative frameworks in the world. Nowadays, AI tools are applied to assist in decision-making in the medical diagnosis of health, banking, law enforcement, education, urban services, and online communication. These systems are able to deal with vast amounts of data, construct obscure patterns, and deliver results quicker than the conventional approaches. Due to their capacity to impact the results that directly involve people and society, AI technologies need to be closely regulated (De Almeida et al., 2021). Regulatory and legal frameworks are required to guarantee that AI systems can operate safely, in an ethical manner, and within the scope of human rights. The necessity of regulation is reinforced by the fact that AI keeps penetrating sensitive areas in which unjust or wrongful judgement may cause significant dangers (Nikolinakos, 2023). Most AI systems are also based on an algorithm trained on data, which in its turn might have historical biases. This may cause discrimination during employment, insurance rates, and criminal risk rating. The regulatory standards should hence impose the disclosure of the manner of decision-making and the assessment of fairness (Pfeiffer et al., 2023).

Another strong piece of reasoning behind the need to regulate AI is the issue of privacy. The latest AI methods require a lot of personal information, such as extensive details of behaviour, location, communication, and online actions

DOI: 10.1201/9781003776659-4

of individuals. In the absence of evident legal protection, users might not have control over the collection and use of their information. Moreover, even more sophisticated AI-driven surveillance will be able to keep an eye on individuals on a scale that jeopardises individual freedom and self-determination. The governments should design powerful data protection policies and ethics to avoid intrusive or unauthorised use of personal information (Oseni et al., 2021). The spreading of AI also defies the traditional legal notions of responsibility and accountability. The automated systems can be independent unlike in manual decision-making where it will be hard to find the person to blame in case of errors. The decision may be related to developers, operators, and end users all, yet one of them might not have complete oversight or control. Regulatory steps should be created to create accountability in case the AI systems harm or breach rights (Novelli et al., 2024).

This accelerated development of AI is even more complicated. The changing face of technologies beats the changing face of policy in that the technologies change before the regulatory framework can adjust its policy. The problem of unequal access to AI also brings up the issue of social and economic inequality. Unless communities are digitally equipped and trained, they might be marginalised in the potential of AI. Simultaneously, automation can be used to decrease employment in areas where the tasks are mechanised. . Such changes demand governance policies that promote equity, diversity, and labour adjustment (Al-Dulaimi & Mohammed, 2025). AI also functions internationally, posing international regulatory risks. There are various legal priorities, cultural values, and enforcement capabilities and this causes countries to have different governance models. To achieve global collaboration, the cross border data flows, the trade regulations, and the ethical application of AI technologies should be discussed on the international level. Laws and regulations thus form a critical aspect of directing AI in the responsible and humanistic use to make sure that the society gains advantages of technological advancements at the least possible harm (Kashefi et al., 2024).

4.2 Principles and Foundations of AI Regulation

4.2.1 Key Regulatory Values: Safety, Fairness, Accountability, Human Rights

The regulation of AI is based on a number of significant values that can give guidance to the development and utilisation of AI systems. Such values will assist in safeguarding people and make AI technologies beneficial in society. Safety is a central value. The AI systems should be dependable and should not do harm. This is relevant in crucial sectors like healthcare, transport, and financial systems. Safety is a matter to be tested, risk-assessed, and under human control and constant monitoring. Regulation will help in safeguarding and putting fail safety measures in place to make AI systems (Gyevnar & Kasirzadeh, 2025). Another value that is important is fairness. Large datasets employed by AI systems are usually biased. Unless unbiased, AI can be used to discriminate against people, according to their race, gender, age, or socioeconomic status. Fairness needs data transparency, judgement of the biasness of algorithms, and periodic audits. The regulation should provide equal treatment, and avoid the further aggravation of the existing social inequalities (Chen et al., 2023).

There must be accountability to establish the person behind the activities of AI systems. With automated decision-making, it is hard to determine who is to be held responsible in the case of something going wrong. Regulatory frameworks entail record keeping, decision description, and definite allocation of responsibility to developers, operators, or institutions. Accountability assures that the damage is correctable (Novelli et al., 2024). The ethical basis of AI regulation consists of human rights. The AI systems shall observe privacy, dignity, equality, and freedom of expression. The regulation avoids the abuse of personal information, stalking, and discrimination. The human rights-based approaches can guarantee that AI is focused on democratic principles and societal good (Randazzo & Hill, 2024).

4.2.2 Risk Based vs. Principle-Based Regulatory Approaches

There are various methods of AI regulation to control risks and ensure responsible development. The risk based method categorises AI systems based on the degree of risk. The systems that are exposed to high risks have strict rules due to the fact that their failure can result in serious damages. These can be medical diagnosis instruments, self-driving cars, and policing systems. These systems need effective control, testing, record keeping, and human monitoring. Light regulation is imposed on the low risk AI systems, e.g., chatbots or recommendation systems. The risk-based model is beneficial to the extent that it imposes proportional requirements, which is why it helps to strike the balance between innovation and safety (Ebers, 2025).

The principled approach places more emphasis on general moral principles than on specific rules. It is very flexible as it gives organisations the chance to apply principles in ways that are context related. The method is applicable with rapidly evolving technologies whereby certain regulations can become obsolete in a short period of time. The principle-based regulation promotes responsibility, fair play, transparency, and safety without limiting innovation. It also enables the organisations to take the initiative in handling ethical issues (Choudhury & Avvari, 2025). The two methods are complementary to each other. The general guidance is given by principles, whereas the specific guidance is offered by risk-based rules, which apply to high impact applications. A great number of states blend these two strategies in order to develop balanced and flexible regulatory systems.

4.2.3 Public vs. Private Sector Roles in Regulation

The regulation of AI includes both governmental and non-governmental participants. Every area of operation has diverse tasks that lead to proper governance. The governments and other regulatory bodies in the public sector develop laws, policies, and rules of AI development. The governments defend the general interest of the people by granting the AI systems to be ethically, legally, and safely satisfactory. They develop the laws on data protection, develop oversight agencies, and enact them. The investigations, received grievances and punishments are also carried out by the public authorities in case of violation. The national strategies, funding schemes, and capacity-building efforts enable governments to benefit the responsible development of AI (Walter, 2024).

The private sector has a significant role in the regulation of AI since, in the majority of AI innovations, the technology companies, research facilities, and industry developers are involved. Such organisations build AI models, gather data, and use AI tools in practical application. They have the mandate of establishing internal systems of governance that tackle risk, equity, privacy, and security. A great number of companies establish ethical audit boards, bias audits, and transparency principles. The actors of the private sector assist in the formulation of regulation as they contribute to technical skills and practical knowledge (Radanliev, 2025).

To have effective AI governance, both the government and the business sector have to work together. Companies depend on clear regulations to be responsible, whereas governments rely on them to know about technical developments. The academia and civil society also play their part in providing research, analysis, and advocacy. The multi-stakeholder collaboration assists in the establishment of balanced regulatory frameworks to benefit the populace and foster innovation at the same time (Sharma & Gupta, 2025).

4.3 Regional Legal Approaches and Governance Models

4.3.1 European Union: EU AI Act and General Data Protection Regulation (GDPR)

The European Union (EU) has come up with one of the most extensive and rigorous methods of AI governance. It has adopted a structure that revolves around safeguarding fundamental rights, safety, and trustworthy AI. The risk-based model applied to AI systems in the EU AI Act predetermines four categories of AI systems, namely, unacceptable risk, high risk, limited risk, and minimal risk. Unacceptable risk systems (social scoring, manipulative AI, etc.) are prohibited. There are strict rules to be adhered to in high risk systems, including those of healthcare, energy, law enforcement, and public administration. These are documentation, transparency, human control, and quality data requirements (Krook et al., 2025).

The GDPR by the EU is also at the centre stage of AI governance. The GDPR establishes powerful data protection, agreement, transparency, and user rights regulations. It provides people with a choice on the way their personal data are gathered and utilised. The automated decision-making systems should be able to explain and enable one to question decisions. The GDPR is a widely regarded international privacy regulatory model and has an impact on AI laws in most countries (Hulok, 2025). This strategy of the EU shows its interest in human rights, responsibility, and trust of society. Nevertheless, critics opine that rigid rules could slow down the pace of innovation and impose compliance costs on the small firms. Nevertheless, the EU has been on the forefront in responsible AI governance at the global level.

4.3.2 United States: Sector Specific and Market-Driven Strategies

The U.S. has a decentralised and market-based strategy to AI regulation. The U.S. has no single federal law, but depends on sector-specific regulations that were developed by various agencies. To illustrate, medical AI is subject to the Food and Drug Administration (FDA), consumer protection, and algorithmic fairness to the Federal Trade Commission (FTC), and autonomous vehicles are under the control of the Department of Transportation. This strategy promotes innovation and enables firms to test out new forms of technologies (Xiao et al., 2025).

The regulatory model of the U.S. is one that is aimed at ensuring economic growth and technological dominance. Self-regulation, voluntary guidelines, and industry standards are important. Internal audits, best practice, and ethical design are usually recommended in organisations. Nonetheless, since there is no federal AI law, there are gaps in regulations. A patchwork of regulations has resulted with a variety of rules having been established by some states, including California, who have their own rules on privacy and accountability. It is also the focus of the U.S. on the competitiveness of the international level. The policies that are frequently discussed are retaining leadership in AI research and avoiding its misuse by foreign actors. As much as the U.S. strategy promotes innovation, there is a notion of weaker protection of privacy, fairness, and accountability (Sloane & Wüllhorst, 2025).

4.3.3 China: State-Driven Governance and Digital Sovereignty

China is a state-based system of governance that employs AI to facilitate national building, government, and social control. The Chinese government is dominant in controlling AI and directions of its development. National security, digital sovereignty, and economic competitiveness are the standards of the regulatory philosophy of China (Zeng, 2022). China has already issued a number of guidelines concerning AI that revolves around safety, algorithm disclosure, and censoring of content. The Algorithm Recommendation Regulation mandates the platforms to render algorithms fair and transparent. The Chinese variant of privacy regulation is the Personal Information Protection Law (PIPL) and it regulates the possibility of collecting and using data. China has also put in place stern facial recognition, internet content, and internet security controls (Calzada, 2022).

Nevertheless, there is also a powerful system of state surveillance and data gathering in China due to its system of governance. The field of AI is applied to social monitoring, administrative control, and security in the public. Critics claim that this model favours the interest of the state and not the privacy of individuals.

Proponents say that it enables the speedy technological expansion and massive adoption of AI systems (Roberts et al., 2021).

4.3.4 Other Regional Examples: UK, Japan, Singapore

There are other models of AI governance that have developed in several other regions.

The United Kingdom has a liberal and innovation based system. It does not enforce stringent laws but instead guides by regulators like the information commissioner's office (ICO). The UK is concerned with ethical values, risk management, and cooperation with the industry (Liddell et al., 2021). Japan has a model of cooperation called Society 5.0 that incorporates AI into the development of society. Japan prioritises security, human dignity, and social good. It has a principle-based regulatory strategy and promotes automation trust (Holroyd, 2022). Singapore encourages a balanced solution in its "Model AI Governance Framework". It offers workable principles on fairness, explainability, and data governance. Singapore pays attention to the industrial preparedness and helps companies by means of the government-led AI projects (Alibašić, 2025). These geographical strategies demonstrate that there is no model of regulation of AI. Every nation is a combination of the values of ethics, economic ambitions, and cultural priorities that help develop its governance policy. Table 4.1 presents the comparison between AI governance models in major regions, which involves regulatory approaches, key features, and major focus areas.

Table 4.1 Comparison of Regional AI Governance Models.

Region	*Regulatory Approach*	*Key Features*	*Focus Area*
European Union	Risk-based, rights centred	Strict rules, GDPR, bans high risk uses	Human rights, accountability
United States	Sector-specific, market driven	Agency-led regulations, innovation focused	Competitiveness, industry autonomy
China	State-driven, sovereignty model	Strong government control, national security	Surveillance, stability, growth
United Kingdom	Flexible, regulator-led	Guidance over strict laws	Innovation and ethical principles
Japan	Principle-based, human centred	"Society 5.0 ", dignity and safety	Social benefit and trust
Singapore	Practical, industry supportive	Model governance framework, pilot programmes	Responsible deployment

4.4 National Case Studies

4.4.1 *Germany: Data Protection and Emerging AI Regulatory Landscape*

The German policy of AI regulation is based on the constitutional adherence of Germany to human dignity and protection of the fundamental rights. Independent data protection authorities perform regulatory supervision on the federal and state (Länder) levels. This decentralised system fosters accountability and subsidises regulatory capacity to suit the sector-specific requirements (Schmidt et al., 2024). Institutional coordination and technical standards are also highlighted through Germany when it comes to governing AI. The standard-setting organisations, research institutions, and industry bodies are involved in the development of transparency, cybersecurity, risk management, and system reliability guidelines. The responsible adoption of AI in areas like manufacturing, mobility, energy, and government are supported by the public funding programmes and innovation programmes (Fraenkel-Haeberle, 2026).

Besides, Germany promotes the consultation procedure and moral reasoning by using advisory councils and committees of experts. These processes keep legal and policy formulations in line with societal values and democracy. Despite the comparatively well established system of governance, there are difficulties in its regular enforcement, serving small and medium-sized businesses with their compliance, and overseeing the more complex AI systems. On the whole, the AI regulatory environment in Germany is still in the developmental stage as the country moves towards addressing changes in technology and AI regulation policies on the European and national scale (Liebig et al., 2024).

4.4.2 *Canada: Responsible Innovation and Transparency Laws*

Canada is known to have an ethical and humanistic attitude to AI governance. The nation focuses on responsible innovation, openness, and respect of individual rights. Canada was the first country to release the Directive on Automated Decision Making, where it introduced a guideline that regulates the use of AI by the government in the world. This guideline demands that AI systems in the public sector should be assessed through algorithmic impacts, transparency reporting, and human oversight (Attard-Frost & Lyons, 2025). Another part of global AI governance is that Canada is participating in Global Partnership on Artificial Intelligence (GPAI). The nation facilitates equity, responsibility, and social good in the use of AI. The Canadian privacy laws such as the personal information protection and electronic documents act (PIPEDA) govern the manner in which organisations process personal information. Modernisation of the privacy laws that Canada is undertaking today is aimed at solving AI specific problems of automated decision-making, algorithmic discrimination, and cross-border data flows (Roberts et al., 2024). The strategy of Canada is the strategy of trust building. It promotes innovation in businesses with a high level of ethical conduct. This regulatory environment is facilitated by public engagement and transparency tools and academic research. It is also investing in AI research hubs in Toronto, Montreal, and Edmonton, which developed a solid ecosystem of responsible AI development (Gherhes et al., 2022).

4.4.3 Australia and Brazil: Developing Governance Structures

Brazil and Australia are two of the new models of governance in the AI world. Regulatory frameworks are being reinforced in both countries in order to deal with the increased use of AI. Australia is focused on risk management, accountability, and safety. Some of the principles addressed in the Australian AI Ethics Framework are fairness, privacy, transparency, and contestability. The government supports ethical policies to companies and protects responsible innovation. Australia is also considering laws involving privacy, rights of consumers, and internet safety in order to deal with the challenge of AI. It has a flexible regulatory environment, and industries have an opportunity to adapt to it without compromising on protection of users (Filgueiras, 2023).

National strategies and legislative reforms are growing AI governance in Brazil. Brazilian Artificial Intelligence Strategy (EBIA) is focused on innovation, education, ethical use, and collaboration with other countries. The General Data Protection Law (LGDP) of Brazil regulates the collection and processing of the data. It is applicable both in the public and the private sector and has regulations on consent, transparency, and user rights. Brazil is also considering novel rules to govern the potential risky AI frameworks and enhance responsibility (Canedo et al., 2022). Infrastructure gaps, enforcement capacity, and awareness of the people are some of the challenges that both Australia and Brazil encounter. Nonetheless, they demonstrate their intentions towards ethical AI and international collaboration in their strategies (Frey & Presidente, 2024).

4.4.4 Lessons Learned from Diverse Regulatory Contexts

A comparison between national strategies brings about a number of lessons. To begin with, it is necessary to have flexible and adaptive regulation since AI technologies change rapidly. Policies need to be revised on a regular basis in the countries to deal with new risks. Second, effective data protection legislation is the basis of secure AI systems. Countries which have good privacy laws are in a position to respond to surveillance, consent, and misuse of data. Third, accountability and transparency play an important role in the development of trust. The impact assessment model of Canada, the rules of documentation of the EU, and the privacy standards of Germany demonstrate that the citizens gain confidence when the AI systems can be understood and explained. Fourth, the government, industry, and academic collaboration will help in better governance. The multi-stakeholder relationships help many states to establish ethical frameworks and technical solutions.

Lastly, the regulatory decisions are influenced by national contexts. There are countries that focus on human rights, whereas there are those that focus on economic growth or national security. Nevertheless, the similarities of all countries lie in having the same objectives: to safeguard citizens, responsible innovation, and make AI a beneficial factor in social and economic progress. Table 4.2 presents a comparative analysis of national AI governance models in Germany, Canada, Australia, and Brazil with the identification of their major features and areas of concentration.

Table 4.2 Comparison of National AI Governance Approaches.

Country	*Key Features*	*Focus Area*
Germany	GDPR and Federal Data Protection Act (BDSG); EU AI Act implementation; National AI Strategy	Fundamental rights protection, risk-based regulation, industrial innovation
Canada	Transparency laws, government AI rules, GPAI	Accountability, fairness, ethical innovation
Australia	AI ethics framework, privacy reforms	Safety, risk management, responsible use
Brazil	National AI strategy, LGPD privacy law	Innovation, data rights, international cooperation

4.5 Enforcement Challenges and Regulatory Gaps

4.5.1 Implementation and Compliance Difficulties

The implementation and compliance have proven to be one of the biggest obstacles to the regulation of AI. The enforcement agencies usually have an insufficient technical capability and resources to assess complicated AI systems even in the presence of legislation. There is a possibility that regulators are fully unfamiliar with the nature of the algorithms, how they process data, and how they make decisions. This makes it hard to assess the compliance of the AI developers and organisations to the regulatory standards. The majority of organisations, particularly the small companies and government institutions with small budgets, find compliance to be time-consuming and expensive. Documentation, bias audits, transparency reports, and risk assessments are some of the requirements that require talented personnel and sophisticated tools. The difficulty in regulatory expectations is that some organisations cannot comprehend regulatory expectations since such rules are not clear, fragmented, or change rapidly (Deshpande, 2024).

The other problem is that most AI systems are black boxes, i.e., the processes that they go through are not easily understandable. Although there are powerful regulations, it will be hard to enforce them when the authorities are not able to interpret or monitor the system. Absence of explicit criteria of explainability also makes compliance monitoring more complex. Organisations might provide that proprietary models can not entirely be disclosed which curbs oversight and responsibility (Hassija et al., 2024). There are also implementation problems in the use of AI in the public sector. Government agencies can implement automated decision instruments without conducting a due evaluation and its effects may be disastrous in the distribution of welfare, in policing, or in immigration evaluations. Unless there is effective internal control, AI in the public sector can cause significant danger to vulnerable populations (Tveita & Hustad, 2025).

4.5.2 Jurisdictional Conflicts and Cross Border Implications

AI systems have a cross-border nature and it raises several legal issues. Various nations have their own privacy regulations, ethical codes, and the risk threshold. In cases where AI tools created in a particular country are implemented in another, there can be a conflict of regulatory standards (De Almeida et al., 2021). As an example, the GDPR and AI Act by the EU established a stringent regulation regarding data security and AI. Non-EU based companies are, however, allowed to adhere to more relaxed or lax rules. In cases where these systems will handle the data of EU citizens, there would be clashes on whose laws to be enforced. This poses a challenge to international companies and makes enforcement a challenge. Another challenge is the cross-border data flows. AI uses extensive datasets that are commonly transferred across countries to store, analyse, and train the models. Certain nations permit free movement of the data and some nations prohibit the movement of the data outside their borders due to security or sovereignty reasons. These disparities complicate the collaboration between countries and might slacken the development of AI (Rong et al., 2025).

Another example of jurisdictional challenge is when detrimental content or biased algorithms are disseminated on the international arena by using digital platforms. One place recommendation algorithm can have an impact on elections, popular opinion, or even consumer behaviour elsewhere. Companies that have operations in more than one legal system are usually difficult to regulate or sanction by regulatory bodies (Kokshagina et al., 2023). New technologies like generative AI act as other sources of intensifying cross border risks. Misinformation created by AI, deepfakes, and hacking can have their source anywhere and influence individuals around the world. Such threats cannot be dealt with by the national authorities alone. The lack of unified international regulations poses major regulatory loopholes and undermines the quality of the entire regulatory environment (Walter, 2024).

4.5.3 Rapid Technological Change vs. Slow Policy Adaptation

The pace of AI technology development is much higher than regulatory ones. New tools, applications, and risks keep coming in without even the lawmakers knowing or being in a position to know how to regulate it. This generates a constant disconnect between law and technological innovation. The AI models are constantly changing, with updates, newly adhered to datasets, and enhanced algorithms. Such changes are capable of changing the behaviour of the systems and existing rules become obsolete. It is not simple to change laws whenever a new model or feature comes up by regulators. Consequently, old regulations might not respond to the new threat of sophisticated deepfakes, intelligent weapons, and big data predictive analytics (Mueller, 2025).

The process of legislation is slow due to the need to debate, consult with the stakeholders, and review of the law. The technology that a regulation is aiming to regulate might have already evolved by the time that regulation is ratified. Such policy time lag undermines policy effectiveness. Firms are also able to take advantage of grey litigations or old legislation to evade responsibility. Another type of risk that has not been yet taken into account by policymakers is the creation of new categories of risk by innovation in AI. In particular, foundation models, as well as generative AI, cast doubt on copyright, misinformation, and content moderation, which cannot be comprehensively covered by current legislative regulations. Organisations can implement these systems without any guidelines or accountable people without updated guidance (Ghosh et al., 2025).

The lack of political awareness is also associated with slow adaptation of the policies. Not all policymakers are highly technical experts in the field of AI, which makes it difficult to establish effective laws. Governments need to depend on professionals, the stakeholders in the industry, and international organisations to keep up to date. Nevertheless, this partnership is time-consuming and can result in uneven policy making (Nordström, 2022). In order to overcome these difficulties, adaptive regulatory frameworks, sandbox settings, and ongoing review are under consideration by numerous countries. These strategies contribute to changing regulations faster and give a chance to test AI applications in an experimental setting. Nevertheless, the implementation is not uniform throughout the world and vast loopholes in the global governing system still exist.

4.6 Harmonization and Global Cooperation

4.6.1 International Standards and Multilateral Agreements

International standards are significant in AI governance. These standards give the principles on safety, data quality, transparency, and accountability. They assist in making various nations observe the same rules despite the fact that they may have different legal systems. Standards also facilitate interoperability, i.e., AI systems written in one area can be utilised in another with significant agreement. Most of these standards are developed by organisations like the international organisation of standardisation (ISO) and the Institute of Electrical and Electronics Engineers (IEEE). The governance of AI globally also needs multilateral agreements. Nations tend to enter into agreements that establish common values and anticipations of responsible AI. Such agreements make countries develop confidence between each other and work together in such areas like research, sharing of technology, and risk management. They also assist in the establishment of international norms, which regulate behaviour in situations where there is a difference in laws (Roberts et al., 2024).

International treaties can be helpful in dealing with information flows, cybercrime, and ethical aspects. Indicatively, data-sharing agreements are designed to allow safeguarding of personal data even when it is received by a different country. Research cooperation agreements enable countries to share knowledge and to eliminate duplication of effort. It is essential to multilaterally coordinate since the risks associated with AI including misinformation on the Internet or cyberattacks can influence international communities (Saeidnia et al., 2025).

4.6.2 Role of Organizations like OECD, UNESCO, G20, and WTO

The international organizations are involved in significant tasks of global AI governance.

The Organisation for Economic Co-operation and Development (OECD) has come up with powerful principles of AI that dwell upon human centred values, transparency, safety, and accountability. These values inform most of the policies in the country and contribute to ethical AI development. OECD also offers research, benchmarks, and policy recommendations to governments (Pappas & Vassilakopoulou, 2025). The initial global agreement on the ethics of AI was developed by the United Nations Educational, Scientific and Cultural Organization (UNESCO). Its focus is on social inclusion, human rights, environmental sustainability, and cultural diversity. Its guidelines are such that it enables AI to benefit all nations including the developing ones that have less technological capacity. UNESCO encourages AI to uphold human dignity as well as safeguard vulnerable communities (Mochizuki et al., 2025).

The G20 nations work together in matters pertaining to global economic governance. The G20 has published the rules of ethical AI and responsible innovation. G20 debates are aimed at finding a balance between economic growth and ethical obligations. The impact of these discussions at the national level is on strategies of the economies which are at the forefront of AI research (Li & Guangwen, 2025). WTO (World Trade Organisation) equally plays a role in governing AI in the world, as it deals with digital trade, cross-border data flows, and technology standards. With the emergence of AI as the focal point of the global markets, WTO systems assist in controlling the commerce of digital products, software, and information services. The negotiations of WTO play a crucial role in achieving equal access to AI technologies and limited barriers impeding global innovation (Qiang & Jing, 2024). These global organisations never impose law, but they establish common norms and expectations. They promote collaboration among nations that adhere to various political systems and economic agendas. They play an important role in establishing a predictable, stable, and ethical global AI ecosystem.

4.6.3 *Building Interoperable and Inclusive Global AI Governance*

One of the challenges is to develop interoperable and inclusive global AI governance. The term interoperability implies that AI systems, regulations, and standards are able to collaborate within countries. International companies will have to deal with conflicting rules without interoperability, and users will have different protection. Nations are currently attempting to work out the systems of governance where various bodies of law will coexist without clamping absolute sameness (Leese, 2024). Inclusive governance allows participation of all the countries, and particularly the developing countries, in decision-making. Several areas do not have the technical skills or financial capability to create powerful AI systems. The world may become more unequal as long as the governance is overtaken by a small group of powerful nations. Expansive collaboration enables every nation to gain access to AI without exploitation and reliance on technology (Effoduh et al., 2024).

In order to achieve inclusive governance, the countries have to exchange best practices, train, and facilitate capacity-building programmes. The sharing of knowledge assists countries to gain local skills in data security, algorithm verification, and AI risk management. Developing countries can be assisted by international financing and collaboration to implement ethical AI systems in medical care, education, agriculture, and government through the implementation of the system (Moon, 2023). There is also the need for transparency in communication amongst governments, industries, researchers, and civil society in collaborative governance. Multi-stakeholder engagement is the way to make sure that the governance is represented by social values and needs of a community. With a number of voices involved, the regulations will be more equal, more realistic, and generally acceptable (Sharma & Gupta, 2025).

Adaptability is another aspect of global governance. AI technologies are rapidly developing, and new threats like deepfakes, autonomous weapons, and generative AI have to be addressed by the governing bodies. The countries require structures which can be revised frequently by working together with countries abroad. Disclosure of risks and new technologies will contribute to raising the resilience of the world (Zaidan & Ibrahim, 2024). Ethical and responsible AI use is facilitated by harmonisation and global cooperation throughout the world. The harmonisation of policies, common standards, and common reactions to world issues are beneficial to countries. Interoperable and inclusive governance will make AI to enhance the well-being of humans, economic growth, and social justice.

4.7 Conclusion

AI has already taken over the social, economic, and political systems of people in different parts of the world, and its fast growth requires efficient legal and regulatory measures. The chapter has demonstrated that various countries and regions are striving to establish governance frameworks that would see AI being secure, equitable, transparent, and responsible. The EU advocates rights-based regulation, the U.S. is more sector and innovation oriented, and China adheres to the state approach that is more concerned with national security and economic dominance. The examples of emerging approaches in Germany, Canada, Australia, and Brazil show how countries can adjust AI governance to the requirements of their localities and priorities in development.

Nevertheless, there are shared issues even though they are different. It is hard to enforce, the movement of data across borders raises legal issues, and technology is changing at a quicker pace than regulation. These problems demonstrate the necessity of international collaboration and unified standards. The protection of human rights, popular trust, and the general availability of AI benefits should continue to be a priority in the governance process.

On the whole, legal and regulatory frameworks can play a crucial role in unleashing AI to ethical and socially viable consequences. The second phase of global governance will involve more adaptable and future receptive regulations and closer cooperation between governments, industry, academia, and civil society. All these measures can aid in making sure that AI does not stop its evolution, but it safeguards people, society, and democratic principles.

References

Al-Dulaimi, A.O.M. and Mohammed, M.A.A.W. (2025). Legal responsibility for errors caused by artificial intelligence (AI) in the public sector. *International Journal of Law and Management*. https://doi.org/10.1108/IJLMA-08-2024-0295.

Alibašić, H. (2025). Harmonizing artificial intelligence (AI) governance: A comparative analysis of Singapore and France's AI policies and the influence of international organization: H. Alibašić. *Global Public Policy and Governance*, 1–21. https://doi.org/10.1007/s43508-025-00116-w.

Attard-Frost, B. and Lyons, K. (2025). AI governance systems: A multi-scale analysis framework, empirical findings, and future directions. *AI and Ethics*, *5*(3), 2557–2604. https://doi.org/10.1007/s43681-024-00569-5.

Calzada, I. (2022). Citizens' data privacy in China: The state of the art of the Personal Information Protection Law (PIPL). *Smart Cities*, *5*(3), 1129–1150. https://doi.org/10.3390/smartcities5030057.

Canedo, E.D., Calazans, A.T.S., Bandeira, I.N., Costa, P.H.T. and Masson, E.T.S. (2022). Guidelines adopted by agile teams in privacy requirements elicitation after the Brazilian general data protection law (LGPD) implementation. *Requirements Engineering*, *27*(4), 545–567. https://doi.org/10.1007/s00766-022-00391-7.

Chen, P., Wu, L. and Wang, L. (2023). AI fairness in data management and analytics: A review on challenges, methodologies, and applications. *Applied Sciences*, *13*(18), 10258. https://doi.org/10.3390/app131810258.

Choudhury, A. and Avvari, V. (2025). Regulatory Frameworks for Autonomous AI: Balancing Innovation and Safety. In: *The Power of Agentic AI: Redefining Human Life and Decision-Making: In Industry 6.0* (pp. 273–289). Cham: Springer Nature Switzerland. https://doi.org/10.1007/978-3-031-89424-4_18.

De Almeida, P.G.R., Dos Santos, C.D. and Farias, J.S. (2021). Artificial intelligence regulation: A framework for governance. *Ethics and Information Technology*, *23*(3), 505–525. https://doi.org/10.1007/s10676-021-09593-z.

Deshpande, A. (2024, April). Regulatory compliance and AI: Navigating the legal and regulatory challenges of AI in finance. In: *2024 International Conference on Knowledge Engineering and Communication Systems* (*ICKECS*) (Vol. 1, pp. 1–5). IEEE. https://doi.org/10.1109/ICKECS61492.2024.10616752.

Ebers, M. (2025). Truly risk-based regulation of artificial intelligence how to implement the EU's AI Act. *European Journal of Risk Regulation*, *16*(2), 684–703. https://doi.org/10.1017/err.2024.78.

Effoduh, J.O., Akpudo, U.E. and Kong, J.D. (2024). Toward a trustworthy and inclusive data governance policy for the use of artificial intelligence in Africa. *Data & Policy*, *6*, e34. https://doi.org/10.1017/dap.2024.26.

Filgueiras, F. (2023). Designing artificial intelligence policy: Comparing design spaces in Latin America. *Latin American Policy*, *14*(1), 5–21. https://doi.org/10.1111/lamp.12282.

Fraenkel-Haeberle, C. (2026). The EU Digital Regulation and Its Impact on Germany. In: *The EU Digital Regulation and Its Impact on Member States* (pp. 7–101). Cham: Springer Nature Switzerland. https://doi.org/10.1007/978-3-032-06490-5_3.

Frey, C.B. and Presidente, G. (2024). Privacy regulation and firm performance: Estimating the GDPR effect globally. *Economic Inquiry*, *62*(3), 1074–1089. https://doi.org/10.1111/ecin.13213.

Gherhes, C., Vorley, T., Vallance, P. and Brooks, C. (2022). The role of system-building agency in regional path creation: Insights from the emergence of artificial intelligence in Montreal. *Regional Studies*, *56*(4), 563–578. https://doi.org/10.1080/00343404.2021.1886273.

Ghosh, A., Saini, A. and Barad, H. (2025). Artificial intelligence in governance: Recent trends, risks, challenges, innovative frameworks, and future directions. *AI & Society*, *Y*, 1–23. https://doi.org/10.1007/s00146-025-02312-y.

Gyevnar, B. and Kasirzadeh, A. (2025). AI safety for everyone. *Nature Machine Intelligence*, 1–12. https://doi.org/10.1038/s42256-025-01020-y.

Hassija, V., Chamola, V., Mahapatra, A., Singal, A., Goel, D., Huang, K., ... & Hussain, A. (2024). Interpreting black-box models: A review on explainable artificial intelligence. *Cognitive Computation*, *16*(1), 45–74. https://doi.org/10.1007/s12559-023-10179-8.

Holroyd, C. (2022). Technological innovation and building a 'super smart' society: Japan's vision of society 5.0. *Journal of Asian Public Policy*, *15*(1), 18–31. https://doi.org/10.1080/17516234.2020.1749340.

Hulok, M. (2025, December). The EU model of AI governance: Regulating artificial intelligence through law and policy. In: *ERA Forum* (pp. 1–21). Berlin/Heidelberg: Springer Berlin Heidelberg. https://doi.org/10.1007/s12027-025-00869-1.

Kashefi, P., Kashefi, Y. and Ghafouri Mirsaraei, A. (2024). Shaping the future of AI: Balancing innovation and ethics in global regulation. *Uniform Law Review*, *29*(3), 524–548. https://doi.org/10.1093/ulr/unae040.

Kokshagina, O., Reinecke, P. C. and Karanasios, S. (2023). To regulate or not to regulate: Unravelling institutional tussles around the regulation of algorithmic control of digital platforms. *Journal of Information Technology*, *38*(2), 160–179. https://doi.org/10.1177/02683962221114408.

Krook, J., Winter, P., Downer, J. and Blockx, J. (2025). A systematic literature review of artificial intelligence (AI) transparency laws in the European Union (EU) and United Kingdom (UK): A socio-legal approach to AI transparency governance. *AI and Ethics*, 1–22. https://doi.org/10.1007/s43681-025-00674-z.

Leese, M. (2024). AI and interoperability. In: *Handbook on Public Policy and Artificial Intelligence* (pp. 146–157). Edward Elgar Publishing. https://doi.org/10.4337/9781803922171.00018.

Li, Y. and Guangwen, Z. (2025). Balancing innovation and accountability: AI's transformative influence on logistics in G20 nations. *Humanities and Social Sciences Communications*, *12*(1), 1–12. https://doi.org/10.1057/s41599-025-05090-6.

Liddell, K., Simon, D.A. and Lucassen, A. (2021). Patient data ownership: Who owns your health? *Journal of Law and the Biosciences*, *8*(2), lsab023. https://doi.org/10.1093/jlb/lsab023.

Liebig, L., Güttel, L., Jobin, A. and Katzenbach, C. (2024). Subnational AI policy: Shaping AI in a multi-level governance system. *AI & Society*, *39*(3), 1477–1490. https://doi.org/10.1007/s00146-022-01561-5.

Mochizuki, Y., Bruillard, E. and Bryan, A. (2025). The ethics of AI or techno-solutionism? UNESCO's policy guidance on AI in education. *British Journal of Sociology of Education*, 1–22. https://doi.org/10.1080/01425692.2025.2502808.

Moon, M.J. (2023). Searching for inclusive artificial intelligence for social good: Participatory governance and policy recommendations for making AI more inclusive and benign for society. *Public Administration Review*, *83*(6), 1496–1505. https://doi.org/10.1111/puar.13648.

Mueller, M.L. (2025). It's just distributed computing: Rethinking AI governance. *Telecommunications Policy*, *49*(3), 102917. https://doi.org/10.1016/j.telpol.2025.102917.

Nikolinakos, N.T. (2023). Ethical principles for trustworthy AI. In: *EU Policy and Legal Framework for Artificial Intelligence, Robotics, and Related Technologies: The AI Act* (pp. 101–166). Cham: Springer International Publishing. https://doi.org/10.1007/978-3-031-27953-9_3.

Nordström, M. (2022). AI under great uncertainty: Implications and decision strategies for public policy. *AI & Society*, *37*(4), 1703–1714. https://doi.org/10.1007/s00146-021-01263-4.

Novelli, C., Taddeo, M. and Floridi, L. (2024). Accountability in artificial intelligence: What it is and how it works. *AI & Society*, *39*(4), 1871–1882. https://doi.org/10.1007/s00146-023-01635-y.

Oseni, A., Moustafa, N., Janicke, H., Liu, P., Tari, Z. and Vasilakos, A. (2021). Security and privacy for artificial intelligence: Opportunities and challenges. *arXiv preprint arXiv:2102.04661*. https://doi.org/10.48550/arXiv.2102.04661.

Pappas, I.O. and Vassilakopoulou, P. (2025). Human Value Alignment in AI. In: *Handbook of Human-Centered Artificial Intelligence* (pp. 1–33). Singapore: Springer Nature Singapore. https://doi.org/10.1080/0144929X.2024.2448719.

Pfeiffer, J., Gutschow, J., Haas, C., Möslein, F., Maspfuhl, O., Borgers, F. and Alpsancar, S. (2023). Algorithmic fairness in AI: An interdisciplinary view. *Business & Information Systems Engineering*, *65*(2), 209–222. https://doi.org/10.1007/s12599-023-00787-x.

Qiang, R.E.N. and Jing, D.U. (2024). Harmonizing innovation and regulation: The EU Artificial Intelligence Act in the international trade context. *Computer Law & Security Review*, *54*, 106028. https://doi.org/10.1016/j.clsr.2024.106028.

Radanliev, P. (2025). Frontier AI regulation: What form should it take? *Frontiers in Political Science*, *7*, 1561776. https://doi.org/10.3389/fpos.2025.1561776.

Randazzo, M.S. and Hill, G. (2024). Human dignity in the age of Artificial Intelligence: An overview of legal issues and regulatory regimes. *Australian Journal of Human Rights*, *30*(3), 386–408. https://doi.org/10.1080/1323238X.2025.2483822.

Roberts, H., Cowls, J., Morley, J., Taddeo, M., Wang, V. and Floridi, L. (2021). The Chinese approach to artificial intelligence: An analysis of policy, ethics, and regulation. In: *Ethics, Governance, and Policies in Artificial Intelligence* (pp. 47–79). Cham: Springer International Publishing. https://doi.org/10.1007/978-3-030-81907-1_5.

Roberts, H., Hine, E., Taddeo, M. and Floridi, L. (2024). Global AI governance: Barriers and pathways forward. *International Affairs*, *100*(3), 1275–1286. https://doi.org/10.1093/ia/iiae073.

Rong, K., Ling, Y., Yang, T. and Huang, C. (2025). Cross-border data transfer: Patterns and discrepancies. *Journal of International Business Policy*, *8*(1), 10–32. https://doi.org/10.1057/s42214-025-00209-7.

Saeidnia, H.R., Hosseini, E., Lund, B., Tehrani, M.A., Zaker, S. and Molaei, S. (2025). Artificial intelligence in the battle against disinformation and misinformation: A systematic review of challenges and approaches. *Knowledge and Information Systems*, *67*(4), 3139–3158. https://doi.org/10.1007/s10115-024-02337-7.

Schmidt, J., Schutte, N.M., Buttigieg, S., Novillo-Ortiz, D., Sutherland, E., Anderson, M., ... & Van Kessel, R. (2024). Mapping the regulatory landscape for artificial intelligence in health within the European Union. *NPJ Digital Medicine*, *7*(1), 229. https://doi.org/10.1038/s41746-024-01221-6.

Sharma, V.C. and Gupta, J.K. (2025). Artificial Intelligence in Construction: Multi-Stakeholder Strategies for Future Development. *International Journal of Construction Education and Research*, 1–25. https://doi.org/10.1080/15578771.2025.2486617.

Sloane, M. and Wüllhorst, E. (2025). A systematic review of regulatory strategies and transparency mandates in AI regulation in Europe, the United States, and Canada. *Data & Policy*, *7*, e11. https://doi.org/10.1017/dap.2024.54.

Tveita, L.J. and Hustad, E. (2025). Benefits and Challenges of Artificial Intelligence in Public Sector: A Literature Review. *Procedia Computer Science*, *256*, 222–229. https://doi.org/10.1016/j.procs.2025.02.115.

Walter, Y. (2024). Managing the race to the moon: Global policy and governance in Artificial Intelligence regulation: A contemporary overview and an analysis of socioeconomic consequences. *Discover Artificial Intelligence*, *4*(1), 14. https://doi.org/10.1007/s44163-024-00109-4.

Xiao, H., Ge, W. and Shi, X. (2025). Policy narratives' salience: A comparative analysis of artificial intelligence policy responsiveness to public attention in China and the United States. *Journal of Comparative Policy Analysis: Research and Practice*, 1–23. https://doi.org/10.1080/13876988.2025.2551038.

Zaidan, E. and Ibrahim, I.A. (2024). AI governance in a complex and rapidly changing regulatory landscape: A global perspective. *Humanities and Social Sciences Communications*, *11*(1). https://doi.org/10.1057/s41599-024-03560-x.

Zeng, J. (2022). *Artificial Intelligence with Chinese characteristics: National Strategy, Security, and Authoritarian Governance*. London: Palgrave Macmillan. https://doi.org/10.1007/978-981-19-0722-7.

5 National AI Strategies
Case Studies in AI Policy Implementation

National approaches to Artificial Intelligence (AI) strategies have taken on a vital role in the direction of how nations begin to embrace AI and regulate it. Governments worldwide are working out the global strategies of supporting innovation, improving governance, and making sure that AI will aid in economic and social development. In this chapter, the author focuses on the case studies of AI policy implementation in the chosen countries and how various national priorities define AI governance. It discusses policy frameworks, institutional arrangements, and strategic endeavours that are employed to ensure ethical, inclusive, and sustainable AI systems. Other obstacles that are typical in this chapter include capacity gaps, regulatory complexity, and lopsided digital readiness. It offers a comparison on the way forward to create responsible and future-oriented AI ecosystems in nations.

5.1 Introduction

Artificial Intelligence (AI) has emerged as a significant force of technology and economic transformation in the world. The nations of all regions are implementing AI to enhance healthcare, education, farming, transport, and government management. This trend of AI-driven world development is a symptom of the increasing popularity of the idea that AI will determine future competitiveness, productivity, and social development (Abbas Khan et al., 2024). Governments appreciate the fact that AI has the capacity to aid the solution of such complicated issues like climate change, disease prediction, urban management, and financial inclusion. Consequently, AI is currently regarded as a technological resource as well as a strategic national resource. Countries are spending on AI research, digital infrastructure, and skill development in order to enhance their ability to be innovative (Alhosani & Alhashmi, 2024). They are also aware that unless efforts are made to coordinate planning, the advantages of AI could be lopsided with some groups or regions being left behind. This international trend demonstrates that the development of AI is not a one-man project; it is under the influence of long-term perspectives and national interests (Shao et al., 2022).

The national AI strategies have a critical role when it comes to how countries handle AI development. These measures give a proper roadmap, which details the national objectives, policy directions, and governance systems of responsible use of AI. They assist governments in making a decision on where they can invest, the areas to focus on, and how they can handle the threats posed by AI

DOI: 10.1201/9781003776659-5

technologies. The national strategy also unites various stakeholders among them government bodies, private companies, university, and civil society organisations. This coordination is necessary since development of AI entails numerous actors, which will need to collaborate to have safe and effective implementation (Demaidi, 2025).

The organisation and the quality of AI ecosystems are also influenced by national strategies. They facilitate establishment of research facilities, technology conglomerates, and networks of innovations. They promote the development of industry through providing incentives, grants, and support of regulation. The ethical principles and data protection rules are present in the strategies of many countries which attempt to make sure that the development of AI is oriented on human rights and democratic values (Papyshev, G., & Yarime, 2023). The other concerns that are addressed by these strategies include digital skills, workforce transition, and access to technology. In the absence of such planning the countries might not be able to create a skilled workforce and may not be able to provide management of social effects like job displacement (Schiff, 2022).

The other significant purpose of national AI strategies is to equip the countries with international collaboration. AI technologies are international, and national policies have an international impact. Strategies assist nations to engage in global discussions on data governance, cybersecurity, standards, and systems of ethical practices. The countries can play a more significant role in global governance by establishing their position in the nation and having international regulations aligned to their interests and concerns (Shi, 2025). National AI strategies nowadays are viewed as key instruments in dictating AI adoption and governance. They offer a long-term orientation, encourage responsible development, and contribute to the widespread distribution of the benefits of AI among the members of society. They also mirror the socio economic background, political ideals, and technological competencies of every country (Djeffal et al., 2022). With the ongoing growth of AI, these are the strategies the innovation ecosystems will be based on, and the opportunities and challenges related to AI-driven development are to be managed in this way.

5.2 Foundations of National AI Policy

5.2.1 Strategic Objectives: Innovation, Competitiveness, Social Benefit

The primary pillar of national AI policy is to come up with a clear strategic objective. These goals are typically innovation oriented, economically competitive, and socially beneficial. Countries consider AI as one of the technologies to strengthen their economies. AI has the potential to make work more productive, lower operational expenses, and develop new business. Thus, the policies of the countries frequently favour AI research and development and the implementation of AI based solutions in various industries (Yang & Turi, 2025). Another important goal is competitiveness. Nations seek to establish themselves as leaders in the development of AI in the world. This needs to be invested in the local talents, research centres, and technology firms. Countries turning into the centres of AI on the global scale will be able to draw foreign investment and develop their technological influence. Other countries specialise in certain areas, including health care, farming, production, or education, to create competitive advantages (Demaidi, 2025).

Social good is also critical. Most national AI strategies focus on the idea of AI enhancing the quality of life and helping to benefit the citizens. Medical diagnosis, climate resilience, transportation systems, and people services can all be made better with the help of AI, to name a few. The national policies promote the application of AI to the solution of social problems like poverty, unequal health, and environmental degradation. Such social orientation makes sure that the development of AI is not reduced to business interests, but it also helps to improve human happiness (Dodhia, 2024).

5.2.2 Ethical and Regulatory Considerations in National Planning

The second basis of national AI policy is ethical and regulatory considerations. AI systems may pose threats to privacy, bias, discrimination, safety, and surveillance. Ethical principles and regulatory frameworks that would enable the responsible development of AI should hence be incorporated into national policies (Kashefi et al., 2024). Values include fairness, transparency, accountability, and respect to human rights which are established through ethical guidelines. Diversity would mean that AI systems do not discriminate against individuals or groups. Transparency means that there must be meaning and explanation of the AI decisions. Accountability will make sure that a person takes responsibility in case of harm caused by AI systems. Human rights safeguards make AI not to breach personal freedoms or conduct an intrusive surveillance (Singh, 2023).

There are also rules of data governance that are considered as regulatory. AI relies on big data, and the governments need to make sure that the personal data is gathered, stored, and utilised conscientiously. Several nations establish legal stipulations like consent, minimalisation of data, and definite rights to users. Cybersecurity also has to be viewed as a regulatory matter as AI systems can be easily manipulated and accessed by unauthorised people (Puthal et al., 2025). The requirement of oversight and audit is also taken into account by the national AI policies. The applications of AI, which are considered to be at risk, can be evaluated, documented, and tested regularly. The use of AI in sensitive areas like healthcare, criminal justice, and public administration may require independent review bodies to monitor their use. The ethical and regulatory actions assist to develop trust in AI systems and make them not contradict the national values (Sharma, 2024).

5.2.3 *Building Capacity through Skills, Infrastructure, and Research Investments*

Capacity building is the third pillar of AI policy at the national level. The use of AI will not be successful without qualified specialists, effective digital infrastructure, and ongoing funding of research. Countries should create the capabilities and mechanisms required to facilitate the development of AI in the long term (Demaidi, 2025). Developing skills is imperative. Machine learning, data science, robotics, and software engineering specialists are required in countries. Concurrently, they require ethical, legal, and policy professionals to provide guidance on responsible governance. Digital education, technical training, and workforce transition are programmes in the national strategies. This will assist workers to adjust to automation, and also makes sure AI advantages are not limited to people without higher abilities (Shi, 2025).

Another important component is infrastructure. AI is based on solid internet connectivity, cloud computing, high performance computing systems, and secure data centres. In the absence of good infrastructure, the development of AI is sluggish and constrained. The national AI policies are also investing in the growth of digital networks, upgrading of computing infrastructure, and cyber resilience. This infrastructure is both in the support of the government and the private sector (Demaidi, 2025). The investment into research enhances the national leadership in AI. Universities, innovation labs, and research institutions are funded by the government to encourage the discovery of science and technological advancement. Collaborative research programmes are intersectoral initiatives that involve the academia, industry, and government agencies in the development of new AI applications. National research centres assist the countries in being involved in the global innovation networks and also contribute to international AI standards (Bazavan & Huidumac-Petrescu, 2022).

Startups and small businesses should also be supported in the process of capacity building. Numerous AI policies on a national level provide grants, tax incentives, and incubation programmes to foster entrepreneurship. Such programmes assist in facilitating the creation of AI solutions by new companies and making them a contributor to the domestic economy (Kim et al., 2025).

5.3 AI for Inclusive Growth

5.3.1 *Vision of "AI for All" and Digital Transformation Goals*

The "AI for All" vision indicates the interest to make sure the AI is accessible to all sectors of the society. The government believes that AI has the capacity to enhance economic growth, raise new working places, and sustainable development. This direction is pointed at by the National Strategy of Artificial Intelligence (NSAI) published by NITI (National Institution for Transforming India) Aayog. It points to priority areas like healthcare, agriculture, education, smart cities, and mobility having high social value that can be created with the help of AI (Agarwal & Nene,

2025). Digital transformation has been the key element in development policy. Digital infrastructure, better connectivity, and digital literacy are the goals of such programmes. The next generation of AI developments is based on these efforts and ensures that these changes can achieve improved governance and more efficient government services. It aims to establish an international AI centre through investing in the domestic talent, data ecosystems, and networks of innovations. This is to ensure growth and decrease disparities between regions and communities. A good percentage of the population resides in the rural regions where access to technological services is minimal. "AI for All" guarantees that the benefits are received by farmers, small business people, students, and underprivileged groups. It not only frames AI as a source of economic opportunity, but it also uses it for social empowerment (Xu et al., 2024).

5.3.2 Government Programs, Missions, and Sectoral Initiatives

The Government has introduced several programmes and missions to facilitate the development of AI. NITI Aayog is a leader in most projects on AI in the country. The National Program of Artificial Intelligence is one of the initiatives that encourage research, innovation, and capacity building. They have introduced pilot projects in agriculture to predict crops and manage pests, in healthcare to diagnose early, and in education to create a personalised learning platform. Planning is also presented at the National AI Portal to facilitate collaboration, knowledge sharing, and skill development. It bridges researchers, startups, and policymakers to enhance the ecosystem of AI. Another programme is Responsible AI for Youth, which educates students in AI, which attracts new talent and innovations (Agarwal & Nene, 2025).

India has a lot to gain through sectoral programmes in AI. Applications of AI in healthcare include screening of tuberculosis, cancer screening, remote monitoring, and telemedicine. These are solutions to the lack of medical professionals and treatment gaps. In farming, AI assists in precision agriculture, irrigation, and farm market prediction to enhance the livelihood of the farmers. In learning, AI applications customise the learning process and assist teachers to assess the achievement of students. It is also making investments in smart cities in which it utilises AI in planning, traffic control, and waste management as well as in energy efficiency (Ali, 2025). Another significant field of AI implementation is the financial industry. There is the popularity of digital payment platforms, fraud detection systems, customer support chatbots, etc. Such programmes as Aadhaar and Unified Payments Interface (UPI) contribute to safe digital identity and financial inclusion of millions of people. It is also increasing innovation in defence and climate resilience. The AIs used in surveillance, disaster prediction systems, and environmental monitoring devices assist in national security and sustainability (Sinanan & McNamara, 2021).

5.3.3 *Institutional Governance and Public-Private Partnerships*

The AI ecosystem relies on robust institutional and governmental cooperation, both in the public and the private sectors. The policymaking, research, and implementation have several institutions involved. NITI Aayog is the hub of strategic planning and pilot projects. The Ministry of Electronics and Information Technology (MeitY) concentrates on the standards of AI, data management, and digital infrastructure. AI adoption is the responsibility of other ministries that provide it in the respective fields like health, agriculture, and education (Ghosh et al., 2025). Innovation and development of advanced technology is supported by research institutions and excellence engineering institutes like the Indian Institute of Technology (IITs) and the Indian Institute of Science (IISc). Such enterprises have specific AI research institutions and training courses. They work together with government bodies and industry associates to create practical uses of AI.

The partnership between the state and companies makes the policy of AI implementation stronger. Technology companies offer technical knowhow, capital, and scaling solution platforms. AI research and exchange of knowledge are facilitated by international partnership with nations like the United States, France, and Japan. The collaborative governance will also make sure that AI solutions are technically valid and consistent with the national objectives (Joshi, 2024). Incubators, innovation hubs, grants, and regulatory support are also among the other ways that aid in startup development. The startups in AI are solving societal issues such as access to healthcare, efficiency, and monitoring of the environment. The competitive advantage with large IT (information technology) service firms enables it to scale AI solutions in the domestic and international markets (Agarwal & Nene, 2025).

Simultaneously, It is working on creating ethical principles to make the use of AI responsible. The debate around privacy, surveillance threats, and algorithmic fairness is taking place. The Digital Personal Data Protection Act (DPDP Act), 2023 enhances the rights and responsibilities of data, which constitute a significant component of AI governance (Khanna & Kotwal, 2025).

5.4 Responsible and Transparent AI Leadership

5.4.1 *Ethical Frameworks and Human Rights Based Regulation*

Canada focuses its AI policies on ethical values and human rights-based governance. The nation is of the opinion that AI must assist human dignity, equity, and democracy. The ethical considerations are incorporated in national regulations and guidelines in the sector of the state. The Directive on Automated Decision Making is one of the most powerful policies that demand openness and responsibility in AI usage by the government. Prior to the implementation of AI systems, government agencies are supposed to conduct Algorithms Impact

Assessment (AIA). These tests measure the possible harms, risk of bias, and effects on the rights of individuals (Hogan & Lasek-Markey, 2024).

The privacy laws in Canada also help in the responsible use of AI. PIPEDA regulates data collection and grants rights to the individuals over their personal information. It demands organisations to make sure of safe data management, legal processing, and consent of the users. Presently, Canada is reforming its privacy system according to the suggested Consumer Privacy Protection Act (CPPA) to cover AI specific issues, including automated decision-making, and algorithmic fairness (Sarabdeen et al., 2022). Canada has significant human-centred governance. The laws must explain how the AI systems arrive at decisions in a clear way particularly when the decision relates to access to services or rights. Ethical design activities in the private sector are also encouraged in Canada. Fairness audits, risk assessment, and transparency reports will be recommended to businesses in order to enhance user trust (Attard-Frost & Lyons, 2025).

5.4.2 Public Sector AI Use and Accountability Mechanisms

The responsible use of AI in the public sector is of high priority in Canada. The AI systems are applied in enhancing public services, easing the administration procedures and decision-making by the government. But these tools are not harmful to people or do not put them in a discriminated position with strict accountability mechanisms. The Directive on Automated Decision making affirms that all sets of AI in the public sector will have human supervision. Risky automated decisions need to be subjected to external scrutiny and offer appeal remedies to the citizens who are impacted (Yuan & Chen, 2025). The government agencies must post information about the AI systems used by them. This openness fosters citizen confidence and enables the citizens to know the impact of automation on service delivery. Procurement guidelines are also used in Canada to make sure that AI systems acquired by the private vendors are ethically sound. The governmental bodies need to ensure that the vendors are practising responsible AI, such as safeguarding vulnerable groups (Hirvonen, 2024).

Civil servants can be trained and made aware by training programmes and awareness campaigns about the dangers and limitations of AI. The government promotes the constant observation of the automated systems so that the performance can be fair and correct in the long run. This will minimise the chances of failures or destructive consequences that might occur. The model of accountability used in Canada shows how robust internal governance can contribute to the safe and ethical implementation of AI in the government. It is also used as a guide by the rest of the world on how to strike a balance between technological efficiencies and democratic checkpoints (Bracci, 2023).

5.4.3 AI Research Hubs and International Cooperation

Canada has developed a good reputation of being a world leader in AI research and innovation. The world leading research institutes, like the Vector Institute,

Mila Quebec AI Institute, and the Alberta Machine Intelligence Institute (AMII) are located in major cities, such as Toronto, Montreal, and Edmonton. These universities undertake graduate courses in machine learning, deep learning, robotics, and ethical AI. They work hand-in-hand with universities, industry, and government organisations. Canada is one of the pioneering nations that put up a national AI strategy, which is based on research and talent development. The strategy assists in scholarships, academic roles, and training to create a powerful AI labour force. The availability of internationally known scholars, including the firsts in the domain of deep learning, has contributed to the enhancement of Canadian power in AI science on the international scope (Madan & Ashok, 2025).

One of the main aspects of the AI leadership in Canada is international cooperation. The nation is part of the Global Partnership on Artificial Intelligence (GPAI) which is an international organisation that advocates responsible building and regulation of AI. Canada collaborates with other countries through GPAI in order to establish ethical standards, capacity building, and collective challenges. Canada is also active in AI projects, both in the OECD and the G7. Such partnerships aid in the harmonization of standards and promote international harmonisation in the areas of fairness, safety, and accountability. Canada is also encouraging the inclusive development of AI through global research and trade of technology with developing nations (Yigitcanlar et al., 2024). With good research capacity and ethical leadership, Canada can be a responsible international player in the development of AI.

5.5 Comparative Evaluation and Emerging Challenges

5.5.1 Differences in Priorities, Governance Styles, and Institutional Strength

National AI strategies are indicative of various priorities. There are countries that specialise in technological leadership and competitiveness in the economy. They make massive investments in research, new ventures, and collaboration with industries. Strong research ecosystems in Canada and Singapore based innovation-oriented governance are examples. Other nations are more interested in social good, and they use AI to enhance social services, agriculture, and health outcomes (Demaidi, 2025).

There is also a wide variation in governance styles:

- The European Union has a stringent right-based approach and has privacy and safety as a priority.
- The United States has a decentralised and market-driven approach, which is more dependent on self-regulation within the industry.
- China is a state-led system that has a predominant goal in terms of national security, economic hegemony, and digital sovereignty.

Such disparities influence the speed at which AI policies are implemented and the risk management process. Nations that have well-developed institutions will be able to implement explicit laws and watch over the AI use. Others can find it difficult because of weak regulatory ability or lack of defined roles among the government agencies. The national AI strategies are influenced by institutional strength. The nations that have highly developed digital infrastructure, autonomous regulators, and have a background of working with AI can implement the innovations of AI in a safer way. Conversely, the emerging economies might have difficulties in adopting ethical and technical protection at all times. The difference leads to an unequal development and various degrees of social trust in AI systems (Langer et al., 2023).

5.5.2 Issues in Implementation: Funding, Skills, and Regional Disparities

Despite the good policies, there are still challenges of implementing them. Numerous nations have a problem with underfunding, particularly AI projects in the state sector. The investments in research and development are long-term projects, yet it is very common that due to budget constraints, large-scale deployment is constrained. Smalls and startup firms might not have access to grants, sophisticated technology, and testing facilities (Yerlikaya & Erzurumlu, 2021). Another significant problem is a lack of qualified specialists. There is demand for AI specialists that outweighs supply, particularly in the developing economies. Its talent is usually concentrated in big cities and the rural or remote areas are abandoned. Training and workforce transition programmes are required in countries to assist people to be adjusted to automation and new job positions. Digital illiteracy also makes the adoption slow and adds to inequality (Sundaram & Wesselbaum, 2025).

Geographical inequalities bring additional hindrances. AI solutions are advantageous in urban settings with great interconnection and infractions. In the meantime, the rural population might not be able to access digital services. Such loopholes may enhance socio economic inequalities unless dealt with using equitable deployment approaches (Sawhney, 2023). There are also regulatory enforcement gaps that have an impact on implementation. However, despite the existence of ethical guidelines, it is important to ensure that they are implemented and monitored through constant checking and auditing and by technical assessment. Most of the regulatory authorities do not have the resources and know how to evaluate sophisticated AI systems. Penalties are also weak or ambiguous and this allows organisations to disregard compliance requirements (Zaidan & Ibrahim, 2024).

The success of implementation depends on the public trust. Citizens might be unwilling to accept AI in healthcare, finance, and government administration, in case they are afraid of being spied upon, abusing their data, and making unjust decisions through AI. Confidence should be established through open communication, social activities, and complaint systems (Robles & Mallinson, 2025). Lastly, there are fast rates of technological change that make implementation difficult. Currently developed policies will not respond to future dangers like advanced deepfakes, autonomous weapons, or mass misinformation. The lack of speed in the adaptation of regulatory regimes will create a loophole in governance where malicious practices may find their way out (Ångström et al., 2023).

5.5.3 *Opportunities for Knowledge Exchange and Policy Alignment*

Nevertheless, collaboration has much opportunity despite the challenges. Nations are able to gain knowledge out of the successes of others and their failures. Distributing best practices of ethical governance, data protection, and AI implementation foster uniformity and minimise repetition of effort. For example:

- India can teach other countries that have development interests in the transformation of the public sector.
- Canadian systems of accountability demonstrate that transparency can build upon the trust of the people.
- The organised pilots programmes in Singapore show the way it is possible to test technologies safely before their full implementation.

The collaboration between different countries assists in alignment of policies and interoperable standards. Such organizations as UNESCO, OECD, and GPAI assist countries to work out the common principles according to the principles of fairness, human rights, and responsible innovation. This harmonisation eliminates regulatory nonconformance and assists firms to conduct operations throughout the world without exposing themselves to non-compliance (Kashyap & Mitra, 2025).

Capacity building is also supported by teamwork. The richer countries and international organisations are able to offer technical support, capacity building, and research grants to the less fortunate countries. This avoids the increasing distance between AI leaders and laggers. Nation countries can collaborate through knowledge exchange in order to deal with global risks. Such problems as cyber threats, algorithmic discrimination, and misinformation need to be addressed in unison. Collaboration can enable countries to come up with more powerful defences and mutual monitoring tools (Tummala et al., 2025). Partnerships between the public and the private generate more opportunities. Governments maintain ethical responsibility, and the industry leaders have high levels of knowledge and tools. Universities assist in research and innovation. Close cooperation between these stakeholders will help to hasten the production of responsible AI and promote the social value of technology (Camilleri, 2024).

5.6 Conclusion

The strategies of national AI have become a significant component of the technological development policies and national policies in most countries. This chapter has explored the way governments develop and use AI plans to facilitate innovation, deliver better services to the population, and become more competitive in the global market. The difference between countries in terms of priorities and models of governance was demonstrated. Adopting inclusive growth is responsible innovation and transparency in AI use. These disparities represent the social needs, economic objectives, and institutional strength of each country.

Although this has improved, there are still significant setbacks. The success of the policy implementation is influenced by the lack of funding, lack of skills, and disparities in the regions. Governments also struggle to keep up with rapid changes in technology to make changes in regulations. Nonetheless, such obstacles open the way to cooperation. One can also learn with the experience of other nations and cooperate to create unified standards and moral systems. On the whole, the chapter underscores the significance of powerful, flexible, and human national policies. The balance that needs to be achieved between technological progress and fairness, accountability, and trust of the population is required in AI governance. Further collaboration, policy education, and capacity development will assist the countries to establish AI ecosystems, which will sustain development and act in the interest of all societal members.

References

Abbas Khan, M., Khan, H., Omer, M.F., Ullah, I. and Yasir, M. (2024). Impact of artificial intelligence on the global economy and technology advancements. In: *Artificial General Intelligence (AGI) Security: Smart Applications and Sustainable Technologies* (pp. 147–180). Singapore: Springer Nature Singapore. https://doi.org/10.1007/978-981-97-3222-7_7.

Agarwal, A. and Nene, M.J. (2025). A five-layer framework for AI governance: Integrating regulation, standards, and certification. *Transforming Government: People, Process, and Policy*, *19*(3), 535–555. https://doi.org/10.1108/TG-03-2025-0065.

Alhosani, K. and Alhashmi, S.M. (2024). Opportunities, challenges, and benefits of AI innovation in government services: A review. *Discover Artificial Intelligence*, *4*(1), 18. https://doi.org/10.1007/s44163-024-00111-w.

Ali, A. (2025). Ethical Implications of Artificial Intelligence: Ensuring Patient Data Security. In: *Transforming Healthcare Sector through Artificial Intelligence and Environmental Sustainability* (pp. 149–164). Singapore: Springer Nature Singapore. https://doi.org/10.1007/978-981-97-9555-0_8.

Ångström, R.C., Björn, M., Dahlander, L., Mähring, M. and Wallin, M.W. (2023). Getting AI implementation right: Insights from a global survey. *California Management Review*, *66*(1), 5–22. https://doi.org/10.1177/00081256231190430

Attard-Frost, B. and Lyons, K. (2025). AI governance systems: A multi-scale analysis framework, empirical findings, and future directions. *AI and Ethics*, *5*(3), 2557–2604. https://doi.org/10.1007/s43681-024-00569-5.

Bazavan, A. and Huidumac-Petrescu, C.E. (2022, March). China's drive for technological leadership in artificial intelligence. Key policies and government-industry integration. In: *International Conference on Business Excellence* (pp. 17–30). Cham: Springer Nature Switzerland. https://doi.org/10.1007/978-3-031-19886-1_2.

Bracci, E. (2023). The loopholes of algorithmic public services: An "intelligent" accountability research agenda. *Accounting, Auditing & Accountability Journal*, *36*(2), 739–763. https://doi.org/10.1108/AAAJ-06-2022-5856.

Camilleri, M.A. (2024). Artificial intelligence governance: Ethical considerations and implications for social responsibility. *Expert Systems*, *41*(7), e13406. https://doi.org/10.1111/exsy.13406.

Demaidi, M.N. (2025). Artificial intelligence national strategy in a developing country. *AI & Society*, *40*(2), 423–435. https://doi.org/10.1007/s00146-023-01779-x.

Djeffal, C., Siewert, M.B. and Wurster, S. (2022). Role of the state and responsibility in governing artificial intelligence: A comparative analysis of AI strategies. *Journal of European Public Policy*, *29*(11), 1799–1821. https://doi.org/10.1080/13501763.2022.2094987.

Dodhia, R. (2024). *AI for Social Good: Using Artificial Intelligence to Save the World*. John Wiley & Sons.

Ghosh, A., Saini, A. and Barad, H. (2025). Artificial intelligence in governance: Recent trends, risks, challenges, innovative frameworks, and future directions. *AI & Society*, 1–23. https://doi.org/10.1007/s00146-025-02312-y.

Hirvonen, H. (2024). Just accountability structures: A way to promote the safe use of automated decision-making in the public sector. *AI & Society*, *39*(1), 155–167. https://doi.org/10.1007/s00146-023-01731-z.

Hogan, L. and Lasek-Markey, M. (2024). Towards a Human Rights-Based Approach to Ethical AI Governance in Europe. *Philosophies*, *9*(6), 181. https://doi.org/10.3390/philosophies9060181.

Joshi, D. (2024). AI governance in India: Law, policy, and political economy. *Communication Research and Practice*, *10*(3), 328–339. https://doi.org/10.1080/22041451.2024.2346428.

Kashefi, P., Kashefi, Y. and Ghafouri Mirsaraei, A. (2024). Shaping the future of AI: Balancing innovation and ethics in global regulation. *Uniform Law Review*, *29*(3), 524–548. https://doi.org/10.1093/ulr/unae040.

Kashyap, A.K. and Mitra, Y.D. (2025). World's First Artificial Intelligence Law: A Human-Centric Model for Strengthening AI Governance. In: *Revolution with Generative AI: Trends and Techniques* (pp. 135–169). Cham: Springer Nature Switzerland. https://doi.org/10.1007/978-3-031-91660-1_8.

Khanna, V. and Kotwal, A. (2025). Examining the significance of the digital personal data protection act, 2023 in the context of the healthcare industry: A comprehensive analysis. *Discover Public Health*, *22*(1), 381. https://doi.org/10.1186/s12982-025-00757-6.

Kim, G.Y., Lee, W.J., Choi, B. and Lew, Y.K. (2025). Fostering collaborative opportunities for AI start-ups: The case of a hybrid business incubator in Seoul. *The Journal of Technology Transfer*, *50*(2), 552–581. https://doi.org/10.1007/s10961-024-10102-9.

Langer, M., König, C.J., Back, C. and Hemsing, V. (2023). Trust in artificial intelligence: Comparing trust processes between human and automated trustees in light of unfair bias. *Journal of Business and Psychology*, *38*(3), 493–508. https://doi.org/10.1007/s10869-022-09829-9.

Madan, R. and Ashok, M. (2025). Making sense of AI benefits: A mixed-method study in Canadian public administration. *Information Systems Frontiers*, *27*(3), 889–923. https://doi.org/10.1007/s10796-024-10475-0.

Papyshev, G. and Yarime, M. (2023). The state's role in governing artificial intelligence: Development, control, and promotion through national strategies. *Policy Design and Practice*, *6*(1), 79–102. https://doi.org/10.1080/25741292.2022.2162252.

Puthal, D., Mishra, A.K., Mohanty, S.P., Longo, A. and Yeun, C.Y. (2025). Shadow AI: Cyber Security Implications, Opportunities, and Challenges in the Unseen Frontier. *SN Computer Science*, *6*(5), 405. https://doi.org/10.1007/s42979-025-03962-x.

Robles, P. and Mallinson, D.J. (2025). Artificial intelligence technology, public trust, and effective governance. *Review of Policy Research*, *42*(1), 11–28. https://doi.org/10.1111/ropr.12555.

Sarabdeen, J., Chikhaoui, E. and Ishak, M.M.M. (2022). Creating standards for Canadian health data protection during health emergency: An analysis of privacy regulations and laws. *Heliyon*, *8*(5). https://doi.org/10.1016/j.heliyon.2022.e09458.

Sawhney, N. (2023). Contestations in urban mobility: Rights, risks, and responsibilities for Urban AI. *AI & Society*, *38*(3), 1083–1098. https://doi.org/10.1007/s00146-022-01502-2.

Schiff, D. (2022). Education for AI, not AI for education: The role of education and ethics in national AI policy strategies. *International Journal of Artificial Intelligence in Education, 32*(3), 527–563. https://doi.org/10.1007/s40593-021-00270-2.

Shao, Z., Yuan, S., Wang, Y. and Xu, J. (2022). Evolutions and trends of artificial intelligence (AI): Research, output, influence, and competition. *Library Hi Tech, 40*(3), 704–724. https://doi.org/10.1108/LHT-01-2021-0018.

Sharma, R. (2024). Governance and Oversight of AI Systems. In: *AI and the Boardroom: Insights into Governance, Strategy, and the Responsible Adoption of AI* (pp. 353–370). Berkeley, CA: Apress. https://doi.org/10.1007/979-8-8688-0796-1_28.

Shi, L. (2025). Global Perspectives on AI Competence Development: Analyzing National AI Strategies in Education and Workforce Policies. *Human Resource Development Review*, 15344843251332360. https://doi.org/10.1177/15344843251332360.

Sinanan, J. and McNamara, T. (2021). Great AI divides? Automated decision-making technologies and dreams of development. *Continuum, 35*(5), 747–760. https://doi.org/10.1080/10304312.2021.1983257.

Singh, T. (2023, October). AI-Driven Surveillance Technologies and Human Rights: Balancing Security and Privacy. In: *International Conference on Smart Systems: Innovations in Computing* (pp. 703–717). Singapore: Springer Nature Singapore. https://doi.org/10.1007/978-981-97-3690-4_53.

Sundaram, A. and Wesselbaum, D. (2025). Economic development reloaded: The AI revolution in developing nations. *New Zealand Economic Papers, 59*(1), 11–17. https://doi.org/10.1080/00779954.2024.2439955.

Tummala, V.S., Burris-Melville, T.S. and Eskridge, T.C. (2025). AI as a Team Member: Redefining Collaboration. *Journal of Leadership Studies, 18*(4), 67–80. https://doi.org/10.1002/jls.70003.

Xu, J., Lee, T. and Goggin, G. (2024). AI governance in Asia: Policies, praxis and approaches. *Communication Research and Practice, 10*(3), 275–287. https://doi.org/10.1080/22041451.2024.2391204.

Yang, X. and Turi, A.N. (2025). The Impact of AI on Economic Growth: A Take for Emerging Economies. In: *Tech Transformation and AI Readiness: Pioneering Paths for the Global South* (pp. 31–38). Cham: Springer Nature Switzerland. https://doi.org/10.1007/978-3-031-73639-1_2.

Yerlikaya, S. and Erzurumlu, Y.Ö. (2021). Artificial intelligence in public sector: A framework to address opportunities and challenges. In: *The Fourth Industrial Revolution: Implementation of Artificial Intelligence for Growing Business Success* (pp. 201–216). https://doi.org/10.1007/978-3-030-62796-6_11.

Yigitcanlar, T., David, A., Li, W., Fookes, C., Bibri, S.E. and Ye, X. (2024). Unlocking artificial intelligence adoption in local governments: Best practice lessons from real-world implementations. *Smart Cities, 7*(4), 1576–1625. https://doi.org/10.3390/smartcities7040064.

Yuan, Q. and Chen, T. (2025). Holding AI-based systems accountable in the public sector: A systematic review. *Public Performance & Management Review*, 1–34. https://doi.org/10.1080/15309576.2025.2469784.

Zaidan, E. and Ibrahim, I.A. (2024). AI governance in a complex and rapidly changing regulatory landscape: A global perspective. *Humanities and Social Sciences Communications, 11*(1). https://doi.org/10.1057/s41599-024-03560-x.

6 Governing AI in the Public Sector
Opportunities and Challenges

Artificial Intelligence (AI) finds more and more acceptance in the government sector in order to make services delivery more effective, decision -making more accurate, and administration more efficient. AI tools are applied in the field of healthcare, transportation, social welfare, taxation, and public safety by the governments. These applications provide great chances to enhance governance and facilitate participation of citizens. Nonetheless, the issues of privacy, algorithmic bias, accountability, and insufficient transparency are also the challenges related to AI in the public sector. Responsible deployment is based on fairness, protection of human rights, and the maintenance of trust of the people. This chapter discusses the advantages and risks of AI in the government processes and the ways to create ethical and reliable AI systems in the public administration.

6.1 Introduction

Artificial Intelligence (AI) is a significant technology in contemporary governance. Governments worldwide are embracing AI systems to improve administrative processes, and to advance the provision of government services. Many spheres of public administration nowadays use AI tools to analyse data, make decisions, and forecast them automatically, and conduct real-time monitoring. Such technologies assist the governments to react better to the social and economic hardships. Digital transformation efforts, growing availability of data, and escalating demands of quicker and more transparent government services have created a surge in AI expansion in government services (Alhosani & Alhashmi, 2024). AI enables governments to process big data and pinpoint trends that can be used to make superior policy choices. An example is that predictive analytics can be used to assist governments predict the outbreak of diseases, manage agricultural resources, or eliminate traffic congestion (Yigitcanla et al., 2024). Automated systems are found to be useful in speeding up application processing in welfare programmes, taxation, and in licensing services. Chatbots will enable citizens to get information about the government and save time waiting to be attended to. The applications demonstrate that AI can lessen the administrative load and enhance the quality of services (Alshahrani et al., 2024).

One of the primary reasons why the use of AI is encouraged in the public sector is the creation of value. Governments are trying to use AI to develop more responsive, efficient, and equitable systems. AI may assist in distributing resources in a more efficient way, discover at-risk populations, and offer prompt support to

DOI: 10.1201/9781003776659-6

their areas when it is most required (Mishra et al., 2024). Use of AI in healthcare aids in early diagnosis and enhanced planning of treatment. AI is used to identify the trends of crime and enhance emergency responses in the field of public safety. In cities, AI is used in the planning of smart cities, managing waste, and monitoring the environment. Such technologies enhance the lives of people and facilitate the sustainability development objectives (Fang et al., 2023).

Another significant goal is modernisation of governance. Conventional administrative methods tend to be arduous, hardcopy, and constrained in carrying out intricate information. Routine work that can be performed with the help of AI systems serves to automatise the routine work and enable human employees to concentrate on those tasks that demand certain judgement and empathy. Governments can re-engineer workflows in order to enhance the accuracy, and minimise human errors. The use of digital platforms with the help of AI allows making more transparent decisions, as citizens can monitor the process of providing services to them (Kovari, 2024).

But there are also new burdens associated with modernisation. Governments should make sure that AI systems are developed and deployed in a manner that does not violate human rights and harbour mistrust among citizens. The decisions of the public sector directly affect the citizens and thus any mistakes or partisan conclusions can cause severe damage. This is why AI regulation within a governmental context needs to be properly planned, monitored, and assessed appropriately. Transparency, fairness, and accountability are the keys to the public accepting AI (Duberry, 2022). The advent of AI into the government system is one of the biggest changes to the functioning of the administration of the government. It is very useful yet it poses new ethical, privacy, and trust-related issues. Knowing the opportunities and threats, governments are able to create policies that can encourage responsible use of AI, and make sure that technological advancement benefits democratic principles and society. AI-driven governance is the future of modernising the service, although it should be applied in a careful manner to bring beneficial results to every citizen (Moon, 2023).

6.2 Applications of AI in Public Administration

6.2.1 AI in Public Service Delivery

AI is applied to enhance the delivery of services to people by automating the routine processes and shortening decision-making. Most of the government services like approvals of social welfare, tax processing, and document verification involve repetitive work. Intelligent systems are able to read the documents, cross check the identities, and verify the eligibility fast. This will save time taken by the citizens to wait as well as save the work of the government employees (Anshari et al., 2025). Virtual assistants and chatbots find their way to government portals to provide answers to the questions and lead a user through a process. They offer 24 hours care and assist citizens to get information without the need to go to the government offices. The use of AI-based translation tools also contributes to breaking the language barrier in the multilingual countries (Chen et al., 2021). Predictive analytics enhances the allocation of resources in key services like transport and collection of waste. Data can be used by governments when planning and predicting peak demand. AI is also used to check infrastructure conditions which enable it to repair them early sabotaging disruption of services (Zong & Guan, 2025). With such applications, AI enhances accessibility, user experiences, and inclusive service delivery to the community.

6.2.2 *Smart Governance and Urban Management*

The concept of smart cities and urban governance are all about AI. The issues that urban areas experience are congestion, pollution, waste management, and energy consumption. AI has the capabilities of gathering information through sensors, cameras, and digital systems and assisting city administrators to gain insight into the changing patterns in real-time (Bosco et al., 2024). During transportation, AI assists smart traffic lights, optimisation of routes, and time schedule of the transport. This lessens the traffic and enhances movement. AI is also useful in monitoring the environment, where it can be used to monitor the quality of air, water, and weather patterns. These insights can guide governments to act rapidly to environmental issues (Luusua et al., 2023).

Intelligent utility systems are the ones that utilise AI in managing the delivery of electricity and water. AI induces demand variability and minimises waste through the distribution of resources. Waste management is enhanced by AI-based sorting, bin tracking, and recycling. Surveillance systems with the involvement of AI help to improve urban safety, detecting abnormal behaviour, or identifying hazards. AI tools can also be used to control street lighting and public areas in order to improve security (Ardabili et al., 2023). Smart governance involves involving citizens in decision -making through digital platforms. Its citizens are able to report on matters, monitor progress, and even access local services online. AI does contribute to this communication and helps to increase trust between the population and governments (Arora et al., 2023).

6.2.3 *AI in Public Health, Policing, and Welfare Systems*

AI has significant advantages to health systems. It is useful in the analysis of medical images, diagnosis of diseases at early stages, and in the process of diagnosis by doctors. In the cases of health emergencies, AI anticipates the spread of the disease, aids in the regulation of hospital resources, and assists in the planning of vaccination. AI is employed by the public health authorities in identifying the outbreaks earlier and responding more efficiently (Wagner et al., 2024). AI is used in policing and in community safety such as crime analysis, emergency response, and surveillance. Predictive policing technologies recognise the locations with high risks and aid in the efficient allocation of security resources. The AI systems will be able to scan the video footage in order to identify dangerous activities, lost individuals, or unauthorised intrusion. Still, such applications need strong control to eliminate discrimination and breach of privacy (Kaufmann, 2024).

Social welfare systems are another area of application of AI. It assists in the identification of citizens who are to receive support programmes, fraud detection, and benefit delivery in good time. Welfare programmes can help governments to comprehend the needs and enhance design of policies. AI can enhance fairness through its use since it minimises obstacles to access by vulnerable groups (Nayak & Tiyadi, 2024). These sensitive sectors, however, need high accountability. The decisions made by AI should be explainable and bias free and should be monitored to detect mistakes. The rights of the citizens should be preserved at all costs.

6.2.4 Digital Government Platforms and Citizen Interaction

The digital platforms powered by AI are changing the interaction between the citizens and the government. E-portals help individuals to order services, follow requests, and get notifications more conveniently. The AIs assist in customising such experiences depending on the users. Another instance of how AI can be used in practice can be illustrated by the recommendation of applicable welfare initiatives or individualized tax filing guidelines (Duberry, 2022). The presence of citizen engagement improves with the help of AI-based data analysis. The governments are able to examine public responses, content in social media, and survey data in order to know the issues of the citizens. This will enable the policymakers to make more responsive decisions (Pislaru et al., 2024).

Transparency is another area where AI is useful because it facilitates the availability of information that has been made public. Improved involvement of people with disabilities or limited literacy is possible with document search tools, automated translation, and speech recognition (Olsen et al., 2024). When it comes to elections or civic consultations, AI is used to facilitate information to voters, to participate in the electoral process, and to keep track of the results of elections. The functions aid in enhancing the democratic processes. However, online communication must be heavily secured to avoid false information, data leaks, or influence on the population. Governments should uphold the trust in the form of transparency and openness on the aspect of how AI systems work (Asimakopoulos et al., 2025).

6.3 Opportunities for Improved Governance

6.3.1 Enhanced Decision-Making and Data-Driven Policy

The benefit of AI in the public sector is one of the most significant ones, and it allows making evidence-based decisions. Health records, taxation systems, transportation networks, and welfare databases are some examples of data generated and stored by governments. AI software processes the data fast and identifies patterns that are not always easy to identify by humans (Arora et al., 2023). AI assists those in policy formulation to know more about social issues. As an example, data analysis can reveal the regions that have more unemployment, those at risk, in case of a disease outbreak, or those with bad infrastructure. The information can be used by governments to establish specific policies which can meet actual needs. Decision-makers can be more effective in policymaking because they could utilise AI insights to make more robust and informed decisions instead of relying solely on traditional approaches (Charles et al., 2022).

AI is also used in real-time decisions. Predictive analytics have the capability to predict upcoming incidents, such as population growth, resource scarcity, or a natural disaster. Early warning allows governments to devise response plans which minimise damages. This renders a more proactive governance and not reactive (Cao, 2023). Moreover, AI provides objective decision support in the case of well-designed systems. It may minimise the errors due to subjectivity of man, fatigue, or misinformation. AI can be used in more uniform and equitable government decisions in areas like environmental management, education planning, and economic policy (Al-Raeei, 2025). However, human judgement has to be involved in the decisions to make sure the context, culture, and values are not violated. AI is a support, and not a substitute, to the policymakers.

6.3.2 Efficiency, Automation, and Reduced Administrative Burden

AI enhances effectiveness in administration as it automates monotonous and time-consuming activities. Governments tend to waste a lot of resources in the processing of documents, responding to inquiries, and in checking information. These tasks can be managed with the help of AI tools quickly and less time is spent on delays and better the satisfaction of the citizens. Automation of things like licensing, approval of social benefits, and identity verification lowers the physical paperwork and physical visits. Citizens are able to get processes through the Internet, and decisions are made quicker. The lack of administrative strain also allows the public employees to concentrate on those jobs that involve showing empathy, reasoning, and communication (Parycek et al., 2024).

AI systems help eliminate bottlenecks in public administration. For example:

- Robotic Process Automation (RPA) can update databases and manage transactions without human effort.
- Chatbots respond instantly to common citizen questions and provide instructions for public services.
- Optical Character Recognition (OCR) digitises documents to improve record-keeping and access.

Cost saving is another factor of efficiency. The saved resources can be directed by governments to improve healthcare services, rural development, and even education. The automation in the digital format will decrease the chances of corruption since there will be minimal human interference in the approval (Abogunrin et al., 2025). Moreover, AI is helpful during crisis resilience. In the case of an emergency like a pandemic, automated systems keep service delivery even when the physical offices are shut down. This guarantees succession of governance and security of the vulnerable groups.

6.3.3 Transparency and Improved Access to Services

One of the major conditions to make the government trustworthy by the people is transparency. AI aids in turning the administrative processes into a clearer and more open one. In a situation where AI-supported systems document decisions, they can be reviewed and audited. It is possible to explain automated decisions to affected citizens by the public authorities (Harrison & Luna-Reyes, 2022). The areas of transparency that AI helps with include budget management, procurement, and welfare distribution. Data dashboards also allow governments to demonstrate their spending and the attainment of programme objectives. Citizens feel confident when they can see and comprehend operations. With the use of AI, access to public services can be improved. Through the use of digital platforms, individuals can request services, get updates, and communicate with the public authorities without necessarily travelling or waiting in line (Lahusen et al., 2024).

This is especially beneficial for:

- Citizens in rural or remote areas;
- Elderly individuals with mobility challenges;
- People with disabilities who need accessible interfaces.

There are AI tools like automatic translators, voice activated systems, which do not respect the language and literacy barrier. Individuals with difficulties in the traditional means of communication have an easy way to access government services. AI also enhances equity in service provision. It is possible to find and stop discriminatory patterns in loan, housing, or welfare applications through the use of algorithms. With proper monitoring, AI can make sure that one is treated equally without consideration of their gender, caste, ethnicity, or income level (Xu et al., 2024). In addition, AI governance should be transparent, which attracts citizens. When they have confidence in the systems of decision-making, people tend to take part in public consultations and offer their feedback. This enhances the democratic process and makes governance more responsive.

6.4 Key Risks and Governance Challenges

6.4.1 Privacy and Surveillance Concerns

AI systems have a tendency to gather and process a lot of information about individuals. The identity systems, healthcare records, welfare databases, and communication networks provide information that is used by the public institutions. In case such data is not controlled appropriately, citizens can lose control over their personal data. Surveillance is one of the issues. Cameras, facial recognition, and surveillance with AI can trace the movements and behaviours. This is beneficial in securing but poses a threat to privacy and freedom without being controlled. Over-monitoring can turn the society into a surveillance state whereby people feel that they are under scrutiny, and they cannot do what they want (Singh, 2023). There are threats of data breaches and cyber attacks. Government databases are vulnerable to hackers. Lack of weak security systems adds vulnerability. AI, in the sector of the public, should consequently adhere to effective data protection guidelines, encryption practices, and restricted access agreements (Herath et al., 2024). Governments have to find equilibrium between the desire to have safety and security and the concern about human rights. To have trust, there must be open communication and consent given by the citizens. The development and deployment of systems should be supported by privacy by design principles.

6.4.2 Algorithmic Bias and Discrimination

The problem of algorithmic bias is acute in AI in the public sector. In case the training data has prejudiced patterns, the AI model will not yield fair outcomes. This has impacts on groups according to race, gender, age, caste, and socioeconomic status. Such biases can deprive vulnerable populations of benefits or opportunities in the context of the work of the public services (Nzobonimpa, 2023).

Examples include:

- Biased crime prediction tools reinforcing stereotypes;
- Welfare eligibility systems excluding deserving applicants;
- Healthcare AI misdiagnosing underrepresented communities.

These harms may enhance inequality and discrimination. The decision-making concerning the issues of the public sector should be impartial and fair, and therefore there should not be any bias in the automated systems. Governments have to embrace checks of fairness, heterogeneous datasets, and evaluations of ethics. Discrimination can be detected at the initial stages by independent audits and monitoring. Human control is needed to make sure AI decisions are legal and ethical. It is also crucial to train public officials to make them understand and solve algorithmic bias (Radanliev, 2025).

6.4.3 Accountability and Explainability Issues

Accountability describes the responsibility of AI decisions. According to traditional public administration, it is the duty of human officials. Nevertheless, AI systems make automatic decisions, and this may cause responsibility to be obscure. Individuals are unaware of whom to hold responsible in case an automated system results in injuries, the refusal to provide city services, or make incorrect assumptions (Novelli et al., 2024). It is also challenging in explainability. Several types of AI models are black boxed, i.e., the process of making decisions is not easily comprehensible. A citizen is not guaranteed to get a clear explanation in case he or she is adversely impacted by an automated decision. It is hard to correct mistakes or dispute this (Von Eschenbach, 2021). Lack of accountability leads to poor trust. The governments should ensure decision processes are documented, audit records are maintained, and avenues of appeal are incorporated by developers and agencies. Explainable AI (XAI) methods assist in making the results more comprehensible. The high risk decisions that concern rights, safety, or welfare should be subject to human review (Hassija et al., 2024). The governance systems should be such that AI systems improve, but do not supersede the responsibility of the populace. Table 6.1 summarises major risks in public sector AI, showing harms and required governance safeguards.

Table 6.1 Key Risks in Public Sector AI Deployment.

Risk Category	*Description*	*Potential Harm*	*Governance Need*
Privacy Violation	Excessive data collection and surveillance	Loss of autonomy, civil liberties threats	Data protection laws, consent rules
Algorithmic Bias	Discriminatory or unfair automated decisions	Inequality and exclusion	Bias audits, fairness checks
Accountability Gap	Unclear responsibility for AI outcomes	Denial of justice, errors remain unchallenged	Clear liability rules, human oversight
Lack of Explainability	Black box decision-making	Reduced trust and transparency	Explainable AI guidelines, appeal mechanisms

6.5 Regulatory and Ethical Governance Mechanisms

6.5.1 Data Protection and Cybersecurity

Data is the core of AI systems. Healthcare services, taxation, identification, or welfare programmes are commonly based on personal information gathered by citizens to avail AI-based services to them in the public sector. In case this data is used wrongly or leaked, it may lead to severe damages. Thus, one of the regulatory requirements is data protection (Androutsopoulou et al., 2025). The governments have to make sure that personal information is gathered legally, and is kept in a secure place, and only used for the intended purpose. There should be clear guidelines regarding the time of accessing data and who should protect the data. Other rights that are commonly contained in data protection laws are the right to consent, right to correct information, and right to restrict the processing (Al-Dulaimi & Mohammed, 2025).

It is also necessary to protect the cybersecurity since the government databases are often attacked by hackers. Hackers can attempt to steal sensitive data or cause havoc with data to disrupt services. Cyber threats are mitigated through such security features as encryption, secure authentication, and periodic testing of vulnerabilities. The public sector organisations should educate officials on the cybersecurity policies and respond to the incident so that they can take immediate measures in case the breach has occurred (Taherdoost, 2025). The protection of data and the security of the computer system eliminate any unauthorised monitoring, identity theft, and abuse. These mechanisms safeguard the rights to privacy and promote popular trust in AI systems led by the government.

6.5.2 Ethical Guidelines and Human Oversight

The ethical values inform the responsible development and practice of AI in the state sector. The governments should guarantee that AI promotes equality, dignity, and human welfare. Values like accountability, non-discrimination, inclusiveness, and transparency are defined by ethical guidelines (Radanliev, 2025). Ethical governance is an important aspect of human control. Although AI is suggested to perform automatic recommendations, in high risk areas of life, such as healthcare, justice, and welfare, people should be left with the final decision. Review of humans would make sure that contextual factors are taken into consideration and automated decisions do not disadvantage people (Ali, 2025a). AI projects may be monitored and independent advice given by ethical decision boards or advisory committees. These teams contribute to solving the problems of prejudice, security, and possible damage. The governments must also train the people who handle AI in ethical conduct, so that they can know the advantages as well as the disadvantages (Ghosh et al., 2025). Ethical governance guarantees that technology does not take human judgement out of the way or diminish the rights of the people. Rather, it encourages responsible innovation and makes AI be in line with the democratic principles and human interests (George & Wooden, 2025).

6.5.3 Algorithmic Auditing and Transparency Tools

Auditing through algorithms is necessary to assess the fairness, accuracy, and safety of the operation of AI systems. Audits include analysis of training data, system output, and pattern of decision-making. They assist in identifying discrimination and systemic mistakes as well as security threats. Auditing can either be in-house or by other external organisations (Nastoska et al., 2025). Explainability is offered by transparency tools. The work of AI systems in the public sector is to be disclosed concerning the functioning of AI systems, the data it uses, and the decision-making process by the public sector organisations. XAI methods are applied to simplify complex models so that the citizens and the government officials can interpret the results (Liu et al., 2025). Openness also involves good communication with the users. When AI is involved in significant decisions, like whether a person qualifies to receive welfare, take a loan, or verify their identity, people should be notified of this activity. They need to be exposed to what decisions are being made and how to question their mistakes (Paris et al., 2025). Accountability is enhanced by open data projects and transparency. Governments are able to make lists of AI systems being used, the outcome of impact assessments, and the description of fairness checks.

Auditing and transparency promotes trust and eliminates the fear of concealed or unjust automation (Balasubramaniam et al., 2023).

6.5.4 Institutional Checks and Legal Safeguards

The legal structures and institutional systems make sure that AI is kept within the correct social control. The governing authorities need to ensure that there is a clear role and responsibilities. Legislation needs to specify the person responsible in case AI systems cause damages or lead to biased results (Al-Dulaimi & Mohammed, 2025).

Legal safeguards may include:

- Appeals processes for citizens affected by automated decisions;
- Requirements for documentation, monitoring, and system validation;
- Penalties for misuse or non-compliance;
- Mandatory human oversight for high risk applications.

Important roles are played by independent regulatory bodies. These bodies oversee AI applications, impose fines, and penetrate complaints. Governments can also bring certification or licensing procedures on high impact AI tools so as to make sure that they are up to the standards needed to be used (Lund et al., 2025). Checks in institutions serve as a way of averting power abuse. They make sure that AI will not be a means of unfair surveillance or discrimination. Laws maintain transparency and accountability in governance, which safeguard citizens against the technological evils. The institutional strength is also promoted by international cooperation. Nations share their experience, embrace international standards, and coordinate legal frameworks to enhance AI safety on the global level. Standardised policies minimise global conflict in regulations and enhance global governance (Kashefi et al., 2024).

6.6 Strengthening Capacity and Public Trust

6.6.1 Workforce Skills and Digital Readiness

The deployment of AI in governments needs a competent employee base. Most of the employees in the government are not conversant with AI systems and might be lacking the technical knowledge to analyse automated decisions. Training programmes are hence necessary. The governments need to invest in digital literacy and data management, as well as simple AI knowledge, at all levels of administration. The officials who supervise the AI systems directly require advanced training. They should be conversant with algorithmic bias, privacy of data, and computer security. The information will assist them in making decisions and identify the possible risks of the deployment of the systems (AbdulKareem & Oladimeji, 2024). It is also digital preparedness which involves the establishment of a conducive work culture. It has to be promoted in learning, innovation, and collaboration in the public institutions. Employees are to feel safe working with digital tools and be able to access technical assistance. Another step that is significant is to recruit AI experts in government positions. Nevertheless, it is difficult to hire and retain quality professionals due to unhealthy competition with the private sector. To overcome this, governments can provide incentives, professional growth, and shared research positions (Johnson et al., 2022). Workforce empowerment also includes infrastructure preparedness. To be able to use AI systems, the office of the government should have a stable internet connection, safe digital environment, and up-to-date hardware. The absence of such resources means that even the most trained workforce will not be able to make full use of AI capabilities (Dehbozorgi et al., 2024).

6.6.2 Citizen Awareness and Participatory Governance

AI and government have to be adopted with the assistance of public trust. Unless citizens comprehend the impact of the AI on the decisions, they can fear the technology or feel that they are not fairly treated. Thus, governments should communicate effectively on the purpose, benefits, and limitations of AI systems (Robles & Mallinson, 2025). The awareness of citizens helps to achieve confidence. The governments may set workshops, public consultations, and online information briefings that will clarify how the AI tools will be applied in fields like welfare distribution, healthcare, and policing. Informed people are more willing to accept automated processes (Alshahrani et al., 2024). Accountability is enhanced in participatory governance. The citizens should be able to challenge automated decisions, seek clarification, and appeal the mistakes. Feedback systems will enable governments to know what is wrong and make systems better. This renders AI governance to be more responsive and democratic (Moon, 2023).

It is also important to be transparent about the use of data. Citizens ought to be aware of the personal information that is being gathered, who will have access to the information, and the duration of storing the information collected. Safeguarding data rights will avoid privacy breaches and enhance better faith in digital governance (Ali, 2025b). Outreach efforts should be based on inclusiveness. There are those people who might not access digital tools or might be lowly digital literate. Governments need to make sure that AI services are affordable to everyone regardless of their disability, rural population, and elderly citizens. Inclusive design promotes equality and prevents digital inequality (Al-Besher & Kumar, 2022).

6.6.3 Collaboration with Industry and Academic Institutions

The successful use of AI in the public sector depends on strong collaboration between government, industry, and academic institutions. Each sector provides unique strengths:

- Industry offers cutting edge technology, innovation capacity, and practical deployment experience.
- Universities and research institutes contribute expertise in AI development, ethics, and governance.

- Government ensures alignment with public values, rights, and national priorities.

The collaboration of government and corporations enables the governments to gain access to sophisticated AI applications and technical advice. A high number of smart city initiatives, health related applications, and cybersecurity systems are collaborating with the services of private technology companies. Cooperation is also beneficial in terms of minimizing expenses by sharing investments (Alshahrani et al., 2024). Research and talent development are facilitated by academic partnerships. Universities aid in the evaluation of AI performance, detect risks related to ethics, and develop guidelines that are responsible in terms of innovation. Training programmes and internships of students contribute to developing the future AI workforce in the public sector (Boobier, 2022).

The cooperation in the international arena is also significant. It is possible to show governments other successful AI projects in other countries. The sharing of knowledge helps in aligning the policies and minimising duplication of efforts. International membership of organisations like OECD, UNESCO, and GPAI is used to influence the international standards and keep their national strategies relevant (Elfert & Ydesen, 2023). The cooperation should be supported by clear roles of governance. The procurement, data sharing, and accountability rules should be provided by the public institutions. This will avoid excessive reliance on the private actors and it will make the public have control in the supplying of essential services.

6.7 Conclusion

AI is changing the administration of the population by making decisions, enhancing efficiency, and gaining access to government services. This chapter clarified the ways that AI can generate significant advantages to society when applied in a reasonable way. It also brought to the fore the main risks that pertain to privacy, discrimination, accountability, and transparency. Good AI in the public sector will necessitate good governance to defend citizens and facilitate trust. All AI implementations should be guided by data protection, cybersecurity, human control, and ethical principles. Fairness and accountability are provided by the use of algorithmic auditing and legal protection.

It is necessary to use a human-centric approach. AI must not override the judgement of public officials instead of aiding them and undermining democracy. People should not be inactive or ignorant. They trust it because of the open communication and right to challenge automated decisions. They should also focus on capacity building and skill development, as well as invest in industry and academic partners with governments. AI governance in the public sector shall be dynamic since technology changes at a very high rate. New structures must work on inclusiveness, transparency, and sustainability in the long run. Governments can create a balance between innovation and powerful safeguards to guarantee that AI enhances civic value, aids in the establishment of equity, and helps build a responsible and trusted administration of governance.

References

AbdulKareem, A.K. and Oladimeji, K.A. (2024). Cultivating the digital citizen: Trust, digital literacy, and e-government adoption. *Transforming Government: People, Process, and Policy*, *18*(2), 270–286. https://doi.org/10.1108/TG-11-2023-0196.

Abogunrin, S., Muir, J.M., Zerbini, C. and Sarri, G. (2025). How much can we save by applying artificial intelligence in evidence synthesis? Results from a pragmatic review to quantify workload efficiencies and cost savings. *Frontiers in Pharmacology*, *16*, 1454245. https://doi.org/10.3389/fphar.2025.1454245.

Al-Besher, A. and Kumar, K. (2022). Use of artificial intelligence to enhance e-government services. *Measurement: Sensors*, *24*, 100484. https://doi.org/10.1016/j.measen.2022.100484.

Al-Dulaimi, A.O.M. and Mohammed, M.A.A.W. (2025). Legal responsibility for errors caused by artificial intelligence (AI) in the public sector. *International Journal of Law and Management*. https://doi.org/10.1108/IJLMA-08-2024-0295.

Alhosani, K. and Alhashmi, S.M. (2024). Opportunities, challenges, and benefits of AI innovation in government services: A review. *Discover Artificial Intelligence*, *4*(1), 18. https://doi.org/10.1007/s44163-024-00111-w.

Ali, A. (2025a). Ethical Considerations and Bias in AI Applications in Healthcare. In: *Artificial Intelligence in Healthcare Information Systems: Security and Privacy Challenges* (pp. 129–146). Cham: Springer Nature Switzerland. https://doi.org/10.1007/978-3-031-84404-1_7.

Ali, A. (2025b). Ethics, Privacy, and Security in Healthcare Informatics. In: *Healthcare Informatics Innovation Post COVID-19 Pandemic* (pp. 180–197). Auerbach Publications.

Al-Raeei, M. (2025). The smart future for sustainable development: Artificial intelligence solutions for sustainable urbanization. *Sustainable Development*, *33*(1), 508–517. https://doi.org/10.1002/sd.3131.

Alshahrani, A., Griva, A., Dennehy, D. and Mäntymäki, M. (2024). Artificial intelligence and decision-making in government functions: Opportunities, challenges, and future research. *Transforming Government: People, Process, and Policy*, *18*(4), 678–698. https://doi.org/10.1108/TG-06-2024-0131

Androutsopoulou, M., Askounis, D., Carayannis, E.G. and Zotas, N. (2025). Leveraging AI for enhanced eGovernment: Optimizing the use of open governmental data. *Journal of the Knowledge Economy*, *16*(3), 12998–13033. https://doi.org/10.1007/s13132-024-02317-w.

Anshari, M., Hamdan, M., Ahmad, N. and Ali, E. (2025). Public service delivery, artificial intelligence, and the sustainable development goals: Trends, evidence, and complexities. *Journal of Science and Technology Policy Management*, *16*(1), 163–181. https://doi.org/10.1108/JSTPM-07-2023-0123.

Ardabili, B.R., Pazho, A.D., Noghre, G.A., Neff, C., Bhaskararayuni, S.D., Ravindran, A., ... & Tabkhi, H. (2023). Understanding policy and technical aspects of AI-enabled smart video surveillance to address public safety. *Computational Urban Science*, *3*(1), 21. https://doi.org/10.1007/s43762-023-00097-8.

Arora, A., Gupta, M., Mehmi, S., Khanna, T., Chopra, G., Kaur, R. and Vats, P. (2023, September). Towards intelligent governance: The role of AI in policymaking and decision support for E-governance. In: *World Conference on Information Systems for Business Management* (pp. 229–240). Singapore: Springer Nature Singapore. https://doi.org/10.1007/978-981-99-8612-5_19.

Asimakopoulos, G., Antonopoulou, H., Giotopoulos, K. and Halkiopoulos, C. (2025). Impact of information and communication technologies on democratic processes and citizen participation. *Societies*, *15*(2), 40. https://doi.org/10.3390/soc15020040.

Balasubramaniam, N., Kauppinen, M., Rannisto, A., Hiekkanen, K. and Kujala, S. (2023). Transparency and explainability of AI systems: From ethical guidelines to requirements. *Information and Software Technology*, *159*, 107197. https://doi.org/10.1016/j.infsof.2023.107197.

Boobier, T. (2022). *AI and the Future of the Public Sector: The Creation of Public Sector 4.0.* John Wiley & Sons.

Bosco, G., Riccardi, V., Sciarrone, A., D'Amore, R. and Visvizi, A. (2024). AI-driven innovation in smart city governance: Achieving human-centric and sustainable outcomes. *Transforming Government: People, Process, and Policy*. https://doi.org/10.1108/TG-04-2024-0096.

Cao, L. (2023). AI and data science for smart emergency, crisis, and disaster resilience. *International Journal of Data Science and Analytics, 15*(3), 231–246. https://doi.org/10.1007/s41060-023-00393-w.

Charles, V., Rana, N.P. and Carter, L. (2022). Artificial Intelligence for data-driven decision-making and governance in public affairs. *Government Information Quarterly, 39*(4), 101742. https://doi.org/10.1016/j.giq.2022.101742.

Chen, T., Guo, W., Gao, X. and Liang, Z. (2021). AI-based self-service technology in public service delivery: User experience and influencing factors. *Government Information Quarterly, 38*(4), 101520. https://doi.org/10.1016/j.giq.2020.101520.

Dehbozorgi, M.H., Rossi, M., Terzi, S., Carminati, L., Sala, R., Magni, F., ... & Rossi, T. (2024, September). AI Education for Tomorrow's Workforce: Leveraging Learning Factories for AI Education and Workforce Preparedness. In: *2024 IEEE 8th Forum on Research and Technologies for Society and Industry Innovation* (*RTSI*) (pp. 677–682). IEEE. https://doi.org/10.1109/RTSI61910.2024.10761217.

Duberry, J. (2022). Artificial intelligence and democracy: Risks and promises of AI-mediated citizen–government relations. In: *Artificial Intelligence and Democracy*. Edward Elgar Publishing. https://doi.org/10.4337/9781788977319.

Elfert, M. and Ydesen, C. (2023). UNESCO, the OECD and the World Bank: A global governance perspective. In: *Global Governance of Education: The Historical and Contemporary Entanglements of UNESCO, the OECD, and the World Bank* (pp. 23–50). Cham: Springer International Publishing. https://doi.org/10.1007/978-3-031-40411-5_2.

Fang, B., Yu, J., Chen, Z., Osman, A. I., Farghali, M., Ihara, I., ... & Yap, P.S. (2023). Artificial intelligence for waste management in smart cities: A review. *Environmental Chemistry Letters, 21*(4), 1959–1989. https://doi.org/10.1007/s10311-023-01604-3.

George, B. and Wooden, O.S. (2025). Ethical AI and Responsible Innovation. In: *AI Empowered: Pioneering African American Entrepreneurship in the Digital Age* (pp. 105–111). Emerald Publishing Limited. https://doi.org/10.1108/978-1-83662-816-320251012.

Ghosh, A., Saini, A. and Barad, H. (2025). Artificial intelligence in governance: recent trends, risks, challenges, innovative frameworks and future directions. *AI & Society*, 1–23. https://doi.org/10.1007/s00146-025-02312-y.

Harrison, T.M. and Luna-Reyes, L.F. (2022). Cultivating trustworthy artificial intelligence in digital government. *Social Science Computer Review, 40*(2), 494–511. https://doi.org/10.1177/0894439320980122.

Hassija, V., Chamola, V., Mahapatra, A., Singal, A., Goel, D., Huang, K., ... & Hussain, A. (2024). Interpreting black-box models: A review on explainable artificial intelligence. *Cognitive Computation, 16*(1), 45–74. https://doi.org/10.1007/s12559-023-10179-8.

Herath, H.M.S.S., Herath, H.M.K.K.M.B., Madhusanka, B.G.D.A. and Guruge, L.G.P.K. (2024). Data protection challenges in the processing of sensitive data. In: *Data Protection: The Wake of AI and Machine Learning* (pp. 155–179). Cham: Springer Nature Switzerland. https://doi.org/10.1007/978-3-031-76473-8_8.

Johnson, B.A., Coggburn, J.D. and Llorens, J.J. (2022). Artificial intelligence and public human resource management: Questions for research and practice. *Public Personnel Management, 51*(4), 538–562. https://doi.org/10.1177/00910260221126498.

Kashefi, P., Kashefi, Y. and Ghafouri Mirsaraei, A. (2024). Shaping the future of AI: Balancing innovation and ethics in global regulation. *Uniform Law Review*, *29*(3), 524–548. https://doi.org/10.1093/ulr/unae040.

Kaufmann, M. (2024). AI in policing and law enforcement. In: *Handbook on Public Policy and Artificial Intelligence* (pp. 295–306). Edward Elgar Publishing. https://doi.org/10.4337/9781803922171.00031.

Kovari, A. (2024). AI for decision support: Balancing accuracy, transparency, and trust across sectors. *Information*, *15*(11), 725. https://doi.org/10.3390/info15110725.

Lahusen, C., Maggetti, M. and Slavkovik, M. (2024). Trust, trustworthiness, and AI governance. *Scientific Reports*, *14*(1), 20752. https://doi.org/10.1038/s41598-024-71761-0.

Liu, X., Huang, D., Yao, J., Dong, J., Song, L., Wang, H., ... & Chu, W. (2025). From Black Box to Glass Box: A Practical Review of Explainable Artificial Intelligence (XAI). *AI*, *6*(11), 285. https://doi.org/10.3390/ai6110285.

Lund, B., Orhan, Z., Mannuru, N.R., Bevara, R.V.K., Porter, B., Vinaih, M.K. and Bhaskara, P. (2025). Standards, frameworks, and legislation for artificial intelligence (AI) transparency. *AI and Ethics*, 1–17. https://doi.org/10.1007/s43681-025-00661-4.

Luusua, A., Ylipulli, J., Foth, M. and Aurigi, A. (2023). Urban AI: Understanding the emerging role of artificial intelligence in smart cities. *AI & Society*, *38*(3), 1039–1044. https://doi.org/10.1007/s00146-022-01537-5.

Mishra, A.K., Tyagi, A.K., Dananjayan, S., Rajavat, A., Rawat, H. and Rawat, A. (2024). Revolutionizing government operations: The impact of artificial intelligence in public administration. *Conversational Artificial Intelligence*, 607–634. https://doi.org/10.1002/9781394200801.ch34.

Moon, M.J. (2023). Searching for inclusive artificial intelligence for social good: Participatory governance and policy recommendations for making AI more inclusive and benign for society. *Public Administration Review*, *83*(6), 1496–1505. https://doi.org/10.1111/puar.13648.

Nastoska, A., Jancheska, B., Rizinski, M. and Trajanov, D. (2025). Evaluating trustworthiness in AI: Risks, metrics, and applications across industries. *Electronics*, *14*(13), 2717. https://doi.org/10.3390/electronics14132717.

Nayak, M. and Tiyadi, J. (2024). Social Welfare and Artificial Intelligence's Role: A Comprehensive Summary of the Study. In: *AI in the Social and Business World: A Comprehensive Approach* (pp. 32–66). Bentham Science Publishers. https://doi.org/10.2174/9789815256864124010l.

Novelli, C., Taddeo, M. and Floridi, L. (2024). Accountability in artificial intelligence: What it is and how it works. *AI & Society*, *39*(4), 1871–1882. https://doi.org/10.1007/s00146-023-01635-y.

Nzobonimpa, S. (2023). Artificial intelligence, task complexity, and uncertainty: Analyzing the advantages and disadvantages of using algorithms in public service delivery under public administration theories. *Digital Transformation and Society*, *2*(3), 219–234. https://doi.org/10.1108/DTS-03-2023-0018.

Olsen, H.P., Hildebrandt, T.T., Wiesener, C., Larsen, M.S. and Flügge, A.W.A. (2024). The right to transparency in public governance: Freedom of information and the use of artificial intelligence by public agencies. *Digital Government: Research and Practice*, *5*(1), 1–15. https://doi.org/10.1145/3632753.

Paris, T., Moon, A. and Guo, J.L. (2025, June). Opening the Scope of Openness in AI. In: *Proceedings of the 2025 ACM Conference on Fairness, Accountability, and Transparency* (pp. 1293–1311). https://doi.org/10.1145/3715275.3732087.

Parycek, P., Schmid, V. and Novak, A.S. (2024). Artificial Intelligence (AI) and automation in administrative procedures: Potentials, limitations, and framework conditions. *Journal of the Knowledge Economy*, *15*(2), 8390–8415. https://doi.org/10.1007/s13132-023-01433-3.

Pislaru, M., Vlad, C.S., Ivascu, L. and Mircea, I.I. (2024). Citizen-centric governance: Enhancing citizen engagement through artificial intelligence tools. *Sustainability*, *16*(7), 2686. https://doi.org/10.3390/su16072686.

Radanliev, P. (2025). AI ethics: Integrating transparency, fairness, and privacy in AI development. *Applied Artificial Intelligence*, *39*(1), 2463722. https://doi.org/10.1080/08839514.2025.2463722.

Robles, P. and Mallinson, D.J. (2025). Artificial intelligence technology, public trust, and effective governance. *Review of Policy Research*, *42*(1), 11–28. https://doi.org/10.1111/ropr.12555.

Singh, T. (2023, October). AI-Driven Surveillance Technologies and Human Rights: Balancing Security and Privacy. In: *International Conference on Smart Systems: Innovations in Computing* (pp. 703–717). Singapore: Springer Nature Singapore. https://doi.org/10.1007/978-981-97-3690-4_53.

Taherdoost, H. (2025). AI for cyber security and cyber security for AI: Complementary role. In: *Artificial Intelligence for Cyber Security and Industry 4.0* (pp. 1–23). CRC Press.

Von Eschenbach, W.J. (2021). Transparency and the black box problem: Why we do not trust AI. *Philosophy & Technology*, *34*(4), 1607–1622. https://doi.org/10.1007/s13347-021-00477-0.

Wagner, J.K., Doerr, M. and Schmit, C.D. (2024). AI governance: A challenge for public health. *JMIR Public Health and Surveillance*, *10*(1), e58358. https://doi.org/10.2196/58358.

Xu, J., Lee, T. and Goggin, G. (2024). AI governance in Asia: Policies, praxis, and approaches. *Communication Research and Practice*, *10*(3), 275–287. https://doi.org/10.1080/22041451.2024.2391204.

Yigitcanlar, T., David, A., Li, W., Fookes, C., Bibri, S.E. and Ye, X. (2024). Unlocking artificial intelligence adoption in local governments: Best practice lessons from real-world implementations. *Smart Cities*, *7*(4), 1576–1625. https://doi.org/10.3390/smartcities7040064.

Zong, Z. and Guan, Y. (2025). AI-driven intelligent data analytics and predictive analysis in Industry 4.0: Transforming knowledge, innovation, and efficiency. *Journal of the Knowledge Economy*, *16*(1), 864–-903. https://doi.org/10.1007/s13132-024-02001-z.

7 Algorithmic Bias and Discrimination
Policy Tools for Mitigation

Discrimination and algorithmic bias have become one of the key issues in the creation and implementation of Artificial Intelligence (AI) systems. AI might perpetuate social inequalities and harm populations susceptible to it when it is trained on biased data or when the algorithms apply unfair decision-making methods. Biased algorithms may affect access to services, job opportunities, access to healthcare services, and legal rights in both the public and the private sphere. Hence, policy instruments and governance systems are required in order to foster transparency, fairness, and accountability. The sources of algorithmic bias, their implications to society, and the present policy measures to detect and mitigate discrimination are discussed in this chapter. It emphasises regulatory approaches, auditing systems, ethics, and inclusive design approaches that contribute to fair and credible AI systems.

7.1 Introduction

The emergence of algorithmic bias is a shifting problem in artificial intelligence (AI) design and application. AI systems process and come up with the decision or prediction in most spheres of everyday life. Nevertheless, biased results can be yielded by the system in case the data or design reflects inequitable tendencies. Such prejudice is usually not planned, yet it may have profound effects. AI applications in education, healthcare, finance, criminal justice, and employment are now in place. Thus, algorithmic bias is a concept that has to be comprehended so that AI can aid the principles of fairness, equality, and trust of the population (Shestakova, 2021). AI is now one of the most important tools of decision-making in contemporary societies. Companies use AI to screen job candidates, grant financial services, and diagnose illnesses, as well as to identify the risk of crimes. These policies have an impact on fundamental opportunities and human rights. In case such processes are guided by biased algorithms, then it is possible that the affected individuals will be discriminated against or excluded (Borgesius, 2025). Prejudice may manifest itself regarding race or gender, age, disability, geographical background, or social economic status. Since the AI systems are capable of performing tasks fast and at a large scale, unfair results can be disseminated in mass and negatively affect dozens or even hundreds of individuals simultaneously (Entschew, 2024).

The practical example of the impact of algorithmic bias on social equity demonstrates itself. Automated screening devices used in the hiring systems often filter out candidates having gaps on their resumes without inquiring about the

DOI: 10.1201/9781003776659-7

feasible reasons of the gap, e.g., childcare, illness. This may also be detrimental to women in instances where gender inequality comes out in patterns of care giving (Panarese et al., 2025). Credit scoring models in the banking sector can be based on past financial records that do not cover underserved or rural areas. This will lead to responsible borrowers being turned away. Within the police, predictive algorithms can also name some neighbourhoods as high risk due to biased historical policing and thus subject them to increased surveillance, thus condensing stereotypes (Gerdon et al., 2022).

Another field where bias is very high is in healthcare. The AI models can perform poorly when the training data is not representative of a diverse population. It could result in medical advice being less precise to the population representatives of the minority groups and endangering their health. These cases demonstrate that algorithmic bias has a potential to increase the existing inequities in society (Agarwal et al., 2023). It is also algorithmic bias that makes people trust technology. When a citizen feels or witnesses unjust auto-made decisions, he/she will lose confidence in the digital governance systems. It becomes hard to be transparent when AI models act as black boxes and therefore make decisions which even designers cannot fully expound on. Such ambiguity brings with itself ethical and legal issues particularly when rights and access to vital services are involved in the decision made (Kordzadeh & Ghasemaghaei, 2022).

The problem of algorithmic bias is not just technical, but also a social and ethical problem. The creation and implementation of AI needs to be equitable from the beginning. The role in combatting AI-based discrimination is taken by policymakers, researchers, developers, as well as communities. Biases require removal through human supervision, variety of data expression, and comprehensive design to enhance fairness. There should also be public involvement where the groups that are impacted have a say in the design and use of the AI systems (Zajko, 2022). The issue of algorithmic bias should be taken seriously since its effects go well beyond technology. It has an impact on actual lives, dictates social results, and shapes the confidence in the social institutions. Knowledge of its causes and consequences assists in correct AI governance and precludes damage to both people and society.

7.2 Sources and Types of Algorithmic Bias

7.2.1 Data Related Bias: Imbalance, Historical Inequalities, and Sampling Errors

The main role of AI decision-making is data. The AI systems are learning trends based on the data and applying them to make predictions. Consequently, data representativeness and quality have a potent impact on the system outcomes. In the case that the dataset is incomprehensive of the population the results can be biased (Chen et al., 2023). One of the problems is usually data imbalance. In the case of under-representation or absence of some groups in the data, the AI will be successful with the majority groups, but not with the minority groups. As an illustration, facial recognition systems primarily trained on images of lighter skinned faces tend to have large error rates with darker skinned faces. This encourages wrong identification and may result in unfair treatment (Mergen et al., 2025). Another significant source of bias is historical inequality. A good number of datasets are indicative of the past human behaviours, social organisation, and discrimination. In the event of skewed data in the past, the AI model can continue to support these disparities rather than address them. To illustrate, recruitment algorithms that are trained on historic recruitment data can be trained to prefer male applicants in case the organisation had previously hired more men. The system perpetuates discrimination on an automatic basis without intervention (Kumar et al., 2025).

Bias can also be brought about by sampling errors. In the case of data gathering on small geographical areas, individual institutions or digital populations, the information might not be representative of other communities of various socioeconomic or demographic categories. Rural areas can be left behind in the provision of public services when the information is centralised in the urban centres. Consequently, AI-based policies can discriminate against one group and leave other groups unaddressed (Varona & Suárez, 2022). The bias in data is hard to trace due to the fact that the datasets look to be objective. Nevertheless, there are social and historical concealed issues still within the data. This renders data auditing, diversity testing, and fairness testing important processes in responsible AI development (Hanna et al., 2025).

7.2.2 Model and Design Bias: Feature Selection and Optimisation Choices

Bias may also take place in development of the models. Although data might be fair, developers may create a discriminatory decision unintentionally. Feature selection is one of these sources. The decision-making variables used in the model are selected by the developers. In case of the inclusion of inappropriate features, biased results can be produced. An example is that a person living within a particular neighbourhood can be described as the neighbourhood being a variable in a loan approval model, which indirectly gives a reflection of race/class divisions. The model can still give disproportionate results in the form of proxy variables even in the absence of sensitive attributes (Li et al., 2025). Fairness is also affected by the optimisation decisions. AI models are typically optimised in terms of accuracy or efficiency. Nonetheless, maximum accuracy may overlook the aspect of whether prediction is just to everyone. A model can be performing very well in general and yet fail among the minorities. Unless fairness is incorporated in the algorithm, inequities may increase (Nagpal et al., 2025).

Fairness is also when model interpretability is adopted. The causes of biased outcomes may be hard to trace in complex black box models like deep neural networks. Lack of transparency enables mistakes to go undetected and they keep causing damage to groups that are affected (Smart & Kasirzadeh, 2025). An unintended personal or cultural assumption may end up in design by developers. This risk is aggravated by a deficiency in development teams. AI products cannot work equally well with various societies when they are developed without taking into account the other viewpoints. Thus, human aspects to design are significant points of bias (Gerlich, 2023).

7.2.3 *Contextual and Operational Bias in Deployment*

However, despite the creation of a model based on balanced data and designed with adequate attention, the bias may manifest itself in the future, as the model is implemented in real-life situations. The performance of AI is affected by operational decisions, conditions of implementation, and social conditions. Contextual bias may occur as a result of the policies and settings of the operations. As an illustration, predictive policing systems guide the police patrols to the high risk neighbourhoods. Nevertheless, in case such regions were once over policed, the model still indicates high risk, which supports a vicious cycle of disproportional surveillance (Panarese et al., 2025). The conditions of deployment are also different. A medical AI system that works well in large hospitals might not be able to work in the same way in small clinics with limited resources. This is because system limitations are immediately translated into inequality in the achievement of health outcomes (Sinha & Lee, 2024).

Human AI interaction might also result in bias. The officials of the community can excessively depend on automated suggestions without doubt of the errors. On the other hand, the lack of trust or poor understanding of the AI tools can result in unequal usage. Both cases may harm justice in decision-making (Chowdhury & Oredo, 2023). There can also be organisational priorities that lead to outcomes. In case an institution is centred on cost reduction, the AI systems may apply efficiency over equity. To illustrate, automated welfare programmes can make benefit reductions to cut on expenditure instead of attending to the needs of individuals. Operational bias may be accrued over time. Small errors can grow and bring significant damages without monitoring and regular assessment. To ensure fairness, it is required to undertake continuous auditing and stakeholder feedback (Nishant et al., 2024).

7.3 Societal and Sectoral Implications

7.3.1 *Effects on Employment, Credit, Policing, Healthcare, and Welfare*

AI is normally applied in job applicant screening and recruitment. The automated recruitment tools scan through resumes, rank, and give suggestions to employers. Assuming that the training data is representative of previous employment trends that discriminated against some segments, there is likelihood of the system excluding women, minorities, and persons with atypical education levels. Consequently, the algorithm can fail to recognise potential in the talented candidates, thereby depriving them of a chance to excel. Discrimination in the employment process can exacerbate the economic disparities (Chen, 2023). Also credit services and financial services have implemented AI in loan approval and credit scoring. The risk is evaluated based on past data, including previous repayment data and geographic data, with the help of algorithms. In cases where the data is used to represent discriminatory lending policies or income disparities, AI can unjustifiably refuse credit to residents of lower income areas or minorities. This impacts their capacity to open business or invest in education or purchase homes, which causes the economical disparities in the long term (Raji et al., 2024).

AI applications can predict crime hotspots, detect suspects, and determine the likelihood of committing crime again in policing and criminal justice. Predictive policing machines can be based on information about locations that have a background of over policing as opposed to the real crime tendencies. This reinforces the stereotypes and results into increased surveillance and arrests within particular communities. The system of judicial bias in legal decision-making, like in sentencing risk assessment, can also affect verdicts. Such results pose a threat to fairness, justice, and human rights (Blount, 2024). Another area of harm of algorithmic bias is healthcare. The diagnostic models that have been trained on small groups of demographics may give unreliable results on less represented groups. Failure to identify medical conditions in some racial or ethnic groups by an AI system can lead to the patients receiving late or wrong treatment. This widens the disparity in health and can lower the lifespan of the at risk populations (Ratwani et al., 2024).

Welfare systems in the government are becoming automated. AI can be applied to determine the eligibility of social benefits or detect fraud. When the system does not understand financial circumstances or is not put into context, the people requiring help might be refused the necessary help. Mistakes in automation of welfare may cause financial strain and poverty to families that are already struggling (Nayak & Tiyadi, 2024). These illustrations demonstrate that algorithmic bias has an impact on critical areas of society. Discriminatory decisions by robots may prevent employment, healthcare, safety, and economic security. Since such services define the quality of life of the people, unjust AI systems may enhance inequality (Ali, 2025).

7.3.2 Marginalisation of Vulnerable and Underrepresented Communities

The biasing of algorithms tends to be applied to the already discriminated population. Biased AI decision-making is more likely to affect minorities, women, the elderly, the disabled, rural citizens, and the poor. When algorithms are trained on information that does not represent or misrepresents these groups, the technology solidifies ways of marginalising those (Mergen et al., 2025). Other communities are not easily visible in digital systems due to lack of technology in them. With the training of AI models, the urban population with digital connectivity is predominant, thus excluding the voices of rural individuals. Majority group optimised services might fail to satisfy the needs of individuals with other languages, cultures, or lifestyles (Calzada & Eizaguirre, 2025).

Structural inequalities can also be portrayed in bias. As an example, when the past data reveals that marginalised populations have lower credit scores because of discrimination, AI picks up this prejudiced assumption too. This implies that technology has the ability to recreate injustice unintentionally (Stypinska, 2023). The weak people can also lack the opportunity to appeal against discriminatory judgements. They might be unaware of the law, be financially unable, or have no technical expertise. This enhances power disparity and obstacles to justice. Prejudice in AI thus does not just make errors. It can positively contribute to marginalisation and inequality by restricting the prospects of the people who are already disadvantaged. Unless it is governed well, AI will be a weapon that enhances social inequalities rather than alleviating those (Garcia et al., 2024).

7.3.3 Loss of Trust in Automated Systems and Public Institutions

Deployment of AI within the society depends on the trust of the population. Individuals lose trust in technology when they feel victimised by the automated judgement or unfairness of the technology. The bad experiences propagate easily via social networks and new media, fostering more fear and opposition to AI (Afroogh et al., 2024). Absence of transparency is one of the key factors. Most AI models cannot be interpreted easily. When governments or businesses are unable to justify the manner in which decisions would be made, the citizens might consider the system as being secretive or manipulative. This undermines not just AI, but also the institutions using AI (Hassija et al., 2024). Prejudice in areas like welfare or policing may hurt the trust of the populace in fairness and justice. Individuals might not use the digital programmes or seek out the services of the population when they believe that the system is discriminatory against them. This may decrease the effectiveness of the social policy and damage social stability (Kordzadeh & Ghasemaghaei, 2022).

There is also low trust in innovation. Consumers can be afraid of being discriminated against, which will make private companies reluctant to embrace AI. Criticism of the technology can be demonstrated by protests or prosecutions that slow down the use of technology in the public sector. Trying to win trust should then be achieved by being responsible in design, allowing open communication, and ensuring good accountability. Building trust in AI is a process that takes time. Technology should ensure that the citizens feel safe and honoured. Governments need to engage communities in decision-making and they need to have systems that will rectify an unjust matter. Through the preservation of trust, AI can be an influential instrument of social good (Luthra et al., 2025).

7.4 Policy and Regulatory Approaches

7.4.1 Legal Frameworks Promoting Fairness and Non-Discrimination

There should be legal safeguards to make sure that automated decisions are not prejudiced against equality and human rights. Anti-discrimination laws already exist in many countries that forbid unfair treatment grounded on race, gender, disability, age, religion, or the socioeconomic status of a person. These legislations also extend to the AI systems. The fairness is also assisted by the laws of data protection by controlling the use and collection of personal information. The General Data Protection Regulation (GDPR) of the European Union enables a person to seek clarifications on algorithmic decisions and have their right to automated profiling dismissed. This will help to introduce transparency and provide more control to users (Abraha, 2023).

However, in some cases, traditional laws do not adequately address AI due to the possibility of discrimination that can be manifested in a hidden way via complex algorithms. As such, there are new legal changes taking place. In certain governments, the deployment of AI in such sensitive fields as policing or welfare will also require algorithmic impact assessments. Explainability and human control requirements in law assist in making sure that AI does not eradicate meaningful accountability (Borgesius, 2025). The regulation of fairness is proactive as opposed to being reactive. Rather than reacting to discrimination after it has taken place, government bodies are demanding that systems be tested on discrimination before utilisation. Such a move insulates people and avoids mass destruction.

7.4.2 International Standards and Principles

International bodies have come up with moral principles that can promote responsible AI use on the international level. These norms assist in harmonising national policies and eliminating ethical discrepancies. OECD Principles on Artificial Intelligence advance human principles, equity, openness, and responsibility. They also urge governments to make sure that AI is socially productive and promotes inclusive development. These principles became the basis of the national AI strategies by many countries (Nikolinakos, 2023). The Recommendation on the Ethics of AI by UNESCO is aimed at safeguarding human rights and cultural diversity. It promotes impartial assessments, inclusion of the populace, and safeguarding of the disadvantaged communities. UNESCO focuses on the fact that AI must not imitate discrimination and place power in the wrong hands (Van Norren, 2023).

The EU AI Act has become one of the most developed regulators in the world. It categorises AI systems based on the degree of risk and establishes rigorous criteria of the high risk applications like law enforcement, hiring, and healthcare. Conformity checks of high-risk systems should be performed, have transparency, and be supervised by humans. Systems that use AI and present too much of a threat to basic rights, including social scoring, are outright prohibited (Hacker,

2023). Multinational standards facilitate uniformity and promote multinational cooperation. They assist governments in cross learning and construct robust, clear, and efficient regulations (Kashefi et al., 2024).

7.4.3 National Level Policies and Enforcement Mechanisms

Different countries are taking various directions to minimise algorithmic bias depending on legislative systems, resources, and social requirements. Other countries are centred on regulations. Canada needs to have automated decision-making systems in the state sector that go through Algorithms Impact Assessments (AIA). The United States has come up with industry-based credit score, employment, and criminal justice guidelines. India is a country that focuses on inclusive approaches and responsible innovation in its current AI policies, particularly in the best interest of the populace (Brandusescu & Sieber, 2025). Government institutions are prioritised in other countries. The AI implementation is controlled by independent oversight authorities, which check the complaints and hold them accountable. Governments perform periodic audits and make organisations record the decision-making process of their systems (Novelli et al., 2024).

Compliance tools are expanding, including:

- Bias detection audits,
- Fairness certification or labelling,
- Mandatory transparency reporting,
- Penalties for discriminatory outcomes.

Civil society organisations and consumer rights groups also support accountability by raising concerns and representing affected populations. This is still difficult to enforce since prejudice may be concealed within the intricate systems. Hence, there is a need to constantly monitor and undergo multidisciplinary reviews. This should be through adjustment of policies in line with the changes in technology to be insured in the long run (Al-Dulaimi & Mohammed, 2025). Table 7.1 defines policy tools that are important in identification, prevention, and correction of algorithmic bias and discrimination.

Table 7.1 Key Policy Approaches for Mitigating Algorithmic Bias.

Policy Tool	*Focus Area*	*Main Goal*	*Example*
Anti-discrimination laws	Rights protection	Prevent unequal outcomes	Equal access laws, hiring fairness rules
Data protection regulation	Data governance	Transparency and user control	GDPR requirements for explainability
Algorithmic impact assessments	Risk screening	Detect harms before deployment	Canada: AIA for public sector AI
Risk-based classification rules	Safety and accountability	Higher standards for high risk sectors	EU AI Act
Oversight bodies and audits	Compliance	Continuous monitoring of fairness	National AI ethics boards

7.5 Technical and Organisational Mitigation Tools

7.5.1 Fairness Metrics and Algorithmic Audits

Fairness metrics are mathematical values that are applied to measure the equality in treatment of different groups by an AI system. These measures compare the error rates, the accuracy of prediction, and decision outcomes among demographic groups, i.e., gender, race, or age. Through the measures of fairness, developers are able to determine whether a model fits a particular group more than the other (Palumbo et al., 2025).

Examples of fairness metrics include:

- **Demographic parity:** Equal outcomes for all groups;
- **Equal opportunity:** Equal true positive rates;
- **Predictive parity:** Equal prediction reliability across groups.

There is no single measure of fairness that would suit every case. Depending on the social environment, the law, and the use of the system, governments and organisations need to select metrics (Pessach & Shmueli, 2022). AI audits are regular assessments of the work of AI. They can assist in identifying bias at pre-deployment and at the continuing use. The audits may be conducted either by the institution or by external professionals. Constant auditing maintains consistency in checking fairness and the risk of discrimination does not grow with time. Audits also enhance transparency and accountability which lead to building up of public trust (Minkkinen et al., 2022).

7.5.2 Bias Detection, Debiasing Techniques, and Explainability Tools

The methods of detecting bias can be used to detect unfair trends in data or model performance. These instruments are used to examine datasets in order to determine missing categories or unbalanced distributions. They also experiment on models to find out whether there are any variations in the results of protected groups. This can eliminate discriminatory effects of AI systems once they have been introduced by early detection (Pagano et al., 2023). The debiasing methods assist in avoiding unfairness. Other techniques add additional examples of underrepresented people to the dataset or eliminate sensitive attributes. Other techniques train models according to the patterns such that they do not associate unfavourable variables with predictions. Outputs are altered through post-processing in order to cut down on disproportionate decisions (Zhou et al., 2021).

Fairness also requires explainability tools. AI models are difficult to interpret as they may be complex. Decisions made using explainable AI (XAI) are more understandable. They indicate what characteristics were taken into consideration and the manner in which the model came to the conclusion. This helps in assuring confidence to the users and enables professionals to consider whether the decisions are just. It also makes people confront automated results in case of error (Minh et al., 2022). High-risk matters like healthcare, policing, or welfare are especially significant when it comes to explainability. People have to know how AI decisions impact their rights. Explainable tools increase the openness of the system and enhance responsible decision-making (Rajendra & Thuraisingam, 2025).

7.5.3 Inclusive Design, Diverse Datasets, and Participatory AI Development

The purpose of inclusive design is to make AI systems representative of the needs of every community. It helps developers to put in mind the experience of individuals having different identities, cultures, and abilities. In case AI tools are created to target a wide audience, equality will become better and social marginalisation will be reduced (Zallio et al., 2025). One of the significant approaches to decrease bias is using different datasets. The data must reflect various groups of people equally. This entails the gathering of information in rural areas, minority languages, the elderly, and the disabled persons. Categories when datasets are composed of different examples, models can be more successful to all. Participatory AI development refers to the community-based approach to designing AI. Citizens and advocacy organisations and domain experts may express their concerns and provide real-life use cases. Their contribution is to determine possible evils and make systems representative of the social values. Engagement enhances legitimacy, trust, and promotes democratic accountability (Bondi et al., 2021).

The companies should also establish policies internally to promote ethical conduct. Such multidisciplinary teams comprising social scientists, policy professionals, and ethicists can be used in identifying risks that technical teams might fail to notice. Accountable governance enhances institutions and better outcomes of fairness (Camilleri, 2024). Table 7.2 summarises the main technical and organisational tools that support fair and transparent AI systems.

Table 7.2 Technical and Organizational Tools for Bias Mitigation.

Tool Category	*Method*	*Purpose*	*Governance Value*
Fairness Metrics	Measure fairness in outputs	Identify unequal outcomes	Supports accountability
Algorithmic Audits	Periodic evaluation of performance	Detect bias and risks	Ensures transparency
Bias Detection	Analyse data/model behaviour	Find unfair patterns early	Prevents discrimination
Debiasing Techniques	Adjust data/model training	Reduce biased decision-making	Improves fairness
Explainability Tools	Make decisions understandable	Enable review and appeals	Protects user rights
Inclusive Design	Consider diverse user needs	Reduce exclusion	Promotes equity

Contd.

Table 7.2 *Contd.*

Tool Category	*Method*	*Purpose*	*Governance Value*
Diverse Datasets	Broader data representation	Improve model performance	Ensures equal access
Participatory Development	Include citizens and experts	Reflect social values	Builds public trust

7.6 Institutional Governance and Cross-Sector Collaboration

7.6.1 Role of Regulators, Civil Society, Academia, and Industry

The regulators are more at the centre of making sure that the AI systems comply with the laws and the ethical requirements. They establish regulations, audit their adherence, and enforce responsibility in the cases of discrimination. Risky AI systems are regulated by regulatory agencies, and can insist on audits, documentation, and authorisation before implementation. They also make sure that the rights of citizens are not violated and that AI does not serve to promote favouritism and unequal consideration (De Almeida et al., 2021). Civil society organisations are the voice of the people particularly the vulnerable or underrepresented groups. They give education on the negative effects and promote openness and fairness. This means that the discussions on ethics will have real-world point of views and various voices because of their involvement. NGOs, digital rights associations, and community activists tend to help people who protest against unjust judgements (LePere-Schloop & Zook, 2023).

Technical research and expertise is provided by academic institutions. Their work is on algorithmic bias, the creation of new fairness tools, and the social effects of technology. The future professionals in AI are also trained in responsible governance in Universities. Independent researchers have the ability of assessing the government and industry systems in order to point out risks. Scientific credibility and objectivity is enhanced through academic participation (Finocchiaro, 2024). The industry factor is significant since most AI technologies are designed and implemented by a company. Companies possess the capital and the technical expertise to introduce innovations in the market. They should be responsible in combatting bias when developing. Most businesses have incorporated boards of ethics, fairness tests, and user reviews in their operations. Scaling of safe and fair solutions of AI requires collaboration in the industry (Sinha & Lee, 2024). These actors collectively have the role of creating a secure and inclusive AI environment.

7.6.2 Transparency Reporting, Risk Assessments, and Oversight Bodies

One of the requirements to minimise algorithmic bias is transparency. By publicly releasing information on the functionality of AI systems, their data sources, and decision-making mechanisms, organisations can be more readily noticed to engage in unethical activities (Balasubramaniam et al., 2023). Transparency reporting can include:

- Descriptions of decision logic in plain language;
- Disclosure of training data characteristics;
- Results of fairness evaluations;
- Records of audit findings.

Public reporting fosters the creation of trust and provision of information to challenge automated results to the citizens. Conscientious deployment requires the use of risk assessments. Developers and policymakers should consider the dangers before implementing an AI system. Reviewing the risk assessments can be used to determine which populations might be impacted out of proportion and whether there are adequate defences. They categorise systems based on the degree of risk and the amount of control to be established (Nordström, 2022).

This is accounted for by oversight bodies. These organisations are keeping an eye on the use of AI and address the grievances of the citizens. Oversight bodies may include:

- National AI regulatory agencies;
- Data protection authorities;
- Ethics boards or commissions;
- Independent review committees.

These organisations are empowered to probe issues, mandate remedial action, or stop destructive systems. Supervision fosters equality and eliminates exploitation. It is necessary to monitor continuously since the bias may develop gradually. Reviewing of systems should be periodically reviewed such that they are always fair as the conditions change. The openness and control promote responsible technological development and assist in keeping the population trustful to automated technologies (Cousineau et al., 2025).

7.6.3 Education, Awareness, and Multi-Stakeholder Partnerships

Successful bias mitigation is essential with the help of education and awareness. The use of AI tools by the public officials should be aware of their strong and weak points. Training programmes can make the employees aware of the situations when the system can be discriminating, and how one can correct them. Education promotes ethical decision-making and good management of systems (Schiff, 2022). Awareness is also needed to ensure the rights of the citizens are safeguarded. Services and opportunities can be explained to the public via outreach programmes on how automated decisions impact services. The understanding of the right to explanation and appeal will help people to fight against unjust results. With increased awareness, there will be less fear of technology and people will participate constructively (Singh, 2023).

Multi-stakeholder alliances enhance governance. Team work enables companies to pool knowledge and resources. Governments can collaborate with universities to carry out fairness assessment or civil society groups to learn the issues in the community. Technology firms can collaborate with regulators to come up with safe systems at the onset. International cooperation also contributes to it. Nations exchange best practices and come up with shared standards and help one another to establish ethical AI capacity (Kashefi et al., 2024). Alliances promote innovation that is socially viable. They make it a collective objective instead of the duty of just one sector to maintain fairness. Through collaboration, the stakeholders contribute to the establishment of strong, flexible, and responsive governance structures that are sensitive to change.

7.7 Conclusion

The problem of algorithmic bias is an important issue with AI systems development and implementation. In case the AIs are based on unjust information or poor design, individual people and communities can be discriminated against and have unequal opportunities. The chapter discussed the primary origins of bias, negative effects of most key sectors, and the necessity to take solid policy actions to ensure the protection of fundamental rights and fairness. The international standards and national governance strategies, as well as legal and ethical frameworks, offer valuable protection. Accountability and accuracy can be facilitated using technical solutions including fairness measures, audits, debiasing, and explainability tools. Inclusive design and incorporating the public in the organisation process are some of the organisational activities that would make AI responsive to diverse social needs.

The mitigation needs to be done in collaboration with the regulators, industry, academia, and civil society. Responsible governance is enhanced by transparency reporting, risk assessment, and oversight bodies. Education and awareness should also be put into effect to bring the officials and citizens into the knowledge about AI systems and difficulty unfair results. In general, algorithmic bias is an important aspect that needs to be addressed to achieve trustful and human-centred AI. Through further cooperation and responsible policymaking, societies will be able to lessen discrimination and have AI contribute to equity and social justice to everyone.

References

Abraha, H. (2023). Regulating algorithmic employment decisions through data protection law. *European Labour Law Journal*, *14*(2), 172–191. https://doi.org/10.1177/20319525231167317.

Afroogh, S., Akbari, A., Malone, E., Kargar, M. and Alambeigi, H. (2024). Trust in AI: Progress, challenges, and future directions. *Humanities and Social Sciences Communications*, *11*(1), 1–30. https://doi.org/10.1057/s41599-024-04044-8.

Agarwal, R., Bjarnadottir, M., Rhue, L., Dugas, M., Crowley, K., Clark, J. and Gao, G. (2023). Addressing algorithmic bias and the perpetuation of health inequities: An AI bias aware framework. *Health Policy and Technology*, *12*(1), 100702. https://doi.org/10.1016/j.hlpt.2022.100702.

Al-Dulaimi, A.O.M. and Mohammed, M.A.A.W. (2025). Legal responsibility for errors caused by artificial intelligence (AI) in the public sector. *International Journal of Law and Management*. https://doi.org/10.1108/IJLMA-08-2024-0295.

Ali, A. (2025). Robotic revolution: Ethical and legal frontiers in healthcare metaverse research. In: *Healthcare Frontiers in the Metaverse* (pp. 209–226). Academic Press. https://doi.org/10.1016/B978-0-443-32998-2.00021-4.

Balasubramaniam, N., Kauppinen, M., Rannisto, A., Hiekkanen, K. and Kujala, S. (2023). Transparency and explainability of AI systems: From ethical guidelines to requirements. *Information and Software Technology*, *159*, 107197. https://doi.org/10.1016/j.infsof.2023.107197.

Blount, K. (2024). Using artificial intelligence to prevent crime: implications for due process and criminal justice. *AI & Society*, *39*(1), 359–368. https://doi.org/10.1007/s00146-022-01513-z.

Bondi, E., Xu, L., Acosta-Navas, D. and Killian, J.A. (2021, July). Envisioning communities: A participatory approach towards AI for social good. In: *Proceedings of the 2021 AAAI/ACM Conference on AI, Ethics, and Society* (pp. 425–436). https://doi.org/10.1145/3461702.3462612.

Borgesius, F.Z. (2025). Discrimination, artificial intelligence, and algorithmic decision-making. *arXiv preprint arXiv:2510.13465*. https://doi.org/10.48550/arXiv.2510.13465.

Brandusescu, A. and Sieber, R.E. (2025). Design versus reality: Assessing the results and compliance of algorithmic impact assessments. *Digital Society*, *4*(2), 64. https://doi.org/10.1007/s44206-025-00221-7.

Calzada, I. and Eizaguirre, I. (2025). Digital inclusion and Urban AI: Strategic roadmapping and policy challenges. *Discover Cities*, *2*(1), 73. https://doi.org/10.1007/s44327-025-00116-9.

Camilleri, M.A. (2024). Artificial intelligence governance: Ethical considerations and implications for social responsibility. *Expert Systems*, *41*(7), e13406. https://doi.org/10.1111/exsy.13406.

Chen, P., Wu, L. and Wang, L. (2023). AI fairness in data management and analytics: A review on challenges, methodologies, and applications. *Applied Sciences*, *13*(18), 10258. https://doi.org/10.3390/app131810258.

Chen, Z. (2023). Collaboration among recruiters and artificial intelligence: Removing human prejudices in employment. *Cognition, Technology and Work*, *25*(1), 135–149. https://doi.org/10.1007/s10111-022-00716-0.

Chowdhury, T. and Oredo, J. (2023). AI ethical biases: Normative and information systems development conceptual framework. *Journal of Decision Systems*, *32*(3), 617–633. https://doi.org/10.1080/12460125.2022.2062849.

Cousineau, C., Dara, R. and Chowdhury, A. (2025). Trustworthy AI: AI developers' lens to implementation challenges and opportunities. *Data and Information Management*, *9*(2), 100082. https://doi.org/10.1016/j.dim.2024.100082,

De Almeida, P.G.R., Dos Santos, C.D. and Farias, J.S. (2021). Artificial intelligence regulation: A framework for governance. *Ethics and Information Technology*, *23*(3), 505–525. https://doi.org/10.1007/s10676-021-09593-z.

Entschew, E.M. (2024). Discriminatory data yields discriminatory systems: When AI biases harm human beings. In: *The Elgar Companion to Applied AI Ethics* (pp. 37–65). Edward Elgar Publishing. https://doi.org/10.4337/9781803928241.00009.

Finocchiaro, G. (2024). The regulation of artificial intelligence. *AI & Society*, *39*(4), 1961–1968. https://doi.org/10.1007/s00146-023-01650-z.

Garcia, A.C.B., Garcia, M.G.P. and Rigobon, R. (2024). Algorithmic discrimination in the credit domain: What do we know about it? *AI & Society*, *39*(4), 2059–2098. https://doi.org/10.1007/s00146-023-01676-3.

Gerdon, F., Bach, R.L., Kern, C. and Kreuter, F. (2022). Social impacts of algorithmic decision-making: A research agenda for the social sciences. *Big Data & Society*, *9*(1), 20539517221089305. https://doi.org/10.1177/20539517221089305.

Gerlich, M. (2023). Perceptions and acceptance of artificial intelligence: A multi-dimensional study. *Social Sciences, 12*(9), 502. https://doi.org/10.3390/socsci12090502.

Hacker, P. (2023). AI regulation in Europe: From the AI Act to future regulatory challenges. *arXiv preprint arXiv:2310.04072*. https://doi.org/10.48550/arXiv.2310.04072.

Hanna, M.G., Pantanowitz, L., Jackson, B., Palmer, O., Visweswaran, S., Pantanowitz, J., ... & Rashidi, H. H. (2025). Ethical and bias considerations in artificial intelligence/machine learning. *Modern Pathology, 38*(3), 100686. https://doi.org/10.1016/j.modpat.2024.100686.

Hassija, V., Chamola, V., Mahapatra, A., Singal, A., Goel, D., Huang, K., ... & Hussain, A. (2024). Interpreting black-box models: A review on explainable artificial intelligence. *Cognitive Computation, 16*(1), 45–74. https://doi.org/10.1007/s12559-023-10179-8.

Kashefi, P., Kashefi, Y. and Ghafouri Mirsaraei, A. (2024). Shaping the future of AI: Balancing innovation and ethics in global regulation. *Uniform Law Review, 29*(3), 524–548. https://doi.org/10.1093/ulr/unae040.

Kordzadeh, N. and Ghasemaghaei, M. (2022). Algorithmic bias: Review, synthesis, and future research directions. *European Journal of Information Systems, 31*(3), 388-409. https://doi.org/10.1080/0960085X.2021.1927212.

Kumar, A., Dhanka, S., Sharma, A., Sharma, A., Nain, M., Kumar, P., ... & Pant, R. (2025). A Comprehensive Review of Bias in AI, ML, and DL Models: Methods, Impacts, and Future Directions. *Archives of Computational Methods in Engineering*, 1–31. https://doi.org/10.1007/s11831-025-10483-6.

LePere-Schloop, M. and Zook, S. (2023). AI governance and civil society: The need for critical engagement. In: *Handbook of Critical Studies of Artificial Intelligence* (pp. 878–889). Edward Elgar Publishing. https://doi.org/10.4337/9781803928562.00087.

Li, D., Tan, Z. and Liu, H. (2025). Exploring large language models for feature selection: A data-centric perspective. *ACM SIGKDD Explorations Newsletter, 26*(2), 44–53. https://doi.org/10.1145/3715073.3715077.

Luthra, A., Dixit, S., Garg, S., Singh, A. and Anchal, M. (2025). Addressing Ethical Considerations and Responsible AI Practices. In: *The ChatGPT Revolution: How Conversational AI is Transforming Customer Service and Business Operations* (pp. 129–149). Emerald Publishing Limited. https://doi.org/10.1108/978-1-83549-852-120251007.

Mergen, A., Çetin-Kılıç, N. and Özbilgin, M.F. (2025). Artificial intelligence and bias towards marginalised groups: Theoretical roots and challenges. In: *AI and Diversity in a Datafied World of Work: Will the Future of Work be Inclusive?* (Vol. 12, pp. 17–38). Emerald Publishing Limited. https://doi.org/10.1108/S2051-233320250000012004.

Minh, D., Wang, H.X., Li, Y.F. and Nguyen, T.N. (2022). Explainable artificial intelligence: A comprehensive review. *Artificial Intelligence Review, 55*(5), 3503–3568. https://doi.org/10.1007/s10462-021-10088-y.

Minkkinen, M., Laine, J. and Mäntymäki, M. (2022). Continuous auditing of artificial intelligence: A conceptualization and assessment of tools and frameworks. *Digital Society, 1*(3), 21. https://doi.org/10.1007/s44206-022-00022-2.

Nagpal, R., Shahsavarifar, R., Goyal, V. and Gupta, A. (2025). Optimizing fairness and accuracy: A Pareto optimal approach for decision-making. *AI and Ethics, 5*(2), 1743–1756. https://doi.org/10.1007/s43681-024-00508-4.

Nayak, M. and Tiyadi, J. (2024). Social Welfare and Artificial Intelligence's Role: A Comprehensive Summary of the Study. In: *AI in the Social and Business World: A Comprehensive Approach* (pp. 32–66). Bentham Science Publishers. https://doi.org/10.2174/97898152568641240101.

Nikolinakos, N.T. (2023). Ethical principles for trustworthy AI. In: *EU Policy and Legal Framework for Artificial Intelligence, Robotics, and Related Technologies-the AI Act* (pp. 101–166). Cham: Springer International Publishing. https://doi.org/10.1007/978-3-031-27953-9_3.

Nishant, R., Schneckenberg, D. and Ravishankar, M.N. (2024). The formal rationality of artificial intelligence-based algorithms and the problem of bias. *Journal of Information Technology*, *39*(1), 19–40. https://doi.org/10.1177/02683962231176842.

Nordström, M. (2022). AI under great uncertainty: Implications and decision strategies for public policy. *AI & Society*, *37*(4), 1703—1714. https://doi.org/10.1007/s00146-021-01263-4.

Novelli, C., Taddeo, M. and Floridi, L. (2024). Accountability in artificial intelligence: What it is and how it works. *AI & Society*, *39*(4), 1871–1882. https://doi.org/10.1007/s00146-023-01635-y.

Pagano, T.P., Loureiro, R.B., Lisboa, F.V., Peixoto, R.M., Guimarães, G.A., Cruz, G.O., ... & Nascimento, E. G. (2023). Bias and unfairness in machine learning models: A systematic review on datasets, tools, fairness metrics, and identification and mitigation methods. *Big Data and Cognitive Computing*, *7*(1), 15. https://doi.org/10.3390/bdcc7010015.

Palumbo, G., Carneiro, D. and Alves, V. (2025). Objective metrics for ethical AI: A systematic literature review. *International Journal of Data Science and Analytics*, *20*(2), 247–267. https://doi.org/10.1007/s41060-024-00541-w.

Panarese, P., Grasso, M.M. and Solinas, C. (2025). Algorithmic bias, fairness, and inclusivity: A multilevel framework for justice-oriented AI. *AI & Society*, 1–23. https://doi.org/10.1007/s00146-025-02451-2.

Pessach, D. and Shmueli, E. (2022). A review on fairness in machine learning. *ACM Computing Surveys* (*CSUR*), *55*(3), 1–44. https://doi.org/10.1145/3494672.

Rajendra, J.B. and Thuraisingam, A.S. (2025). The role of explainability and human intervention in AI decisions: Jurisdictional and regulatory aspects. *Information & Communications Technology Law*, 1–32. https://doi.org/10.1080/13600834.2025.2537514.

Raji, A.A.H., Alabdoon, A.H.F. and Almagtome, A. (2024, April). AI in credit scoring and risk assessment: Enhancing lending practices and financial inclusion. In: *2024 International Conference on Knowledge Engineering and Communication Systems* (*ICKECS*) (Vol. 1, pp. 1–7). IEEE. https://doi.org/10.1109/ICKECS61492.2024.10616493.

Ratwani, R.M., Sutton, K. and Galarraga, J.E. (2024). Addressing AI algorithmic bias in health care. *Jama, 332*(13), 1051–1052. doi:10.1001/jama.2024.13486.

Schiff, D. (2022). Education for AI, not AI for education: The role of education and ethics in national AI policy strategies. *International Journal of Artificial Intelligence in Education*, *32*(3), 527–563. https://doi.org/10.1007/s40593-021-00270-2.

Shestakova, V. (2021). Best practices to mitigate bias and discrimination in artificial intelligence. *Performance Improvement*, *60*(6), 6–11. https://doi.org/10.1002/pfi.21987.

Singh, T. (2023, October). AI-Driven Surveillance Technologies and Human Rights: Balancing Security and Privacy. In: *International Conference on Smart Systems: Innovations in Computing* (pp. 703–717). Singapore: Springer Nature Singapore. https://doi.org/10.1007/978-981-97-3690-4_53.

Sinha, S. and Lee, Y.M. (2024). Challenges with developing and deploying AI models and applications in industrial systems. *Discover Artificial Intelligence*, *4*(1), 55. https://doi.org/10.1007/s44163-024-00151-2.

Smart, A. and Kasirzadeh, A. (2025). Beyond model interpretability: Socio-structural explanations in machine learning. *AI & Society*, *40*(4), 2045–2053. https://doi.org/10.1007/s00146-024-02056-1

Stypinska, J. (2023). AI ageism: A critical roadmap for studying age discrimination and exclusion in digitalized societies. *AI & Society*, *38*(2), 665–677. https://doi.org/10.1007/s00146-022-01553-5.

Van Norren, D.E. (2023). The ethics of artificial intelligence: UNESCO and the African Ubuntu perspective. *Journal of Information, Communication, and Ethics in Society*, *21*(1), 112–128. https://doi.org/10.1108/JICES-04-2022-0037.

Varona, D. and Suárez, J.L. (2022). Discrimination, bias, fairness, and trustworthy AI. *Applied Sciences*, *12*(12), 5826. https://doi.org/10.3390/app12125826.
Zajko, M. (2022). Artificial intelligence, algorithms, and social inequality: Sociological contributions to contemporary debates. *Sociology Compass*, *16*(3), e12962. https://doi.org/10.1111/soc4.12962.
Zallio, M., Ike, C.B. and Chivăran, C. (2025). Designing Artificial Intelligence: Exploring Inclusion, Diversity, Equity, Accessibility, and Safety in Human-Centric Emerging Technologies. *AI*, *6*(7), 143. https://doi.org/10.3390/ai6070143.
Zhou, Y., Kantarcioglu, M. and Clifton, C. (2021). Improving fairness of AI systems with lossless de-biasing. *arXiv preprint arXiv:2105.04534*. https://doi.org/10.48550/arXiv.2105.04534.

8 Data Governance and Privacy in the Age of AI

The concept of data governance and privacy protection has become one of the central concerns in the era of Artificial Intelligence (AI). AI systems are based on big datasets of personal and sensitive information to make decisions and predict actions as well as to provide public and private services. Nevertheless, there are risks of unauthorised access, surveillance, profiling, and discrimination that are worsening with the reconstruction of data usage. There is a need to have strong governance structures that can ensure data collection, sharing, and processing is done in a responsible manner, and the rights of individuals are upheld. This chapter discusses the fundamental principles of data governance, the major privacy dilemmas that arise as a result of AI technologies, and regulatory strategies embraced in various locations. It further examines some of the practical solutions, including consent management, data minimisation, anonymisation, and safe data infrastructure to facilitate ethical and trustful AI ecosystems.

8.1 Introduction

In the era of Artificial Intelligence (AI), data is one of the most valuable resources. Contemporary AI systems use extensive and diverse sets of data to understand patterns and make predictions as well as assist in decision-making. The daily activities are monitored by government departments, businesses, and social networks that convey large volumes of data in real time (Verma & Singhal, 2023). Such data contains individuals, location history, financial history, health records, and online communications. AI can utilise this data to advance services, make them more efficient, and develop new innovations. AI systems cannot operate without big and properly organised datasets. Data is thus at the centre of development, correctness, as well as dependability of AI apps in various industries (Sarker, 2022).

Data significance in AI-based systems is increasing due to the high level of penetration of digital technologies into our daily lives. There is always the generation of real-time data in smartphones, sensors, online platforms, and smart devices. It allows AI systems to keep an eye on health, traffic, support customers, and personalise digital experiences (Chander et al., 2022). Data is used by business organisations to know how consumers behave and by governments to develop public services. Quality data enhances forecasts, minimises mistakes, and evidence use in policymaking. With the growing infiltration of AI in society, there is a growing demand to have greater and more sustained data. This introduces new

DOI: 10.1201/9781003776659-8

possibilities of innovation and also imposes new duties of protection of data (Kumar et al., 2024).

Meanwhile, there is an increase of privacy issues in digital societies. The high frequency of gathering and distributing personal information poses threats of abuse, intrusion, and monitoring. People are not aware of how their data are gathered, with what purposes they are used, and who can access them. AI systems have the ability to assemble various sources of data to form comprehensive profiles of people, which can be on an unconscious or even unwillful scale. Such profiling can be used to affect employment, credit, healthcare or government services. Loss of control over their data endangers the privacy and autonomy of the individuals (Grey & Segerie, 2025).

There is also the likelihood of mass violations of privacy with AI technologies. Breaching of information has become a regular occurrence and hackers focus on targeting sensitive data held by businesses. Moreover, AI systems are able to draw conclusions about the personal information based on the apparently innocent data (Mühlhoff, 2023). As an example, algorithms can be used to predict health, political preferences, or personal habits based on the browsing history or social media activity. These risks present some serious ethical and legal issues. Individuals might feel that they are under constant surveillance in the online world and this influences their operation and lacks trust in institutions (Menard & Bott, 2025).

The issue of privacy is especially acute due to the fact that AI systems are able to make decisions directly affecting the rights and opportunities. The decisions can be unjust in case information is false or prejudiced. People cannot fight to have automated decisions as they do not know how the system functions. Such a non-transparency undermines accountability. It also creates more fear of the abuse of personal information by the government, corporations, or third parties (Martin & Zimmermann, 2024). Hence, effective data governance infrastructure is necessary. To safeguard people in AI-driven societies, data collection must be done responsibly, stored safely, consent obtained in a clear manner, and transparently. To ensure that the people can trust the AI systems, privacy protection should be part of the design and functionality of these systems. One of the most important challenges of digital governance is balancing the positive aspect of AI with the safety of the rights of the individuals (Ghosh et al., 2025).

8.2 Principles of Data Governance

8.2.1 User Data Rights: Ownership, Access, and Consent

The most important aspect of gaining trust in AI systems is transparency. Companies that create and implement AI have a role to play in clarifying the role of such systems. They are also supposed to give information on how decisions are made, the source of the data, and the risks that can occur as a result of automated decisions being made. Transparency enables people to know when AI systems are being accessed and also determine whether the decision generated is just, legal, and warranted (Lund et al., 2025). Accountability is also supported by straightforward and available information. People can monitor the performance of an AI system better when they have knowledge on how it works, as they can ask questions, appeal unfair decisions, and seek redressal. The lack of transparency means that the automated systems can be used without being subject to scrutiny by the population, which is more likely to result in discrimination, abuse, and violation of rights (Park & Young Yoon, 2025).

The advocacy and activism are significant in safeguarding digital rights in the era of AI. Human rights and digital rights activists as well as civil society organisations observe the application of AI technologies and attract attention to malicious actions. They report on and investigate instances of algorithmic discrimination, mass surveillance, and infringement of privacy. These organisations also advocate those people and groups that have suffered negatively due to automated systems (Gregory, 2023). There are various developments that have been brought about through advocacy. They are like publicly revealing surveillance technologies, limits or prohibitions on facial recognition technologies in a number of cities, and expanded application of fairness testing and transparency reports in organisations. Advocacy has also impacted in intensifying the rights to privacy and data protection by enacting new laws and regulations (Shaban, 2025).

The media is also quite important in creating awareness. Investigative journalism will be able to expose unseen dangers and discriminatory effects of AI systems within the institutions of the general population and the state. Journalists play a role in informing society and bringing about a healthy debate through public reporting (Leiser, 2022). Collectively, activism, transparency, and advocacy put pressure on governments and companies to be responsible. They confirm the idea that technological innovation should not violate human dignity, civil liberties, and basic rights.

8.2.2 Data Quality, Accuracy, and Integrity

The quality of data is an important aspect ofAI e systems performance and reliability. AI e models rely on information to acquire patterns and make a decision. In case the data processed is of low quality, the results generated by the AI systems will also be unreliable or even dangerous. Data governance is thus an important aspect that needs stiff measures to make data accurate, complete, and relevant to its intended use (Nguyen et al., 2024). The aspect of accuracy is the degree to which data is accurate in reflecting reality. The personal and institutional information should be accurate and up to date. The updates must be done regularly to reflect the changes in the situations of a person, including the employment status, financial situation, or health facts. Misleading data will result in wrong automatic decision-making, which can do severe damage in such sensitive fields as medical diagnosis, credit evaluation, or the services of the population (Aldoseri et al., 2023).

The other aspect of data quality is completeness. All the relevant information must be incorporated in the data sets and they must reflect different groups in the society. In cases of missing or underrepresentation of particular groups, AI systems can yield biased or unjust outputs. This underrepresentation can contribute to the current inequalities and decrease the impartiality of automated judgements. Representative and inclusive data ensures better reliability and equity of the AI systems (Panarese et al., 2025). Data integrity can be defined as the safety of data against unauthorised alteration, manipulation, or corruption. Data must always be reliable and stable during the lifecycle. Any change in the information should be permitted, documented, and traceable. Data changes are well documented and facilitate transparency and accountability, particularly in systems that are based on large and complex data (Akhtar et al., 2024).

Data standards must be high and this can only be achieved through quality control measures. These controls involve checking of validation, mixed data sampling, and data performance monitoring. Periodic audits are used to detect the mistakes and flaws in datasets. Quality data enhances fairness, accuracy, and reliability within the AI systems. Organisations can help to ensure the safe, efficient, and fair use of AI technologies by ensuring the quality, accuracy, and integrity of data (Chen et al., 2023).

8.2.3 Security, Accountability, and Risk Management

Responsible data governance and AI systems are based on security. With more and more sensitive information being gathered and processed by organisations, the chances of unwarranted access, data theft, and misuse also increase. Effective security procedures would be required to secure individual and institutional data. Such measures encompass encryption, secure data storage, access controls, and frequent security auditing. Their joint efforts are aimed at averting cyber attacks and minimising possible damage to people and businesses (Werder et al., 2022). Responsibility is also a critical aspect of the regulation of AI and data systems. Organisations should be responsible in the manner data is gathered, processed, and utilised. Legal and ethical standards are supposed to be observed by both the private and the public institutions. Organisations should also assign clear roles and responsibilities in order to determine whose roles are aimed at managing the data, making decisions, and responding to issues. The lack of accountability can result in the perpetuation of bad practices, loss of trust, and risk of rights abuse (Stahl, 2023).

By preventing future problems, risk management aids in security and accountability by identifying the possibility of potential problems. Risk assessments should be conducted on AI systems before they are put into practice and during the period of operation. Such tests analyse the probability of data intrusions, the potential consequences of algorithm errors, and potential injuries to personalities and society. A particular focus should be placed on risks that happen to marginalised or vulnerable groups in a disproportionate manner. Maximum risk management involves possession of contingency planning. Companies are to work out the emergency response strategies to respond to data breaches or failures of their systems. When such a situation occurs, the affected persons should be notified early enough and corrective measures implemented to contain the damages. Openness in events assists in upholding trust and conducive accountability (Steimers & Schneider, 2022). Security, accountability, and risk management are three elements that constitute the basis of reliable AI governance. They assist in mitigating harm, upholding individual rights, and making sure that the data practices are equitable, trustworthy, and socially useful.

8.2.4 Transparency and Ethical Data Stewardship

Transparency is a vital value embedded in the management of data and how AI systems work. By sharing data practices, organisations enable people to better comprehend the way automated decisions are being determined. Open systems assist in establishing trustworthiness and lessen the doubt of using the personal data (Walmsley, 2021). Transparent communication involves organisations communicating in a clear manner about what data is gathered, why it is gathered, and how the decisions that are made as a result may impact on people. This data must be displayed in an understandable and easy to comprehend language. The more the users are aware of the data practices, the better they can make informed decisions regarding the need to share their personal data and how to do it. Transparency also helps in accountability as it enables the data practices to be scrutinised and challenged (Kovari, 2024).

Ethical data stewardship is the role of organisations to handle data in a manner that considers human dignity and basic rights. It is a concept of fairness, non-discrimination, and respect towards cultural and social diversity. Individuals or groups should not be exploited, manipulated, and taken unfair advantage by using data. Ethical stewardship demands that data utilisation must be consistent with social principles and laws (Buijsman, 2024). People should consider data minimisation as one of the key elements of ethical data stewardship. The data must only be collected by the organisations that have a definite and legal purpose. The reduction in data collection minimises the chances of misuse, unauthorised access, breach of data, and re-identification. It also promotes the use of more responsible and careful data handling (Hosseini Tabaghdehi & Ayaz, 2025).

Long-term effects of data usage are also to be taken into consideration when it comes to ethical stewardship. The designers and developers of AI systems must keep in mind the possible unintended effects and future threats of information practices. To facilitate such a process, organisations are advised to put in place an oversight structure like ethics committees, oversight boards, or stakeholder feedback mechanisms. These systems give the possibility to conduct a constant assessment and advancement according to moral principles and social demands (Marwala, 2024). Ethical data stewardship and transparency are two very close terms. By making people think that their data is processed in a responsible and ethical way, people are more likely to accept AI systems. This trust promotes the uses of AI technologies in society that are responsible and beneficial.

8.3 AI Driven Privacy Challenges

8.3.1 Surveillance, Profiling, and Behavioural Prediction

AI has increased the power of governments and companies to monitor and scrutinise human actions. Internet gadgets, cameras, and the internet are continuously collecting information on people. This information is processed by AI systems and they determine the identity of people, their activities, and where they move. It brings about the prospect of total monitoring (Fontes et al., 2022). Facial recognition systems are able to scan the population areas and monitor individuals without their consent. The technologies behind smart cities track people movement, safety, and transportation. AI enables employers to monitor productivity of workers. Such practices can enhance efficiency or security, but they can also take away individual liberty and privacy (Elmi, 2025).

Online, profiling is the norm. Artificially intelligent algorithms read the history of purchases and browsing history and create detailed profiles of likes, preferences, and habits based on them. They might be used to affect job advertisements, insurance costs, or service eligibility. Profiling can give unfair results when information is full of stereotypes. Another issue is behaviour forecasting. AI can predict the actions of individuals in the future, including the way they will vote or pay a loan back. These forecasts can be applied to personalised persuasion or discrimination. People might feel manipulated by decisions concerning them without any consultations (Cao, 2022). Surveillance and profiling combined pose a greater threat to the manipulation, unequal treatment, and loss of personal autonomy in digital societies (Botes, 2023).

8.3.2 Data Breaches, Misuse, and Cyber Threats

The systems of AI need to be supported by extensive data sets. Cyber attackers are lured to these huge data storage facilities. One instance of data breach can reveal the personal data of millions of people. The stolen data can be financial documents, health information, family records, and accurate location information. Misuse of this information may result in serious harm like identity theft, financial fraud, and impersonation (Bécue et al., 2021). The rise in cyber threats has also been caused by the fast development of AI technologies. The AI tools allow cybercriminals to orchestrate attacks in an automated fashion, develop phishing messages that sound convincing, and detect vulnerabilities in digital systems. These hi-tech methods have increased the occurrence of cyber attacks and their ability to avoid detection. Simultaneously, a number of organisations do not have a robust security infrastructure. This issue mostly occurs in small organisations and in developing countries, where resources and technical know-how can be in short supply (Dai & Boroomand, 2022).

Extrinsic attacks do not necessarily lead to data breaches. Human mistakes may result in accidental exposure of data through poor passwords, system misconfiguration, or neglect to upgrade old software. Such errors will cause loopholes in security that can be exploited by attackers. Lack of proper data management heightens the chances of intrusion and loss of data (De Azambuja et al., 2023). There is also misuse of data in the organisations. The employees with access to sensitive information can misuse information either with intentions or unintentionally. Individual information can be discriminated upon, harassed, or other people targeted unfairly. In other instances, information gathered to serve the people can be distributed to the other companies without appropriate permission and knowledge of the user. Organisations can also store personal data without need or utilise it in other purposes that were not initially revealed (Zhang et al., 2022).

These threats demonstrate that the problem of data protection is not only technical but also a question of social trust. As long as people think that their personal information is not safe, they might not use online services and they will not easily accept AI-driven innovations. Data protection practices should therefore be strong to ensure that people have confidence and the development of AI is responsible.

8.3.3 Risks of Re-Identification and Sensitive Data Exposure

Anonymisation is a common factor that ensures privacy reinforcement, but it does not ensure safety. AIs are able to re-identify individuals through connecting anonymity data to additional datasets. Even a few location points or records of the activities can be enough to identify who a person is. This puts risk to people whose personal behaviours should be confidential due to safety or health reasons or due to the law (Gangavarapu, 2025). Medical conditions, genetic information, mental health records, political opinions, religion, and biometric identifiers are sensitive data. When such data is exposed, it may bring about discrimination, societal stigma, or personal injuries. Here are some examples illustrating how employers might discriminate against the workers in case they obtain the information about a medical condition. The insurance companies are allowed to increase the price depending on the forecasted health risks (Ford et al., 2025).

Even AI models can be sensitive information sources. Machine learning systems may at times learn information about training data. In dealing with users, they can end up disclosing personal information. This form of breach of privacy is not easily noticed. The likelihood of re-identification increases in case the organisations have access to excessive information. Integrating behavioural monitoring, use of social media, and use of a smart device provides AI with a strong capability to predict individual traits. These inferences can be very secretive although one did not present them in goodwill (Manzanares-Salor et al., 2024). In order to minimise exposure, organisations should employ very strong protection measures like differential privacy, high access control, and frequent risk evaluation. However, most institutions are not yet capable or even aware of such protection.

8.4 Regulatory and Policy Frameworks

8.4.1 GDPR and Data Protection in the European Union

The General Data Protection Regulation (GDPR) is considered to be one of the most comprehensive data protection laws across the globe. It was implemented to enhance the security of personal information and provide individuals with more control over the collection and use of their personal information. The regulation concerns all organisations that handle personal information of persons residing in the European Union, irrespective of the geographical location of the organisation. The scope here may be described as global due to the digital data flows (Labadie & Legner, 2023). GDPR creates a number of significant rights of individuals. These rights are the right to know what personal data organisations have about them, and the right to be corrected or to complete inaccurate information. An individual also has the right to demand the removal of his personal information commonly known as the right to be forgotten. Moreover, GDPR grants the liberty to disagree with some types of automatic decision-making, particularly when these decisions have serious consequences on the recipients (Vukovic et al., 2022).

There are explicit liabilities of organisations in the regulation. One should only gather personal information for specific, legitimate, and legal reasons. Organisations must not engage in the collection of unnecessary data and should also be careful to have data not used in a manner that is not within the original intent of the data collection. In instances where organisations do not enforce the provisions of GDPR, they are subject to very high financial penalties. For data protection, there are such fines that should promote seriousness (Ruohonen & Hjerppe, 2022).

GDPR further assumes that the organisation should have proper security measures to prevent the unauthorised access, loss or misuse of the personal data. Audits and risk assessment should be done regularly to facilitate continuous compliance. In other instances, companies are required to have a Data Protection Officer who will be in charge of practising data protection and complying with the legal requirements (Shukla et al., 2022). An issue of note in GDPR is its focus on data minimisation and privacy by design. This means that privacy protection must be enforced in technologies at the very beginning of their creation. GDPR has made an impact on the global data protection legislations and has been a good example of privacy regulation in the era of AI.

8.4.2 Data Governance in the United States and California CCPA

In the United States, data governance is not a unified law of data protection but instead, it is a sectoral approach which is fragmented. There are various privacy laws applied to different industries. As an example, medical, banking, and education institutions have a legal framework of their own. This system portrays a market-based approach where innovation, business fluidity is highly valued by regulation uniformity. One of the biggest data protection trends in the United

States is the California Consumer Privacy Act (CCPA). The law gives the people of California significant rights regarding their personal information. Among others, these rights are the right to information about personal data that companies are collecting and the use of the data. People can also demand that their personal data should be removed and that they should not have their personal information sold to third parties. These provisions are used to enhance transparency and consumer control (Sargiotis, 2024).

The CCPA mostly concerns the large scale corporations and technology enterprises that gather and process a lot of personal information. The law mandates organisations that it applies to have accessible privacy notices. Such notices should detail the practice of data collection and its users about their rights. These requirements enable the CCPA to enhance accountability within data-driven business models (Julakanti et al., 2025). Data governance in the wider U.S. context is much dependent on industry self-regulation and consumer protection. Although this method is flexible, it has received a lot of criticism in that it creates loopholes in privacy protection. The privacy standards in different states and sectors are varied and thus are not uniformly enforced. Consequently, this can lead to the fact that different levels of protection can be given to individuals in relation to their location or the kind of data (Kuzio et al., 2022).

The application of AI in the non-governmental sector is also of concern. Firms are able to obtain precise behavioural information which can be used in advertising, profiling, and personalisation without robust consent rights. On this note, policymakers have started debating the necessity to have a law on data protection on a federal level. Nevertheless, the regulation of data in the United States is less integrated and comprehensive than the system of the European Union (Mallet, 2025).

8.4.3 DPDP Act and Emerging AI Specific Laws

India has developed digital services and the use of AI at an alarming pace. It has one primary data protection law, the Digital Personal Data Protection (DPDP) Act, 2023. It controls the way personal information is gathered, stored, and distributed. The Act is applicable to the government and the organisations in the private sector (Khanna & Kotwal, 2025).

Key principles include:

- Lawful and transparent data processing;
- Consent-based data collection;
- Reasonable security safeguards;
- Rights to access, correct, and erase personal data.

The DPDP Act creates the Data Protection Board of India, which oversees the compliance and addresses the complaints. It also permits data transfers across borders provided that certain conditions are met. Spreading AI specific regulations is also investigated. Guidelines on responsible AI are under development by NITI Aayog and the Ministry of Electronics and Information Technology (MeitY) in terms of fairness, safety, and inclusiveness. It is focused on creating public value by means of AI in healthcare, agriculture, and education, and it also tackles the issue of surveillance, data misuse, and discrimination (Xu et al., 2024). It is an extremely diverse nation, and there are differences in digital penetration rates, thus a powerful enforcement and awareness initiative is required to secure successful privacy protection.

8.4.4 Role of Global Guidelines and Multilateral Cooperation

AI and data flows work beyond the national boundaries. That is why collaboration at the global level is a key to successful data management and moral regulation of AI. International organisations are also significant in that they formulate common principles and guidelines that states can consider, in the process of establishing their national laws and policies. These international systems are used to enhance uniformity, justice, and safeguarding of human rights in the world (Ala-Pietilä & Smuha, 2021). International guidelines are designed to assist countries in solving the most frequent issues regarding the protection of data, its accountability, and ethical utilisation of AI. In case of alignment of standards in various regions, organisations find it easy to do business in other countries without having to grapple with contradictory regulations. This consistency also aids in minimising legal uncertainty to the businesses and responsible innovation (Nuño-Santana, 2024).

Multilateral cooperation will be particularly beneficial to the emerging and developing economies. These countries can be in a position to acquire technical expertise, best practices, and capacity-building initiatives through global partnerships. The international cooperation also enhances the capacity of the states to counter cross border cyber threats, data breaches, and AI technologies abuse (Natorski, 2024). Others are influential frameworks that have been formulated by several international organisations which dictate ethical AI and data governance. These programmes focus on collective values and action. Table 8.1 outlines key contributions by key international organisations in terms of global governance of AI and data.

Table 8.1 Major international organisations influential initiatives.

Organization	*Guideline / Framework*	*Focus Area*
OECD	AI Principles	Human-centred values, fairness, accountability
UNESCO	Recommendation on the Ethics of AI	Human rights, cultural diversity, inclusive governance
G20 and G7	Digital Economy and AI Policy Statements	Innovation, interoperability, safe cross-border data flows
Global Privacy Assembly	Data protection coordination	Collaboration among national regulators

These multilateral structures are usually based on the principles of respect to human rights, openness in automated decision-making, and responsibility to the adverse consequences. They also emphasise that there is a need to safeguard the weak and oppressed against technology discrimination and abuse. International collaboration is needed as well to deal with common threats like disinformation, unethical surveillance, and discriminatory profiling. These problems cannot be handled by an individual nation. Conscientious AI and data governance then requires values and standards coordination and inter-country action (Natorski, 2024).

8.5 Strategies for Responsible Data Management

8.5.1 Consent Management and Data Minimisation

Consent management also guarantees that the individuals are in control of their personal information. In collecting data, organisations should educate the users about the intended use of data processing, people who will access the data, and duration of storage. The consent should be voluntary, transparent and withdrawable. This brings openness and gives individuals the opportunity to participate in the decision making of their data (Andreotta et al., 2022). AI systems tend to operate based on constant streams of data, and consent is more complicated. Consent dashboards, preference settings, and clear notices should therefore be used by organisations that enable users to change preferences. They should not be dark pattern designs in which the user is coerced into providing information. Unless there is some form of deceit, consent is not to be concealed in thick legal papers or solicited in ambiguous terms (Chen et al., 2023).

Data minimisation minimises the risk of privacy because of the amount of data gathered. One should only collect information that is required for a particular purpose. Gathering additional field information enhances susceptibility in case of violations or abuse. As an illustration, a fitness app will not need to have access to the contacts to offer health related advice. By reducing data collection, organisations will reduce the possible harm and enhance privacy law compliance (Goldsteen et al., 2022).

8.5.2 Anonymisation, Encryption, and Secure Infrastructures

Anonymisation is a method which eliminates pieces of identities like name, address, or phone number to maintain privacy. It gives the organisations the opportunity to conduct research and innovation with data and minimise the probability of damaging people. Nonetheless, the anonymisation should be thoroughly planned since AI may occasionally rediscover people when they relate data between datasets. Thus, anonymisation is to be used together with other measures (Koyuncu & Altaher, 2025). Encryption can secure data by transforming it to unreadable codes which can only be accessed with due authorisation. The encryption should be implemented when storing data as well as when transmitting data over networks. Having a strong encryption also ensures that even after the system is accessed by hackers and unauthorised people, they cannot see the sensitive information. This is relevant to medical records, billing, and government records.

Cyber attacks and unauthorised access can only be prevented by having secure data infrastructures. Such tools as firewalls, multi factor authentication, biometric access controls, and intrusion detection systems should be used by organisations. Periodical cyber security updates and training of employees to prevent errors. Cloud environments should also be scrutinised to arrive at the level of ensuring that they meet the laws of data protection, particularly when crossing borders of countries (Luqman et al., 2024). Secure management includes data retention regulations. Unnecessary storage of personal information should be avoided. Data that is not required should be removed through secure means of deletion. This will avoid unauthorised recovery or reusing of sensitive information. With the combination of anonymisation, encryption, and secure infrastructures, organisations would be able to reduce the threat of privacy to a large extent even though the data can be used to develop AI (Vardalachakis et al., 2024).

8.5.3 Privacy by Design, Audits, and Impact Assessments

Privacy by design is a method which considers privacy protection in technology at the initial phases of its development. Rather than treating the issue of privacy when they have already been harmed, this method attempts to avert risks by coming up with a very keen system design. Privacy by design focuses on restricting collection of data, exposure of data, and the introduction of high security levels as a standard practice. Privacy must not be a feature of technology but an option (Mooradian et al., 2025). This strategy will also promote early moral consideration in the development of systems. It is believed that privacy risks should be taken into account by designers and developers prior to the deployment of AI systems. Secure default settings prevent the need to take extra action since the users are assured of maximum privacy protection. Privacy can be incorporated in the design of a system to minimise the chances of data abuse, unauthorised access, and high scale breaches of privacy (Almeida et al., 2025).

As a factor of determining the adherence of AI systems to legal and ethical standards, audits are significant. Audits have the capacity to evaluate the methods of collecting data, consent processes, accuracy of data, and the equitability of the results. They are also able to look into the effectiveness of the existing safeguards in preserving the privacy of users. Audits can be done by third party organisations that are independent or in-house. Regular audit is used to detect flaws at an early stage and preclude serious violations prior to the emergence. Accountability and public trust are further enhanced when the result of the audit is transparent (Yadav & Ansari, 2025).

Impact assessments are formal assessments on the possible risks of AI systems. These tests are performed prior to the deployment of the systems and after they have been deployed. DPIA is a mandatory framework of data protection assessment for a variety of laws, among them the General Data Protection Regulation. Impact assessments address potential injuries to people, threats of discrimination, surveillance or profiling, as well as measures that would reduce such a threat. They also assess the proportions of possible advantages of the AI system compared to its potential damages (Kasirzadeh & Clifford, 2021). Facial recognition, predictive policing, and automated welfare decisions are a few examples of high-risk applications where impact assessments are particularly vital. They facilitate wise decision-making by organisations and regulators. Collectively, privacy by design and audits, and data impact assessment encourage ethical, transparent, and responsible data governance across the AI lifecycle (Abhivardhan, 2025).

8.6 Conclusion

The age of AI requires the regulation of data and their privacy. The increasing power and popularity of AI systems rely on massive data sets of personal data. This poses great advantages to society, but also brings serious threats in the form of surveillance, profiling, data breach, and revelation of sensitive information. They need robust governance systems that will facilitate responsible and ethical management of personal data. This is reflected in global privacy and data protection laws like the GDPR, CCPA, and DPDP Act in which express international interest in the right to privacy. Nevertheless, the issue of laws should be a continuous process with the advancement of AI skills. Practical means of harm reduction and building trust in the community are responsible data management practices, such as consent control, data minimisation, secure infrastructures, anonymisation techniques, privacy by design, and frequent audits. Data governance is primarily aimed at striking a balance between change and safeguarding of individual rights. The field of AI will keep on reshaping the life of people, industrial sectors, and government services. Good governance is what will make such developments pro-social without undermining the autonomy, dignity, and freedom. Creating a human-centred and transparent data governance ecosystem is necessary to create a future where AI will be trusted and helpful to everyone.

References

Abhivardhan. (2025). Data Governance. In: *Handbook of Human-Centered Artificial Intelligence* (pp. 1–61). Singapore: Springer Nature Singapore. https://doi.org/10.1007/978-981-97-8440-0_62-2.

Akhtar, M.A.K., Kumar, M. and Nayyar, A. (2024). Transparency and accountability in explainable AI: Best practices. In: *Towards Ethical and Socially Responsible Explainable AI: Challenges and Opportunities* (pp. 127–164). Cham: Springer Nature Switzerland. https://doi.org/10.1007/978-3-031-66489-2_5.

Ala-Pietilä, P. and Smuha, N.A. (2021). A framework for global cooperation on artificial intelligence and its governance. In: *Reflections on Artificial Intelligence for Humanity* (pp. 237–265). Cham: Springer International Publishing. https://doi.org/10.1007/978-3-030-69128-8_15.

Aldoseri, A., Al-Khalifa, K.N. and Hamouda, A.M. (2023). Re-thinking data strategy and integration for artificial intelligence: Concepts, opportunities, and challenges. *Applied Sciences*, *13*(12), 7082. https://doi.org/10.3390/app13127082.

Almeida, R., Freitas, A., Silva, T., Dias, D., Lacroix, J., De Lathauwer, I., ... & Conceição, L. (2025, June). Integrating Privacy by Design Principles into AI-Driven Systems for Human Activity and Health Monitoring. In: *International Conference on Human-Computer Interaction* (pp. 23–41). Cham: Springer Nature Switzerland. https://doi.org/10.1007/978-3-031-92840-6_2.

Andreotta, A.J., Kirkham, N. and Rizzi, M. (2022). AI, big data, and the future of consent. *AI & Society*, *37*(4), 1715–1728. https://doi.org/10.1007/s00146-021-01262-5.

Bécue, A., Praça, I. and Gama, J. (2021). Artificial intelligence, cyber-threats and Industry 4.0: Challenges and opportunities. *Artificial Intelligence Review*, *54*(5), 3849–3886. https://doi.org/10.1007/s10462-020-09942-2.

Botes, M. (2023). Autonomy and the social dilemma of online manipulative behavior. *AI and Ethics*, *3*(1), 315–323. https://doi.org/10.1007/s43681-022-00157-5.

Buijsman, S. (2024). Transparency for AI systems: A value-based approach. *Ethics and Information Technology*, *26*(2), 34. https://doi.org/10.1007/s10676-024-09770-w.

Cao, L. (2022). AI in finance: Challenges, techniques, and opportunities. *ACM Computing Surveys (CSUR)*, *55*(3), 1–38. https://doi.org/10.1145/3502289.

Chander, B., Pal, S., De, D. and Buyya, R. (2022). Artificial intelligence-based internet of things for industry 5.0. In: *Artificial Intelligence-based Internet of Things Systems* (pp. 3–45). Cham: Springer International Publishing. https://doi.org/10.1007/978-3-030-87059-1_1.

Chen, P., Wu, L. and Wang, L. (2023). AI fairness in data management and analytics: A review on challenges, methodologies, and applications. *Applied Sciences*, *13*(18), 10258. https://doi.org/10.3390/app131810258.

Dai, D. and Boroomand, S. (2022). A review of artificial intelligence to enhance the security of big data systems: State-of-art, methodologies, applications, and challenges. *Archives of Computational Methods in Engineering*, *29*(2), 1291–1309. https://doi.org/10.1007/s11831-021-09628-0.

De Azambuja, A.J.G., Plesker, C., Schützer, K., Anderl, R., Schleich, B. and Almeida, V.R. (2023). Artificial intelligence-based cyber security in the context of industry 4.0: A survey. *Electronics*, *12*(8), 1920. https://doi.org/10.3390/electronics12081920.

Elmi, M. (2025). Faces and places: Navigating the cross-border legal challenges of AI facial recognition technologies. *AI and Ethics*, *5*(5), 5453–5466. https://doi.org/10.1007/s43681-025-00787-5.

Fontes, C., Hohma, E., Corrigan, C.C. and Lütge, C. (2022). AI-powered public surveillance systems: Why we (might) need them and how we want them. *Technology in Society*, *71*, 102137. https://doi.org/10.1016/j.techsoc.2022.102137.

Ford, E., Pillinger, S., Stewart, R., Jones, K., Roberts, A., Casey, A., ... & Nenadic, G. (2025). What is the patient re-identification risk from using de-identified clinical free text data for health research?. *AI and Ethics*, 1–14. https://doi.org/10.1007/s43681-025-00681-0.

Gangavarapu, R. (2025). Invisible Exposure: The Privacy Risks of AI Models. In: *Mastering AI Governance: A Guide to Building Trustworthy and Transparent AI Systems* (pp. 47–55). Cham: Springer Nature Switzerland. https://doi.org/10.1007/978-3-031-93681-4_5.

Ghosh, A., Saini, A. and Barad, H. (2025). Artificial intelligence in governance: Recent trends, risks, challenges, innovative frameworks, and future directions. *AI & Society*, 1–23. https://doi.org/10.1007/s00146-025-02312-y.

Goldsteen, A., Ezov, G., Shmelkin, R., Moffie, M. and Farkash, A. (2022). Data minimization for GDPR compliance in machine learning models. *AI and Ethics*, *2*(3), 477–491. https://doi.org/10.1007/s43681-021-00095-8.

Gregory, S. (2023). Fortify the truth: How to defend human rights in an age of deepfakes and generative AI. *Journal of Human Rights Practice*, *15*(3), 702–714. https://doi.org/10.1093/jhuman/huad035.

Grey, M. and Segerie, C.R. (2025). The AI Risk Spectrum: From Dangerous Capabilities to Existential Threats. *arXiv preprint arXiv:2508.13700*. https://doi.org/10.48550/arXiv.2508.13700.

Hosseini Tabaghdehi, S.A. and Ayaz, Ö. (2025). AI ethics in action: A circular model for transparency, accountability, and inclusivity. *Journal of Managerial Psychology*. https://doi.org/10.1108/JMP-03-2024-0177.

Julakanti, S.R., KiranmayeeSattiraju, N.S. and Julakanti, R. (2025). Data protection through governance frameworks. *arXiv preprint arXiv:2502.10404*. https://doi.org/10.48550/arXiv.2502.10404.

Kasirzadeh, A. and Clifford, D. (2021, July). Fairness and data protection impact assessments. In: *Proceedings of the 2021 AAAI/ACM Conference on AI, Ethics, and Society* (pp. 146–153). https://doi.org/10.1145/3461702.3462528.

Khanna, V. and Kotwal, A. (2025). Examining the significance of the digital personal data protection act, 2023 in the context of the healthcare industry: A comprehensive analysis. *Discover Public Health, 22*(1), 381. https://doi.org/10.1186/s12982-025-00757-6.

Kovari, A. (2024). AI for decision support: Balancing accuracy, transparency, and trust across sectors. *Information, 15*(11), 725. https://doi.org/10.3390/info15110725.

Koyuncu, H. and Altaher, R. (2025). Classification of data anonymization techniques. In: *Artificial Intelligence for Cyber Security and Industry 4.0* (pp. 57–96). CRC Press. https://doi.org/10.48550/arXiv.2402.00896.

Kumar, S., Verma, A.K. and Mirza, A. (2024). *Digital Transformation, Artificial Intelligence and Society*. Springer. https://doi.org/10.1007/978-981-97-5656-8.

Kuzio, J., Ahmadi, M., Kim, K.C., Migaud, M.R., Wang, Y.F. and Bullock, J. (2022). Building better global data governance. *Data & Policy, 4*, e25. https://doi.org/10.1017/dap.2022.17.

Labadie, C. and Legner, C. (2023). Building data management capabilities to address data protection regulations: Learnings from EU-GDPR. *Journal of Information Technology, 38*(1), 16–44. https://doi.org/10.1177/02683962221141456.

Leiser, M.R. (2022). Bias, journalistic endeavours, and the risks of artificial intelligence. In: *Artificial Intelligence and the Media* (pp. 8-32). Edward Elgar Publishing. https://doi.org/10.4337/9781839109973.00007.

Lund, B., Orhan, Z., Mannuru, N.R., Bevara, R.V.K., Porter, B., Vinaih, M.K. and Bhaskara, P. (2025). Standards, frameworks, and legislation for artificial intelligence (AI) transparency. *AI and Ethics*, 1–17. https://doi.org/10.1007/s43681-025-00661-4.

Luqman, A., Mahesh, R. and Chattopadhyay, A. (2024). Privacy and security implications of cloud-based AI services: A survey. *arXiv preprint arXiv:2402.00896*. https://doi.org/10.48550/arXiv.2402.00896.

Mallet, P. (2025). Comparative Analysis of Data Privacy Legislation: Convergence and Divergence between the GDPR and CCPA. In: *Tech Fusion in Business and Society* (pp. 465–475). Springer, Cham. https://doi.org/10.1007/978-3-031-84636-6_40.

Manzanares-Salor, B., Sanchez, D. and Lison, P. (2024). Evaluating the disclosure risk of anonymized documents via a machine learning-based re-identification attack. *Data Mining and Knowledge Discovery, 38*(6), 4040–4075. https://doi.org/10.1007/s10618-024-01066-3.

Martin, K.D. and Zimmermann, J. (2024). Artificial intelligence and its implications for data privacy. *Current Opinion in Psychology, 58*, 101829. https://doi.org/10.1016/j.copsyc.2024.101829.

Marwala, T. (2024). Transparency Versus Truth. In: *The Balancing Problem in the Governance of Artificial Intelligence* (pp. 69–85). Singapore: Springer Nature Singapore. https://doi.org/10.1007/978-981-97-9251-1_5.

Menard, P. and Bott, G.J. (2025). Artificial intelligence misuse and concern for information privacy: New construct validation and future directions. *Information Systems Journal, 35*(1), 322–367. https://doi.org/10.1111/isj.12544.

Mooradian, N., Franks, P.C. and Srivastav, A. (2025). The impact of artificial intelligence on data privacy: A risk management perspective. *Records Management Journal, 35*(2), 147–159. https://doi.org/10.1108/RMJ-06-2024-0013.

Mühlhoff, R. (2023). Predictive privacy: Collective data protection in the context of artificial intelligence and big data. *Big Data & Society, 10*(1), 20539517231166886. https://doi.org/10.1177/20539517231166886.

Natorski, M. (2024). Compromise in multilateral negotiations and the global regulation of artificial intelligence. *Democratization, 31*(5), 1091–1116. https://doi.org/10.1080/13510347.2024.2351583.

Nguyen, T.H., Saghir, A., Tran, K.D., Nguyen, D.H., Luong, N.A. and Tran, K.P. (2024). Safety and Reliability of Artificial Intelligence Systems. In: *Artificial Intelligence for Safety and Reliability Engineering: Methods, Applications, and Challenges* (pp. 185–199). Cham: Springer Nature Switzerland. https://doi.org/10.1007/978-3-031-71495-5_9.

Nuño-Santana, F.E. (2024). International Cooperation, Multilateralism, and Civil Society in the Face of the Technological Revolution 4.0. In: *International Relations and Technological Revolution 4.0: World Order, Power, and New International Society* (pp. 173–187). Cham: Springer Nature Switzerland. https://doi.org/10.1007/978-3-031-66750-3_11.

Panarese, P., Grasso, M.M. and Solinas, C. (2025). Algorithmic bias, fairness, and inclusivity: A multilevel framework for justice-oriented AI. *AI & Society*, 1–23. https://doi.org/10.1007/s00146-025-02451-2.

Park, K. and Young Yoon, H. (2025). AI algorithm transparency, pipelines for trust not prisms: Mitigating general negative attitudes and enhancing trust toward AI. *Humanities and Social Sciences Communications, 12*(1), 1–13. https://doi.org/10.1057/s41599-025-05116-z.

Ruohonen, J. and Hjerppe, K. (2022). The GDPR enforcement fines at glance. *Information Systems, 106*, 101876. https://doi.org/10.1016/j.is.2021.101876.

Sargiotis, D. (2024). Legal and regulatory considerations in data governance. In: *Data Governance: A Guide* (pp. 445–466). Cham: Springer Nature Switzerland. https://doi.org/10.1007/978-3-031-67268-2_15.

Sarker, I.H. (2022). AI-based modeling: Techniques, applications, and research issues towards automation, intelligent, and smart systems. *SN Computer Science*, 3(2), 158. https://doi.org/10.1007/s42979-022-01043-x.

Shaban, A. (2025). Digital Rights, Digital Representation, and Digital Justice: Towards Digital Democracy and Freedom of Expression. In: *Digital Geographies: Theory, Space, and Communities: A Machine-Generated Literature Review* (pp. 765–899). Singapore: Springer Nature Singapore. https://doi.org/10.1007/978-981-97-4734-4_7.

Shukla, S., George, J.P., Tiwari, K. and Kureethara, J.V. (2022). Data security. In: *Data Ethics and Challenges* (pp. 41–59). Singapore: Springer Singapore. https://doi.org/10.1007/978-981-19-0752-4_3.

Stahl, B.C. (2023). Embedding responsibility in intelligent systems: From AI ethics to responsible AI ecosystems. *Scientific Reports, 13*(1), 7586. https://doi.org/10.1038/s41598-023-34622-w.

Steimers, A. and Schneider, M. (2022). Sources of risk of AI systems. *International Journal of Environmental Research and Public Health, 19*(6), 3641. https://doi.org/10.3390/ijerph19063641.

Vardalachakis, M., Tampouratzis, M., Papadakis, N. and Vasilakis, M. (2024, May). The Future of Privacy: A Review on AI's Role in Shaping Data Security. In: *2024 5th International Conference in Electronic Engineering, Information Technology and Education (EEITE)* (pp. 1–8). IEEE. https://doi.org/10.1109/EEITE61750.2024.10654397.

Verma, A. and Singhal, N. (2023, September). Integrating Artificial Intelligence for Adaptive Decision-Making in Complex System. In: *International Conference on Advances in Data-*

driven Computing and Intelligent Systems (pp. 95–105). Singapore: Springer Nature Singapore. https://doi.org/10.1007/978-981-99-9521-9_8.

Vukovic, J., Ivankovic, D., Habl, C. and Dimnjakovic, J. (2022). Enablers and barriers to the secondary use of health data in Europe: General data protection regulation perspective. *Archives of Public Health, 80*(1), 115. https://doi.org/10.1186/s13690-022-00866-7.

Walmsley, J. (2021). Artificial intelligence and the value of transparency. *AI & Society, 36*(2), 585–595. https://doi.org/10.1007/s00146-020-01066-z.

Werder, K., Ramesh, B. and Zhang, R. (2022). Establishing data provenance for responsible artificial intelligence systems. *ACM Transactions on Management Information Systems (TMIS), 13*(2), 1–23. https://doi.org/10.1145/3503488.

Xu, J., Lee, T. and Goggin, G. (2024). AI governance in Asia: Policies, praxis, and approaches. *Communication Research and Practice, 10*(3), 275–287. https://doi.org/10.1080/22041451.2024.2391204.

Yadav, A. and Ansari, M.T.J. (2025). Managing privacy and innovation in AI-enhanced legal services: Addressing data protection challenges and ethical considerations. *AI and Ethics*, 1–14. https://doi.org/10.1007/s43681-025-00745-1.

Zhang, Z., Ning, H., Shi, F., Farha, F., Xu, Y., Xu, J., ... & Choo, K.K.R. (2022). Artificial intelligence in cyber security: Research advances, challenges, and opportunities. *Artificial Intelligence Review, 55*(2), 1029–1053. https://doi.org/10.1007/s10462-021-09976-0.

9 AI and Human Rights
Safeguarding Civil Liberties in Automated Systems

Artificial intelligence (AI) is a growing influence on the decisions that influence civil liberties, social rights, and democracies. It is true that AI systems potentially bring tremendous advantages to governance, security, and provision of services to the population; however, they also threaten basic human rights. The automated decision-making may result in discrimination, exclusion, surveillance, and intrusion of privacy where the systems are not designed well or are not well controlled. The chapter explores the association of AI and human rights, and it faces prominent aspects like fairness, equality, freedom of speech, due process, and right to privacy. It also examines international human rights norms, regulation, and accountability systems that can assist in protecting people in AI-driven worlds. The chapter focuses on the significance of human-centric AI and high supervision to safeguard civil liberties.

9.1 Introduction

Artificial Intelligence (AI) is becoming popular to facilitate and mechanise decision-making in most sectors of society. AI systems help governments, corporate entities, and government agencies to make predictions, categorise information, and make critical decisions. Such choices affect the access of people to jobs, education, medical services, financial services, and welfare. Police, surveillance, border control, and court systems are also done by AI. Consequently, the problem of AI has a direct and substantial effect on human rights' protection. The design and governance of automated systems that define the opportunities and freedoms in life have to be highly safeguarded in rights-based approaches (Alshahrani et al., 2024). The emergence of AI in decision-making has both opportunities and threats. On the one hand, AI has the potential to enhance efficiency, pattern recognition, human error minimisation, and help ensure more impartial decisions are made in case of responsible usage. As an illustration, AI can assist in bias discovery during the recruitment process or enhance the distribution of social services (Kahraman, 2025). Alternatively, AI systems may also result in discrimination and unfair treatment and exclusion when they are based on biased information or are poorly designed. Social inequality can be reproduced, stereotypes can be reinforced, and it may discriminate against vulnerable groups through automated decision-making. These consequences raise questions about such basic values as equality, dignity, and justice (Varona & Suárez, 2022).

DOI: 10.1201/9781003776659-9

The issue of civil liberties has also been on the rise because AI is increasingly integrated in online spaces. Most AI systems are running in modes that cannot be understood by the people. People are not always aware of how their data is processed, what an automated decision entails, and how to dispute an automated decision. This is an accountability weakness due to lack of transparency. It is more difficult to recognise errors, pernicious consequences or infringing rights when decisions are opaque. In other situations, AI can control the behaviour of individuals without their awareness by serving personalised content, targeted advertisements, or even doing predictive profiling (Duberry, 2022). One of the biggest concerns in AI societies is surveillance. Advanced sensors, facial recognition systems, and predictive analytics enable one to monitor the movements and activity of people continuously. Although these tools can be used to enhance security, it can also restrict privacy, freedom of expression, and right to protest (Saheb, 2023). Too much surveillance may develop an atmosphere of fear and intimidate individuals against exercising their rights. Computerised surveillance systems can also create false identifications of people, and individuals wrongly suspected or punished. These dangers demonstrate that the efficacy of technologies is unable to substitute basic safeguards of civil freedoms (Singh, 2023).

The other problem is the increased use of AI in government and policing. It can be through automated decision systems that can impact sentencing recommendations, bail determinations, fraud detection, or welfare eligibility. Unless such systems are transparent and also can be reviewed by humans, then there might not be any possible way of appealing to decisions made. This compromises the due process and the right to a fair and responsible procedure. AI should not thus substitute but assist human judgement on issues that concern rights and freedoms (Kumar & Choudhury, 2023). On the whole, the growing adoption of AI in decision-making requires a high priority on human rights. Protecting civil liberties through regulations, ethical construction, and proper regulation is essential. AI systems should be constructed and implemented in a manner that considers equality, privacy, autonomy as well as justice. With the development of more automated systems in societies, provision of protection to human rights should be one of the primary concerns (Amariles & Baquero, 2023).

9.2 Human Rights at Stake in AI Systems

9.2.1 Equality and Non-Discrimination

One of the human rights principles is equality. It should treat all people equally, and give them the same opportunities irrespective of gender, race, ethnicity, disability, religion among other personal traits. In reality, though, AI technologies may threaten this ideology when they replicate or exacerbate social inequalities that are already there. The AI systems are trained on previous data. When such data is an indication of discrimination or social prejudice in the past, there is a chance that the social level AI models will also be discriminatory. Indicatively, AI-based recruitment systems can be biased towards men in cases where previous decisions in hiring were discriminatory against women. On the same note, facial recognition technologies tend to be inaccurate when it comes to people of dark colour due to the lack of diversity in the training sets. Predictive policing systems can also work against the minority community in that crime data is biased by previous discriminatory policing modes (Akhtar et al., 2024).

These consequences are not necessarily premeditated yet they can be very damaging. With automated decision-making systems, they can be used on a large scale usually impacting many people simultaneously, and this implies that the bias may be passed on. Also, AI systems can result in discrimination that is hard to detect. Most AI models have their decision-making processes that are complex and opaque. The non-transparency of this fact makes it difficult to comprehend how certain decisions were made or even to demonstrate the fact of discrimination (Çetin Kumkumoğlu & Kemal Kumkumoğlu, 2023). The non-discriminatory and popular character of algorithmic discrimination poses great concerns on equality and non-discriminatory issues. In response to these risks, the active protection of equality should be observed during the design, development, and deployment of AI systems. Such measures as fairness testing, representative and diverse dataset, frequent audits, and explicit accountability mechanisms are crucial. Moreover, robust legal and regulatory frameworks are required so that citizens could also have a viable recourse in case the AI systems infringe their right to equal treatment (Giovanola & Tiribelli, 2023).

9.2.2 Privacy and Personal Autonomy

One of the fundamental human rights is privacy which is associated with dignity and freedom. It helps people to be safeguarded against unwanted encroachment into their personal lives. To make predictions or provide services, AI systems can regularly gather and process great amounts of personal information. Such information can contain sensitive information like their location, health records, their finances, and their personal relations (Vaassen, 2022). In cases where organisations gather information without being well informed or keeping it in unsecured locations, privacy abuse may take place. AI technologies applied to track or monitor behaviour may restrict individual agency by shaping the behaviour of people and their self-expression. People can experience being followed all the time and can evade behaviours that they think will be negatively evaluated by the functioning of automated systems (Elliott & Soifer, 2022).

The use of AI in profiling can also influence individual autonomy in that what individuals are allowed to have is determined in advance by it. As an example, the algorithms can conceal job opportunities or loans of some people on the basis of predictions, which are made out of their data. These manipulative forces undermine individualism and critical choices (del Valle & Lara, 2024). Thus, the necessity to protect privacy aspects (i.e., control of consent, encrypted information storage, surveillance restriction, etc.) ensures that personal autonomy can be maintained in AI settings.

9.2.3 Freedom of Expression and Access to Information

Freedom of expression is a human right, which facilitates the freedom of communication, democratic action, and cultural and creative growth. It enables people to exchange ideas, get information, and engage in the discussion. The digital era has been characterised by the significant role of AI when it comes to the creation of online information environments. The content moderation, recommendation algorithms, as well as automated filtering are widespread AI systems that have a significant impact on the content users view, share, and discuss online (Jougleux, 2022). The AI-driven content moderation systems are created to identify and eliminate objectionable or unlawful material. Nevertheless, such systems tend to fail to differentiate between illegal content and free speech. Since AI does not have complete awareness of social, cultural, and context, it can end up censoring authentic speech. These mistakes may curtail freedom of expression and restrain some voices particularly those of minority or marginalized groups (De Vries, 2022).

Recommendation systems have an influence on the freedom of speech and access to information as well. Most of these systems tend to promote content that is captivating and makes the user engage. This leads to the possibility that content with sensational, emotionally evocative, or biased content will be encouraged more often than balanced and reliable information. The practice may undermine the discourse of the people and result in the proliferation of misinformation and disinformation (Mueller, 2025). Access to information is also formed by personalisation. The AI systems can usually match the content according to the likes and internet activity of a user. Although this may enhance the user experience, it may also form filter bubbles. In these settings, the users are generally exposed to the opinions that support their pre-existing beliefs. This eliminates access to a variety of views and diminishes the capacity to make informed opinions (Ozmen Garibay et al., 2023).

In other countries, the AI technologies allow the governments to spy on the online space and ban speech that criticises the authorities. These practices are a big menace to democratic principles and an endangering factor to safety of human rights (Peron et al., 2025). In a bid to protect freedom of speech, AI systems should be open, responsible, and have regulations. These frameworks must honour cultural diversity, allow a healthy debate, and guard access to a variety of information and reliable facts (Cheong et al., 2025).

9.2.4 Due Process and Justice in Automated Decisions

Due process is a means of ensuring fairness in decisions which affect legal rights. People are supposed to be able to learn what decisions to make, dispute them, and human review in case required. The field of application of AI is growing in law enforcement, sentencing suggestions, credit ratings, and welfare provision. These are life and death choices and they need to be considered (Suksi, 2021). The automated systems can refuse service, label people as suspicious, or decide on their eligibility of benefits without any significant clarification. The fact that the people are being negatively influenced means that they will not know how to challenge the result. The absence of transparency reduces accountability and justice. Errors in criminal justice use, e.g., predictive policing or risk assessment systems, can be deadly. In case the AI systems err and discriminate against people based on biased data, they will not be able to escape more surveillance or even more severe legal cases. These dangers put the notions of fairness and equality before the law into the test (Blount, 2024).

Effective due process requires:

- Human oversight of automated systems;
- Right to explanation for automated decisions;
- Appeal mechanisms that allow individuals to contest errors;
- Clear accountability, specifying who is responsible for the outcomes.

When due process is protected, AI can support more accurate and timely decision-making without compromising justice (Barysė & Sarel, 2024).

9.3 Sources of Rights Violations in AI

9.3.1 Biased Data and Discriminatory Algorithms

The AI systems attend to the trends in the data. In case the information is biased towards historical disparities or social stereotypes, the system can reproduce and enhance the discrimination. Most data sets have gender, racial, socioeconomic, and geographic imbalances. As a result of such data being used to make automated decisions, certain groups can be unfairly treated (Varona & Suárez, 2022).

For example:

- Hiring algorithms may prefer male candidates if trained on past hiring records that favoured men.
- Medical AI tools may misdiagnose women or minority groups if trained mainly on data from other populations.
- Credit scoring models may deny loans to people living in low-income neighbourhoods due to biased financial data.

Prejudice is also caused by the model choice. The features that developers choose may be used to indirectly indicate features like race or religion that had been protected. Moreover, the optimisation to efficiency, as opposed to equity, can be made by algorithms, resulting in detrimental trade offs that favour discriminatory choices against specific groups. Vulnerable communities are the ones that are most susceptible to biased systems and the victims do not have the capability to detect it or challenge it. It then leads to fairness testing, a variety of data sources, and robust regulation as a means of safeguarding equality (Borgesius, 2025).

9.3.2 *Lack of Transparency and Explainability*

A large number of AI systems are black boxes. They also arrive at predictions and decision making processes which are complex in nature and may be hard to be understood by even the developers. Whenever automated decisions affect the people, they tend not to know how the system arrived at its conclusion. Such transparency is undermining trust and minimal accountability (Balasubramaniam et al., 2023).

Opacity becomes especially dangerous in high stakes areas such as:

- Judicial decision support;
- Credit and insurance evaluation;
- Child protection and welfare allocation;
- University admissions and job selection.

Unless explainable, people will not be able to appeal against unjust decisions or seek redress. Absence of rationality also makes it impossible to determine whether a system is discriminative or inaccurate to regulators. Others conceal details of the systems deliberately to safeguard business. As much as intellectual property rights are essential, secrecy may hinder accountability of sensitive applications to the public. AI systems should offer meaningful explanations to the affected people in order to safeguard human rights. The independent evaluators, human supervisors, and the public who are necessary should be able to see the decision-making rules and risk factors where necessary (Hussain & Hussain, 2025).

9.3.3 *Excessive Surveillance and Profiling*

AI allows strong surveillance systems that may pose a threat to privacy and freedom. The cameras, online behaviour, biometrics, and wearable technologies form sources of gathered information by surveillance systems. This data is analysed using profiling tools in order to make future behaviour predictions and influence (Fontes et al., 2022).

Examples include:

- Facial recognition systems tracking people in public spaces;
- Social media monitoring to identify political beliefs;
- Predictive policing tools focusing on specific neighbourhoods;
- Behavioural analytics predicting employee productivity.

These technologies can enhance security or convenience and at the same time limit civil liberties. Citizens are unlikely to voice their opinions or get involved in protests in the case they believe that their activities are under surveillance. The AI system may cause wrongful suspicion and discrimination due to poor judgements. Profiling can also restrict the provision of important services since people are grouped according to stereotypes. As an illustration, they might lock out certain users who do not get housing opportunities or job offers due to system forecasting an adverse result that is not factual. Excessive surveillance will transform a democratic society into a managed one, where individuals become deprived of autonomy and dignity. There is a need to have strong legal checks and balances that would not allow surveillance technologies to undermine basic freedoms (Singh, 2023).

9.3.4 Weak Accountability Mechanisms

The responsible use of AI systems requires accountability. Nevertheless, there are numerous AI systems that are implemented without defined accountability frameworks. In the case of harm, it is usually hard to determine the person responsible. The developers can argue that the system was used improperly by users and the organisations can use the fact that the technology is complex. This ambiguity permits the abuse of human rights to take place, without any meaningful penalty (Novelli et al., 2024). Poor accountability systems can be particularly visible in the automated decision-making systems. In most situations, those who are subjected to these systems have no chance to oppose or make questions concerning the decisions made regarding them. There are usually no clear procedures of complaints or appeals. The government can also use AI technologies without proper legal protection or control. Simultaneously, the considerations of efficiency, minimising costs, and speed may be prioritised by the private companies instead of morality and the protection of human rights (Lechterman, 2022).

There are AI systems that provide no meaningful human review of the judgement provided by the system. This especially is a problem in the high risk areas of welfare distribution, immigration control, law enforcement, and national security. When people are unjustly deprived of social benefits or unjustly declared as a threat to security, they do not know who has made this decision and how to address the issue. This scenario compromises due process and fairness, and access to justice (Cheong, 2024). In order to deliver on these difficulties, effective accountability systems are needed in the whole AI lifecycle. Developers, deployers, and users of AI systems should be assigned clear roles and responsibilities. High-risk applications should have human supervision to enable the automated decisions to be reviewed and re-done. There should also be good redress mechanisms that can enable individuals to oppose harmful decisions and avail redress (Slota et al., 2023). Secondly, self-auditing and regulation implementation is required to control AI systems and make them compliant with law and ethical requirements. These technologies become more likely to work safely, transparently, and respecting rights in case the institutions take over the responsibility for the results of AI systems (Mikalef et al., 2022).

9.4 International Human Rights Standards and Legal Frameworks

9.4.1 UN Guiding Principles and Digital Rights Charters

The United Nations (UN) is in the forefront in advancing the idea of rights-based approach to digital technologies. The UN framework of human rights focuses on equality, dignity, privacy, expression of freedom, and due process. These are relevant to the implementation of AI. According to the UN Guiding Principles on Business and Human Rights, companies must observe human rights, prevent discrimination, and carry out due diligence. These guidelines urge companies to assess risks prior to applying AI systems and to offer redress in case of damage (Shaelou & Razmetaeva, 2023). Reports on AI and human rights have also been issued by the UN High Commissioner on Human Rights (UNHCR). Discriminatory profiling, mass surveillance, and no disclosed automated decisions are among the threats pointed out by these reports. According to them, restrictions to high-risk AI applications, including real-time biometric policing in the streets, are recommended. It is a requirement of digital rights charters, such as the principles of the UN Internet Governance Forum or the Global Digital Compact, to be fair, transparent, and empowering users. These charters advocate unrestricted availability, privacy, and ethical application of technology. Together, UN systems stress that AI should be in line with the predetermined human rights at all times (Wörsdörfer, 2025).

9.4.2 OECD, UNESCO, and EU Approaches to Rights-Based AI

A number of organisations in the world and within the region give advice on ethical and rights-based governance of AI. In 2019, the Organisation for Economic Co-operation and Development (OECD) presented the OECD AI Principles. These values emphasise inclusive growth, people focused values, transparency, strength, and responsibility. They call on governments to evaluate the social cost of AI and to avoid the situation when systems infringe on civil liberties (Nguyen et al., 2023). In 2021, UNESCO accepted the Recommendation on the Ethics of AI. It emphasises on human rights, diversity, sustainability, and cultural respect. Another aspect that UNESCO focuses on is the necessity to safeguard vulnerable populations and provide equality in automatic judgements. Member states undertake to establish ethical supervision institutions, transparency devices, and robust regulation mechanisms (Nguyen et al., 2023).

One of the most powerful models of AI governance is the European Union (EU) model. The EU Charter of Fundamental Rights defends the rights of privacy, non-discrimination, and expression. The rights promoted by the General Data Protection Regulation (GDPR) are access to data, correction, and opposition to automated decisions (Shaelou & Razmetaeva, 2023). The new EU AI Act categorises AI systems based on their risk and provides strict conditions to the high risk systems that are employed in the fields of policing, employment, education, and public services. It bans AI systems that are deemed to be a threat to human rights like social scoring and some biometric surveillance. The EU model is broadly considered as an international standard of the protection of rights (Szostek & Prabucki, 2025).

9.4.3 National Laws Protecting Civil Liberties in AI Deployments

The laws have been implemented in many countries to guarantee that civil liberties are not violated by AI systems. The methods differ, but some of the most popular ones are to preserve privacy, avoid discrimination, and be accountable.

- The United States has no federal law on AI, however, there exist sector specific laws that safeguard some rights. The Civil Rights Act and Fair Credit Reporting Act restrict automated decision discrimination. Another initiative that has arisen at the White House is the Blueprint to an AI Bill of Rights which proposes concepts of safe systems, protection against algorithmic discrimination, and human alternatives to automated decisions (Cheong et al., 2025).
- The GDPR along with the Federal Data Protection Act (BDSG) of Germany protect the privacy and provide the rights to access, correct, and delete personal data, unlawful processing protection as well. Moreover, the national AI strategy in Germany suggests credible and user-friendly AI, focusing on the protection of fundamental rights, technological advancement, and responsible use in the whole range of the economic realm (Hornuf et al., 2023).
- The Brazilian General Data Protection Law contains robust rights oriented points, like the right to an explanation of automated decision (Domínguez Hernández et al., 2026).
- The proposed Artificial Intelligence and Data Act (AIDA) in Canada is expected to oversee high impact AI systems, and mitigate the potential risks associated with discrimination, surveillance and harmful automated decision-making (Brandusescu & Sieber, 2025).

These national laws are varied, but all of them have the same commitment of safeguarding individuals against unfair or intrusion AI practices. Table 9.1 provides the summary of the major international and national frameworks that are aimed at safeguarding human rights and civil liberties in the context of AI governance.

Table 9.1 Key International and National Frameworks for Rights-Based AI.

Body/Region	*Framework/Law*	*Primary Rights Protected*
United Nations	UN Guiding Principles, Digital Rights Charters	Equality, privacy, due process
OECD	OECD AI Principles	Transparency, accountability
UNESCO	Ethical AI Recommendation	Human dignity, cultural rights
European Union	GDPR, EU AI Act	Privacy, fairness, expression
United States	AI Bill of Rights (Blueprint)	Autonomy, anti-discrimination
Germany	Federal Data Protection Act (BDSG); GDPR implementation; EU AI Act enforcement	Privacy, data protection, human dignity

9.5 Governance Strategies and Safeguards

9.5.1 Human Oversight and Accountability Frameworks

AI systems cannot be deemed completely trustworthy and objective and, thus, require human supervision. Machine learning tools have the potential to err, incorrectly interpret information, or cause prejudice to society. Human decision-makers should not be left behind particularly in high-risk scenarios that impact rights and freedoms (Holzinger et al., 2025).

Oversight ensures that:

- People can review automated decisions;
- Harmful outcomes can be corrected quickly;
- Responsibility remains clearly assigned;
- Fundamental rights are protected above technical efficiency.

Some of the examples of such areas in need of vigorous supervision are law enforcement, immigration control, healthcare related decisions, and public service availability. With this in consideration, humans should sanction significant decisions as opposed to letting AI systems run on their own. Accountability structures assist in supervision, by identifying those in charge in the occurrence of harm. Such frameworks give responsibilities to policy authorities, operators, and developers. They need to be documented on the design, training, and utilisation of AI systems as well. With the accountability records, organisations will be able to provide answers to the questions concerning why the decisions are made and the rights violations will not go without the answers. Accountability should be clear so as to enhance trust in automated systems by the population. It guarantees people that their rights are important and that the concerned parties will respond to harm by systems (Sayles, 2024).

9.5.2 Impact Assessments, Audits, and Redress Mechanisms

Impact assessment is used by organisations to determine risks prior to the implementation of AI systems. They consider the possibility of a system to benefit some groups of people or infringe essential rights. In case of the detection of risks, the system needs to be altered or observed more attentively. The most common tools are the human rights impact assessment and the algorithmic impact assessment (AIA) (Stahl et al., 2023).

Impact assessments encourage organisations to:

- Consider the social context of AI deployment;
- Identify discrimination risks in advance;
- Apply safety measures before harm occurs;
- Make decisions that balance benefits and rights.

The other significant protection is audits. They include testing and checking of AI systems on a continuous basis to identify errors or bias. Audits can be conducted within or by third parties. Periodic audits are used to make sure that systems are not biased or inaccurate during the period of use. They also give evidence of the adherence to legal and ethical standards (Kazim et al., 2021). Redress schemes allow an individual to appeal automated decisions. Individuals should be aware of how to demand clarifications and how to rectify errors which influence their opportunities of securing employment, credit, health, or justice (Pi & Proctor, 2025). Redress mechanisms may include:

- Complaint procedures;
- Human review panels;
- Appeals systems for automated decisions;
- Compensation for damage caused by AI errors.

People might get hurt without seeking any redress. Protections should therefore make systems not only monitored, but also to be sensitive to the concerns of the people.

9.5.3 Ethical Design and Rights-Based Development Approaches

Ethical design integrates human values into all stages of AI development. Developers must consider fairness, privacy, inclusiveness, and transparency from the initial planning process. Human rights must not be considered only after deployment; they must guide the technology lifecycle (Smuha, 2021).

Rights-based development approaches encourage:

- Using diverse and representative datasets;
- Testing for harmful outcomes before deployment;
- Avoiding excessive surveillance and manipulation;
- Ensuring accessible information about system functions.

The principle of inclusive design is significant. The teams are to be multidisciplinary, i.e., comprising social scientists, lawyers, and representatives of communities. Engagement of communities involved in consultation assists in the identification of issues that might have been neglected by technical developers. The involvement also provides the citizens with a voice in making decisions concerning their day to day lives (Hogan & Lasek-Markey, 2024). User empowerment is also a part of ethical design. By clarifying, offering permission choices, and privacy settings, one will be able to make decisions concerning their data. Automated systems must enable users to rectify mistakes and protest against automatic decisions in case they are hurt. The transparency tools help in developing rights-based development as the internal processes are revealed. This enables the organisations to identify problems at an early stage and modify their design as well. It also enables regulators and the general population to assess systems in regard to being ethical (Prabhakaran et al., 2022).

9.6 Collaborative Responsibility and Societal Awareness

9.6.1 Role of Governments, Industry, Civil Society, and Communities

Governments lead in legislation and policies through which the civil liberties are safeguarded in automated systems. They need to be in control of risky AI applications, hold them accountable, and establish mechanisms to control the same. The state also has the role of offering control in sensitive subjects like policing, administration of welfare, and border control. When the governments embrace AI judiciously, they provide good examples to other sectors (Moon, 2023). Most AI systems are developed by industry organisations, and thus they are very influential in the rights protection. The firms should adhere to morality and carry out risk analysis before introducing AI products. They ought to have internal review boards, which would examine the issue of fairness, protection of privacy, and harm. Innovation should not undermine dignity and equality, so that the developers of technologies should take care of it (Dunleavy & Margetts, 2025).

The civil society organisations back the interests of the people by keeping track of AI use in the society. They create awareness of the bad ways, defend vulnerable populations, and seek increased protection. They are involved to make sure that social issues are incorporated in the policymaking. The human rights associations, digital rights activists, and journalists are significant contributors to exposing the abuses and holding the institutions to account (LePere-Schloop & Zook, 2023). Stakeholders are also communities and individuals. Automated decisions directly affect them. They should be involved to learn about the challenges in the actual world and make sure AI systems satisfy the needs of the society. The voices of communities are used to formulate solutions of cultural, social, and economic diversity (Bélisle-Pipon et al., 2023). The cooperation between all these actors creates a more involved and accountable AI governance model.

9.6.2 Human Rights Education and Public Participation

The age of automation requires the protection of rights through the use of public awareness. Citizens should be aware of the functioning of AI systems, the data they analyse, and the impact of rights and opportunities they have. In the absence of this information, citizens will not be aware when harm is being conducted or the way to behave (Gentelet & Mizrahi, 2024). In digital literacy, human rights education should be incorporated. The schools, universities, government departments, and companies should educate people to recognise threats to privacy, discrimination, and unethical surveillance. Transparency can be ensured because citizens are empowered to demand it and challenge unjustified automated decisions (Schiff, 2022).

The citizen involvement enhances democratic accountability. When individuals are given chances to express their concerns, institutions are able to develop systems that would depict values of the society. There are mechanisms like community forums, public consultations, and feedback platforms which aid in the identification of risks at an early stage. Other groups that face a higher risk of being impacted by biased algorithms or intrusive surveillance, especially the marginalised groups, are particularly valuable participants in the process (Zidouemba, 2025). Learning and involvement mean that AI is not created in a vacuum of society. Rather, the technology is changing based on the contribution of the masses and control, and the governance is more acceptable and responsible.

9.6.3 Transparency, Activism, and Advocacy for Digital Rights

The most important aspect of gaining trust in AI systems is transparency. Companies that create and implement AI have a role to play in clarifying the role of such systems. They are also supposed to give information on how decisions are made, the source of the data, and the risks that can occur as a result of automated decisions being made. Transparency enables people to know when AI systems are being accessed and also determine whether the decision generated is just, legal and warranted (Cheong, 2024). Accountability is also supported by straightforward and available information. People can monitor the performance of an AI system better when they have knowledge on how it works, as they can ask questions, appeal unfair decisions, and seek redress. The lack of transparency means that the automated systems can be used without being subject to scrutiny by the population, which is more likely to result in discrimination, abuse, and violation of rights (Olsen et al., 2024).

The advocacy and activism are significant in safeguarding digital rights in the era of AI. Human rights and digital rights activists as well as civil society organisations observe the application of AI technologies and attract attention to malicious actions. They report on and investigate instances of algorithmic discrimination, mass surveillance, and infringement of privacy. These organisations also advocate those people and groups that have suffered negatively due to automated systems (Gregory, 2023). There are various developments that have been brought about through advocacy. They are like publicly revealing surveillance technologies, limits, or prohibitions on facial recognition technologies in a number of cities, and expanded application of fairness testing and transparency reports in organisations Advocacy has also impacted in intensifying the rights to privacy and data protection by enacting new laws and regulations (Bakiner, 2023).

The media is also quite important in creating awareness. Investigative journalism will be able to expose unseen dangers and discriminatory effects of AI systems within the institutions of the general population and the state. Journalists play a role in informing society and bringing about a healthy debate through public reporting (Stray, 2021). Collectively, activism, transparency, and advocacy puts pressure on governments and companies to be responsible. They confirm the idea that technological innovation should not violate human dignity, civil liberties, and basic rights.

9.7 Conclusion

The role of AI is transforming the way decision-making takes place in contemporary societies. This gives numerous chances to service improvement, reinforced governance, and growth. Nevertheless, AI technologies may lead to severe damages as well when they subvert equality, privacy, freedom of speech, and due process. These are the inherent rights of humanity and democracy. Thus, the protection of civil liberties should be among the main priorities in AI development and implementation. Biased information, transparency, over-surveillance, and poor accountability are primary causes of human rights infringements in automated systems. The international frameworks, regional and national laws are very guiding, though they need to be well-enforced and constantly adapted. The harm is averted with the help of the governance strategies of human oversight, independent audits, impact assessments, and redress mechanisms. Protection is enhanced by ethical design, community awareness, and participation of the people. The responsible AI involves the cooperation between governments, industry, civil society, and individuals. Societies should be able to benefit from automation of the computing world without having to give up any of the values of the civil liberties by ensuring that all aspects of the AI lifecycle are respected by human rights values. It is imperative to create trusted, fair, and responsible AI systems to frame the future in which technology is used to promote justice and human wellbeing to everyone.

References

Akhtar, M.A.K., Kumar, M. and Nayyar, A. (2024). Ensuring Fairness and Non-discrimination in Explainable AI. In: *Towards Ethical and Socially Responsible Explainable AI: Challenges and Opportunities* (pp. 165–192). Cham: Springer Nature Switzerland. https://doi.org/10.1007/978-3-031-66489-2_6.

Alshahrani, A., Griva, A., Dennehy, D. and Mäntymäki, M. (2024). Artificial intelligence and decision-making in government functions: Opportunities, challenges, and future research. *Transforming Government: People, Process, and Policy, 18*(4), 678–698. https://doi.org/10.1108/TG-06-2024-0131.

Amariles, D.R. and Baquero, P.M. (2023). Promises and limits of law for a human-centric artificial intelligence. *Computer Law & Security Review, 48*, 105795. https://doi.org/10.1016/j.clsr.2023.105795.

Bakiner, O. (2023). The promises and challenges of addressing artificial intelligence with human rights. *Big Data & Society, 10*(2). https://doi.org/10.1177/20539517231205476.

Balasubramaniam, N., Kauppinen, M., Rannisto, A., Hiekkanen, K. and Kujala, S. (2023). Transparency and explainability of AI systems: From ethical guidelines to requirements. *Information and Software Technology, 159*, 107197. https://doi.org/10.1016/j.infsof.2023.107197.

Barysė, D. and Sarel, R. (2024). Algorithms in the court: Does it matter which part of the judicial decision-making is automated?. *Artificial Intelligence and Law, 32*(1), 117–146. https://doi.org/10.1007/s10506-022-09343-6.

Bélisle-Pipon, J.C., Monteferrante, E., Roy, M.C. and Couture, V. (2023). Artificial intelligence ethics has a black box problem. *AI & Society, 38*(4), 1507–1522. https://doi.org/10.1007/s00146-021-01380-0.

Blount, K. (2024). Using artificial intelligence to prevent crime: Implications for due process and criminal justice. *AI & Society*, *39*(1), 359–368. https://doi.org/10.1007/s00146-022-01513-z.

Borgesius, F.Z. (2025). Discrimination, artificial intelligence, and algorithmic decision-making. *arXiv preprint arXiv:2510.13465*. https://doi.org/10.48550/arXiv.2510.13465.

Brandusescu, A. and Sieber, R.E. (2025). Missed opportunities in AI regulation: Lessons from Canada's AI and data act. *Data & Policy*, *7*, e40. doi:10.1017/dap.2025.17.

Çetin Kumkumoğlu, S. and Kemal Kumkumoğlu, A. (2023). Rethinking Non-discrimination Law in the Age of Artificial Intelligence. In: *Algorithmic Discrimination and Ethical Perspective of Artificial Intelligence* (pp. 33–53). Singapore: Springer Nature Singapore. https://doi.org/10.1007/978-981-99-6327-0_3.

Cheong, B.C. (2024). Transparency and accountability in AI systems: Safeguarding wellbeing in the age of algorithmic decision-making. *Frontiers in Human Dynamics*, *6*, 1421273. https://doi.org/10.3389/fhumd.2024.1421273.

Cheong, I., Caliskan, A. and Kohno, T. (2025). Safeguarding human values: Rethinking US law for generative AI's societal impacts. *AI and Ethics*, *5*(2), 1433–1459. https://doi.org/10.1007/s43681-024-00451-4.

De Vries, K. (2022). Let the robot speak! AI-generated speech and freedom of expression. In: *YSEC Yearbook of Socio-Economic Constitutions 2021: Triangulating Freedom of Speech* (pp. 93–115). Cham: Springer International Publishing. https://doi.org/10.1007/16495_2021_38.

del Valle, J.I. and Lara, F. (2024). AI-powered recommender systems and the preservation of personal autonomy. *AI & Society*, *39*(5), 2479–2491. https://doi.org/10.1007/s00146-023-01720-2.

Domínguez Hernández, A., Perini, A.M., Hadjiloizou, S., Borda, A., Mahomed, S. and Leslie, D. (2026). Towards a sociotechnical ecology of artificial intelligence: Power, accountability, and governance in a global context. *AI and Ethics*, *6*(1), 43. https://doi.org/10.1007/s43681-025-00902-6.

Duberry, J. (2022). Artificial intelligence and democracy: Risks and promises of AI-mediated citizen–government relations. In: *Artificial Intelligence and Democracy*. Edward Elgar Publishing. https://doi.org/10.4337/9781788977319.

Dunleavy, P. and Margetts, H. (2025). Data science, artificial intelligence, and the third wave of digital era governance. *Public Policy and Administration*, *40*(2), 185–214. https://doi.org/10.1177/09520767231198737.

Elliott, D. and Soifer, E. (2022). AI technologies, privacy, and security. *Frontiers in Artificial Intelligence*, *5*, 826737. https://doi.org/10.3389/frai.2022.826737.

Fontes, C., Hohma, E., Corrigan, C.C. and Lütge, C. (2022). AI-powered public surveillance systems: Why we (might) need them and how we want them. *Technology in Society*, *71*, 102137. https://doi.org/10.1016/j.techsoc.2022.102137.

Gentelet, K. and Mizrahi, S.K. (2024). A Human-Centered Approach to AI Governance: Operationalizing Human Rights through Citizen Participation. In: *Human-Centered AI* (pp. 215–230). Chapman and Hall/CRC.

Giovanola, B. and Tiribelli, S. (2023). Beyond bias and discrimination: Redefining the AI ethics principle of fairness in healthcare machine-learning algorithms. *AI & Society*, *38*(2), 549–563. https://doi.org/10.1007/s00146-022-01455-6.

Gregory, S. (2023). Fortify the truth: How to defend human rights in an age of deepfakes and generative AI. *Journal of Human Rights Practice*, *15*(3), 702–714. https://doi.org/10.1093/jhuman/huad035.

Hogan, L. and Lasek-Markey, M. (2024). Towards a Human Rights-Based Approach to Ethical AI Governance in Europe. *Philosophies*, *9*(6), 181. https://doi.org/10.3390/philosophies9060181.

Holzinger, A., Zatloukal, K. and Müller, H. (2025). Is human oversight to AI systems still possible?. *New Biotechnology*, *85*, 59–62. https://doi.org/10.1016/j.nbt.2024.12.003.

Hornuf, L., Mangold, S. and Yang, Y. (2023). Data protection law in Germany, the United States, and China. In: *Data Privacy and Crowdsourcing: A Comparison of Selected Problems in China, Germany, and the United States* (pp. 19–79). Cham: Springer Nature Switzerland. https://doi.org/10.1007/978-3-031-32064-4_3.

Hussain, A. and Hussain, A. (2025). Transparency and accountability: Unpacking the real problems of explainable AI. *AI & Society*, 1–2. https://doi.org/10.1007/s00146-025-02302-0.

Jougleux, P. (2022). Freedom of expression and the rise of AI. In: *Facebook and the (EU) Law: How the Social Network Reshaped the Legal Framework* (pp. 213–245). Cham: Springer International Publishing. https://doi.org/10.1007/978-3-031-06596-5_8.

Kahraman, Ö.F. (2025). AI and Decision Making. *Theoretical and Empirical Researches in Urban Management*, *20*(2), 81–103. https://www.jstor.org/stable/27384084.

Kazim, E., Denny, D.M.T. and Koshiyama, A. (2021). AI auditing and impact assessment: According to the UK information commissioner's office. *AI and Ethics*, *1*(3), 301–-310. https://doi.org/10.1007/s43681-021-00039-2.

Kumar, S. and Choudhury, S. (2023). Normative ethics, human rights, and artificial intelligence. *AI and Ethics*, *3*(2), 441–450. https://doi.org/10.1007/s43681-022-00170-8.

Lechterman, T.M. (2022). The concept of accountability in AI ethics and governance. In: *The Oxford Handbook of AI Governance*, 164–182. https://doi.org/10.1093/oxfordhb/9780197579329.001.0001.

LePere-Schloop, M. and Zook, S. (2023). AI governance and civil society: The need for critical engagement. In: *Handbook of Critical Studies of Artificial Intelligence* (pp. 878–889). Edward Elgar Publishing. https://doi.org/10.4337/9781803928562.00087.

Mikalef, P., Conboy, K., Lundström, J.E. and Popovič, A. (2022). Thinking responsibly about responsible AI and 'the dark side' of AI. *European Journal of Information Systems*, *31*(3), 257–268. https://doi.org/10.1080/0960085X.2022.2026621.

Moon, M.J. (2023). Searching for inclusive artificial intelligence for social good: Participatory governance and policy recommendations for making AI more inclusive and benign for society. *Public Administration Review*, *83*(6), 1496–1505. https://doi.org/10.1111/puar.13648.

Mueller, M.L. (2025). It's just distributed computing: Rethinking AI governance. *Telecommunications Policy*, *49*(3), 102917. https://doi.org/10.1016/j.telpol.2025.102917.

Nguyen, A., Ngo, H.N., Hong, Y., Dang, B. and Nguyen, B.P.T. (2023). Ethical principles for artificial intelligence in education. *Education and Information Technologies*, *28*(4), 4221–4241. https://doi.org/10.1007/s10639-022-11316-w.

Novelli, C., Taddeo, M. and Floridi, L. (2024). Accountability in artificial intelligence: What it is and how it works. *AI & Society*, *39*(4), 1871–1882. https://doi.org/10.1007/s00146-023-01635-y.

Olsen, H.P., Hildebrandt, T.T., Wiesener, C., Larsen, M.S. and Flügge, A.W.A. (2024). The right to transparency in public governance: Freedom of information and the use of artificial intelligence by public agencies. *Digital Government: Research and Practice*, *5*(1), 1–15. https://doi.org/10.1145/3632753.

Ozmen Garibay, O., Winslow, B., Andolina, S., Antona, M., Bodenschatz, A., Coursaris, C., ... & Xu, W. (2023). Six human-centered artificial intelligence grand challenges. *International Journal of Human–Computer Interaction*, *39*(3), 391–437. https://doi.org/10.1080/10447318.2022.2153320.

Peron, A.E.D.R., Almstadter Mattar de Magalhães, D. and Caetano, G.F. (2025). Beyond digital repression: Techno-authoritarianism in radical right governments. *Cogent Social Sciences*, *11*(1), 2528457. https://doi.org/10.1080/23311886.2025.2528457.

Pi, Y. and Proctor, M. (2025, January). Toward empowering AI governance with redress mechanisms. In: *Cambridge Forum on AI: Law and Governance* (Vol. 1, p. e24). Cambridge University Press. https://doi.org/10.1017/cfl.2025.9.

Prabhakaran, V., Mitchell, M., Gebru, T. and Gabriel, I. (2022). A human rights-based approach to responsible AI. *arXiv preprint arXiv:2210.02667*. https://doi.org/10.48550/arXiv.2210.02667.

Saheb, T. (2023). Ethically contentious aspects of artificial intelligence surveillance: A social science perspective. *AI and Ethics*, *3*(2), 369–379. https://doi.org/10.1007/s43681-022-00196-y.

Sayles, J. (2024). Human Oversight of AI Systems. In: *Principles of AI Governance and Model Risk Management: Master the Techniques for Ethical and Transparent AI Systems* (pp. 267–276). Berkeley, CA: Apress. https://doi.org/10.1007/979-8-8688-0983-5_12.

Schiff, D. (2022). Education for AI, not AI for education: The role of education and ethics in national AI policy strategies. *International Journal of Artificial Intelligence in Education*, *32*(3), 527–563. https://doi.org/10.1007/s40593-021-00270-2.

Shaelou, S.L. and Razmetaeva, Y. (2023, December). Challenges to Fundamental Human Rights in the age of Artificial Intelligence Systems: Shaping the digital legal order while upholding Rule of Law principles and European values. In: *ERA Forum* (Vol. 24, No. 4, pp. 567–587). Berlin/Heidelberg: Springer Berlin Heidelberg. https://doi.org/10.1007/s12027-023-00777-2.

Singh, T. (2023, October). AI-Driven Surveillance Technologies and Human Rights: Balancing Security and Privacy. In: *International Conference on Smart Systems: Innovations in Computing* (pp. 703–717). Singapore: Springer Nature Singapore. https://doi.org/10.1007/978-981-97-3690-4_53.

Slota, S.C., Fleischmann, K.R., Greenberg, S., Verma, N., Cummings, B., Li, L. and Shenefiel, C. (2023). Many hands make many fingers to point: Challenges in creating accountable AI. *Ai & Society*, *38*(4), 1287–1299. https://doi.org/10.1007/s00146-021-01302-0.

Smuha, N.A. (2021). Beyond a human rights-based approach to AI governance: Promise, pitfalls, plea. *Philosophy & Technology*, *34*(Suppl 1), 91–104. https://doi.org/10.1007/s13347-020-00403-w.

Stahl, B.C., Antoniou, J., Bhalla, N., Brooks, L., Jansen, P., Lindqvist, B., ... & Wright, D. (2023). A systematic review of artificial intelligence impact assessments. *Artificial Intelligence Review*, *56*(11), 12799–12831. https://doi.org/10.1007/s10462-023-10420-8.

Stray, J. (2021). Making artificial intelligence work for investigative journalism. *Algorithms, Automation, and News*, 97–118. https://doi.org/10.1080/21670811.2019.1630289.

Suksi, M. (2021). Administrative due process when using automated decision-making in public administration: Some notes from a Finnish perspective. *Artificial Intelligence and Law*, *29*(1), 87–110. https://doi.org/10.1007/s10506-020-09269-x.

Szostek, D. and Prabucki, R.T. (2025). High-risk AI systems. In: *The European Artificial Intelligence Act: Promises and Perils?* (pp. 157–180). Cham: Springer Nature Switzerland. https://doi.org/10.1007/978-3-031-98406-8_7.

Vaassen, B. (2022). AI, opacity, and personal autonomy. *Philosophy & Technology*, *35*(4), 88. https://doi.org/10.1007/s13347-022-00577-5.

Varona, D. and Suárez, J.L. (2022). Discrimination, bias, fairness, and trustworthy AI. *Applied Sciences*, *12*(12), 5826. https://doi.org/10.3390/app12125826.

Wörsdörfer, M. (2025). AI ethics and ordoliberalism 2.0: Towards a 'Digital Bill of Rights'. *AI and Ethics*, *5*(1), 507–525. https://doi.org/10.1007/s43681-023-00367-5.

Zidouemba, M.T. (2025). Governance and artificial intelligence: The use of artificial intelligence in democracy and its impacts on the rights to participation. *Discover Artificial Intelligence*, *5*(1), 12. https://doi.org/10.1007/s44163-025-00229-5.

10 AI and the Future of Work
Labour Policy and Workforce Readiness

Artificial Intelligence (AI) is revolutionising the workplace, working arrangements, and the labour market in the global scene. The high skill jobs and routine jobs are undergoing reshaping through automation, intelligent systems, and advanced robotics that provide new opportunities and uncertainty to the workers. The chapter discusses the effects of AI on the dynamics of the workforce, including job displacement, skill transformation, and the rise of digital labour ecosystems. It discusses some of the issues that are central to labour policy, including the protection of employment, equitable pay, and rights of workers in the algorithmic management world. Also, the chapter indicates the measures that can be taken to prepare the workforce by reskilling, lifelong learning, and inclusive labour reforms. This is aimed at humanising the future of work by ensuring that AI can boost productivity to the fullest without negatively affecting social equity.

10.1 Introduction

Artificial Intelligence (AI) is contributing to a significant change in the system of work and employment. Smart machines, high level algorithms, and robots are gaining significance as constituents of the contemporary working environment. To enhance productivity, organisations are increasingly turning to AI to curb the costs of operations and increase their efficiencies. Therefore, automated systems now support or substitute several job activities that were once performed manually. This change brings drastic alteration in the model of the labour market worldwide (Malik et al., 2022). AI has taken over numerous industries. Robots in the manufacturing industry are used to carry out activities like packing and assembly. AI has applications in healthcare diagnosis, treatment planning, and patient monitoring. Alpha In the financial industry, algorithms are used to identify fraud, risk, and aid in financial decision-making. Digital learning platforms are used to educate students, and these platforms modify educational contents to suit them. The AI is applied in the retail and logistics sector to optimise the supply chain, personalised marketing, and fast customer service (Javaid et al., 2022). These two demonstrate that AI does not belong to any particular sector, but is transforming the overall economy.

The transformation is accompanied with new opportunities. AI technologies present a challenge to find specialised skills in the field of data science, robotics support, user experience design, and system maintenance. The AI development, cybersecurity, and digital entrepreneurship spheres are developing new industries

DOI: 10.1201/9781003776659-10

(Gruetzemacher & Whittlestone, 2022). Automation can decrease hazardous or physically strenuous labour, enhancing safety and wellbeing of the employees. AI innovation can also enhance productivity and economic expansion, enhancing country competitiveness at the international level (Abbas Khan et al., 2024). But there is a concern also with the shift. Among the most popular risks, there is job displacement. Employees of routine, low skill, or repetitive jobs have a possibility of getting lower jobs since machines replace them. This shift would exacerbate the income inequality provided that workers are not offered retraining or skill development opportunities. The level of disruption will affect some areas and communities more than others, based on their economic organisation and preparedness to use digital technology (Lokesh et al., 2024).

The other issue of great concern is the evolving workplace management. AI tools are becoming more popular in overseeing the productivity of workers, scheduling, and measuring worker performance. Although they can assist in having a better organisation, it can also lead to a decrease in autonomy and create stressful work settings. The absence of transparency in algorithmic management may result in an unfair treatment in case employees do not know how algorithms are formed about them (Li, 2024). Platform and gig work is also changing employment relations. Most gig workers lack protection afforded to traditional workers including stable income, health care, and social security. AI-based systems delegate the work, define the rates, and impose the performance policies without adequate human controls. This poses a challenge of labour rights and fair working conditions (Pradhan & Saxena, 2023). Thus, opportunities and risks must be taken into account in the future of work. The evolution of the labour force is a positive prospect, but the change must be managed carefully so that everyone could be the beneficiary of technological progress.

10.2 Impact of AI on Employment

10.2.1 Job Creation vs. Job Displacement

AI influences employment to a considerable extent. It is not only able to generate new jobs, but it also replaces old jobs. New employment opportunities are found in technical areas in large numbers. These are: data science, machine learning engineering, and cybersecurity. These jobs demand technical expertise and great educational experiences. Moreover, AI evolution has resulted in the emergence of new jobs in the non-technical division. These are such as AI ethics, system monitoring, and user experience design. Such positions help to use AI technologies responsibly and efficiently (Rawashdeh, 2025). Companies that move towards AI tend to be more competitive and productive. Greater efficiency will allow lowering costs and enhancing the quality of service. Due to this, businesses can increase their activities. This growth may result in economic development and the establishment of new forms of jobs. By doing so, AI can be beneficial to the field of labour markets (Balakumar et al., 2024).

Nevertheless, AI leads to job displacement, as well. Most vulnerable jobs include routine and repetitive jobs. These tasks can be executed faster and with precision by machines and automated systems than human beings. These are assembly line work, data entry work, setting schedules, and simple customer service. Employees in such jobs have a greater challenge of unemployment. They might not be able to transition to new positions without adequate training (Khogali & Mekid, 2023). AI does not have evenly distributed impacts on employment. New opportunities are more likely to be enjoyed by highly skilled workers. On the contrary, workers with low skills can be more challenged. Unless support is offered, job displacement may become a source of rising income inequality. Industries and governments make a significant contribution towards this problem. There is a need to invest in education, reskilling, and career transition programmes. The issue of creating a number of jobs is not the only problem, but the quality of jobs and the equal opportunity to access the new employment opportunities (Bankins et al., 2024).

10.2.2 Changing Roles in Different Sectors

AI is not necessarily job killers. It transforms the way work is done on most occasions. The roles of a job do not necessarily vanish. AI systems assist the employees by making them more accurate, faster, and decisive. Most sectors still need human participation though (Ramachandran et al., 2022). There are also AI applications used in the medical field to help physicians and nurses identify ailments and medical information. These systems are able to work with large volumes of information in a short period of time. They assist in the detection of patterns that might be quite unnoticeable to human beings. Despite this support, patient care is still granted by the healthcare professionals. Human judgement, empathy, and moral decision are equally vital in medical practice (Lee & Yoon, 2021).

AI and digital technologies assist educators in the field of education to make learning individual. With Adaptive Learning systems, it is possible to modify content according to the performance of the students. These aids are in the evaluation and planning of lessons. Nevertheless, instructors still support students and motivate them. Social development and emotional support depends on human interaction (Zhang & Zhang, 2024). AI technologies are applicable in agriculture to track crops, examine soils, and water management. The farmers apply data-driven tools to enhance productivity and minimise waste. Manual work and human control is required nevertheless. Farmers use opinion and local wisdom in making decisions (Patel et al., 2025).

Due to such changes, numerous jobs turn out to be hybrid ones. These functions are a combination of human efforts and machine support. Employees should be more digitally literate and technologically conscious. Also of importance is problem solving. Such skills as creativity, communication, and emotional intelligence become valuable. These human skills cannot be easily substituted by machines. Industries change at varying rates. The fields that embrace AI faster are technology based. During the use of AI, the traditional industries might be slower. However, every industry needs to anticipate the changes in the organisation of workflows, organisational structure, and training of professionals. These transformations require one to constantly learn to keep up with them (Babashahi et al., 2024).

10.2.3 Rise of Automation, Robotics, and Digital Labour Markets

Automation and robotics are becoming common in the manufacturing industry as well as the service industry. The assembly, packaging, and quality control are done with a high degree of precision by robots. Robotic warehouses are effective in the movement of goods with minimum human intervention. The robotic processes automation (RPA) takes care of the paperwork, accounting, and other daily digital activities in offices (William et al., 2023). Increases in digital labour markets are also increasing. Platform work encompasses ride hailing, delivery, online freelancing, and micro tasks, e.g., data labelling. Such positions are usually automated by AI algorithms that distribute tasks, analyse performance, and pay. Online labour markets offer freedom and autonomy to the employees. Nevertheless, they also create an issue of job security, fair wages, and workers' rights (Langmann & Turi, 2022).

AI opens opportunities for remote work globally, but it also adds competition among workers worldwide. The standards of payment can become very different, and not all workers will get legal safeguards. The policymakers need to overcome these challenges by formulating labour laws that are best fitted to the digital employment patterns (Abbas Khan et al., 2024). Table 10.1 illustrates major positive and negative impacts of AI on employment as job creation, job roles, automation, and digital labour.

Table 10.1 Summary of AI's Impact on Employment.

Impact Area	*Positive Effects*	*Negative Effects*
Job creation	New roles in tech and support sectors	Unequal access to high skill jobs
Job displacement	Efficiency and productivity gains	Loss of routine and low skill jobs
Changing roles	Humans focus on higher value tasks	Pressure to learn new skills
Automation and robotics	Safety improvements and reduced manual labour	Fewer traditional manufacturing jobs
Digital labour platforms	Flexible work, global opportunities	Insecure work, low protection and pay

10.3 Skills Transformation and Workforce Readiness

10.3.1 New Skill Requirements in AI-Enabled Industries

AI alters the job descriptions in most industries. The work activities are becoming more engaging with the digital systems. The employees should be familiar with the functioning of automated tools. They should also have the ability to read the data and the system outputs. These skills are now necessary at the workplaces. Some of the AI-related jobs require technical expertise. The software development and system maintenance depends on the programming knowledge. Data analytics are abilities to process large amounts of data and assist workers in decision-making. Cybersecurity skills are required to defend the digital systems. Robotics maintenance and machine learning skills are also becoming necessary. The positions require one to work logically and to have good knowledge of sophisticated technologies (Miglani & Khandelwal, 2025).

Nevertheless, not every single job of the future demands higher level coding. Most jobs are based on how people use their skills which are not readily substituted by AI. These are problem solving skills and critical thinking skills. Team work and effective communication are also significant in teamwork environments. Leadership proficiencies are useful in organisational coordination and decision-making. The decision that affects critical outcomes should be ethically evaluated in the case of AI systems (Theben et al., 2025). In most sectors, human-centred skills are still needed. Social services, education, and healthcare rely on emotional knowledge and communication with other individuals. Originality and cultural awareness is appreciated in the creative industries. Machines can hardly copy these qualities. Consequently, human skills remain a major factor in the labour market (Ozmen Garibay et al., 2023).

Hybrid skills are getting quite useful. Employees need to integrate professional expertise and digital applications usage. One can see this trend in finance, agriculture, journalism, and logistics. The employees themselves can observe and control the systems better when they are aware of the influence of AI systems on the decision-making process. Being able to collaborate with intelligent machines is already one of the determinants of professional success. The industries that have implemented AI therefore require continuous learning and skill development (Rodgers et al., 2023).

10.3.2 Reskilling and Lifelong Learning Strategies

Employees with shifting jobs because of automation need to re skill to meet the requirements of the updated job descriptions. Lack of opportunities to train will expose many individuals to the threat of job displacement and chronic unemployment. Reskilling courses enable employees to move to new positions that offer them greater job security and future prospects (Goel et al., 2024). It is also necessary to engage in lifelong learning. In dynamic technological settings, knowledge is obsolete very fast. The employees are forced to keep on updating their skills so that they can remain relevant. Accessible and affordable learning opportunities should be offered to governments and companies by way of vocational training, online learning, apprenticeship, and workplace development programmes.

It is especially significant to support mid-career workers. Unless guided, older workers might find it hard to adjust to new technologies. Retraining should be promoted by providing financial support, professional counselling, and accommodating course designs by the public policies. Academic institutions have to liaise with the business world to make learning programmes relevant to the present labour market (Pradhan & Saxena, 2023). Employers are also very important. Skilled workers are beneficial to companies which are supposed to invest in training to facilitate transformation within the company. Employees can acquire new skills and trust in new technology with the aid of internal training programmes, mentorship, and job rotation. An effective reskilling programme would lead to a decrease in inequality as all employees would have access to opportunities, irrespective of their backgrounds, age, and location. It makes the benefits of AI common to society instead of the few (Li, 2024).

10.3.3 Enhancing Digital Literacy and Adaptability

In the era of AI, digital literacy has become an essential precondition. Digital systems are essential in the day to day work of workers; they need to know how to operate. This encompasses the familiarity with the manner of data collection, storage, and processing. The workers should also be aware of the impact of algorithms on making decisions and results. This type of knowledge would enable people to apply technology in a safe and responsible manner. It also helps them adapt better to new digital tools at the work place (Parra-Valencia & Massey, 2023). Digital literacy is beyond mere technical prowess. Data privacy and online security awareness are also included. Employees should be made aware of how they should safeguard both personal and organisational information. They must be aware of online dangers like misappropriation of data and cyber dangers. Another thing is ethical use of technology. The employees must be capable of recognising instances where automated decision-making seems wrong or unjust. This consciousness gives workers the ability to challenge and report possible issues (Naamati-Schneider & Alt, 2024).

Another necessary skill in AI sensitive settings is flexibility. AI evolves quickly and transforms the work process rather often. Consequently, employees have to be ready to use new systems and to revise their competencies. Career development in the long run is supported by flexibility and openness to change. Curiosity and lifelong learning can keep people relevant in the constantly evolving workplaces. Fast adapting workers are in a better position to deal with disruptions in the economy and technology (Strielkowski et al., 2025). Educational institutions are important in the development of these skills. They need to encourage digital readiness at a young age in schools and universities. The curriculum is expected to focus on problem solving and critical thinking. There should also be responsible and ethical use of technology. To avoid social inequality, equal access to digital education should be provided. Societies that are poorly equipped digitally need further assistance. Equal access to digital resources will make sure that everyone can enjoy technological advancement (Tiernan et al., 2023).

10.4 Labour Policy and Workers' Rights in the AI Era

10.4.1 Fair Wages and Employee Protections

One of the key principles of labour rights is fair wages. Proper remuneration of workers should be offered. This principle is applicable on the individual employee or the one who is working with automated systems. The wage structure can, however, be influenced by the introduction of AI. Digital and technical employees have high skills, and hence they are paid higher. Low skilled workers on the contrary can be exposed to low wage increases or job instability. This situation may augment earnings disparity in the labour market (Hamilton et al., 2023). The use of AI also has the potential to change the way wages are set. Other organisations have automated systems to aid in wage setting. These systems process performance measures and productivity. They usually aim at cutting labour and enhancing efficiency. Such systems can cause unequal remuneration without proper supervision. They can also lower wages without any justifiable reason. This is why transparency is required. Employees are supposed to know how their salaries are computed. They are also supposed to be given a right to challenge and rectify wrong or biased decisions (Deranty & Corbin, 2024).

Technological change should not undermine the protections of employees. AI is to be employed to make working conditions better. It must not diminish the safety and employment of workers. The chances of safety risks are high in workplaces where humans work together with machines. There should be proper equipment and training by employers. There are also needs for clear emergency procedures in technology intensive environments (Getman et al., 2025). Workers are also safeguarded by public policy. The labour laws should keep up with the emerging types of work. Such laws must introduce equality and discourage discrimination. Close securities make sure that employees are not regarded as fungible resources. Technological advancements must be a good thing to every employee. Sustainable and inclusive economic development requires fair salaries and safe working environments (Santoni de Sio et al., 2024).

10.4.2 Algorithmic Management and Workplace Surveillance

There is an increased use of AI in management in the workplace. Employers use AI in recruitment, time management, performance appraisal, and monitoring employees. This is what is referred to as algorithmic management. There are the systems that have the capacity to enhance efficiency and cut on the administrative work load. Nevertheless, they also give severe doubts concerning workers' rights and well-being when they are out of regulation (Zhang et al., 2025). Workplace surveillance is one of the significant areas of concern. Other organisations are utilising sensors, cameras, and digital tracking systems to track the movements of the workers. There are others that track the keystroke, screen time, and Internet usage. In other instances, productivity is measured by collecting biometric data. Decisions regarding discipline or dismissal can also be made by the automated systems using performance scores. The practices may severely diminish the privacy of the employees (Howard, 2022).

Too much surveillance is psychologically stressing. Employees can experience permanent stress since their performances are constantly measured. The risk of errors can grow. This climate may damage psychological well-being and result in lower satisfaction at the workplace. More so, decisions made through algorithms can hardly be comprehended. Employees are not aware of the calculation of performance scores. They also might not know data that is utilised in such systems. Consequently, this makes it hard to appeal against unjust or wrong judgments (De Stefano & Taes, 2023). These are several risks that should be dealt with in labour policy. There must be regulations that give a clear explanation of automated decisions which influence employment results. The quantity and nature of the data gathered should be limited. Personal information that is sensitive should be preserved. Disciplinary measures and firing decisions should be under human control. Monitoring systems should also be introduced before they are introduced to workers (Mettler, 2024). There should be a balance between efficiency and respect for human dignity. There should be fair management practices supported by technology. Workers should be treated as persons, having their rights and duties. They are not to be minimised to data points in the automated systems.

10.4.3 Social Protection Frameworks for Gig and Platform Workers

Online labour markets have altered conventional employment. Ride hailing services, food delivery websites, and online freelancing sites are popular. Such platforms provide easy employment. Nevertheless, they transform the relations between workers and employers as well. Most of the platform workers group themselves as independent contractors as opposed to employees. Due to this category, they frequently do not have fundamental labour rights (Divya & Barani, 2024). Platform workers typically lack the type of benefits that are typical in normal jobs. These are the health insurance, minimum wage, paid leave, and pension contributions. This has left most of the workers without financial security. The income can be changing according to the demand and rules on platforms. This aspect makes economically vulnerable people who depend on platform work as their primary income source (Sieker, 2022).

AI is a key factor in controlling platform workers. They are used in algorithms to allocate tasks, wage calculation, and performance measurement of the workers. The existence of an automated system also monitors activity levels. There is the risk that workers could lose employment after being labelled by an algorithm as being inactive or low performing. These are decisions which are not usually explained. In most instances, employees cannot counter or correct such results. Transparency is deficient, which generates power inequalities between platforms and workers (De Stefano & Doellgast, 2023). These new ways of working have to be adjusted to social protection systems. Platform workers should have minimum wages guaranteed by public policy. The workers should have insurance cover that will take care of their accidents and work risks. There should also be access to unemployment benefits and social security programmes. The rights of the platform workers should be legalised. These involve the rights to form unions and collective bargaining (Duggan et al., 2023).

Companies that work on the digital platform and governments have a joint responsibility to enhance working conditions. There should be co operation to develop equitable rules. Dynamism should be encouraged by digital labour. Meanwhile, it should safeguard the stability of workers, their dignity, and general welfare. Table 10.1 summarises the primary risks to workers' rights in AI-driven workplaces and the policy needed to address each challenge.

Table 10.1 Key Labour Policy Challenges in the AI Era.

Challenge Area	*Main Concerns*	*Policy Needs*
Fair wages	Wage inequality, automated pay decisions	Transparent wage systems and equal pay protections
Algorithmic management	Lack of privacy, biased performance evaluations	Human oversight and limits on workplace surveillance
Gig and platform labour	Low protection, unstable income	Social security inclusion and labour rights recognition

10.5 Industry, Government, and Institutional Roles

10.5.1 Public Private Partnerships for Workforce Development

The role of the public private partnership is significant in the era of AI workforce development. The high rate of technological change presents new skills. It is not only the governments that can act positively to these changes. There are also restrictions in the private industries that are not guided by the policy and the support of the people. Partnership between the state and the non-state actors can address such challenges (Prasad et al., 2024). A major advantage of the public private partnerships is the enhanced fit between education and the labour market requirements. Firms will have the capacity to communicate about new positions and competencies. The knowledge aids the training institutions to design pertinent programs. These efforts can be supported by governments by means of funding and policy reforms. Access to training opportunities is also enhanced by investment in digital infrastructure (Tanveer et al., 2025).

One of the significant results of such cooperation is joint training. Such efforts can involve apprenticeship and internship. Learning modules related to the industries enable workers to gain practical experience. The participants are able to develop theoretical knowledge in practice. The method will enhance employability and minimise mismatches. Employees are in a better position to work AI jobs (Rotatori et al., 2021). Partnership with the government is particularly useful when there is a rapid process of automation in one area. There are tremendous changes in work processes of manufacturing, logistics, finance and health care. Workers impacted by automation can be assisted by the targeted training programs. These programmes assist employees in settling in new positions in industries or between industries (Cismas & Dumitru, 2023).

Corporation complements social inclusion too. Advanced training is usually unavailable in rural places and under-served communities. Local learning facilities and online educational sources may be offered through the efforts of public private efforts. Such initiatives cut down inequality in the region and increase the job opportunities. Workforce development is enhanced when the two sectors are responsible. In general, the partnerships between the government and the business contribute to sustainable economic growth. They are useful in ensuring that workers acquire relevant skills. Collective responsibility enhances equal opportunity and sustainability in the labour markets (Campion et al., 2022).

10.5.2 Education System Reforms and Vocational Training

The education systems should be prepared to fit in the requirements of an AI-enabled economy. Due to traditional education systems, the academic content of schools is often concerned with theory, as opposed to skills. The contemporary work environments demand not only digital skills but also excellent problem solving skills. AI literacy, data skills, and computational thinking must be introduced in schools, colleges, and universities (Southworth et al., 2023). Digital literacy needs to be introduced at an early stage of education and promote curiosity, creativity, and collaboration. There should be interdisciplinary programmes in higher education that are interlaced between technology and social sciences and humanities as well as ethics. This assists students in gaining knowledge about the advantages and the impact of AI on society (Kafai & Proctor, 2022).

Vocational training is also necessary to equip employees who have knowledge of automation. Polytechnic and technical institutions should also renew their curricula with the help of robotics maintenance, cybersecurity, digital and advanced manufacturing methods skills. Modular learning pathways and short-term certification courses can assist those workers that are required to revise the skills and maintain the employment (Yu & Guo, 2023). One of the issues that are significant to lifelong development is flexible learning opportunities. Online learning platforms, micro credentials, and training in the workplace provide individuals with a liberty to learn at their own capacity. These opportunities can be made available more by financial support measures like training vouchers and government subsidies, especially to low income workers and rural workers (Chiu et al., 2024). Education and training system reforms are the key elements of making sure that workers do not lose their competitiveness and their faith in labour markets of the future.

10.5.3 Ethical Employment and Responsible Automation Policies

Responsible automation is an endeavour to apply AI in possibilities that help workers. Technology must augment human work as opposed to substituting workers blindly. Ethical employment practices should concentrate on social and human consequences of automation. Employers ought to engage workers in strategising automation plans. Communication early will help to decrease uncertainty and fear. Retraining opportunities should also be provided to the workers prior to the occurrence of major job changes (Santoni de Sio, 2024). Fairness and transparency should be applied when making automation decisions. The companies will have to justify the introduction of automation and its impact on the job roles. Technology should result in productivity that should be shared with employees. The working processes should not be changed without fair wages being maintained. Career development and skills advancement should also be given to the employees. Workplaces that are dependent on digital management systems should avoid discrimination (Camilleri, 2024).

The uses of algorithmic systems in the task assignment and performance evaluation are growing. Such systems should be friendly and responsible. The automated tools used by employers should be clarified to the workers. Audits should be performed regularly in order to identify errors and bias. The workers should be informed in a clear way about the decision making procedure. The right to appeal to automated results should be available to them. Decisions that have grave consequences should be reviewed by humans (Chang & Ke, 2024). Another important principle is respect for privacy. The operations of monitoring are to be confined to the essential work related operations. The overstepping of personal behaviour by the employer should be shunned. The standards of data protection should be observed (Elliott & Soifer, 2022).

Responsible automation is facilitated by social dialogue. There should be labour unions, worker groups, and community groups included in the formation of the policies. Their participation assists in safeguarding the rights and dignity of the workers. Governments also are at the heart of it. Technology use should be made responsible with the help of policy frameworks. Such frameworks should restrict intrusive behaviour and need human supervision in applications with high risks. Ethical labour practices enhance stability in the labour market. When the workers feel appreciated, they would be more accepting of new technologies. Responsible automation is beneficial to long-term innovation and social trust (Iphofen & Kritikos, 2021).

10.6 Inclusive and Equitable Future of Work

10.6.1 Tackling Inequality and Digital Divides

Digital divide is an issue of concern in most societies. The availability of digital solutions and good internet facilities is not uniform. The novel technologies tend to be widespread in the city and affluent zones. However, individuals in rural or low income areas usually do not have adequate digital infrastructure. This is constrained by lack of access to the digital economy. Digital illiteracy is also a hindrance. Those who do not feel comfortable with the use of technology might not be able to enjoy digital services and job opportunities (Kitsara, 2022). Inequality can also be further enhanced by the use of AI. New digital jobs are more likely to be benefiting high skilled workers. Employees of low skill or routine jobs are more exposed to the threat of job insecurity. Low levels of education and inability to access technology make them less flexible. This leads to the possibility of increasing income and employment disparities. Gender inequality can also grow when women are less likely to access education on technologies and digital professions. People with disabilities can be further challenged when digital systems are not made to be accessible (Hammerschmidt et al., 2025).

To reduce inequality, there must be concentrated and inclusive policies. Governments need to spend on digital infrastructure in low density and isolated regions. Education, training, and employment are all dependent on reliable internet access. Public investment assists in the establishment of equal initial conditions. Schools also can contribute to bridging the digital divide. Digital tools and other entry level skills in technology should be accessible in schools and training centres. Practices are supposed to be in favour of lifelong learning and digital confidence (Lazanyuk et al., 2025). Specific programmes should also be used to facilitate inclusion. Women, minorities, and the disadvantaged groups are supposed to be encouraged to apply in technology-related areas. The digital tools should be accommodating to people with disabilities through the availability of accessible design standards. Social inclusion is enhanced by having equal access to digital opportunities. It also enhances economic resilience. Sustainable development in the era of AI requires the need to address digital divides (Bentley et al., 2024).

10.6.2 Supporting Vulnerable and Displaced Workers

Jobs can be displaced as a result of automation and AI. Employees who are displaced because of technological revolution need powerful support structures. The loss of jobs is usually a source of economic and emotional strain. It is also able to lower self-confidence and social participation. Displaced workers can be unemployed over a long period without any proper help. There are some groups that are more susceptible to job displacement. These are low skilled labour and the elderly employees. There are also increased risks among informal workers and other workers who engage in physically demanding work. Low level of education and lack of mobility gives these workers a hard time moving into new positions.

Consequently, it might lead to the growth of inequality in case support measures are not provided (Plikas et al., 2023).

It is the role of the governments and employers to assist the affected workers. Programmes of reskilling and up-skilling are necessary. Such programmes assist employees in acquiring the new skills in the new jobs. There is also the need for income support in the case of transition. The temporary financial aid assists employees with their fundamental needs when they are searching for new jobs. With career counselling, workers can be guided with regard to finding the right job. Job placement programmes have the potential to match workers to jobs (Idrisi et al., 2024). Older and mid-career workers have a need to have flexible learning options. The training programmes must be available and flexible. Continued participation can be facilitated by online and part-time formats of learning. These strategies alleviate education and skills training barriers.

To be in line with the evolving labour markets, social protection systems should be increased. The work should also be covered, and gig employment and platform employment should also be included. The traditional employment contracts should not only be used to determine access to health insurance, paid leaves pensions and unemployment benefits. Economic security is facilitated by equal protection (Kong et al., 2023). Social level programmes also contribute significantly. Mentorship and skills building programmes can be offered by the local organisations. Cooperation with labour unions makes worker views to be taken into consideration when designing the policies. Employees who are displaced should be supported to avoid poverty. It also reinforces the belief of the population towards technological advancement and social security (Aly, 2022).

10.6.3 Global Cooperation and Policy Harmonization

The labour markets on the national level are impacted by AI. It does not influence one country or a territory. Consequently, international collaboration is required to defend the workers around the globe. Labour standards may vary widely across countries without common policies. Strong protections may be practised in some regions, and weak rules may be permissible in others. The imbalance may lead to an unfair competition and put workers at the risk of being exploited (Alibašić, 2025). International and local organisations are significant in the coordination of the labour policy. The international labour organisation upholds international labour rights and fair working conditions. It is used to give directions on fair employment practices within the evolving labour markets. The G20 promotes collaboration between the great economies. It facilitates policy discussion in the areas of employment and technological change. The OECD also carries out research and policy suggestions on skills development and adjustment to the labour market. The European Union promotes geographical integration by common rules and labour policies (Roberts et al., 2024).

There are some areas that policy harmonisation should do. The safety of workers in workplaces where AI is in place is necessary. The labour based on digital and platform should be subject to fair employment criteria. Skill and professional qualifications that are recognised internationally have the potential to enhance movement of workers. The ethical application of automation and monitoring technologies are also to be encouraged. Transparency and accountability can be achieved with the help of clear standards (von Ingersleben-Seip, 2023). Of particular interest is aid to developing countries. The adoption of AI is not very responsible in many low income countries. Financial aid and technical aid can be given by developed nations. Local capacity is built with the aid of technology transfer and knowledge sharing. Such activities decrease inequality in the world and promote inclusive development. AI can also help in achieving common wealth when nations collaborate. Planned strategies make sure that the technological advancements are used to the advantage of employees throughout. International collaboration makes the international labour system fair, stable, and trustworthy (Zaidan & Ibrahim, 2024).

10.7 Conclusion

AI is revolutionising the world of work. It is a new source of innovations, productivity, as well as economic development, and it is redefining skills and labour patterns along with workplace designs. Simultaneously, AI presents the issue of work displacement, inequality, digital communities, and the change in labour rights. Such developments must be well planned and provide powerful labour laws that safeguard employees and allow environmentally conscious technology development. Human-centred methods are necessary in order to make the benefits of automation fairly distributed. To train workers to work in AI-enabled industries, reskilling, lifelong learning, and becoming digital is required. There should be coordination between governments, industry, and educational facilities to develop an inclusive workforce development system. Worker protection is further enhanced by ethical employment practices, fair wages, and clear algorithmic management. The future of work is based on an international collaboration, a levelled access to digital resources, and a robust social safety net. With a focus on fairness, dignity, and mobility, societies will be able to create an AI-driven work environment that promotes economic development as well as social welfare.

References

Abbas Khan, M., Khan, H., Omer, M.F., Ullah, I. and Yasir, M. (2024). Impact of artificial intelligence on the global economy and technology advancements. In: *Artificial General Intelligence (AGI) Security: Smart Applications and Sustainable Technologies* (pp. 147–180). Singapore: Springer Nature Singapore. https://doi.org/10.1007/978-981-97-3222-7_7.

Alibašić, H. (2025). Harmonizing artificial intelligence (AI) governance: A comparative analysis of Singapore and France's AI policies and the influence of international organization: H. Alibašić. *Global Public Policy and Governance*, 1–21. https://doi.org/10.1007/s43508-025-00116-w.

Aly, H. (2022). Digital transformation, development, and productivity in developing countries: Is artificial intelligence a curse or a blessing? *Review of Economics and Political Science*, *7*(4), 238–256. https://doi.org/10.1108/REPS-11-2019-0145.

Babashahi, L., Barbosa, C.E., Lima, Y., Lyra, A., Salazar, H., Argôlo, M., ... & Souza, J.M.D. (2024). AI in the workplace: A systematic review of skill transformation in the industry. *Administrative Sciences*, *14*(6), 127. https://doi.org/10.3390/admsci14060127.

Balakumar, A., Sawant, P.D., Nimma, D., Khan, S.A. and Siddiqua, A. (2024, November). Impact of AI-Driven Automation on Job Displacement and Skill Development: A Societal Perspective. In: *2024 IEEE Silchar Subsection Conference* (*SILCON 2024*) (pp. 1–5). IEEE. https://doi.org/10.1109/SILCON63976.2024.10910660.

Bankins, S., Ocampo, A.C., Marrone, M., Restubog, S.L.D. and Woo, S.E. (2024). A multilevel review of artificial intelligence in organizations: Implications for organizational behavior research, and practice. *Journal of Organizational Behavior*, *45*(2), 159–182. https://doi.org/10.1002/job.2735.

Bentley, S.V., Naughtin, C.K., McGrath, M.J., Irons, J.L. and Cooper, P.S. (2024). The digital divide in action: How experiences of digital technology shape future relationships with artificial intelligence. *AI and Ethics*, *4*(4), 901–915. https://doi.org/10.1007/s43681-024-00452-3.

Camilleri, M.A. (2024). Artificial intelligence governance: Ethical considerations and implications for social responsibility. *Expert Systems*, *41*(7), e13406. https://doi.org/10.1111/exsy.13406.

Campion, A., Gasco-Hernandez, M., Jankin Mikhaylov, S. and Esteve, M. (2022). Overcoming the challenges of collaboratively adopting artificial intelligence in the public sector. *Social Science Computer Review*, *40*(2), 462–477. https://doi.org/10.1177/0894439320979953.

Chang, Y. L. and Ke, J. (2024). Socially responsible artificial intelligence empowered people analytics: A novel framework towards sustainability. *Human Resource Development Review*, *23*(1), 88–120. https://doi.org/10.1177/15344843231200930.

Chiu, T.K., Ahmad, Z., Ismailov, M. and Sanusi, I.T. (2024). What are artificial intelligence literacy and competency? A comprehensive framework to support them. *Computers and Education Open*, *6*, 100171. https://doi.org/10.1016/j.caeo.2024.100171.

Cismas, L.M. and Dumitru, C. (2023). Investing in Social and Intellectual Capital: A Public–Private Partnership Issue. In: *Cooperation and Enlargement: Two Challenges to be Addressed in the European Projects: 2022* (pp. 301–324). Cham: Springer Nature Switzerland. https://doi.org/10.1007/978-3-031-42253-9_15.

De Stefano, V. and Doellgast, V. (2023). Introduction to the Transfer special issue. Regulating AI at work: Labour relations, automation, and algorithmic management. *Transfer: European Review of Labour and Research*, *29*(1), 9–20. https://doi.org/10.1177/10242589231157656.

De Stefano, V. and Taes, S. (2023). Algorithmic management and collective bargaining. *Transfer: European Review of Labour and Research*, *29*(1), 21–36. https://doi.org/10.1177/10242589221141055.

Deranty, J.P. and Corbin, T. (2024). Artificial intelligence and work: A critical review of recent research from the social sciences. *AI & Society*, *39*(2), 675–691. https://doi.org/10.1007/s00146-022-01496-x.

Divya, S. and Barani, G. (2024). An Evaluation of Social Protection Measures for Gig Workers: A Pilot Study. In: *Organization, Purpose, and Values* (pp. 143–165). Routledge.

Duggan, J., Carbery, R., McDonnell, A. and Sherman, U. (2023). Algorithmic HRM control in the gig economy: The app-worker perspective. *Human Resource Management*, *62*(6), 883–899. https://doi.org/10.1002/hrm.22168.

Elliott, D. and Soifer, E. (2022). AI technologies, privacy, and security. *Frontiers in Artificial Intelligence*, *5*, 826737. https://doi.org/10.3389/frai.2022.826737.

Getman, A.P., Yaroshenko, O.M., Dmytryk, O.O., Tykhonovych, O.Y. and Hryn, D.V. (2025). The role of artificial intelligence and algorithms in the working conditions formation. *AI & Society*, *40*(5), 3909–3917. https://doi.org/10.1007/s00146-024-02160-2.

Goel, A., Dede, C., Garn, M. and Ou, C. (2024). AI-ALOE: AI for reskilling, upskilling, and workforce development. *AI Magazine*, *45*(1), 77–82. https://doi.org/10.1002/aaai.12157.

Gruetzemacher, R. and Whittlestone, J. (2022). The transformative potential of artificial intelligence. *Futures*, *135*, 102884. https://doi.org/10.1016/j.futures.2021.102884.

Hamilton, L., Elliott, D., Quick, A., Smith, S. and Choplin, V. (2023). Exploring the use of AI in qualitative analysis: A comparative study of guaranteed income data. *International Journal of Qualitative Methods*, *22*. https://doi.org/10.1177/16094069231201504.

Hammerschmidt, T., Stolz, K. and Posegga, O. (2025). Bridging the gap: Inequalities that divide those who can and cannot create sustainable outcomes with AI. *Behaviour & Information Technology*, 1–30. https://doi.org/10.1080/0144929X.2025.2500451.

Howard, J. (2022). Algorithms and the future of work. *American Journal of Industrial Medicine*, *65*(12), 943–952. https://doi.org/10.1002/ajim.23429.

Idrisi, M.J., Geteye, D. and Shanmugasundaram, P. (2024). Modeling the complex interplay: Dynamics of job displacement and evolution of artificial intelligence in a socio-economic landscape. *International Journal of Networked and Distributed Computing*, *12*(2), 185–194. https://doi.org/10.1007/s44227-024-00025-0.

Iphofen, R. and Kritikos, M. (2021). Regulating artificial intelligence and robotics: Ethics by design in a digital society. *Contemporary Social Science*, *16*(2), 170–184. https://doi.org/10.1080/21582041.2018.1563803.

Javaid, M., Haleem, A., Singh, R.P. and Suman, R. (2022). Artificial intelligence applications for industry 4.0: A literature-based study. *Journal of Industrial Integration and Management*, *7*(01), 83–111. https://doi.org/10.1142/S2424862221300040.

Kafai, Y.B. and Proctor, C. (2022). A revaluation of computational thinking in K–12 education: Moving toward computational literacies. *Educational Researcher*, *51*(2), 146–151. https://doi.org/10.3102/0013189X211057904.

Khogali, H.O. and Mekid, S. (2023). The blended future of automation and AI: Examining some long-term societal and ethical impact features. *Technology in Society*, *73*, 102232. https://doi.org/10.1016/j.techsoc.2023.102232.

Kitsara, I. (2022). Artificial intelligence and the digital divide: From an innovation perspective. In: *Platforms and Artificial Intelligence: The Next Generation of Competences* (pp. 245–265). Cham: Springer International Publishing. https://doi.org/10.1007/978-3-030-90192-9_12.

Kong, J.D., Fevrier, K., Effoduh, J.O. and Bragazzi, N.L. (2023). Artificial intelligence, law, and vulnerabilities. In: *AI and Society* (pp. 179–196). Chapman and Hall/CRC.

Langmann, C. and Turi, D. (2022). *Robotic Process Automation* (*RPA*): *Digitization and Automation of Processes*. Springer Books. https://doi.org/10.1007/978-3-658-38692-4.

Lazanyuk, I.V., Eyeberdiyeva, M.M. and Diaz, M.H.A.Z. (2025). AI and the Digital Divide: Challenges and Opportunities. In: *Management of Digital Technologies in the Innovative Economy* (pp. 283–288). https://doi.org/10.1007/978-3-031-83331-1_46.

Lee, D. and Yoon, S.N. (2021). Application of artificial intelligence-based technologies in the healthcare industry: Opportunities and challenges. *International journal of Environmental Research and Public Health*, *18*(1), 271. https://doi.org/10.3390/ijerph18010271.

Li, L. (2024). Reskilling and upskilling the future-ready workforce for industry 4.0 and beyond. *Information Systems Frontiers*, *26*(5), 1697–1712. https://doi.org/10.1007/s10796-022-10308-y.

Lokesh, G.R., Harish, K.S., Sangu, V.S., Prabakar, S., Kumar, V.S. and Vallabhaneni, M. (2024, April). AI and the future of work: Preparing the workforce for technological shifts and skill evolution.

In: *2024 International Conference on Knowledge Engineering and Communication Systems (ICKECS)* (Vol. 1, pp. 1–6). IEEE. https://doi.org/10.1109/ICKECS61492.2024.10616486.

Malik, N., Tripathi, S.N., Kar, A.K. and Gupta, S. (2022). Impact of artificial intelligence on employees working in industry 4.0 led organizations. *International Journal of Manpower*, *43*(2), 334–354. https://doi.org/10.1108/IJM-03-2021-0173.

Mettler, T. (2024). The connected workplace: Characteristics and social consequences of work surveillance in the age of datafication, sensorization, and artificial intelligence. *Journal of Information Technology*, *39*(3), 547–567. https://doi.org/10.1177/02683962231202535.

Miglani, M. and Khandelwal, K. (2025). The future of workforce development: Leveraging AI-enabled skills inference for employee preparedness. *Development and Learning in Organizations: An International Journal*. https://doi.org/10.1108/DLO-02-2025-0049.

Naamati-Schneider, L. and Alt, D. (2024). Beyond digital literacy: The era of AI-powered assistants and evolving user skills. *Education and Information Technologies*, *29*(16), 21263–21293. https://doi.org/10.1007/s10639-024-12694-z.

Ozmen Garibay, O., Winslow, B., Andolina, S., Antona, M., Bodenschatz, A., Coursaris, C., ... & Xu, W. (2023). Six human-centered artificial intelligence grand challenges. *International Journal of Human–Computer Interaction*, *39*(3), 391–437. https://doi.org/10.1080/10447318.2022.2153320.

Parra-Valencia, J.A. and Massey, M.L. (2023). Leveraging AI tools for enhanced digital literacy, access to information, and personalized learning. In: *Managing Complex Tasks with Systems Thinking* (pp. 213–234). Cham: Springer Nature Switzerland. https://doi.org/10.1007/978-3-031-40635-5_9.

Patel, A., Shukla, C., Trivedi, A., Balasaheb, K.S. and Sinha, M.K. (2025). Smart Farming: Utilization of Robotics, Drones, Remote Sensing, GIS, AI, and IoT Tools in Agricultural Operations and Water Management. In: *Integrated Land and Water Resource Management for Sustainable Agriculture* (Vol. 1, pp. 127–151). Singapore: Springer Nature Singapore. https://doi.org/10.1007/978-981-97-9796-7_8.

Plikas, J.H., Trakadas, P. and Kenourgios, D. (2023, September). Assessing the ethical implications of artificial intelligence (AI) and machine learning (ML) on job displacement through automation: A critical analysis of their impact on society. In: *International Conference on Frontiers of Artificial Intelligence, Ethics, and Multidisciplinary Applications* (pp. 313–325). Singapore: Springer Nature Singapore. https://doi.org/10.1007/978-981-99-9836-4_24.

Pradhan, I.P. and Saxena, P. (2023). Reskilling workforce for the Artificial Intelligence age: Challenges and the way forward. In: *The Adoption and Effect of Artificial Intelligence on Human Resources Management, Part B* (pp. 181–197). Emerald Publishing Limited. https://doi.org/10.1108/978-1-80455-662-720230011.

Prasad, K.R., Karanam, S.R., Ganesh, D., Liyakat, K.K.S., Talasila, V. and Purushotham, P. (2024). AI in public-private partnership for IT infrastructure development. *The Journal of High Technology Management Research*, *35*(1), 100496. https://doi.org/10.1016/j.hitech.2024.100496.

Ramachandran, K.K., Mary, A.A.S., Hawladar, S., Asokk, D., Bhaskar, B. and Pitroda, J.R. (2022). Machine learning and role of artificial intelligence in optimizing work performance and employee behavior. *Materials Today: Proceedings*, *51*, 2327–2331. https://doi.org/10.1016/j.matpr.2021.11.544.

Rawashdeh, A. (2025). The consequences of artificial intelligence: An investigation into the impact of AI on job displacement in accounting. *Journal of Science and Technology Policy Management*, *16*(3), 506–535. https://doi.org/10.1108/JSTPM-02-2023-0030.

Roberts, H., Hine, E., Taddeo, M. and Floridi, L. (2024). Global AI governance: Barriers and pathways forward. *International Affairs*, *100*(3), 1275–1286. https://doi.org/10.1093/ia/iiae073.

Rodgers, W., Murray, J.M., Stefanidis, A., Degbey, W.Y. and Tarba, S.Y. (2023). An artificial intelligence algorithmic approach to ethical decision-making in human resource management processes. *Human Resource Management Review*, *33*(1), 100925. https://doi.org/10.1016/j.hrmr.2022.100925.

Rotatori, D., Lee, E.J. and Sleeva, S. (2021). The evolution of the workforce during the fourth industrial revolution. *Human Resource Development International*, *24*(1), 92–103. https://doi.org/10.1080/13678868.2020.1767453.

Santoni de Sio, F. (2024). Artificial intelligence and the future of work: Mapping the ethical issues. *The Journal of Ethics*, *28*(3), 407–427. https://doi.org/10.1007/s10892-024-09493-6.

Santoni de Sio, F., Almeida, T. and Van Den Hoven, J. (2024). The future of work: freedom, justice and capital in the age of artificial intelligence. *Critical Review of International Social and Political Philosophy*, *27*(5), 659–683. https://doi.org/10.1080/13698230.2021.2008204.

Sieker, F. (2022). Platform work and access to social protection across major European countries. *Journal of International and Comparative Social Policy*, *38*(3), 193–207. https://doi.org/10.1017/ics.2022.13.

Southworth, J., Migliaccio, K., Glover, J., Glover, J.N., Reed, D., McCarty, C., ... & Thomas, A. (2023). Developing a model for AI Across the curriculum: Transforming the higher education landscape via innovation in AI literacy. *Computers and Education: Artificial Intelligence*, *4*, 100127. https://doi.org/10.1016/j.caeai.2023.100127.

Strielkowski, W., Grebennikova, V., Lisovskiy, A., Rakhimova, G. and Vasileva, T. (2025). AI-driven adaptive learning for sustainable educational transformation. *Sustainable Development*, *33*(2), 1921–1947. https://doi.org/10.1002/sd.3221.

Tanveer, U., Hoang, T.G., Ishaq, S. and Khalid, R.U. (2025). Public-private partnerships as catalysts for digital transformation and circular economy: Insights from developing countries. *Technological Forecasting and Social Change*, *219*, 124270. https://doi.org/10.1016/j.techfore.2025.124270.

Theben, A., Plamenova, N. and Freire, A. (2025). The "new currency of the future": A review of literature on the skills needs of the workforce in times of accelerated digitalisation. *Management Review Quarterly*, *75*(1), 495–526. https://doi.org/10.1007/s11301-023-00387-9.

Tiernan, P., Costello, E., Donlon, E., Parysz, M. and Scriney, M. (2023). Information and Media Literacy in the Age of AI: Options for the Future. *Education Sciences*, *13*(9), 906. https://doi.org/10.3390/educsci13090906.

von Ingersleben-Seip, N. (2023). Competition and cooperation in artificial intelligence standard setting: Explaining emergent patterns. *Review of Policy Research*, *40*(5), 781–810. https://doi.org/10.1111/ropr.12538.

William, P., Tidake, V.M., Thorat, S.R. and Verma, A. (2023). Future of digital work force in robotic process automation. *Robotic Process Automation*, 297–314. https://doi.org/10.1002/9781394166954.ch20.

Yu, H. and Guo, Y. (2023, June). Generative artificial intelligence empowers educational reform: Current status, issues, and prospects. In: *Frontiers in Education* (Vol. 8, p. 1183162). Frontiers Media SA. https://doi.org/10.3389/feduc.2023.1183162.

Zaidan, E. and Ibrahim, I.A. (2024). AI governance in a complex and rapidly changing regulatory landscape: A global perspective. *Humanities and Social Sciences Communications*, *11*(1). https://doi.org/10.1057/s41599-024-03560-x.

Zhang, J. and Zhang, Z. (2024). AI in teacher education: Unlocking new dimensions in teaching support, inclusive learning, and digital literacy. *Journal of Computer Assisted Learning*, *40*(4), 1871–1885. https://doi.org/10.1111/jcal.12988.

Zhang, M.M., Cooke, F.L., Ahlstrom, D. and McNeil, N. (2025). The Rise of Algorithmic Management and Implications for Work and Organisations. In: *New Technology, Work, and Employment*. https://doi.org/10.1111/ntwe.12343.

11 AI Governance in Critical Sectors
Health, Education, and Finance

Artificial Intelligence (AI) is a fast spreading innovation, which is becoming more and more entrenched into key industries, including health, education, and finance, affecting vital services and day-to-day decision-making processes. These industries rely on trust, accuracy, and high ethical principles and proper AI governance is vital. The chapter is an analysis of AI and its role in transforming diagnosis, the treatment system, learning systems, financial transactions, and risk assessment. It outlines major governance issues such as privacy of data, fairness, trustworthiness, and responsibility. Regulatory schemes, institutional protection, and industry specific issues are also surveyed in the chapter that influence responsible AI implementation. Comparing the governance requirements of health, education, and finance, the chapter reveals those strategies that make AI enhance the quality of services and safeguard the interests of the population and reduce harm.

11.1 Introduction

Artificial Intelligence (AI) is fast emerging as an element of a necessary service throughout the globe. It is employed to aid in decision-making, automation of complex processes, as well as enhancement of the provision of both public and private services. AI is applied in healthcare institutions to help diagnose, plan treatment, and manage the hospital (Maleki Varnosfaderani & Forouzanfar, 2024). AI-based learning technologies in schools and universities are used to facilitate individualised learning and student measurement. Financial institutions use AI to detect fraud, score credit, AI trading, and customer services. Such applications demonstrate that AI does not exist as an experimental research anymore, but it actively participates in the industries which directly influence human well-being and financial stability (Aldoseri et al., 2024).

The expansion of the use of AI in such key areas has numerous advantages. It has the potential to make work easier, minimise human mistakes, and assist organisations to handle big volumes of information within a short period. The accessibility to the services can be improved using AI, particularly in the regions with scarce human resources (Jarrahi et al., 2023). As an example, remote health monitors can be useful with patients that are in remote locations and smart tutoring systems can assist students with unique learning needs. AI in finance will be used to stop fraud and enhance risk management, which makes financial security better in the case of individuals and businesses (Mishra, 2023). Nonetheless, the application of AI to potentially hazardous industries also creates new governance

DOI: 10.1201/9781003776659-11

issues. The consequences of the decision made by AI can be severe in regard to health, education, and financial stability of people. Incorrect diagnosis of a disease, the suggestion of inequitable education opportunity, or rejection of credit based on biased data can be detrimental to an AI system in the long term. Such industries deal with very sensitive personal data as well and thus privacy and data security are important. There is a need to have a strong governance to make sure that AI systems are safe, fair, and transparent (Ghosh et al., 2025).

Sector-based governance is significant as different fields are characterised by various risks, rules, and ethical demands. As an illustration, the medical field requires high level safety standards and privacy of patient information. Discrimination in learning areas should be eliminated through equal access and protection of the learning process. Finance should guarantee consumer protection, avoid exploitation and stability of the market. The same model of governance will not be able to cater to the unique requirements of various sectors. The policies should be customised to the context, the objectives, and the risks that are in each area (Goos & Savona, 2024).

One of the success factors of AI implementation is public trust. The more people believe that the systems are developed in a responsible manner and are controlled by taking care, the more they will accept AI-enabled services. Trust is formed when one is familiar with the idea that AI results are vulnerable to explanations and corrections in case of issues. Hence, human control is still an important aspect of governance patterns. AI must assist professionals, and not take their decisions out of their hands during emergencies (Robles & Mallinson, 2025).

The growing use of AI in vital services demonstrates the necessity of good governance systems. These should entail legal laws, ethics, accountability, and risk reduction measures. Governance must promote innovation and safeguard human rights and the interest of the people. What has been learnt in one industry can be used to make improvements in others, but one must be very adaptable in order to meet the challenges that are specific to different sectors (Zhao & Gómez Fariñas, 2023).

11.2 AI in Healthcare

11.2.1 Clinical Decision Support and Diagnostics

The clinical decision support and medical diagnostics have been broadly embracing AI. The systems help healthcare workers to make the right timely decisions. AI technology uses big data and medical records and can give valuable information to physicians. They are usually utilised in medical imaging, disease risk forecasting, treatment suggestions, and patient monitoring (Ouanes & Farhah, 2024). The radiology images that can be studied by machine learning models include X-rays, CT scans, and MRI images. Early symptoms of diseases, such as cancer and neurological disorders, can be observed with the help of these models. The electrocardiogram (ECG) data is also analysed using AI systems. They aid in the detection of heart rhythm defects and other heart related disorders. AI could be used to decrease the number of human errors and enhance the results of patients by assisting doctors with their diagnosis (El-Kareh & Sittig, 2022).

Telemedicine and remote healthcare are other elements of AI. Smart sensors and wearable devices can record real-time information on vital signs, including the heart rate, blood pressure, and oxygen levels. These systems have the ability to notify the healthcare providers in case some abnormal pattern is identified. The method enables permanent tracking of the patient even beyond the conventional hospitals. This is particularly useful to patients residing in rural or underserved regions where there is limited access to medical experts (Perez et al., 2025). Although these benefits exist, AI systems have to be properly tested and verified to be used in clinical practice. Unqualified or prejudiced models could produce faulty or dangerous suggestions. Healthcare is one of the fields where mistakes can be severe to patients. Thus, AI tools must have transparency, reliability, and accuracy (Kovari, 2024). Human doctors still should not be substituted by AI. Rather, it must be practised as a clinical judgement aiding technology. Medical practitioners need to be held accountable to make ultimate medical decisions. With an appropriate integration of AI, efficiency can be enhanced without compromising patient safety and ethics (Khera et al., 2023).

11.2.2 Patient Data Governance and Confidentiality

Medical facilities have a lot of sensitive patient information. This information comprises electronic health records, genetic, and behavioural records. AI systems are usually developed and trained using such information. The use of patient data needs to be highly regulated to earn privacy and responsible data use (Ali, 2025a). The term data governance is used to refer to the regulations that inform the processes of patient data collection, storage, distribution, and processing. Patients are entitled to know what they do with their personal information. They are to be made aware of the essence of data collection and the involvement of AI technologies. Informed consent is a choice given to individuals on whether their data can be utilised in clinical care, research, or building systems (Zhang & Zhang, 2023).

Health data can be very harmful when accessed or misused without the correct authority. Disclosure of medical data can result in discrimination at work, insurance, or even social life. As such, the healthcare organisations are required to use powerful security measures. Data breach should be prevented by ensuring the storage of data is secure, communication is encrypted, and access is restrained (Alonso & Siracuse, 2023). In research and AI training, privacy threats are most often minimised by anonymising the data. Nevertheless, anonymised data can still be re-identified in case of a combination with other datasets. Risk assessment and continuous monitoring are needed. Being in line with the data protection laws and transparency, enhances trust and promotes the ethical use of AI in healthcare (Khan et al., 2025).

11.2.3 *Ethical Issues: Safety, Bias, and Accountability*

AI and its application in healthcare have some significant ethical concerns. The most important of these problems is the patient's safety. Clinical decisions that involve AI systems direct human health. Any malfunction of the system or wrong suggestion can lead to severe damage. It is due to this reason that AI tools require rigorous clinical verification prior to their implementation. There is also a need to ensure long-term safety and reliability through continuous testing and performance monitoring (Hanna et al., 2025). Another significant issue of medical AI systems is bias. AI models are learning patterns based on historical data. Provided that this data does not reflect different groups of patients, the system can generate biased or inaccurate outcomes. As an illustration, an AI system which was conditioned largely on the data of a particular ethnic group might not diagnose diseases accurately in other groups. This issue can increase current health inequalities and decrease trust in digital healthcare solutions (Ali, 2025b).

The issue of accountability is also one of the central aspects of using AI in medical decision-making. When the results of AI systems affect the clinical results, it may prove hard to establish who is responsible in case of mistakes or injuries. Responsibility can be carried by the health profession, technology developers. or healthcare institutions. In the absence of clear rules, there is no clear accountability. Thus, the governance systems should have clear definitions of the roles, responsibilities, and legal liability (Lechterman, 2022). Transparency is significant in dealing with accountability. The process of generating recommendations should be explained by AI systems. There must be human supervision at every phase of AI application. The healthcare practitioners will need to process and certify the outputs of AI before the final decision (Hussain & Hussain, 2025). The ethical governance systems must encourage fairness, transparency, and respect towards the rights of the patients. The engagement of the population in the policy making process could be used to make AI technologies more reflective of societal values. Ethical principles should be high to promote safe and responsible AI application in the medical field in the best interest of patients (Khan et al., 2025).

11.2.4 *Regulatory and Institutional Safeguards*

The healthcare sector is a much regulated sector since the decisions made in the field of healthcare involve human lives. The application of the eHealth AI should be regulated. Medical AI systems are not approved before they are evaluated by medical authorities. Such analyses are directed towards safety, accuracy, effectiveness, and reliability. Regulatory acceptance can be used to make sure that AI technologies do not put patients in an unplanned danger (Zhang & Zhang, 2023). Healthcare facilities are also significant in the governance of AI. Internal oversight mechanisms need to be developed within the hospitals, clinics, and research centres. Ethical issues associated with AI systems are reviewed by ethics committees. Risk management teams establish possible failures in the system and safety concerns. Trial monitoring and real-world applications are monitored by clinical review boards (You et al., 2025).

It is necessary to conduct regular performance assessments and audits following the deployment of AI systems. Such reviews are used to identify flaws, bias, or other surprises in the long run. There are ethical rules of responsible AI use, which are established by international organisations, including the World Health Organisation and the Organisation for Economic Co-operation and Development. Healthcare professional education and training is needed. Effective safety measures safeguard patients and ethical and responsible use of AI in healthcare (Wagner et al., 2024).

11.3 AI in Education

11.3.1 Personalized Learning and Adaptive Systems

AI aids in customised learning in learning. Personalised learning is based on individual student needs responding to teaching techniques. AI technology uses the data of students to determine learning patterns, strengths, and weaknesses. According to this analysis, the teaching strategies and learning material can be modified to accommodate each learner (Kaswan et al., 2024). Smart tutoring systems track the performance of students. Such systems will offer customised feedback and recommendations to learning. Learners with weaknesses in certain areas are given more explanations and practice tasks. The better achieving students receive more challenging assignments to aid in further learning. Auto feedback assists students to identify errors and gain clarity (Laak & Aru, 2025).

Adaptive learning platforms also help teachers to deal with a classroom that has varying levels of learning. AI e devices are used to systematise the learning resources and monitor the student's progress. Automated grading saves the time of routine tests. This will enable teachers to concentrate on student development and mentoring (Strielkowski et al., 2025). AI technologies enhance accessibility with the help of assistive devices to students with disabilities. Nevertheless, the teachers should be actively engaged in order to encourage creativity and social learning (Kooli & Chakraoui, 2025).

11.3.2 Data Privacy and Student Profiling Concerns

Technology systems based on AI e in education depend on extensive data about students. This information consists of school performance, learning patterns, school attendance, and other learning styles. The process of gathering and processing this information brings forth the issue of privacy and data security in a serious manner. Several students and parents might not be well-informed on what kind of data is gathered and the ways to use it in the future (Kamenskih, 2022). Without the proper measures to protect student information, it can be abused. One can use educational data to classify or profile students in a manner that is unjust or inaccurate. In a case where AI systems form student profiles, a threat of stereotyping negative ideas exists. To illustrate, when a student is classified as low performing, it can have an effect on the treatment of the student either by the teachers or the institution or the systems. This may restrict access to learning and demotivate. This profiling may result in self-fulfilment, which has an impact on the long term educational process (Prinsloo et al., 2022).

Another significant issue is data security. It may lead to sensitive student data such as academic history and behavioral data being disclosed during a data breach. Publication of such information can be detrimental to the future education or job of the students. Young learners and children are especially susceptible due to the inability to secure their personal information and comprehend the threats in the long term (Sajja et al., 2025). These risks require tough policies on data governance. Learning institutions need to come up with explicit guidelines of data collection, storage, and utilisation. Students or parents need to be informed to give their consent before confidential data is collected. The schools are also supposed to use secure data systems and access information by authorised members only (Marshall et al., 2022). The students and parents should be allowed to view their data and demand corrections in case information is not correct. They are also supposed to be allowed to restrict, or even deny, sharing data where feasible. The governance of education data should focus on the safety of students and ethical use of data and should also contribute to responsible innovation (Demartini et al., 2024).

11.3.3 Equity, Access, and Digital Divides

AI can be used to enhance education and learning outcomes. Nevertheless, when it is not implemented with caution, it can create more inequalities. There are a large number of students in low income, rural, and remote areas who have no access to reliable internet access, digital devices, and basic digital skills. The students will not be able to utilise the AI-based learning tools without these resources. It leads to the digital divide where certain groups of people have access to sophisticated educational technologies (Bulathwela et al., 2024). Agreement of access is significantly caused by economic inequality. Schools that are underfunded usually do not have electronic infrastructure and current learning resources. Consequently, the learners in such institutions might lag behind their counterparts in institutions that are better off. There are also other issues such as social and gender inequalities. Under-represented girls and students can possibly be less exposed to digital learning resources, particularly in the field of science and technology. Equitable AI in the field of education requires inclusive design. Inequality can be reduced by investing in infrastructure, training of teachers, and available learning platforms (Assefa et al., 2025).

11.3.4 Governance Standards for Responsible EdTech

Education is a very important factor to personal growth and future. This is why the use of educational technologies requires high standards of governance. The ethical principles applied to AI systems in the field of education should be clear and should safeguard the rights and welfare of students. Qualified management assists in making sure that technology assists in learning in an amicable and secure way (Kousa & Niemi, 2023). One of the major ideas of responsible educational technology is transparency. Students and their families are expected to be aware of the functioning of AI systems and the way of making decisions. Explanations are important to develop trust and enable users to doubt or criticise automated results. Transparency also contributes to knowledgeable consent and sensible technological utilization (Hillman, 2023).

The other requirement is accountability. Learning institutions should make it a point that human supervision is at the heart of key academic decisions. AI must be used with teachers, not to replace them. The teachers and school leaders should also be accountable to grade, assess and learn pathways (Porayska-Pomsta, 2024). Equity is necessary to avoid discrimination. Systems based on AI should be tested on a regular basis to eliminate bias. Algorithms are not supposed to discriminate against students according to gender, socioeconomic status, ethnicity, and disability. Constant observation can be used to provide equality of treatment and learning environments. Another big issue is safety. AI in education should ensure that the content that students get is beneficial and that it helps maintain psychological health. Systems must be that stimulate good learning processes but not too much pressure or negative labelling (Schiff, 2022).

Educational technologies must be audited on a regular basis by the policy frameworks. Data retention, sharing of student data with third parties, and commercial use of student information should have clear rules. The student data, such as targeted advertising, or profiling should not be abused by the government without consent (Li & Zhang, 2025). Teachers, parents, and students should be included in the decisions to be made in education. Their participation makes technology be in line with cultural values and educational objectives. Global bodies like UNESCO and OECD offer solutions on ethical and fair EdTech utilization. These guidelines need to be nationalized to meet local requirements (Mochizuki et al., 2025).

11.4 AI in Finance

11.4.1 Automated Decision-Making in Lending, Insurance, and Trading

Automated decision-making systems are very common in the financial sector. Lending and insurance as well as financial trading are significant areas of AI application. They are systems that process big data volumes to help in making quick and effective decisions (Wu et al., 2025). In the field of lending and credit scoring, AI technology analyses loan applications based on their income, credit history, and payment discipline. The automated process saves on administration expenses and decision time. It also enables the financial institutions to deal with numerous applications effectively. Nevertheless, when the data is inaccurate or the assumptions are influenced, there are chances of rejection of the loan unfairly. This can cause a decline in confidence of automated financial services (Maple et al., 2023).

AI is applied in insurance companies to evaluate risk and claims. AI technologies process the health data, accident records, and property data. These systems are assistive in pricing of insurance and in fraud detection. Although accuracy leads to efficiency, theoretical historical data can create unjust treatment of a particular group of people (Eling et al., 2022). In the financial market, algorithmic trading systems trade at a high rate. These systems have the ability to enhance liquidity although they may result in higher volatility of the market. To make accountability, to preserve equity and stability human control is required (Sukma & Namahoot, 2025).

11.4.2 Fraud Detection, Risk Scoring, and Compliance Systems

Fraud detection and financial risk management involve the use of AI. The AI systems are deployed by the financial institution to track the high number of transactions in real-time. The systems compare behavioural patterns to detect any unusual or suspicious behaviour. These activities can be a sign of fraud or identity theft or even money laundering. This is because early detection enables the banks to respond promptly and minimise financial losses. It also serves to safeguard the customers and ensure financial service trust is not lost (Narender & Anand, 2025). Risk scoring is also a common use of AI. Machine learning models determine credit risk, investment risk, and market volatility. These systems take real -time data and update risk assessment. The correct risk scoring is used by the financial institutions to make quality lending and investment decision-making. It also promotes financial stability in that it is able to determine the risks that are about to cause significant failures (Giudici et al., 2024).

The other important area where AI is used is compliance with financial regulations. Anti-money laundering and knowing your customer laws are some of the legal requirements that compliance systems based on AI can support. The systems automatically examine extensive datasets which would otherwise be hard to review effectively by human analysts. The AI tools prevent unlawful financial operations by detecting suspicious transactions and confirming the details of the customer. They also assist the regulators and institutions to comply with legal requirements (Mirishli, 2025). Although these advantages exist, AI systems are prone to flaws or miscalculations. False warnings on fraud may lead to freezing of accounts or delays in transactions. These practices may inconvenience the customers and destroy trust. Wrong risk ratings can also cause unjust financial limitations (Aljunaid et al., 2025).

This is why systems of governance are necessary. The financial institutions should have specified ways of overturning automated decisions. Mechanisms of appealing and human checking should be available to the customers. This requires transparency and accountability so that there is fairness and consumer rights are safeguarded. The use of AI can enhance financial security without undermining trust and regulation (Ridzuan et al., 2024).

11.4.3 Bias, Transparency, and Consumer Protection

Financial AI systems rely on the information inputted to them. AI models can replicate or amplify existing discrimination in case historical financial information harbours some biased tendencies. Some of them can be branded high risk due to their little history of credit or disproportionate access to financial services. This can result in a financial exclusion cycle and minimise the equal access to economic opportunities (Aldboush & Ferdous, 2023). Automated financial systems may be biased in lending, insurance, and credit scoring. Individuals facing financial disadvantages in the long term may be experienced when it comes to poor results in an unfair manner. These results pose serious moral and social issues. To this end, it is necessary to make financial institutions proactive in detecting and eliminating bias in AI models. Testing and evaluation should be done frequently to make sure that all the consumers are treated fairly (Maple et al., 2023).

The other significant problem with AI-based financial systems is transparency. Most of the algorithms are intricate and hard to comprehend. Consequently, consumers are not able to know the reasons why a loan application was declined and the way a credit score was determined. Such deficiency of clarity of explanations can create low confidence in financial institutions. It also does not allow people to know how to better their financial condition (Lopez & Garza, 2023). Close consumer protection policies are needed to deal with these challenges. Financial systems should have equitable access to financial products and services. When automated decision-making systems are involved, it should be made clear by the institutions concerned. Consumers should be given the freedom to access, challenge, and make corrections to false financial information. The use of sensitive personal characteristics to profile should be limited or avoided (Adanyin, 2024).

Automated financial decision-making still requires human control. Banking institutions should permit human representatives to step in to prevent the damage of automated results. Auditing ethics procedures must be performed on a frequent basis in order to identify discrimination and unjust influences. Ethical governance can facilitate consumer safety and promote openness, fairness, and trust in AI-based financial systems (Awosika et al., 2024).

11.3.4 Regulatory Requirements and Oversight Bodies

The reason why the financial sector is controlled is that it has a direct influence on the national economies and personal welfare. Governments and regulators have intensified supervision as more people in the financial sector increasingly adopt AI. The use of AI systems is only supervised by financial regulatory bodies and central banks. They are to make sure that they comply with the consumer protection laws, anti-money laundering and know your client laws, data protection regulations, and ethical guidelines (Deshpande, 2024). There are many regulatory practices that are applied to AI-based financial systems. The accountability rules of the algorithms demand transparency in the automated decisions. There is model risk management advice that evaluates the validity and dependability of AI systems. There are financial products that are supported by AI and need to be licensed prior to entering the market. Automated decision-making and regulatory review also demand audit trails to record them (Ridzuan et al., 2024). International cooperation is also significant since there are numerous financial services that are conducted internationally. The internal governance structure is also expected to be in place in financial institutions. The regulated balance will safeguard consumers and embrace innovation and trust in AI-driven finance (Mirishli, 2025).

11.5 Cross Sector Governance Challenges

11.5.1 Algorithmic Bias and Discrimination Risks

The key problem with the governance of AI is algorithmic bias. The AI systems are trained on past information. In case such data has unfair tendencies, social disparities, or stereotypes, then the system can replicate or reinforce such issues. Subsequently, AI based decisions may discriminate against some individuals or groups (Moussawi et al., 2024). Bias affects many sectors. AI systems designed to process biased credit reports can discriminate against certain groups of people in the financial sector. In the context of healthcare, patients who belong to underrepresented communities might not be diagnosed using the diagnostic tools as accurately as they are in other patients, resulting in the delay or incorrect treatment. Student profiling systems can be a barrier in education because the learners will be classified on the basis of incomplete or biased information (Varona & Suárez, 2022).

Unequal results enhance social inequalities and diminish the confidence towards automated systems. It is hard to detect bias since most of the AI models are not transparent and are complex. They should use regular testing and auditing to determine the presence of unfair outcomes. Fairness can be enhanced with the help of various and representative datasets. The systems of governance should put fairness at the forefront and human control to make amends on negative decisions (Pfeiffer et al., 2023).

11.5.2 Data Privacy, Security, and Consent Management

AI systems are dependent on big data. A lot of such data sets include personal sensitive information. Medical records, financial information, and academic achievement are some of the personal topics about a person. The information could be of great detriment to individuals and organisations in case of an unauthorised access or misuse (Andreotta et al., 2022). Good data privacy is a strong aspect that must be applied in the governance of AI. The use of personal data should be done and taken care of. Companies are expected to establish clearly the intent of data gathering, and restrict the data usage to authorised processes. People are to be aware of the way their data are stored, analysed, and disseminated. Effective communication enables users to know the dangers and advantages of using data (Mooradian et al., 2025).

One of the components of data privacy is consent management. The consent should be significant, free, and comprehensible. Users need to have the freedom to determine whether their information may be used for a particular purpose. They ought also to be allowed to give their consent whenever they want. The systems should not ignore these decisions and cease to use the information in case of withdrawal of consent (Golda et al., 2024). The other significant challenge of AI systems is cybersecurity. Due to the sensitive and valuable information that AI platforms handle, cyber attacks are common in the platforms. Cybercrime can provide sensitive information and destroy confidence in it. Institutions should establish a good level of security, which involves encryption, access controls, and frequent security updates. Constant monitoring will allow identifying the threat beforehand and minimising the possible harm (Chen et al., 2024).

There should also be clear incidence response and reporting procedures. Organisations should be fast and open when security incidents arise. It must have governance structures that establish responsibility on data protection and security management. Frequent audits can be used to ensure that the privacy and security standards are followed. Protection of privacy has to be one of the priorities during the whole AI lifecycle. The individual rights should not be compromised by efficiency and convenience. Effective governance encourages trust, responsibility, and ethical application of AI technologies (Selvarajan et al., 2023).

11.5.3 Lack of Explainability and Trust

Most AI systems are complicated and difficult to comprehend. These systems are said to be black boxes as no one can be certain of how they do their decision-making process. Explainability is particularly relevant where AI is applicable in fields of action that have direct influence on human lives like in healthcare, education, and government services. People have the privilege to understand the way decisions are made and the reason why certain outcomes are the case (Ferrario & Loi, 2022). Explainability can decline trust in AI systems in the case of a lack of it. In cases where users are not able to comprehend or question automated decisions, they can get a feeling of exclusion or being uncertain. Such a scenario may cause it to be resistant to the use of AI technologies. Weak accountability is also supported by limited explainability. In case of mistakes, the responsibility is hard to trace or rectify mistakes (de Brito Duarte et al., 2023). Explainable AI is meant to enhance transparency by making the decision easier to comprehend. Both professionals and the victims do not fail to comprehend how the system operates with clear and valuable explanations. Governance structures are supposed to demand plain and straightforward explanations. The use of AI by humans and the involvement of the population also enhance the trust and ethical use of AI (Baron, 2025).

11.5.4 Need for Harmonized Ethical Principles

AI-based systems are being applied more and more across national borders, as well as in various sectors. Such systems are usually international, yet the ethical standards and regulations across countries and industries are quite different. This inconsistency introduces vulnerabilities of protection and doubt to users. Indicatively, the laws of data privacy could be strict in a given region and lax in another. Consequently, consumers of the same online service can have varying protection cover depending on their geographical location (Kashefi et al., 2024). Convergent moral values are significant to deal with these issues. Global norms aid in the creation and application of AI systems in a reasonable and ethical way. Some of the common ethical principles are fairness, transparency, accountability, safety, and respect of human rights. When these principles are coordinated at the regional level, they give a better direction to governments, companies, and institutions (Nikolinakos, 2023).

Transnational organizations are crucial towards enhancing moral conformity. Governments like UNESCO, OECD, or the European Union have come up with recommendations towards credible and human friendly AI. Such frameworks are meant to minimise damage, guard users, and enhance trust with automated systems by the general population (Todorova et al., 2023). These attempts notwithstanding, global harmonisation is hard. Nations are varied in terms of legal frameworks, culture, and economic interests. Other governments are interested in promoting innovation and fast technological development. Other ones have more focus on the protection of privacy, social benefit and the rights of consumers. Due to these distinctions, complete standardisation might not be a possibility (Tidjon & Khomh, 2022).

Communication and collaboration is thus imperative. The governments, the leaders of the industries, the researchers, and the civil society organisations have to collaborate to create mutual approaches. Balanced principles must be permissive, but with main ethical safeguards.

Innovation should not be restricted through harmonisation. Rather, it is expected to offer a steady ethical basis. Responsible development of AI can be buttressed by strong and mutual principles that can benefit human beings and societies worldwide (Jedlickova, 2024).

11.6 Sector Specific Regulatory Frameworks

11.6.1 Health: HIPAA, GDPR, and Medical Device Regulations

Healthcare is among the most highly controlled industries due to the personal information that it deals with as well as the decisions that have a direct impact on human lives. To keep the data secure and patients safe, AI systems applied to healthcare should be based on powerful legal and ethical principles. The Health Insurance Portability and Accountability Act (HIPAA) in the United States defines the standards of the protection of patient health information. HIPAA stipulates healthcare organisations to maintain a secure place of storing medical data and that access of data should be restricted to authorised employees. It also controls the sharing of health information. Hospital based AI systems, including diagnostic tools or patient monitoring systems, should be able to meet the following requirements when handling medical data. Lack of compliance with HIPAA regulations may lead to legal fines and loss of credibility (Pantanowitz et al., 2024).

The General Data Protection Regulation (GDPR) in the European Union gives high level protection to personal data. Under the GDPR, informed consent needs to be explicit and voluntary when gathering health data. It further puts a stress on minimisation of data, i.e., only data required should be gathered. People are entitled to their data, to amend or even to have it erased. The developers of AI should need to make sure that health data utilised in research or model training is anonymised or pseudonymised to circumvent privacy threats (Pecchia, 2024). It is common to categorise medical AI systems as medical devices. These are clinical decision support systems, diagnostic algorithms, and robots used in surgery. They are considered as medical devices, and before using them in clinical trials, they have to be subjected to stringent tests. These technologies are evaluated by regulatory bodies like the U.S Food and Drug Administration (FDA) and the European Medicines Agency (EMA). They evaluate safety, accuracy, effectiveness and risks (Ajmal et al., 2025). These regulatory standards assist in making AI systems in healthcare safe, reliable, and transparent. Intense regulation not only shields the patients, but also contributes to responsible innovation in medical technology.

11.6.2 Education: Student Data Protection and Platform Accountability

The educational system is becoming more and more digital and based on tools of AI. Examples of such technologies include personalised learning, assessment of students and administration. Since students represent a vulnerable group, the protection of the data is crucial. Educational data usually has personal facts, academic data, and behavioural facts, which should be treated with care (Filgueiras, 2024). In America, the Family Educational Rights and Privacy Act safeguard the education records of students. The law controls the prohibited sharing of data and protects the students and parents right of accessing and rectifying educational data. On the same note, similar data protection regulations are found in most other countries. These laws demand school authorities and technology vendors to ensure that they protect student information and utilise it efficiently (Alam, 2023).

The EdTech systems should act ethically in gathering and processing of student data. Schools have the role of ensuring that AI devices utilised in classrooms do not adopt unfair profiling or biased recommendations. The consent management particularly applies to the case of minors who might not comprehend the way their data is gathered and utilised in detail. Consent should, whenever possible, be taken by parents or guardians (Chan, 2023). One of the main features of responsible EdTech usage is platform accountability. The technology providers should be open regarding the data gathering procedures, algorithms, and collaboration with the third parties. School authorities and governments must also do a regular audit of educational technology vendors. Clear standards can be used to ensure the AI systems serve the learning objectives without jeopardising the rights and well-being of the students (Bogina et al., 2022).

11.6.3 Finance: KYC/AML Rules, Audit Trails, and Algorithmic Oversight

The financial sector is very sensitive as any mistake, malpractices, or any other observed malfunctions can have an impact on people, organisations, and the economy of a country. That is why the introduction of AI into the world of finance is highly regulated. The AI systems also need to be in line with legal positions on identity verification, preventing fraud, and financial risks management (Johora et al., 2024). The basis of financial regulation is Know Your Customer and Anti-Money Laundering rules. These regulations compel the financial institutions to check the identity of the customers and trace their transactions in case of any suspicious activity. The AI systems assist with these activities by analysing massive amounts of transaction data and identifying patterns which are unusual. This enhances the speed of detection of fraud and illegal practices by banks. Nevertheless, AI tools have to work within the limits of the law and ethics. Wrong predictions or models that are poorly constructed can lead to wrongful investigations or freezing of accounts. These consequences may be harmful to consumers and decrease the confidence in the financial institutions (Horobets et al., 2025).

AI use in finance should be responsible, which is possible only through audit trails. Financial institutions have to record the process of making automated decisions. These are the documentation of the utilised data, training of models, and risk evaluation techniques. Audit trails enhance transparency and enable the regulators to assess decisions and recognise mistakes or malpractices. Accountability can hardly be realised without documentation (Fritz-Morgenthal et al., 2022). Automated trading, credit rating, and insurance pricing are some of the fields where algorithmic oversight is of significant importance. AI systems have the ability to operate fast and at scale, creating greater efficiency and risk. Securities regulators and central banks restrict high risk automation and insist that key decisions be monitored by humans. Explainability requirements also contribute to transparency and protection of the consumers (Ridzuan et al., 2024). Intense regulation would safeguard users, ensure the financial system remains stable, and promote confidence in AI-based financial systems.

11.6.4 Role of National and International Standards

National governments formulate laws and regulations according to the local values, priorities and social needs. These legislations deal with country specific risks of AI. Nevertheless, there are numerous AI systems that work internationally. This is why the national laws should be in line with international standards so as to have uniform and efficient administration. The international organisations are significant in the creation of global AI standards. Ethical principles and technical rules on responsible AI usage are set by such institutions as OECD, UNESCO, the international organisation of standardisation and the European Union. These models ensure transparency, accountability, fairness, safety, and human rights (Lund et al., 2025).

The international standards facilitate uniformity in data protection and digital governance. They are used to defend personal data internationally and make international digital services secure. Balanced standards eliminate regulatory competition and create confidence in the population. The consistency between domestic and international regulations helps responsible innovation and global collaboration (Schiff, 2022). Table 11.1 summarises major regulations and governance priorities for using AI in healthcare, education, and finance.

Table 11.1 Key Regulatory Focus across Critical Sectors.

Sector	*Primary Regulations*	*Main Governance Focus*
Healthcare	HIPAA, GDPR, medical device approvals	Data privacy, patient safety, clinical accuracy
Education	FERPA, student data laws, EdTech policies	Child privacy, fair assessments, platform accountability
Finance	KYC/AML rules, algorithmic supervision	Consumer protection, risk management, transparency

11.7 Frameworks for Responsible and Inclusive AI Deployment

11.7.1 Safety, Accountability, and Human Oversight Mechanisms

The AI systems, working in high risk conditions need safety as a key feature. There should be no harm to AI in hospitals, schools, and financial markets when it comes to making mistakes or untested choices. The safety measures should consist of constant system analysis, practical testing, and updating. Monitoring of systems must be done to ensure that performance is correct in the long run (Holzinger et al., 2025). The concept of accountability implies that decisions along with their support or creation by AI should be accounted to someone. There should be well-established roles in the management of AI systems in institutions. In cases of negative results, one must be able to determine who failed and what went wrong. Accountability frameworks can also contain records of model design, decision records, and audit trails (Sayles, 2024).

Human monitoring is critical as human beings introduce moral judgement, compassion, and contextual knowledge. AI is supposed to assist human professionals instead of overriding them in the process of making important decisions. Physicians will have to examine AI written diagnoses. Digital learning recommendations need to be deciphered by teachers. Automated trading systems have to be monitored by financial managers. The mechanisms of humans in the loop allow the verification of the decisions and remedy the errors before the damage is done (Kyriakou & Otterbacher, 2023). Accountable deployment presupposes the institutions to have the proper balance between automation and human control. This has made sure that technology is an instrument of empowerment and not a means of uncontrolled risk (Tsamados et al., 2025).

11.7.2 Stakeholder Engagement and Public Participation

AI governance should have the interests and rights of all the stakeholders. Such stakeholders are users, workers, citizens and communities impacted by AI systems. Within the context of healthcare, patients are supposed to know how AI tools can affect the diagnosis, treatment, and care decisions. Effective communication will enable patients to make decisions. In teaching, assessment of digital learning platforms should be done in collaboration with teachers, learners, and families. Their contribution means that technology is useful in achieving learning objectives and student wellness. In the field of finance, the consumers are required to be given transparent data on the processes of automated systems to evaluate the applications and take decisions (Wilson, 2022). People should be involved in the development of trust and accountability. Individuals will feel more confident in AI implementation when they are discussed about its use, which will lead them to trust the technology and the organisations implementing it. The community feedback has the ability to determine ethical risks that could be missed by the developers or policy makers. This feedback is particularly relevant to the protection of vulnerable groups (Marmolejo-Ramos et al., 2022).

The inclusion of different stakeholders works towards inequality reduction. It makes sure that AI systems are used to the benefit of the people and not to the benefit of commercial or institutional purposes. Participation also facilitates fairness since different views are given the opportunity to influence the process of making decisions (Chong et al., 2026).

The stakeholder engagement may be in very many ways. These are citizen consultations on emerging technologies, citizen advisory groups, and open dialogues on the risks and benefits. Another way of reinforcing governance is by working with civil society organisations and advocacy groups. Responsible development and use of AI can be supported with the help of participatory governance models. They assist in matching AI systems with the value of society and democracy (Pislaru et al., 2024).

11.7.3 Interoperability, Transparency, and Impact Assessments

Interoperability guarantees the smooth work of the AI systems with other technologies and data sources. Patient records should be available and safe in various hospitals and online platforms in the field of healthcare. Learning tools should fit the classroom technologies in education without causing discontinuity. In the financial sector, information should be shared safely among the systems to avoid fraud or financial misconducts. Interoperability standards facilitate efficiency, consistency, and data protection (Nilsson et al., 2024). The other essential requirement is transparency. The AI systems should be comprehensible to system users, regulators, and decision-makers. Transparency is not always about letting all the lines code out. Rather, it involves giving substantive explanations regarding the way algorithms work, the data that they take into consideration and the decision-making process. Open systems promote responsibility and equality (Leese, 2024). Impact assessments are essential before deploying AI in critical sectors. These assessments evaluate:

- Risks to privacy;
- Bias and discrimination concerns;
- Effects on user rights and social well-being;
- Safety and security vulnerabilities.

Impact assessments can be performed at pre-implementation (ex-ante), at the time of deployment or at the time of observable outcomes in reality. Their use aids the institutions in spotting the possible harms in their early stages and putting mitigation measures in place. In specific jurisdictions high risk AI applications have to be submitted to an Algorithmic Impact Assessment (AIA) or Data Protection Impact Assessment (DPIA). Such tools reinforce control and show the adherence to legal and ethical regulation (Aloisi et al., 2025).

11.8 Conclusion

The use of AI in the provision of such vital services like healthcare, education, and finance is becoming more significant. Such industries directly influence human well-being, personal rights, and economic safety. Thus, the AI systems applied in these spheres are to be controlled by an excellent level of ethical standards, efficient laws, and institutional control. Ethical AI governance means that technology enhances the quality of the services and safeguards themselves, equity, privacy, and confidence of the people. The risks in each sector are specific and need specific policies and protection. Healthcare requires clinical judgement and tight management of confidential information regarding a patient. Education should be fair in assessment of students and well-established anti-profiling rules. Finance should have transparency in automatic decisions and dependable mechanisms to avoid fraud and market imbalance. Meanwhile, cross-sector issues like bias, misuse of data, and lack of explainability should be resolved by merging ethical standards. In the future, governments, industries, educators, healthcare practitioners, and civil society should work together to overcome irresponsible and exclusive use of AI. AI would empower the state services, promote human rights, and help to create a more balanced and reliable digital future with the right governance structures.

References

Adanyin, A. (2024). Ethical AI in retail: Consumer privacy and fairness. *arXiv preprint arXiv:2410.15369*. https://doi.org/10.48550/arXiv.2410.15369

Ajmal, C.S., Yerram, S., Abishek, V., Nizam, V.M., Aglave, G., Patnam, J.D., ... & Srivastava, S. (2025). Innovative approaches in regulatory affairs: Leveraging artificial intelligence and machine learning for efficient compliance and decision-making. *The AAPS Journal*, *27*(1), 22. https://doi.org/10.1208/s12248-024-01006-5.

Alam, A. (2023). Developing a curriculum for ethical and responsible AI: A university course on safety, fairness, privacy, and ethics to prepare next generation of AI professionals. In: *Intelligent Communication Technologies and Virtual Mobile Networks* (pp. 879–894). Singapore: Springer Nature Singapore. https://doi.org/10.1007/978-981-99-1767-9_64.

Aldboush, H.H. and Ferdous, M. (2023). Building trust in fintech: An analysis of ethical and privacy considerations in the intersection of big data, AI, and customer trust. *International Journal of Financial Studies*, *11*(3), 90. https://doi.org/10.3390/ijfs11030090.

Aldoseri, A., Al-Khalifa, K.N. and Hamouda, A.M. (2024). AI-powered innovation in digital transformation: Key pillars and industry impact. *Sustainability*, *16*(5), 1790. https://doi.org/10.3390/su16051790.

Ali, A. (2025a). Ethical Considerations and Bias in AI Applications in Healthcare. In: *Artificial Intelligence in Healthcare Information Systems: Security and Privacy Challenges* (pp. 129–146). Cham: Springer Nature Switzerland. https://doi.org/10.1007/978-3-031-84404-1_7.

Ali, A. (2025b). Ethics, Privacy, and Security in Healthcare Informatics. In: *Healthcare Informatics Innovation Post COVID-19 Pandemic* (pp. 180–197). Auerbach Publications.

Aljunaid, S.K., Almheiri, S. J., Dawood, H. and Khan, M. A. (2025). Secure and transparent banking: explainable AI-driven federated learning model for financial fraud detection. *Journal of Risk and Financial Management*, *18*(4), 179. https://doi.org/10.3390/jrfm18040179.

Aloisi, A., Joppe, A. and Abraha, H. (2025). From 'general' to 'context-specific' data protection for workers: Insights from the EU rules on platforms, algorithmic management, and AI systems. *European Labour Law Journal*, *16*(4), 538–564. https://doi.org/10.1177/20319525251375031.

Alonso, A. and Siracuse, J.J. (2023, September). Protecting patient safety and privacy in the era of artificial intelligence. In: *Seminars in Vascular Surgery* (Vol. 36, No. 3, pp. 426–429). WB Saunders. https://doi.org/10.1053/j.semvascsurg.2023.06.002.

Andreotta, A.J., Kirkham, N. and Rizzi, M. (2022). AI, big data, and the future of consent. *AI & Society*, *37*(4), 1715–1728. https://doi.org/10.1007/s00146-021-01262-5

Assefa, Y., Gebremeskel, M.M., Moges, B.T., Tilwani, S.A. and Azmera, Y.A. (2025). Rethinking the digital divide and associated educational in (equity) in higher education in the context of developing countries: The social justice perspective. *The International Journal of Information and Learning Technology*, *42*(1), 15–32. https://doi.org/10.1108/IJILT-03-2024-0058.

Awosika, T., Shukla, R.M. and Pranggono, B. (2024). Transparency and privacy: The role of explainable AI and federated learning in financial fraud detection. *IEEE Access*, *12*, 64551–64560. https://doi.org/10.1109/ACCESS.2024.3394528.

Baron, S. (2025). Trust, explainability, and AI. *Philosophy & Technology*, *38*(1), 4. https://doi.org/10.1007/s13347-024-00837-6.

Bogina, V., Hartman, A., Kuflik, T. and Shulner-Tal, A. (2022). Educating software and AI stakeholders about algorithmic fairness, accountability, transparency, and ethics. *International Journal of Artificial Intelligence in Education*, *32*(3), 808–833. https://doi.org/10.1007/s40593-021-00248-0.

Bulathwela, S., Pérez-Ortiz, M., Holloway, C., Cukurova, M. and Shawe-Taylor, J. (2024). Artificial intelligence alone will not democratise education: On educational inequality, techno-solutionism, and inclusive tools. *Sustainability*, *16*(2), 781. https://doi.org/10.3390/su16020781.

Chan, C.K.Y. (2023). A comprehensive AI policy education framework for university teaching and learning. *International Journal of Educational Technology in Higher Education, 20*(1), 38. https://doi.org/10.1186/s41239-023-00408-3.

Chen, Y. and Esmaeilzadeh, P. (2024). Generative AI in medical practice: In-depth exploration of privacy and security challenges. *Journal of Medical Internet Research, 26*, e53008. https://doi.org/10.2196/53008.

Chong, T., Yu, T., Keeling, D.I., de Ruyter, K. and Hilken, T. (2026). Stakeholder engagement with AI service interactions. *Journal of Product Innovation Management, 43*(1), 31–56. https://doi.org/10.1111/jpim.12786.

de Brito Duarte, R., Correia, F., Arriaga, P. and Paiva, A. (2023). AI trust: Can explainable AI enhance warranted trust? *Human Behavior and Emerging Technologies, 2023*(1), 4637678. https://doi.org/10.1155/2023/4637678.

Demartini, C.G., Sciascia, L., Bosso, A. and Manuri, F. (2024). Artificial intelligence bringing improvements to adaptive learning in education: A case study. *Sustainability, 16*(3), 1347. https://doi.org/10.3390/su16031347.

Deshpande, A. (2024, April). Regulatory compliance and AI: Navigating the legal and regulatory challenges of AI in finance. In: *2024 International Conference on Knowledge Engineering and Communication Systems* (*ICKECS*) (Vol. 1, pp. 1–5). IEEE. https://doi.org/10.1109/ICKECS61492.2024.10616752.

Eling, M., Nuessle, D. and Staubli, J. (2022). The impact of artificial intelligence along the insurance value chain and on the insurability of risks. *The Geneva Papers on Risk and Insurance-Issues and Practice, 47*(2), 205–241. https://doi.org/10.1057/s41288-020-00201-7.

El-Kareh, R. and Sittig, D.F. (2022). Enhancing diagnosis through technology: Decision support, artificial intelligence, and beyond. *Critical Care Clinics, 38*(1), 129. https://doi.org/10.1016/j.ccc.2021.08.004.

Ferrario, A. and Loi, M. (2022, June). How explainability contributes to trust in AI. In: *Proceedings of the 2022 ACM Conference on Fairness, Accountability, and Transparency* (pp. 1457–1466). https://doi.org/10.1145/3531146.3533202.

Filgueiras, F. (2024). Artificial intelligence and education governance. *Education, Citizenship and Social Justice, 19*(3), 349–361. https://doi.org/10.1177/17461979231160674.

Fritz-Morgenthal, S., Hein, B. and Papenbrock, J. (2022). Financial risk management and explainable, trustworthy, responsible AI. *Frontiers in Artificial Intelligence, 5*, 779799. https://doi.org/10.3389/frai.2022.779799.

Ghosh, A., Saini, A. and Barad, H. (2025). Artificial intelligence in governance: recent trends, risks, challenges, innovative frameworks, and future directions. *AI & Society*, 1–23. https://doi.org/10.1007/s00146-025-02312-y.

Giudici, P., Centurelli, M. and Turchetta, S. (2024). Artificial Intelligence risk measurement. *Expert Systems with Applications, 235*, 121220. https://doi.org/10.1016/j.eswa.2023.121220.

Golda, A., Mekonen, K., Pandey, A., Singh, A., Hassija, V., Chamola, V. and Sikdar, B. (2024). Privacy and security concerns in generative AI: A comprehensive survey. *IEEE Access, 12*, 48126–48144. https://doi.org/10.1109/ACCESS.2024.3381611.

Goos, M. and Savona, M. (2024). The governance of artificial intelligence: Harnessing opportunities and mitigating challenges. *Research Policy, 53*(3), 104928. https://doi.org/10.1016/j.respol.2023.104928.

Hanna, M.G., Pantanowitz, L., Jackson, B., Palmer, O., Visweswaran, S., Pantanowitz, J., ... & Rashidi, H. H. (2025). Ethical and bias considerations in artificial intelligence/machine learning. *Modern Pathology, 38*(3), 100686. https://doi.org/10.1016/j.modpat.2024.100686.

Hillman, V. (2023). Bringing in the technological, ethical, educational, and social-structural for a new education data governance. *Learning, Media and Technology, 48*(1), 122–137. https://doi.org/10.1080/17439884.2022.2052313.

Holzinger, A., Zatloukal, K. and Müller, H. (2025). Is human oversight to AI systems still possible?. *New Biotechnology*, *85*, 59–62. https://doi.org/10.1016/j.nbt.2024.12.003.

Horobets, N., Reznik, O., Maliyk, V., Vyhivskyi, I. and Bobrishova, L. (2025). Artificial intelligence technologies in banking: Challenges and opportunities for anti-money laundering in the context of EU regulatory initiatives. *Journal of Money Laundering Control*. https://doi.org/10.1108/JMLC-03-2025-0041.

Hussain, A. and Hussain, A. (2025). Transparency and accountability: Unpacking the real problems of explainable AI. *AI & Society*, 1–2. https://doi.org/10.1007/s00146-025-02302-0.

Jarrahi, M.H., Askay, D., Eshraghi, A. and Smith, P. (2023). Artificial intelligence and knowledge management: A partnership between human and AI. *Business Horizons*, *66*(1), 87–99. https://doi.org/10.1016/j.bushor.2022.03.002.

Jedlickova, A. (2024). Ensuring ethical standards in the development of autonomous and intelligent systems. *IEEE Transactions on Artificial Intelligence*, *5*(12), 5863–5872. https://doi.org/10.1109/TAI.2024.3387403.

Johora, F.T., Hasan, R., Farabi, S.F., Alam, M.Z., Sarkar, I. and Al Mahmud, A. (2024, June). AI advances: Enhancing banking security with fraud detection. In: *2024 First International Conference on Technological Innovations and Advance Computing* (*TIACOMP*) (pp. 289–294). IEEE. https://doi.org/10.1109/TIACOMP64125.2024.00055.

Kamenskih, A. (2022). The analysis of security and privacy risks in smart education environments. *Journal of Smart Cities and Society*, *1*(1), 17–29. https://doi.org/10.3233/SCS-210114.

Kashefi, P., Kashefi, Y. and Ghafouri Mirsaraei, A. (2024). Shaping the future of AI: Balancing innovation and ethics in global regulation. *Uniform Law Review*, *29*(3), 524–548. https://doi.org/10.1093/ulr/unae040.

Kaswan, K.S., Dhatterwal, J.S. and Ojha, R.P. (2024). AI in personalized learning. In: *Advances in Technological Innovations in Higher Education* (pp. 103–117). CRC Press.

Khan, M.M., Shah, N., Shaikh, N., Thabet, A. and Belkhair, S. (2025). Towards secure and trusted AI in healthcare: A systematic review of emerging innovations and ethical challenges. *International Journal of Medical Informatics*, *195*, 105780. https://doi.org/10.1016/j.ijmedinf.2024.105780.

Khera, R., Simon, M.A. and Ross, J.S. (2023). Automation bias and assistive AI: Risk of harm from AI-driven clinical decision support. *Jama*, *330*(23), 2255–2257. doi:10.1001/jama.2023.22557.

Kooli, C. and Chakraoui, R. (2025). AI-driven assistive technologies in inclusive education: Benefits, challenges, and policy recommendations. *Sustainable Futures*, *10*, 101042. https://doi.org/10.1016/j.sftr.2025.101042.

Kousa, P. and Niemi, H. (2023). AI ethics and learning: EdTech companies' challenges and solutions. *Interactive Learning Environments*, *31*(10), 6735–6746. https://doi.org/10.1080/10494820.2022.2043908.

Kovari, A. (2024). AI for decision support: Balancing accuracy, transparency, and trust across sectors. *Information*, *15*(11), 725. https://doi.org/10.3390/info15110725.

Kyriakou, K. and Otterbacher, J. (2023). In humans, we trust: Multidisciplinary perspectives on the requirements for human oversight in algorithmic processes. *Discover Artificial Intelligence*, *3*(1), 44. https://doi.org/10.1007/s44163-023-00092-2.

Laak, K.J. and Aru, J. (2025). AI and personalized learning. *Educational Technology & Society*, *28*(4), 133–150. https://www.jstor.org/stable/48839360.

Lechterman, T.M. (2022). The concept of accountability in AI ethics and governance. *The Oxford Handbook of AI Governance* (pp. 164–182). Oxford University Press.

Leese, M. (2024). AI and interoperability. In: *Handbook on Public Policy and Artificial Intelligence* (pp. 146–157). Edward Elgar Publishing. https://doi.org/10.4337/9781803922171.00018.

Li, Z. and Zhang, W. (2025). Technology in education: Addressing legal and governance challenges in the digital era. *Education and Information Technologies*, *30*(7), 8413–8443. https://doi.org/10.1007/s10639-024-13036-9.

Lopez, A. and Garza, R. (2023). Consumer bias against evaluations received by artificial intelligence: The mediation effect of lack of transparency anxiety. *Journal of Research in Interactive Marketing*, *17*(6), 831–847. https://doi.org/10.1108/JRIM-07-2021-0192.

Lund, B., Orhan, Z., Mannuru, N.R., Bevara, R.V.K., Porter, B., Vinaih, M.K. and Bhaskara, P. (2025). Standards, frameworks, and legislation for artificial intelligence (AI) transparency. *AI and Ethics*, 1–17. https://doi.org/10.1007/s43681-025-00661-4.

Maleki Varnosfaderani, S. and Forouzanfar, M. (2024). The role of AI in hospitals and clinics: Transforming healthcare in the 21st century. *Bioengineering*, *11*(4), 337. https://doi.org/10.3390/bioengineering11040337.

Maple, C., Szpruch, L., Epiphaniou, G., Staykova, K., Singh, S., Penwarden, W., ... & Avramovic, P. (2023). The AI revolution: Opportunities and challenges for the finance sector. *arXiv preprint arXiv:2308.16538*. https://doi.org/10.48550/arXiv.2308.16538.

Marmolejo-Ramos, F., Workman, T., Walker, C., Lenihan, D., Moulds, S., Correa, J.C., ... & Sonna, B. (2022). AI-powered narrative building for facilitating public participation and engagement. *Discover Artificial Intelligence*, *2*(1), 7. https://doi.org/10.1007/s44163-022-00023-7.

Marshall, R., Pardo, A., Smith, D. and Watson, T. (2022). Implementing next generation privacy and ethics research in education technology. *British Journal of Educational Technology*, *53*(4), 737–755. https://doi.org/10.1111/bjet.13224.

Mirishli, S. (2025). Regulating Ai In Financial Services: Legal Frameworks and Compliance Challenges. *arXiv preprint arXiv:2503.14541*. https://doi.org/10.48550/arXiv.2503.14541.

Mishra, S. (2023). Exploring the impact of AI-based cyber security financial sector management. *Applied Sciences*, *13*(10), 5875. https://doi.org/10.3390/app13105875.

Mochizuki, Y., Bruillard, E. and Bryan, A. (2025). The ethics of AI or techno-solutionism? UNESCO's policy guidance on AI in education. *British Journal of Sociology of Education*, 1–22. https://doi.org/10.1080/01425692.2025.2502808.

Mooradian, N., Franks, P.C. and Srivastav, A. (2025). The impact of artificial intelligence on data privacy: A risk management perspective. *Records Management Journal*, *35*(2), 147–159. https://doi.org/10.1108/RMJ-06-2024-0013.

Moussawi, S., Deng, X. and Joshi, K.D. (2024). AI and Discrimination: Sources of Algorithmic Biases. *ACM SIGMIS Database: The DATABASE for Advances in Information Systems*, *55*(4), 6–11. https://doi.org/10.1145/3701613.3701615.

Narender, M. and Anand, A.J. (2025). Artificial Intelligence in Financial Fraud Detection. In: *Handbook of AI-Driven Threat Detection and Prevention* (pp. 193–207). CRC Press.

Nikolinakos, N.T. (2023). Ethical principles for trustworthy AI. In: *EU Policy and Legal Framework for Artificial Intelligence, Robotics, and Related Technologies: The AI Act* (pp. 101–166). Cham: Springer International Publishing. https://doi.org/10.1007/978-3-031-27953-9_3.

Nilsson, J., Javed, S., Albertsson, K., Delsing, J., Liwicki, M. and Sandin, F. (2024). Ai concepts for system of systems dynamic interoperability. *Sensors*, *24*(9), 2921. https://doi.org/10.3390/s24092921.

Ouanes, K. and Farhah, N. (2024). Effectiveness of artificial intelligence (AI) in clinical decision support systems and care delivery. *Journal of Medical Systems*, *48*(1), 74. https://doi.org/10.1007/s10916-024-02098-4.

Pantanowitz, L., Hanna, M., Pantanowitz, J., Lennerz, J., Henricks, W.H., Shen, P., ... & Rashidi, H.H. (2024). Regulatory aspects of artificial intelligence and machine learning. *Modern Pathology*, *37*(12), 100609. https://doi.org/10.1016/j.modpat.2024.100609.

Pecchia, L., Maccaro, A., Matarrese, M.A., Folkvord, F. and Fico, G. (2024). Artificial Intelligence, data protection, and medical device regulations: Squaring the circle with a historical perspective in Europe. *Health and Technology*, *14*(4), 663–670. https://doi.org/10.1007/s12553-024-00878-z.

Perez, K., Wisniewski, D., Ari, A., Lee, K., Lieneck, C. and Ramamonjiarivelo, Z. (2025, February). Investigation into application of AI and telemedicine in rural communities: A systematic literature review. In: *Healthcare* (Vol. 13, No. 3, p. 324). MDPI. https://doi.org/10.3390/healthcare13030324.

Pfeiffer, J., Gutschow, J., Haas, C., Möslein, F., Maspfuhl, O., Borgers, F. and Alpsancar, S. (2023). Algorithmic fairness in AI: An interdisciplinary view. *Business & Information Systems Engineering*, *65*(2), 209–222. https://doi.org/10.1007/s12599-023-00787-x.

Pislaru, M., Vlad, C.S., Ivascu, L. and Mircea, I.I. (2024). Citizen-centric governance: Enhancing citizen engagement through artificial intelligence tools. *Sustainability*, *16*(7), 2686. https://doi.org/10.3390/su16072686.

Porayska-Pomsta, K. (2024). A manifesto for a pro-actively responsible AI in education. *International Journal of Artificial Intelligence in Education*, *34*(1), 73–83. https://doi.org/10.1007/s40593-023-00346-1.

Prinsloo, P., Slade, S. and Khalil, M. (2022). The answer is (not only) technological: Considering student data privacy in learning analytics. *British Journal of Educational Technology*, *53*(4), 876–893. https://doi.org/10.1111/bjet.13216.

Ridzuan, N.N., Masri, M., Anshari, M., Fitriyani, N.L. and Syafrudin, M. (2024). AI in the financial sector: The line between innovation, regulation, and ethical responsibility. *Information*, *15*(8), 432. https://doi.org/10.3390/info15080432.

Robles, P. and Mallinson, D.J. (2025). Artificial intelligence technology, public trust, and effective governance. *Review of Policy Research*, *42*(1), 11–28. https://doi.org/10.1111/ropr.12555.

Sajja, R., Sermet, Y., Cwiertny, D. and Demir, I. (2025). Integrating AI and learning analytics for data-driven pedagogical decisions and personalized interventions in education. *Technology, Knowledge, and Learning*, 1–31. https://doi.org/10.1007/s10758-025-09897-9.

Sayles, J. (2024). Human Oversight of AI Systems. In: *Principles of AI Governance and Model Risk Management: Master the Techniques for Ethical and Transparent AI Systems* (pp. 267–276). Berkeley, CA: Apress. https://doi.org/10.1007/979-8-8688-0983-5_12.

Schiff, D. (2022). Education for AI, not AI for education: The role of education and ethics in national AI policy strategies. *International Journal of Artificial Intelligence in Education*, *32*(3), 527–563. https://doi.org/10.1007/s40593-021-00270-2.

Selvarajan, S., Srivastava, G., Khadidos, A.O., Khadidos, A.O., Baza, M., Alshehri, A. and Lin, J.C.W. (2023). An artificial intelligence lightweight blockchain security model for security and privacy in IIoT systems. *Journal of Cloud Computing*, *12*(1), 38. https://doi.org/10.1186/s13677-023-00412-y.

Strielkowski, W., Grebennikova, V., Lisovskiy, A., Rakhimova, G. and Vasileva, T. (2025). AI-driven adaptive learning for sustainable educational transformation. *Sustainable Development*, *33*(2), 1921–1947. https://doi.org/10.1002/sd.3221.

Sukma, N. and Namahoot, C.S. (2025). Enhancing trading strategies: A multi-indicator analysis for profitable algorithmic trading. *Computational Economics*, *65*(6), 3807–3840. https://doi.org/10.1007/s10614-024-10669-3.

Tidjon, L.N. and Khomh, F. (2022). The different faces of AI ethics across the world: A principle-to-practice gap analysis. *IEEE Transactions on Artificial Intelligence*, *4*(4), 820–839. https://doi.org/10.1109/TAI.2022.3225132.

Todorova, C., Sharkov, G., Aldewereld, H., Leijnen, S., Dehghani, A., Marrone, S., ... & Gargiulo, F. (2023, December). The European AI tango: Balancing regulation innovation and competitiveness. In: *Proceedings of the 2023 Conference on Human Centered Artificial Intelligence: Education and Practice* (pp. 2–8). https://doi.org/10.1145/3633083.3633161.

Tsamados, A., Floridi, L. and Taddeo, M. (2025). Human control of AI systems: From supervision to teaming. *AI and Ethics*, *5*(2), 1535–1548. https://doi.org/10.1007/s43681-024-00489-4.

Varona, D. and Suárez, J.L. (2022). Discrimination, bias, fairness, and trustworthy AI. *Applied Sciences*, *12*(12), 5826. https://doi.org/10.3390/app12125826.

Wagner, J.K., Doerr, M. and Schmit, C.D. (2024). AI governance: A challenge for public health. *JMIR Public Health and Surveillance*, *10*(1), e58358. https://doi.org/10.2196/58358.

Wilson, C. (2022). Public engagement and AI: A values analysis of national strategies. *Government Information Quarterly*, *39*(1), 101652. https://doi.org/10.1016/j.giq.2021.101652.

Wu, M., Subramaniam, G., Li, Z. and Gao, X. (2025). Using AI Technology to Enhance Data-Driven Decision-Making in the Financial Sector. In: *Artificial Intelligence-Enabled Businesses: How to Develop Strategies for Innovation* (187–207). https://doi.org/10.1002/9781394234028.ch11.

You, Z., Wang, Y. and Xiao, Y. (2025). Analysing the Suitability of Artificial Intelligence in Healthcare and the Role of AI Governance. *Health Care Analysis*, 1–33. https://doi.org/10.1007/s10728-025-00514-5.

Zhang, J. and Zhang, Z.M. (2023). Ethics and governance of trustworthy medical artificial intelligence. *BMC Medical Informatics and Decision Making*, *23*(1), 7. https://doi.org/10.1186/s12911-023-02103-9.

Zhao, J. and Gómez Fariñas, B. (2023). Artificial intelligence and sustainable decisions. *European Business Organization Law Review*, *24*(1), 1–39. https://doi.org/10.1007/s40804-022-00262-2.

12 AI and Democracy
Disinformation, Manipulation, and Electoral Integrity

Artificial Intelligence (AI) is now a powerful tool in political communication and public discourse. The use of AI can complement a democratic process by enhancing access to information, but poses severe threats to elections and the trust of citizens. Disinformation is created and disseminated quickly and with the help of automated systems via social media, and sometimes it is directed to certain audiences with manipulative political messages. Deepfakes, bots, and micro targeting can alter the perception of the voters and interfere with informed decision-making. These difficulties cast doubts on transparency, accountability, and fair digital politics. This chapter examines how AI supported disinformation and manipulation pose a threat to the democratic values, and discusses governance practices, regulatory actions, and international cooperation that are needed to ensure the protection of free elections and the security of democratic processes.

12.1 Introduction

Artificial intelligence (AI) has become one of the core elements of political communication in the digital society. The use of AI in social media and online news systems is significant to arrange information, suggest what to read, and predetermine what users watch. AI-based tools help political actors reach out to voters, draw conclusions about them, and develop targeted campaign messages (Battista & Mangone, 2025). Smarter and more rapid engagement is possible due to the automated communication technologies of chatbots, natural language processing tools, and audience analytics. AI thus has potential to enhance the involvement, accessibility of information, and participation of citizens in the democratic endeavours (López-López et al., 2023). Meanwhile, the high usage of AI in political realms poses significant threats. The takeover of AI systems can be used to generate and disseminate fake information faster than ever before. Social media algorithms tend to feature sensational or emotionally charged content since it receives more of their attention, whether or not it is accurate or not. This will promote quick spread of rumours, false assertions, and conspiracy theories. The development of deepfakes that produce realistic but false images, audio, or videos of people in the population is also facilitated by AI. This information may lose voters, damage reputations, and interfere with political stability (Islam et al., 2024).

Online discussions are manipulated by automated accounts (such as bots and organised networks of fake identities). Such systems give the impression of popular opinion and propagate polarising messages. Due to the fact that AI is able

DOI: 10.1201/9781003776659-12

to process personal data and make predictions about the behaviour pattern, the level of political persuasion is more targeted and less noticeable (Williamson & Prybutok, 2024). Micro targeting is the delivery of various messages to various people, sometimes by their vulnerabilities, personal bias, or even by their emotions. This unseen force is harmful to transparency and can make elections less fair as voters are not equally exposed to political information (Romanishyn et al., 2025). Echo chambers can also be strengthened through AI and make them more polarising. Algorithms give preference to similar content as that has already been viewed by the users, restricting their exposure to different points of view and effective discussions. In the worst situations, AI-driven content might advance hate speech, extremism, and harassment of individuals or groups. Constant exposure to distorted information may destroy confidence in democratic institutions, independent media, and an election system itself (Coeckelbergh, 2023).

All these issues are even intensified when foreign participants use AI to meddle in the political game. External actors can seek to influence voter attitudes, lower trust in the election process, or disrupt governance through cyberattacks, fake news campaigns, or influence operations. There is the need to protect digital systems and infrastructures against manipulation in safeguarding democratic procedures (Hajli et al., 2022). Although these dangers exist, AI can also be useful in empowering democracy. Responsible use of AI can enhance transparency, detecting misinformation, aiding the process of verification, and tracking election integrity (Shin & Shin, 2025). It is capable of popularising the services that are provided by the government and enable citizens to influence decision-making in a more convenient way. To make sure that AI does not compromise the democratic values, policymakers, civil society, and technology experts should collaborate and strive to see that AI reinforces these values (Romanishyn et al., 2025).

12.2 AI-Driven Disinformation Ecosystems

12.2.1 Automated Content Creation and Deepfakes

AI allows people to generate political messages automatically with the minimum human input. False news articles, counterfeit political quotes, and convincing posts on social networks may be created in large quantities using natural language generation software. Such messages can be perceived to be credible since AI can replicate writing styles and tones of emotions. After being produced, the content rapidly disseminates through digital media exposing high numbers of people to it before the fact checking organisations can react (Ghiurău & Popescu, 2024). The other significant threat is the Deepfake technology. It applies AI to produce highly realistic videos or audio recordings to depict things that people did not say or do. Deepfakes have the potential to ruin the reputation and cause confusion among the population and affect the confidence of voters in politics. As an example, a deepfake of an election candidate admitting that he/she has committed a crime or has expressed dangerous opinions could alter voter opinion immediately. With the advancement of deepfakes, it is hard to differentiate between fake information and reality among the average user (Zhang et al., 2025). Automated disinformation campaigns are bad since they can be increased ad infinitum. AI does not need a break, salary, and emotional incentive. Once it is deployed, it will constantly generate fake content, bombing platforms and viewers with fake news (Busacca & Monaca, 2023).

12.2.2 Bots, Fake Accounts, and Coordinated Manipulation

Bots are automated online accounts that are supposed to act as actual users. They are able to like, repost, follow political leaders, and engage in online debates. Such activities render bots to look human. When these bots are used in large numbers, they may give the illusion that a specific opinion is supported by many people. This social media artificial popularity can drive the trending topics on social media. Consequently, news outlets should also be able to pay more attention to these issues (Hajli et al., 2022). Political stories are commonly enhanced by bots. They are capable of circulating certain messages in a repetitive and fast manner. Political opponents are also attacked using them. As an example, to silence critics, bots can send thousands of aggressive or threatening messages. This act can make individuals not give their views online (Khaund et al., 2021).

Another significant instrument of manipulation on the internet is fake accounts. Such accounts can be managed by humans or they can be backed by AI programmes. The counterfeit accounts usually masquerade as normal citizens, activists, or journalists. They will win trust and credibility by pretending to be real users. In case of a great number of false accounts sharing the same message, people can think that the message is the real opinion of the masses (Ienca, 2023). This is referred to as coordinated inauthentic behaviour. It entails sets of accounts collaborating to share the same stories. Some of the elections in the world have employed such strategies. They aim to impact the discourse of the people, disseminate misinformation, and propagate propaganda (Grimme et al., 2022).

Well-coordinated networks usually work in critical political times. These occasions are during election days, political debates, and during major social or economic crises. Throughout these seasons, individuals could be scared, angry, or confused. These emotions are exploited by the manipulators to disseminate radical or distorted stories (Romanishyn et al., 2025). AI enhances the rate and magnitude of these processes. The production and distribution of content is fast. This increases detection and elimination challenges. Governments and social media sites lack the capacity to react in time. Consequently, dangerous material might be propagated to a very large extent before it is curtailed (Makhortykh et al., 2022).

12.2.3 Micro Targeting and Personalized Political Persuasion

AI examines personal data on scale, such as the activity on a web page, their social media habits, location data, and demographics. This enables political advertisers to come up with very personal messages. Micro targeting aims to capitalise on the beliefs, fears, or biases of a person to sway the political choices. Diverse users can get various versions of political messages, specifically designed to their psychological profile (Druckman, 2025). Although micro targeting has the potential of enhancing voter turnout, it has been an ethical issue. The voters might not know that they are being targeted according to their personal vulnerabilities. They could assume that everybody is seeing the same data in reality political messages are broken and concealed. This non-transparency is detrimental to the democratic fairness as it does not allow transparent debate and mutual understanding (Saifeddine & Abdellatif Chakor, 2024).

The persuasion that is based on AI is usually more emotional than factual. Fear, anger, and outrage are much more viral online. This may enhance political division and intolerance to contrary views. One-on-one disinformation may also deceive certain groups of citizens into accepting false statements on candidates or rules of an election or vote. Voting behaviour affects the legitimacy of election results when it is misinformed (Dhawan & Hegelich, 2022). Besides, micro targeting can be done by non-democratic bodies within the country, such as foreigners and unrestrained corporate bodies. This raises the danger of unobtrusive influence within national politics (Baines et al., 2025).

11.3 Societal and Political Impacts

11.3.1 Influence on Voter Behaviour and Public Opinion

Political messages produced by AIs tend to be targeted at certain emotions and beliefs. Such messages have the ability to influence voters in their perceptions towards candidates, political parties, as well as the public policies. Voters can be influenced by the effects of fake news when false information spreads faster than the verified information. This interferes with the democratic expectation of citizens making informed votes (Kamal & Kaur, 2025). Micro targeted persuasion is the application of personal data to find out emotional triggering. It is possible that voters can get political advertisements that can be exploited either through fear, anger, or hope. Other messages can be sensitive like religion, migration, and security. Due to the personalised character of the messages, they are not necessarily exposed to a wider audience discourse. This decreases political campaigning transparency and influences electoral fairness (Neyazi et al., 2025).

AI-generated content may also deteriorate voter turnout by disseminating misinformation related to voting regulations of discouragement of the political system. There may be certain groups that are targeted with the aim of suppressing their participation. Say, minority communities can get counterfeit messages stating that their vote is not going to count. Equal democratic participation is disturbed by such manipulation (Jungherr, 2023). When disinformation is exploited to form opinions rather than fact, then the quality of a popular debate is weakened by a lack of rationality and high emotion. The citizens are deprived of the power to be critical in their assessment of policies. The voter behaviour will be erratic and based on misinformation and not actual issues that are problematic to society (Wong, 2025).

11.3.2 *Erosion of Trust in Institutions and Media*

Democracy requires people to trust the government institutions. Governments, election organisations, and courts, the media and other institutions depend on the confidence of the people to run efficiently. The disinformation emitted through AI undermines this trust by proposing misleading and false information. Whenever individuals are subjected to mixed messages they tend to be lost. The lack of clarity complicates the determination of quality information (Gundu, 2024). When people start losing trust in the authorities and in the opinions of experts, they can start distrusting the official sources. Even the correct information can be doubted or dismissed. This uncertainty may eventually result in an overall lack of trust in authority. The citizens will lose trust in the institutions that conduct governance and communication to the people (Sahebi & Formosa, 2025).

The problem is further enhanced by deepfake technology. Deepfakes can be defined as fake pictures, videos, or audio words that look real. Their dissemination leads to the questioning of the authenticity of visual and audio evidence by people. Consequently, actual evidence can be overruled to be counterfeit. This state of affairs leads to a phenomenon that is commonly referred to as truth, decay. The truth decay declines the capacity of the institutions to communicate effectively and clearly with people (Masood et al., 2023). Journalists, scientists, and election officials are often the victims of disinformation campaigns. These groups are very instrumental in the provision of correct information. As their credibility is destroyed, people have lesser understanding of critical issues. False accusations, conspiracy theories, and deceptive assertions on elections can harm trust in democracy. More specifically, the credibility of the election results can be undermined by misleading information regarding the number of votes (Robertson & Ridge-Newman, 2022).

The loss of trust is not something that has long-term implications. The citizens who lose trust in the institutions might stop participating in civic activities. They can also gain positiveness towards extremist or anti-democratic movements. Trust is a quality that is hard to regain after it is destroyed. Constant exposure to misinformation brings about mistrust (Wong et al., 2024). In the absence of trust there is limited cooperation between the citizens and the state. Democratic societies require common facts and confidence in each other. Trust is lost, and the social cohesiveness is undermined. This complicates the process of making a decision collectively and endangers the sustainability of the democratic systems (Feher et al., 2024).

11.3.3 *Polarisation, Hate Speech, and Civic Unrest*

AI-driven disinformation tends to foster radical opinions and enhance political polarisation. The algorithms that are used by social media are designed to deliver content that provokes powerful emotional responses. The content of such is usually anger, fear, or hostile content towards conflicting groups. Consequently, individuals are presented with views that only support their ideologies in an ideological echo chamber (Burton, 2023). The polarisation separates the society into opposite factions that regard one another as adversaries as opposed to being fellow citizens. The process of political disagreement turns personal, unfriendly rather than honourable and constructive. Decision-making in society becomes a fight rather than a problem. It renders political compromise challenging and undermines democratic ideas of governance (Rodilosso, 2024).

Hate speech can also be propagated against some communities by disinformation campaigns. The vulnerable groups can be accused of economic, political, or even social issues. AI will be able to spread bigotry and discriminatory narratives very quickly. These messages can encourage harassment, violence, or discrimination on the Internet as well as the real world (Vasist et al., 2024). Civic unrest may arise when the false reports provoke citizens to protest or be aggressive due to misinformation. The rumours of election fraud, health emergencies, or security threats may gather masses behind them into a war with the authorities or other citizens. Such occurrences disrupt the stability of society and undermine social cohesion (Coeckelbergh, 2025).

11.4 Threats to Electoral Integrity

11.4.1 Manipulation of Election Campaigns and Debates

AI has changed political campaigns. Although it may be useful in making parties realise the needs of its voters, it can also be abused to influence opinion. AI will produce misleading statements, counterfeit promises, and misdirecting attacks on political candidates. This information would go viral via social media and create a negative perception among people (Safiullah & Parveen, 2022). Deepfakes form a very severe threat. AI may create videos in which candidates can say things they did not. Such videos might be shown in debates or even on the eve of the election, and it will be difficult to make corrections. Such material can cast unfavourable doubts in voters even after they are proven to be fake (Islam et al., 2024).

The organisation of the campaign debates is also affected by AI. Artificial support of some opinions can be flooded into online discussions by bots and organised networks. This distorts social opinion as extreme or unpopular views seem to be more prevalent. The artificial noise may make real citizens pressured, intimidated by that noise, or misled (Auliya et al., 2025). Micro targeting is an AI-driven process that sends personalised political messages to individual people. These messages can tap into emotions of fear, anger, or insecurity. The information does not reach all the voters which compromises equity and open discussion. The hidden message enables the campaigns to present conflicting or misguided statements, and yet they go scot free. Election campaign manipulation lowers transparency, undermines informed judgement, and creates uneven political landscape (Ienca, 2023).

11.4.2 Interference through Foreign Influence Operations

AI is increasingly becoming popular in the activities of foreign influence to tamper with the elections of other nations. These are operations that are to be used to sabotage democratic systems. Their main goals include reducing the degree of trust of the people, disintegrate societies, and influence the political outputs. With the help of AI, the operations become more efficient as it provides the opportunity to create content and share in mass. The flow of information across national borders may be performed cheaply in a short amount of time (Islam et al., 2024). The foreign players normally propagate artificial information with the use of bots and fake accounts. They are false or exaggerated information about political candidates, government policies, or elections. When repeated severally, such messages can affect the opinion of the people. It also spreads radical or polarising opinions in some of its activities. This strategy increases the level of social tension and polarization of the political situation in the target country (Hajli et al., 2022).

The other method is targeted online advertising. AI can be used to determine the voting behaviours and to target the vulnerable groups by foreign groups. They then have their sights on customised messages that are supposed to control emotions or ideologies. Such messages may be fear-based or hate-based or mistrust. By this, there is an opportunity to manipulate certain groups of voters easily (Saifeddine & Abdellatif Chakor, 2024). AI also supports advanced cyberattacks. Attempts to hack political party systems or campaign databases can be made by foreign hackers. They are allowed to steal personal correspondence, such as internal reports or emails. Through such information, leaked reputations can be destroyed and a controversy can be created in the society. The attack on cyber can also disrupt the campaign and undermine the confidence in the electoral security (Sanders & Schneier, 2021).

In addition, the foreign actors have the capability of assaulting journalists, activists, and social media influencers. AI-generated messages have the ability to imitate human writing style and language of the area. This makes it difficult to involve foreign people. Media reporting or discussion may be trying to be manipulated through such messages. The issue of a threat of foreign influence is vital to the sovereignty of a country. They interfere with the citizens in their freedom of choice of political choices. The activities interfere with the democratic processes and undermine the trust that the people have in the elections and leadership by spreading false information and causing instabilities (Vacarelu, 2023).

11.4.3 Risks to Voter Registration, Election Infrastructure, and Digital Platforms

Election systems are becoming more and more digital based. Electronic devices enhance efficiency, accessibility, and speed in the electoral processes. It is also more digitalised, however, posing new security risks. Attackers can use AI to capitalise on the vulnerability of election infrastructure. These are risks to voter registration, voting technology, and online platforms (Adeleke, 2025). Sensitive personal information is stored in voter registration databases. This data consists of names, addresses, and identification. In case cyberattacks are aimed at such systems, data can be modified or destroyed. Qualified citizens can be stricken off voting lists or be placed on wrong polling lists. These shocks may deny voters an opportunity to vote. Even partial interference may cause confusion and low turnout of voters (Islam et al., 2024).

There are also security challenges on electronic voting machines. Unless these machines are well guarded, they can easily be tempered with. AI may be used to assist attackers in discovering weaknesses in the systems more effectively. Going to the voting machine with the wrong votes or changing the figures can be done with a tampered voting machine. Although there might not have been any real manipulation, the perception that the machines are not safe may decrease the trust of the election outcomes (Duberry, 2022). Another point of interest is election-related websites and communication systems. Vital information is available to voters through official websites. This involves the time and place of voting and the process. These websites can be overloaded with AI-supported attacks, including distributed denial of service attacks. Voters can also fail to get the right information when sites are down. This can demotivate the engagement or dependency on untrustworthy sources (Dad & Khan, 2023).

Online platforms are also very essential in influencing information among voters. The use of social media and search algorithms affects the content that users watch. The recommendation system based on AI can promote misleading or false data without a purpose. This would involve wrong voting directives or falsified candidate tales. Voters should not be misinformed or discouraged when there is harmful content that can spread fast (Asimakopoulos et al., 2025). Secure and transparent digital systems are needed in order to protect election integrity. Effective cybersecurity controls and management are necessary. Unless properly safeguarded, AI powered dangers may interfere with the electoral system and reduce the trust of citizens in democratic organisations (Jungherr, 2023).

12.5 Regulatory, Legal, and Governance Responses

12.5.1 National Regulations on Political Advertising and Platform Accountability

Nations are developing regulations to govern political advertisement in the online space. The laws on conventional political advertising were made to be used in the television, radio, and the print. They never expected AI-based micro targeting or covert political persuasion. Thus, the new legislation should guarantee the transparency and traceability of the digital campaign content (Bogiatzis-Gibbons, 2024). Political advertisements should also have clear labels of the sponsors in many countries. Certain governments require that political advertisement budgets and messages be publicised in databases. Transparency also makes the voters know the reason why they are viewing some content and by whom they are being swayed (Nitzberg & Zysman, 2022).

Together with platform accountability, it is growing. The social media firms have now been called upon to be more vigilant in monitoring the political content. Certain nations penalise the platforms in case they do not take down dangerous disinformation promptly. The platforms will have to evaluate the coordinated manipulation, fake accounts, and automated amplification tools. They should also provide news on political activity to regulators and researchers (Mökander & Floridi, 2022). The governments are contemplating the limitation of micro targeting. Restraints on using sensitive personal information (religion, ethnicity, or illness, etc.) will diminish unfair strategies of influence. These regulations aid in the equal political contribution and minimise some manipulation in the shadows (Percy et al., 2022).

12.5.2 Global Initiatives and Democratic Safeguards

The use of AI to interfere with elections is an international problem. It is not weighed down by national boundaries. Foreign actors have the ability to transmit disinformation and sway opinions anywhere. Due to this fact, it is impossible to solve the issue individually. The democratic systems need to be safeguarded through international cooperation. Numerous global organisations and alliances are collaborating in an effort to develop common standards and reactions. The attempts are meant to lessen the negative impact of AI on democracy. The EU has proposed codes of practices to curb the proliferation of fake news on the internet. It has also developed very solid data protection regulations in the form of the General Data Protection Regulation. Such precautions contribute to the security of data of the user and prevent abuse in the case of political campaigns (Roberts et al., 2024).

Cooperation is also encouraged by other international communities. The G7 and the G20 promote cooperation in the field of cybersecurity and responsible political communication. Such forums enable nations to exchange information, best practices, and organise responses to digital threats. The United Nations is significant in advocating world standards. It endorses digital rights standards and ethical use of AI. These principles would make sure that the new technologies do not violate human rights and democratic values (Jelinek et al., 2021). There must also be democratic protections on both national and international levels. Election commissions are independent bodies that aid in the supervision of elections. Safe election systems will minimise the chances of interference. Transparency and accountability are backed by legal protections of journalists and civil societies. These are actors who explore and uncover election manipulations. Another important aspect of world governance is education. Digital literacy programmes assist citizens to be aware of fake or misrepresenting information. A less educated populace is less susceptible to influence. Civil society groups play a role in fact checking a story, and generating awareness (Dame Adjin-Tettey, 2022). International collaboration also assists in bringing more superior technologies that enhance democracy, versus undermining it. Collective accountability is very vital to the safety of democratic institutions across the world (Cupać et al., 2024).

12.5.3 Transparency, Auditing, and Oversight Mechanisms

A degree of transparency is required to identify any manipulation of AI and be accountable. The political actors should give information on the instances of using AI tools in messaging, profiling, or decision-making. Places should be shown to expose the ways in which their algorithms suggest political content and filter harmful posts (Cheong, 2024). Auditing processes assist in measuring AI systems to be fair and safe. Data sources, algorithmic processes, and content distribution patterns can be analysed by independent experts. Bias, misinformation networks, and ill-intentioned design decisions are identified during the regular audits before they can inflict severe damage (Cen & Alur, 2024).

Legal rights to challenge automated political decisions are also considered to be some of the oversight mechanisms. The users should have a way of rectifying themselves when they feel that they have been discriminated against or that they have been denied the opportunity to access valuable information (Balasubramaniam et al., 2022). The governments can also create autonomous regulatory institutions that monitor digital political life. These bodies would create enforcement of rules of the election, investigate malpractices, and enforce violations. Monitoring will make sure that technology corporations do not abuse their power over the mass discourse (Lund et al., 2025). Combined, auditing, transparency, and oversight mechanisms will protect the democratic values and preserve the public trust. Table 12.1 reflects governance techniques, which will facilitate fair elections and minimise AI-controlled manipulation of political systems.

Table 12.1 Key Governance Approaches for AI in Elections.

Governance Focus	*Example Measures*	*Main Goals*
Political Advertising Regulation	Labels, spending transparency, ad databases	Voter awareness and fairness
Platform Accountability	Removal obligations, penalties, monitoring systems	Reduced spread of disinformation
Global Democratic Safeguards	International cooperation, cybersecurity	Protection from foreign interference
Oversight Mechanisms	Algorithm audits, user rights, regulatory bodies	Transparency and accountability

12.6 Strengthening Democratic Resilience

12.6.1 Media Literacy, Civic Education, and Public Awareness

A good democracy needs the presence of educated citizens who are able to think critically on political information. AI propagated disinformation is fast and it usually looks credible. In the absence of media literacy, individuals might find it difficult to distinguish between fake assertions or other manipulative information. Media literacy is an education that enables people to understand how to judge sources of information, determine the content validity, and understand when they are being manipulated emotionally. It also promotes responsible sharing in the online platforms (Tiernan et al., 2023). Civic education enhances the knowledge of the democratic institutions, electoral processes, and individual rights. It is by knowing the working of elections that people will not be easily misled by false claims that affect the confidence of the system. Civic education also leads to positive involvement in the public discussion and does not encourage violence or hatred (von Gillern et al., 2022). Education of the citizens about the dangers of deepfakes, bots, micro targeting, and opinion manipulation may be held among the citizens through the public awareness campaigns. Such campaigns can either be done on TV, schools, universities, community, and online platforms. All groups such as older adults and rural populations that might lack experience with digital should also be aware of the efforts (Tinmaz et al., 2023). Media literacy and civic knowledge can help citizens avoid manipulation and make sound political decisions.

12.6.2 Role of Independent Fact Checking and Civil Society

The independent fact-checking organisations are vital in safeguarding the democratic systems. They have the primary duty of verifying political assertions and statements of the population. They also analyse speeches, campaign messages, and web content to determine their accuracy. False or misleading information disseminated is rectified by evidence-based fact checkers. This process assists the citizens to have a better idea of the intricate political matters. Credible information makes the voters make decisions based on facts other than manipulation (Shin & Shin, 2025). Viral rumours and coordinated disinformation are also investigated by the fact checkers. Lots of fake statements go viral on the Internet and social media. Fact-checking organisations minimise the impact of this content by determining the sources and trends of such material. Their efforts make the communication with people more transparent and make people trust confirmed information (Cazzamatta & Sarısakaloğlu, 2025).

The civil society organisations also play a role in the integrity of elections. These organisations keep an eye on political advertisement and campaigning activities. They examine voter manipulation with the use of digital tools. They also disclose their findings to the people or the authorities where they can be addressed when they discover unethical or illegal practices. By doing so, civil society will be seen as the watchdog body of both political actors and technologies (Lewkowicz & Lewczuk, 2023). There is a special significance of cooperation between civil society groups, journalists, researchers, and educators. False information is viral and slow reaction may contribute to more damage. Collaborative networks enable professionals to exchange information, tools, and analysis effectively. Partnerships of this kind enhance quicker identification and reaction of misinformation. Digital platforms are also obligated to help in these endeavours. The dissemination of disputed information can be constrained by labelling it and deemphasising the false information (Jaakkola, 2022).

Vulnerable groups are also safeguarded by the civil society organisations. These groups are usually manipulated and harassed. The advocacy organisations offer education, legal, and community programmes. These initiatives encourage digital safety, inclusion and equality (Sénit & Biermann, 2021). Civil society is powerful and active which enhances the robustness of democracy. It encourages transparency, accountability, and awareness to society. Civil society contributes to keeping the trust towards the operational and democratic institutions and processes through fact checking and civic participation (Lall, 2025).

12.6.3 Technological Solutions for Detection and Prevention

AI may be applied to generate threats as well as diminish them. The technological instruments are useful in identifying and mitigating AI-driven elections' interruptions. Detection systems can be automated to detect fake accounts and organised networks of bots. These systems process vast amounts of data in a fast manner. With the help of frequency of posting, pattern of interaction, and account behaviour, machine learning models can differentiate between human users and automated activity. Harmful accounts can be restricted or closed after being detected (Kumar, 2022). Another defence is the deepfake detection technologies. These tools are used to analyse images, videos, and audio recordings in order to detect the manipulation. They investigate facial expressions, voice patterns, and visual discrepancies on the pixel level. In case artificial content is identified, automated warnings may be sent. These warnings contribute to the rapid reaction of journalists, digital platforms, and the population. Early news coverage minimises the chances of fake news going viral (Pachimatla et al., 2024).

Political messaging and online advertising are also monitored by use of monitoring systems. Algorithms can monitor the process of distributing and targeting political content. This enhances visibility of digital campaigning. These trends can be examined by researchers and regulators to reveal unethical behaviour, which may include misleading advertisements or unfair targeting of certain groups. This kind of oversight facilitates political communication accountability (Azgin & Kiralp, 2024). To secure election infrastructure, it is important to have cybersecurity technologies. AI systems have the ability to survey networks on abnormal operations. Such anomalies can be evidence of hacking or access to the systems. This will result in the authorities responding in time before they cause any serious damage. Secure systems can safeguard the voter registration databases, voting machines, and election websites (Marwala, 2023).

Certain safeguards are also implemented on the digital platforms. These are the minimisation of the exposure of harmful material and mass sharing. Social media can seek identity verification of political advertisers and warn of suspicious activity. It can be done so that it minimises manipulation and enhances trust (Wörsdörfer, 2026). Detection and prevention tools, however, need to be updated on a regular basis. Disinformation actors evolve fast in relation to new defences. There is a need to continue with innovation and collaboration among the technology firms, government, and civil society. These should also not violate the privacy and human rights to uphold democratic values.

12.7 Conclusion

AI has altered the role of political communication and posed new difficulties to the democratic societies. As much as AI has the capacity of supporting participation and enhancing information accessibility, it also facilitates the processes of disinformation and manipulation on a massive scale, as well as covert influence. These dangers undermine sound decision-making and put the bases of electoral integrity at risk. The presence of deepfakes, bots, micro targeting, and coordinated propaganda networks manipulate the opinion of the population and decrease the level of trust towards institutions, media, and democratic processes. Polarisation, hate speech, and the risk of civic war are also further fuelled by AI-induced manipulation.

Democratic security needs to be safeguarded by robust legal systems, clear regulations, and accountable platform regulation. To solve the cross border interference and encourage moral digital political communication, national and international collaboration is necessary. Media literacy should enable citizens by creating civic education and awareness. Civil society, autonomous fact checkers, and other academic institutions are instrumental in keeping an eye on political information and raising a finger about the activities that are dangerous. Deepfake detection and bot identification technology as well as election infrastructure security are also important. Democratic resilience relies on human-centric based governance that values fairness, transparency, and accountability. Regulation, education, and innovation can help societies to protect electoral integrity and enhance democracy in the era of AI.

References

Adeleke, F. (2025). Reinstating trust in elections in the era of artificial intelligence and emerging technologies. *Data & Policy*, *7*, e38. https://doi.org/10.1017/dap.2025.14.

Asimakopoulos, G., Antonopoulou, H., Giotopoulos, K. and Halkiopoulos, C. (2025). Impact of information and communication technologies on democratic processes and citizen participation. *Societies*, *15*(2), 40. https://doi.org/10.3390/soc15020040.

Auliya, S.F., Kudina, O., Ding, A.Y. and Van de Poel, I. (2025). AI versus AI for democracy: Exploring the potential of adversarial machine learning to enhance privacy and deliberative decision-making in elections. *AI and Ethics*, *5*(3), 2801–2813. https://doi.org/10.1007/s43681-024-00588-2.

Azgin, B. and Kiralp, S. (2024). Surveillance, disinformation, and legislative measures in the 21st century: AI, social media, and the future of democracies. *Social Sciences*, *13*(10), 510. https://doi.org/10.3390/socsci13100510.

Baines, P., Harris, P., Hejlova, D. and Panagopoulos, C. (Eds.). (2025). *The Sage Handbook of Political Marketing*. SAGE Publications Limited.

Balasubramaniam, N., Kauppinen, M., Hiekkanen, K. and Kujala, S. (2022, March). Transparency and explainability of AI systems: Ethical guidelines in practice. In: *International Working*

Conference on Requirements Engineering: Foundation for Software Quality (pp. 3–18). Cham: Springer International Publishing. https://doi.org/10.1007/978-3-030-98464-9_1.

Battista, D. and Mangone, E. (2025). Technological Culture and Politics: Artificial Intelligence as the New Frontier of Political Communication. *Societies*, *15*(4), 75. https://doi.org/10.3390/soc15040075.

Bogiatzis-Gibbons, D.J. (2024, June). Beyond Individual Accountability: (Re-) Asserting Democratic Control of AI. In: *Proceedings of the 2024 ACM Conference on Fairness, Accountability, and Transparency* (pp. 74–84). https://doi.org/10.1145/3630106.3658541.

Burton, J. (2023). Algorithmic extremism? The securitization of artificial intelligence (AI) and its impact on radicalism, polarization and political violence. *Technology in Society*, *75*, 102262. https://doi.org/10.1016/j.techsoc.2023.102262.

Busacca, A. and Monaca, M.A. (2023). Deepfake: Creation, purpose, risks. In: *Innovations and Economic and Social Changes due to Artificial Intelligence: The State of the Art* (pp. 55–68). Cham: Springer Nature Switzerland. https://doi.org/10.1007/978-3-031-33461-0_6.

Cazzamatta, R. and Sarısakaloğlu, A. (2025). Mapping global emerging scholarly research and practices of AI-supported fact-checking tools in journalism. *Journalism Practice*, 1–23. https://doi.org/10.1080/17512786.2025.2463470.

Cen, S.H. and Alur, R. (2024, October). From transparency to accountability and back: A discussion of access and evidence in AI auditing. In: *Proceedings of the 4th ACM Conference on Equity and Access in Algorithms, Mechanisms, and Optimization* (pp. 1–14). https://doi.org/10.1145/3689904.3694711.

Cheong, B.C. (2024). Transparency and accountability in AI systems: Safeguarding wellbeing in the age of algorithmic decision-making. *Frontiers in Human Dynamics*, *6*, 1421273. https://doi.org/10.3389/fhumd.2024.1421273.

Coeckelbergh, M. (2023). Democracy, epistemic agency, and AI: Political epistemology in times of artificial intelligence. *AI and Ethics*, *3*(4), 1341–1350. https://doi.org/10.1007/s43681-022-00239-4.

Coeckelbergh, M. (2025). Politiquette: Liberalism, identity, and free speech on AI-powered digital social media. *Ethics and Information Technology*, *27*(4), 56. https://doi.org/10.1007/s10676-025-09872-z.

Cupać, J., Schopmans, H. and Tuncer-Ebetürk, İ. (2024). Democratization in the age of artificial intelligence: Introduction to the special issue. *Democratization*, *31*(5), 899–921. https://doi.org/10.1080/13510347.2024.2338852.

Dad, N. and Khan, S. (2023). Reconstructing elections in a digital world. *South African Journal of International Affairs*, *30*(3), 473–496. https://doi.org/10.1080/10220461.2023.2265886.

Dame Adjin-Tettey, T. (2022). Combating fake news, disinformation, and misinformation: Experimental evidence for media literacy education. *Cogent Arts & Humanities*, *9*(1), 2037229. https://doi.org/10.1080/23311983.2022.2037229.

Dhawan, S. and Hegelich, S. (2022). From outside in: Profiling, persuasion, and political opinion in the age of big data. In: *Digital Phenotyping and Mobile Sensing: New Developments in Psychoinformatics* (pp. 151–169). Cham: Springer International Publishing. https://doi.org/10.1007/978-3-030-98546-2_10.

Druckman, J.N. (2025). Persuasive political targeting. In: *The Handbook of Personalized Persuasion* (pp. 236–259). Routledge.

Duberry, J. (2022). Artificial intelligence and democracy: Risks and promises of AI-mediated citizen–government relations. In: *Artificial Intelligence and Democracy*. Edward Elgar Publishing. https://doi.org/10.4337/9781788977319.

Feher, K., Vicsek, L. and Deuze, M. (2024). Modeling AI Trust for 2050: Perspectives from media and info-communication experts. *AI & Society*, *39*(6), 2933–2946. https://doi.org/10.1007/s00146-023-01827-6.

Ghiurău, D. and Popescu, D.E. (2024). Distinguishing reality from AI: Approaches for detecting synthetic content. *Computers*, *14*(1), 1. https://doi.org/10.3390/computers14010001.

Grimme, C., Pohl, J., Cresci, S., Lüling, R. and Preuss, M. (2022, October). New automation for social bots: From trivial behavior to AI-powered communication. In: *Multidisciplinary International Symposium on Disinformation in Open Online Media* (pp. 79–99). Cham: Springer International Publishing. https://doi.org/10.1007/978-3-031-18253-2_6.

Gundu, T. (2024). Combating Trust Erosion. *Journal of Information Warfare*, *23*(2), 95–108. https://www.jstor.org/stable/27384397.

Hajli, N., Saeed, U., Tajvidi, M. and Shirazi, F. (2022). Social bots and the spread of disinformation in social media: The challenges of artificial intelligence. *British Journal of Management*, *33*(3), 1238–1253. https://doi.org/10.1111/1467-8551.12554.

Ienca, M. (2023). On artificial intelligence and manipulation. *Topoi*, *42*(3), 833–842. https://doi.org/10.1007/s11245-023-09940-3.

Islam, M.B.E., Haseeb, M., Batool, H., Ahtasham, N. and Muhammad, Z. (2024). AI threats to politics, elections, and democracy: A blockchain-based deepfake authenticity verification framework. *Blockchains*, *2*(4), 458–481. https://doi.org/10.3390/blockchains2040020.

Jaakkola, M. (2022). Journalists as media educators: Journalistic media education as inclusive boundary work. *Journalism Practice*, *16*(6), 1265–1285. https://doi.org/10.1080/17512786.2020.1844040.

Jelinek, T., Wallach, W. and Kerimi, D. (2021). Policy brief: The creation of a G20 coordinating committee for the governance of artificial intelligence. *AI and Ethics*, *1*(2), 141–150. https://doi.org/10.1007/s43681-020-00019-y.

Jungherr, A. (2023). Artificial intelligence and democracy: A conceptual framework. *Social Media+ Society*, *9*(3), 20563051231186353. https://doi.org/10.1177/20563051231186353.

Kamal, R. and Kaur, J. (2025). Artificial intelligence and electoral decision-making: Analyzing voter perceptions of AI-driven political Ads. In: *Recent Advances in Sciences, Engineering, Information Technology and Management* (pp. 890–896). CRC Press.

Khaund, T., Kirdemir, B., Agarwal, N., Liu, H. and Morstatter, F. (2021). Social bots and their coordination during online campaigns: A survey. *IEEE Transactions on Computational Social Systems*, *9*(2), 530–545. https://doi.org/10.1109/TCSS.2021.3103515.

Kumar, Y. (2022). AI techniques in blockchain technology for fraud detection and prevention. In: *Security Engineering for Embedded and Cyber-physical Systems* (pp. 207–224). CRC Press.

Lall, R. (2025). Making global governance accountable: Civil society, states, and the politics of reform. *American Journal of Political Science*, *69*(1), 96–117. https://doi.org/10.1111/ajps.12824.

Lewkowicz, J. and Lewczuk, A. (2023). Civil society and compliance with constitutions. *Acta Politica*, *58*(1), 181–211. https://doi.org/10.1057/s41269-022-00240-z.

López-López, P.C., Barredo-Ibáñez, D. and Jaráiz-Gulías, E. (2023). Research on Digital Political Communication: Electoral Campaigns, Disinformation, and Artificial Intelligence. *Societies*, *13*(5), 126. https://doi.org/10.3390/soc13050126.

Lund, B., Orhan, Z., Mannuru, N.R., Bevara, R.V.K., Porter, B., Vinaih, M.K. and Bhaskara, P. (2025). Standards, frameworks, and legislation for artificial intelligence (AI) transparency. *AI and Ethics*, 1–17. https://doi.org/10.1007/s43681-025-00661-4.

Makhortykh, M., Urman, A., Münch, F.V., Heldt, A., Dreyer, S. and Kettemann, M.C. (2022). Not all who are bots are evil: A cross-platform analysis of automated agent governance. *New Media & Society*, *24*(4), 964–981. https://doi.org/10.1177/14614448221079035.

Marwala, T. (2023). Cybersecurity in politics. In: *Artificial Intelligence, Game Theory and Mechanism Design in Politics* (pp. 135–155). Singapore: Springer Nature Singapore. https://doi.org/10.1007/978-981-99-5103-1_9.

Masood, M., Nawaz, M., Malik, K.M., Javed, A., Irtaza, A. and Malik, H. (2023). Deepfakes generation and detection: State-of-the-art, open challenges, countermeasures, and way forward. *Applied Intelligence*, *53*(4), 3974–4026. https://doi.org/10.1007/s10489-022-03766-z.

Mökander, J. and Floridi, L. (2022). From algorithmic accountability to digital governance. *Nature Machine Intelligence*, *4*(6), 508–509. https://doi.org/10.1038/s42256-022-00504-5.

Neyazi, T.A., Khai Ee, T. and Kuru, O. (2025). Campaign Deepfakes and Affective Polarization: The Role of Artificial Intelligence in Campaigns in Shaping Voter Attitudes. *Social Science Computer Review*, 08944393251362247. https://doi.org/10.1177/08944393251362247.

Nitzberg, M. and Zysman, J. (2022). Algorithms, data, and platforms: The diverse challenges of governing AI. *Journal of European Public Policy*, *29*(11), 1753–1778. https://doi.org/10.1080/13501763.2022.2096668.

Pachimatla, D., Kilari, R., Ranitha, I.B., Ranaveer, I., Rao, K.S. and Renuka, K. (2024, March). Advanced Algorithms to Detect and Prevent the Spread of Manipulated Images and Videos Using Deep Learning and AI. In: *International Conference on Recent Trends in Machine Learning, IOT, Smart Cities and Applications* (pp. 415–427). Singapore: Springer Nature Singapore. https://doi.org/10.1007/978-981-97-8865-1_35.

Percy, C., Dragicevic, S., Sarkar, S. and d'Avila Garcez, A. (2022). Accountability in AI: From principles to industry-specific accreditation. *AI Communications*, *34*(3), 181–196. https://doi.org/10.3233/AIC-210080.

Roberts, H., Hine, E., Taddeo, M. and Floridi, L. (2024). Global AI governance: Barriers and pathways forward. *International Affairs*, *100*(3), 1275–1286. https://doi.org/10.1093/ia/iiae073.

Robertson, C. and Ridge-Newman, A. (2022). The potential of artificial intelligence to rejuvenate public trust in journalism. In: *Futures of Journalism: Technology-Stimulated Evolution in the Audience-News Media Relationship* (pp. 127–142). Cham: Springer International Publishing. https://doi.org/10.1007/978-3-030-95073-6_9.

Rodilosso, E. (2024). Filter bubbles and the unfeeling: How AI for social media can foster extremism and polarization. *Philosophy & Technology*, *37*(2), 71. https://doi.org/10.1007/s13347-024-00758-4.

Romanishyn, A., Malytska, O. and Goncharuk, V. (2025). AI-driven disinformation: Policy recommendations for democratic resilience. *Frontiers in Artificial Intelligence*, *8*, 1569115. https://doi.org/10.3389/frai.2025.1569115.

Safiullah, M. and Parveen, N. (2022). Big data, artificial intelligence, and machine learning: A paradigm shift in election campaigns. In: *The New Advanced Society: Artificial Intelligence and Industrial Internet of Things Paradigm* (pp. 247–261). https://doi.org/10.1002/9781119884392.ch11.

Sahebi, S. and Formosa, P. (2025). The AI-mediated communication dilemma: Epistemic trust, social media, and the challenge of generative artificial intelligence. *Synthese*, *205*(3), 1–24. https://doi.org/10.1007/s11229-025-04963-2.

Saifeddine, S. and Abdellatif Chakor, M. (2024, April). Systematic Literature Reviews in Political Marketing: Behavior, Influence, and Trust in the Era of Big Data and Artificial Intelligence. In: *The International Workshop on Big Data and Business Intelligence* (pp. 112–126). Cham: Springer Nature Switzerland. https://doi.org/10.1007/978-3-031-65018-5_11.

Sanders, N.E. and Schneier, B. (2021). Machine learning featurizations for AI hacking of political systems. *arXiv preprint arXiv:2110.09231*. https://doi.org/10.48550/arXiv.2110.09231.

Sénit, C.A. and Biermann, F. (2021). In whose name are you speaking? The marginalization of the poor in global civil society. *Global Policy*, *12*(5), 581–591. https://doi.org/10.1111/1758-5899.12997.

Shin, E.Y. and Shin, D. (2025). Trustworthy AI and the governance of misinformation: Policy design and accountability in the fact-checking system. In: *Transforming Government: People, Process, and Policy* (pp. 1–19). https://doi.org/10.1108/TG-09-2025-0273.

Tiernan, P., Costello, E., Donlon, E., Parysz, M. and Scriney, M. (2023). Information and Media Literacy in the Age of AI: Options for the Future. *Education Sciences*, *13*(9), 906. https://doi.org/10.3390/educsci13090906.

Tinmaz, H., Fanea-Ivanovici, M. and Baber, H. (2023). A snapshot of digital literacy. *Library Hi Tech News*, *40*(1), 20–23. https://doi.org/10.1108/LHTN-12-2021-0095.

Vacarelu, M. (2023). Malicious use of artificial intelligence in political campaigns: Challenges for international psychological security for the next decades. In: *The Palgrave Handbook of Malicious Use of AI and Psychological Security* (pp. 203–230). Cham: Springer International Publishing. https://doi.org/10.1007/978-3-031-22552-9_8.

Vasist, P.N., Chatterjee, D. and Krishnan, S. (2024). The polarizing impact of political disinformation and hate speech: A cross-country configural narrative. *Information Systems Frontiers*, *26*(2), 663–688. https://doi.org/10.1007/s10796-023-10390-w.

von Gillern, S., Gleason, B. and Hutchison, A. (2022). Digital citizenship, media literacy, and the ACTS Framework. *The Reading Teacher*, *76*(2), 145–158. https://doi.org/10.1002/trtr.2120.

Williamson, S.M. and Prybutok, V. (2024). The era of artificial intelligence deception: Unraveling the complexities of false realities and emerging threats of misinformation. *Information*, *15*(6), 299. https://doi.org/10.3390/info15060299.

Wong, L.W., Tan, G.W.H., Ooi, K.B. and Dwivedi, Y. (2024). The role of institutional and self in the formation of trust in artificial intelligence technologies. *Internet Research*, *34*(2), 343–370. https://doi.org/10.1108/INTR-07-2021-0446.

Wong, W. (2025). Trends in Political Science Research: Artificial Intelligence and Voter Disinformation. *International Political Science Abstracts*, *75*(2), 205–222. https://doi.org/10.1177/00208345251339324.

Wörsdörfer, M. (2026). Ten reasons why: The case for more and better AI regulation. *AI and Ethics*, *6*(1), 62. https://doi.org/10.1007/s43681-025-00865-8.

Zhang, Y., Pang, Z., Huang, S., Wang, C. and Zhou, X. (2025). Unmasking AI-created visual content: A review of generated images and deepfake detection technologies. *Journal of King Saud University Computer and Information Sciences*, *37*(6), 148. https://doi.org/10.1007/s44443-025-00154-8.

13 The Role of International Organisations in AI Governance

Artificial Intelligence (AI) is now a powerful tool in political communication and The international organisations are also very important in determining the AI governance of the world as AI keeps affecting the societies, economies, and policies of the people spread across borders. No country can effectively regulate AI technologies since they work in the global arena and cannot be regulated through individual countries. International institutions offer arenas of collaboration, creation of standards, and regulation of responsible AI applications. They assist in upholding ethical values, protection of human rights and safety all over the world. Organisations like the United Nations, OECD, UNESCO, and alliances in various regions come up with guidelines, policy frameworks, and collaboration projects that help in enhancing fairness, accountability, and transparency in AI. This chapter discusses their inputs, issues, and prospects of ensuring inclusive and harmonised AI governance by countries.

13.1 Introduction

Artificial Intelligence (AI) is a disruptive technology that is increasingly gaining power in the world. It has found extensive applications in the field of healthcare, finance, education, transportation, and public administration. The AI systems are used to enhance efficiency, automatise work, and assist in making complex decisions. They also help in conducting scientific studies, economic growth, and new communications. Since AI becomes viral across the borders on a global digital platform and data exchange, it is not confined to the effects of a country (Girasa, 2025). The global nature of AI creates both significant opportunities and serious risks. The opportunities are the use of AI to solve climate problems, forecast natural cataclysms, enhance medical diagnosis, and inclusive economic development. Meanwhile, AI poses threats in the areas of privacy loss, discrimination by algorithms, cybercrime, monitoring, job instability, and fake news. These issues may be manifested across different countries simultaneously. In cases of failure or harm of an AI system, the effect of the same can be far reaching beyond the country of creation (Tampubolon & Tampubolon, 2025).

Digital technologies rely on global services of data, hardware, software, and network clouds. A trained model developed in a country can be used in a different country. The information gathered among users in most of the regions is usually manipulated by firms that have their operations worldwide. Such strong interconnection makes regulation even more complex. The local laws that are

DOI: 10.1201/9781003776659-13

based on national interest cannot completely cover the cross border activities like disinformation campaigns, cyber attacks by foreign countries, and the overall use of predictive algorithms in business and social services (Afzal, 2024). International politics is also affected by the creation and implementation of AI. Countries are racing to be on top of AI innovation, research, and technology infrastructure. This is competition which defines the world power relations and it has influence on the way nations structure their systems of governance (Marwala, 2023). The national values and priorities may cause differences in policy, including human rights centric strategies that are highly regulated in some countries and more state controlled in others. These differences bring in loopholes and contradictions in the international application of AI tools (Küçükuncular, 2026).

Shared governance is thus necessary to ensure unity and collaboration within the AI ecosystem. The international bodies offer negotiation, exchange of knowledge, and standard setting platforms. They promote communication among governments, technology/research organisations and civil societies. Through these deliberations, shared values of responsible AI application such as transparency, safety, accountability, and respect of human rights are formed. They also help in the establishment of ethical principles and technical standards that could be used in a standard manner across the borders (Gill & Germann, 2022).

The cooperation of countries on the international level enhances the response to the emerging risks. It will permit collaborative work in the field of cybersecurity, risk analysis, and the identification of unethical practices. Capacity building initiatives assist developing countries to embrace AI in a safe manner and be involved in international digital advancement. Multilateral governance promotes the balanced approach where technological advancement is combined with social and ethical aspects (Natorski, 2025). An international aspect of AI regulation is critical in the process of making technology helpful to the global population. The ability to coordinate among countries aims at taking advantage of opportunities together and minimises risks as a result of joint policy formulation (Walter, 2024).

13.2 Global Governance Landscape for AI

13.2.1 Multilateral Coordination and Shared Responsibility

The key characteristic of global AI governance is multilateral coordination. The risks associated with AI are applicable to various industries and cyber attacks, online manipulation, surveillance, as well as algorithmic bias, and impact many countries simultaneously. These risks cannot be handled by one government. International cooperation is the process that allows nations to collaborate in order to develop shared rules, control non-compliance, and decrease cross border damage (Roberts et al., 2024). There are numerous multilateral forums in the form of many international organisations that include the United Nations, OECD, UNESCO as well as regional organisations. . They are organised through inviting policymakers, researchers, civil society, and technology companies to deliberate on common issues. Through these forums countries are able to come up with coherent policies and prevent side by side or even conflicting policies. By coordinating the efforts of countries, the control of the movement of information in the world, control over AI corporations, and safe innovation will be facilitated (Natorski, 2024).

It is also critical to have shared responsibility as AI has an effect on the global markets, security conditions, and human rights. The task of ensuring ethical use of AI is the responsibility of all countries irrespective of their size or affluence. The developed countries are anticipated to assist the developing countries to build capacity through imparting knowledge, technology, and training. This would minimise the gaps in the world and we would make sure that the world benefits from AI and does not miss out (Nuño-Santana, 2024). Multilateral coordination is also useful to control the tensions of geopolitics. Coupled with globalisation and competition among the nations in dominance in AI research and infrastructure, cooperative governance offers a platform of negotiation and conflict mitigation. This coordination enhances stability in the world and leads to a safer future of the digital world (Olugbade, 2025).

13.2.2 Themes of Ethics, Trust, and Human Rights

Global AI governance is based on ethics, trust, and human rights. Ethical governance is one of the ways to make sure that AI systems do not violate human dignity and social values. The international organisations advance the concepts of fairness, accountability, transparency, safety, and privacy. These principles present an overall basis upon which the countries can make changes into their own legal systems (Birkstedt et al., 2023). Another significant theme is trust. People will never accept AI because they will not trust that technologies will be used in a responsible manner by the societies. The global governance systems strive to establish a reliable AI through advancing transparency in algorithm design, responsible data use, and informing on risks. Trust is also based on whether AI systems are not discriminative and destructive bias. To avoid inequitable results, the international organisations promote the utilisation of various data, the effect evaluations, and surveillance tools (Camilleri, 2024).

The protection of human rights is the focal point of international governance. AI systems affect the freedom of expression, privacy, equality, and access to information, among other rights. According to international standards, AI cannot be utilised to infringe human rights or do harmful surveillance. There is the discussion on restricting intrusive data gathering, avoiding discrimination, and providing due process to automated decision-making (David et al., 2024). The human rights-based approach assists in guarding the vulnerable groups. International governance promotes the use of policies that mitigate the existence of digital differences as well as equal access to the benefits of AI. Ethical and rights oriented models hold policymakers and technology firms accountable in creating AI that benefits social welfare instead of harming it (Corrêa et al., 2023).

13.2.3 *Increasing Role of Digital Diplomacy*

Digital diplomacy is emerging as a key instrument in the development of AI governance across the world. Conventional diplomacy was based on political deals, commerce, and security. On the one hand, diplomacy currently faces the need to deal with digital technologies, algorithms, data flows, and cybersecurity. Digital diplomacy is used to negotiate the rules of AI implementation, exchange the technical expertise, and establish strategic alliances between countries (Roumate, 2022). Digital diplomacy enables states to express their interests in global technology debate. Indicatively, nations discuss the data protection, responsible AI implementation, and digital trade standards across borders. Governments can bring up the issue of foreign surveillance, misinformation, and malicious applications of AI through diplomacy (Roberts et al., 2023).

Digital diplomacy is also facilitated by technology companies. Due to the fact that most AI tools are created by multinational corporations, the governments have to negotiate with them in the context of diplomatic talks. The dialogue between the government and the businesses can be used to establish a common sense of ethical obligations and regulatory demands (Bjola & Manor, 2025). Peace and security are also the concerns of digital diplomacy. AI technologies have the ability to affect military systems, cybersecurity actions, and international conflict. Diplomatic treaties can minimise the chance of applying AI to war or spying. The debate on AI safety, checkpoints, and responsible innovation assists in developing trust between countries (Radanliev, 2025).

Moreover, digital diplomacy helps in the development of the world. Countries also work with each other to exchange AI expertise, research, and technical expertise. Such collaborations enable the poor countries to be part of the AI economy and develop domestic capabilities. Digital diplomacy also promotes collaboration in the field of scientific studies, climate modelling, health technologies, and the management of disasters (Sepasspour, 2023). The relations in the international arena are progressively being tied to the way of managing digital technologies by the countries. Because of this, diplomatic institutions need to evolve to learn AI, conclude agreements, and assist with coordination on the international level (Huang, 2025).

13.3 United Nations and Human Centric AI Governance

13.3.1 *UN Guiding Principles on Ethics and Human Rights*

The United Nations is keen on ensuring that AI upholds international human rights law at all times. These rights encompass equality rights, privacy rights, freedom of expression rights, and the right against discrimination. Some of the ethical concepts promoted by the UN are fairness, accountability, transparency, and safety. These ethics are followed by governments and technology enterprises in order to create and implement AI systems in a responsible manner (Lane, 2023). The Human Rights Council of the UN has expressed concern over the use of AI in surveillance, profiling, as well as predictive policing. Automation can either heighten discrimination or offend privacy. The UN proposes security measures to make sure that no AI system is used to harm people and limit civil liberties. This encompasses explicit guidelines on how the data is being safeguarded, transparency in algorithms, and human control (Corrêa et al., 2023).

Inclusion is also an ethical requirement that is promoted by the UN. AI should be beneficial to every individual irrespective of their gender, age, disability, race, or economic status. The approach to inclusivity will help to minimise worldwide disparities and avoid any reinforcement of historical discrimination by AI systems. The UN urges countries to implement legislations that promote equal access to technological advancements and safeguard the vulnerable groups against technological abuse (Camilleri, 2024).

13.3.2 SDGs and AI for Sustainable Development

The United Nations Sustainable Development Goals (SDGs) give a worldwide idea of peace, prosperity, and environmental safeguards. When applied in a responsible manner, AI can achieve most of these objectives. In the example, AI helps pursue SDG 3 (Good Health and Well-Being) through better disease diagnosis, epidemic tracking, and health logistics assistance. It promotes SDG 13 (Climate Action) with climate modelling, early warning, and environmental observation. AI is also used in SDG 4 (Quality Education) by providing personalised learning resources and online platforms that increase access to learning content (Gohr et al., 2025). Nonetheless, the UN cautions that AI may also cripple sustainability in case risks are overlooked. The uncontrolled automation can lead to worsening economic inequality or the depletion of job opportunities because algorithms can be utilized to enlarge the existing disparities. Those countries which do not have digital infrastructure can stay behind, increasing disparities in the development of the world. Inclusive digital transformation is thus a priority of the UN in relation to sustainable development. These involve investment in digital infrastructure, AI education and ethical data governance (Madavarapu et al., 2024).

AI has to be in line with the SDGs so that positive long-term results can be achieved. The UN stimulates governments to incorporate sustainability objectives in national AI policies. It is also willing to assist developing nations by providing them with training programmes, financial assistance, and technical collaborations in order to enable them to apply AI to realise their development goals (Kulkov et al., 2024).

13.3.3 Roles of ITU, UNDP, OHCHR in AI Governance

The efforts of the UN in AI governance are performed by several special agencies, each of which brings a certain angle. International Telecommunication Union (ITU) is a significant actor in establishing technical standards within the global environment. It works on AI interoperability guidelines, infrastructure security guidelines, and digital connectivity guidelines. Also at ITU is the annual summit of AI for Good whereby innovators and policymakers convene to talk about useful AI applications in health, agriculture, climate, and education (Taylor, 2025). The United Nations Development Programme (UNDP) deals with AI as an economic and social development. It guides governments on how to plan national AI policies, enhance digital capabilities, as well as develop governance systems. Another study that UNDP undertakes is the role of AI in inequality, workforce, and administration. The agency assists low and middle income nations to contribute to global AI innovation by training, providing resources and collaborating with them (Kong et al., 2023).

The human rights implication of AI systems is observed by the Office of the High Commissioner of Human Rights (OHCHR). It also explores the situations in which AI can cause harm to individuals or disregard liberties, including discriminative algorithms or invasive surveillance technology. OHCHR collaborates with the governments to set rights based AI laws. It also promotes openness and responsibility in autonomous decision-making (Strange & Tucker, 2024). With the joint efforts of ITU, UNDP, and OHCHR, the global governance of AI has a powerful institutional base. Their joint effort will guarantee the technical, ethical, and social inclusiveness of AI development.

13.3.4 UN Led Global Dialogues and Capacity Building Initiatives

The UN helps in international discussion of AI governance by conferences, expert groups, and policy consultations. Such discussions enable countries to exchange best practices, harmonise regulatory policies, and deliberate on new risks. The developed countries can assist other countries in knowing about new technologies whereas developing countries demonstrate their demands to have equal access (Misuraca et al., 2024). One of the priorities of the UN is capacity building. There are a large number of countries that do not have technical skills, internet infrastructure, or funding to control AI. The UN provides advisory services, digital literacy programmes, workshops, and training programmes. Such initiatives will enhance the national AI preparedness and make sure that weaker economies are not lagged behind in international AI development (Natorski, 2025).

Another way in which the UN facilitates cross-border cooperation is through research networks and collaboration with universities, civil societies as well as the private sector. Such partnerships widen world knowledge and assist countries to react promptly to novel AI dilemmas (Calderaro, 2025). The UN promotes openness in the development of AI by sponsoring open data programmes, ethical reporting standards, and algorithmic disclosure guidelines. This enhances responsibility and boosts the confidence of AI systems internationally (Yilma, 2025). Table 13.1 provides some of the significant UN initiatives that would facilitate international collaboration, ethical standards, and inclusive human-based governance in the field of AI development.

Table 3.1 UN Contributions to Human Centric AI Governance.

UN Focus Area	*Main Actions*	*Governance Outcomes*
Ethical & Human Rights Principles	Guidelines, rights oversight, non-discrimination	Protection of dignity and equality
Sustainable Development	AI for SDGs, inclusive digital transformation	Social progress and reduced inequality
Institutional Support (ITU, UNDP, OHCHR)	Standards, capacity-building, rights monitoring	Responsible and coordinated global governance
Global Cooperation & Capacity	Dialogues, training, partnerships	Stronger national readiness and shared benefits

13.4 OECD, UNESCO, and Regional Governance Efforts

13.4.1 OECD AI Principles and Global Policy Alignment

The OECD was one of the first bodies to publish comprehensive AI governance principles. These principles highlight five major ideas (Erkkilä, 2023):

- AI should support human-centred values and fairness;
- AI systems should be transparent and explainable;
- Safety, robustness, and security must be ensured;
- Accountability should be guaranteed;
- Inclusive growth and well-being should be promoted.

The OECD AI Principles have been incorporated in over 40 countries. These consist of the G20 and other countries that are in partnership. The principles form the basis of writing of their own national AI strategies by many nations. Consequently, there has been increased harmonisation of policies across the globe. Research and sharing of data is also encouraged in the OECD. It has established the OECD.AI Policy Observatory that gathers data on national AI policies, regulatory experiments, and innovation programmes. Through this platform, governments are able to learn about each other, and keep track of the global progress (Roberts et al., 2024). The risk of fragmented regulation is minimised with the aid of the OECD principles. When numerous countries are guided by the same principles, AI companies can be provided with more definite expectations and motivated to be responsible (Huang et al., 2024).

13.4.2 UNESCO Recommendation on Ethics of AI

UNESCO is concerned with the ethical side of AI. UNESCO has, in 2021, embraced the Recommendation on the Ethics of Artificial Intelligence, which is the first international framework endorsed by approximately 200 states. It focuses on equality, cultural diversity, human rights, and peace (Van Norren, 2023).

UNESCO calls for:

- Elimination of algorithmic bias and discrimination;
- Protection of privacy and personal data;
- Environmental sustainability in AI development;
- Ethical oversight in high-risk AI applications;
- Public participation in AI governance.

Educational programmes are also encouraged by UNESCO to make citizens aware about the risks and benefits of AI use. It promotes gender equity in the AI-related areas and contributes to the representation of under-represented populations in the policymaking process. The recommendation guides governments in formulation of laws countrywide. It also impacts the technology developers through responsible innovation and responsibility (Bean et al., 2025).

13.4.3 European Union and Regional Policy Leadership

The European Union (EU) is a leader in strong and rights-based AI governance. The EU has introduced major regulations such as:

- General Data Protection Regulation (GDPR) for data rights;
- Digital Services Act for platform accountability;
- EU AI Act for risk based regulation of AI systems.

The EU is more concerned with human rights, security, and ethical management. The use of AI with high risks to the rights of the community, e.g., facial recognition, predictive policing, etc. should be heavily controlled, transparently reported, and supervised by humans (Justo-Hanani, 2022). The EU also spends on research and collaborative innovation with schemes such as Horizon Europe. Such developments are meant to enhance AI potentials, but the technology should be used to promote democracy. Through this, the EU has become an example to other nations that are formulating the same policies. Its management promotes international conformity to high ethical standards (Brandão, 2024).

13.4.4 Regional Cooperation in Africa, Asia Pacific, and Latin America

The Global South is also increasingly operating AI governance within regional alliances.

The African Union (AU) is developing a continental AI strategy that is aimed at development, social good, and digital inclusion. It notes that local capacity should be developed, they should not be dependent on foreign technologies, and human rights must be safeguarded in automated systems (Effoduh et al., 2024). There is collaboration in the Asian Pacific region via the ASEAN, APEC, and national alliances. These organisations venture into digital governance, cybersecurity, and responsible innovation. Examples of countries with good national AI policies are Japan, South Korea, and Singapore, which impact the alignment of the region (Keith, 2024).

In Latin America, agencies such as the Inter-American Development Bank (IDB) are funding AI governance on social protection, equitable access, and improving the delivery of services to the population. Brazil, Chile, and Mexico are some of the countries that have started to embrace ethical AI concepts in the administration (Zambrano et al., 2021). Regional cooperation assists nations to exchange knowledge, develop digital infrastructure, and develop frameworks in accordance with the values and economic conditions of the region. It also enhances the shared decision-making at the global level. Table 13.2 gives an overview of key international and regional bodies influencing AI governance via standards, ethical frameworks, and collaborative efforts.

Table 13.2 Major International and Regional AI Governance Efforts.

Organisation/ Region	*Key Governance Actions*	*Focus Areas*
OECD	Global AI principles, policy monitoring	Fairness, accountability, policy alignment
UNESCO	Ethical AI recommendation, education	Human rights, inclusion, sustainability
European Union	GDPR, EU AI Act, oversight systems	Safety, transparency, rights protection
Africa / Asia Pacific / Latin America	Regional strategies and cooperation networks	Capacity-building, development, digital inclusion

13.5 International Standards and Technical Frameworks

13.5.1 ISO, IEC, and IEEE Standards

The International Organization of Standardization (ISO) and the International Electrotechnical Commission (IEC) collaborate in AI standards by having a joint technical committee (ISO/IEC JTC 1/SC 42). This body develops international guidelines on what AI is and how it ought to be handled at its lifecycle. Such standards enable the policymakers to formulate effective legislation since they contain technicalities that capture current scientific knowledge (Oviedo et al., 2024).

ISO/IEC standards address areas such as:

- AI terminology and classification;
- System performance and testing methods;
- Data quality and bias mitigation;
- Transparency and documentation practices;
- Robustness and resilience of models.

These guidelines are used by companies and governmental organisations to adopt AI in harmless and regular manners. They also facilitate international trade as companies will be able to design the products that will be used in various markets with the same demands. The Institute of Electrical and Electronics Engineers

(IEEE) comes up with standards that are concerned with the societal and ethical effects of AI. IEEE focuses on human rights, safety, and responsibility of the people. Among its most significant contributions, one can note the Ethically Aligned Design framework that provides reasonable advice to engineers and designers (Agarwal & Nene, 2025).

IEEE standards encourage:

- Clear explanation of AI decisions;
- Protection of user privacy;
- Respect for human autonomy;
- Prevention of discriminatory outcomes;
- Responsible control of autonomous systems.

Robotics, autonomous vehicles, and intelligent sensors are some of the emerging technologies that use IEEE standards. Together, the ISO/IEC and the IEEE standards are the pillars of technical governance in AI. They foster trust and make systems constructed based on shared global values.

13.5.2 Safety, Interoperability, and Risk Management Guidelines

The AI systems should be accessible and be safe to operate in various settings and to everyone. Security protocols can be used to avoid accidents and adverse consequences. They make AI act in a predictable manner even in the case of a change in conditions. To deal with the failures, risk testing and tests every so often are needed in order to detect the weak points (Yang, 2023).

Safety guidelines include:

- Robustness against errors and malicious attacks;
- Secure handling of sensitive data;
- Fail safe mechanisms in critical applications like transportation and healthcare;
- Human supervision in high risk systems.

Another standardisation goal is interoperability. The AI products should be compatible with one another, even when they are manufactured by the different companies or implemented in the varied nations. Interoperability avoids market fragmentation and is beneficial to technological collaborations (Wirtz et al., 2022).

Examples include:

- Common data formats that allow information sharing;
- Standard communication protocols among devices;
- Compatibility across cloud infrastructures and networks.

Risk management models assist organisations to prepare against the possibility of issues in the area of AI implementation. These models involve the systematic assessment mechanisms to find, quantify, and limit risks. They advise that they should be constantly monitored since there are chances of increased risks post deployment as systems learn and modify. Most importantly, risk management should be considered in systems that have effects on human rights, national governance, or public security. Safety, interoperability, and risk management are preventive controls that societies are safe, and AI is trustworthy (Sayles, 2024).

13.5.3 Role of Industry Consortia in Standard Setting

The technological firms and individual partnerships have significant influence on AI standards since they have direct access to extensive systems and real-life information. Their real-world experience can be used to spot problems that otherwise would not be realised in the laboratory development. The role of industry in furthering innovation also quickens the process since innovation takes the form of standards that capture technological advancement in a fast manner (von Ingersleben-Seip, 2023).

Several industry consortia contribute to AI governance, including:

- Global Partnership on AI (GPAI);
- Partnership on AI (PAI);
- OpenAI collaborative governance initiatives;
- Sector specific alliances in finance, healthcare, and cybersecurity.

Their work focuses on:

- Best practices for ethical development;
- Tools to reduce algorithmic bias and improve explainability;
- Guidelines for safe deployment of AI in public services;
- Sharing research, knowledge, and training resources;
- Cooperation between companies, universities, and policymakers.

Pilot projects are also conducted by groups in the industry to experiment with governance approaches under actual conditions. Such pilots give evidence to the regulators to come up with more effective laws. The partnership between the public and the private enhances the governance through integration of social and legal views with technical knowledge (Cantero Gamito & Marsden, 2024). Responsibility is however also needed in dependence on industry consortia. Business interests might take precedence over the business, and therefore the policy makers should make sure that the standards they assist in formulating are pro-democratic and conducive to the welfare of the people (Cantero Gamito, 2024).

13.6 Cooperation Mechanisms and Policy Harmonization

13.6.1 Cross Border Data Governance Frameworks

AI depends on data greatly, and a part of the data is obtained, processed, and stored across the borders. The national laws contrast on privacy, security, and data transfer have posed a challenge in companies and institutions that conduct business internationally. Cross-border data governance systems seek to overcome such problems by establishing common rules that ensure safety in the transfer of data between the nations. Such structures help build trust since the standards of data protection will be high even at the point where the information is transferred across jurisdictions (Marcucci et al., 2023). Certain geographical areas value stringent privacy restrictions whereas others emphasise more on facilitating digital trade and economic development. Regardless of such variations, various nations are becoming aware of the necessity of consistent systems within which there is a safeguard of individual rights and encouragement of creativity (Kuzio et al., 2022). These contracts can be used to avoid data misuse, lower legal risks in business, and establish environments that are predictable when developing AI. They are also conducive to global collaboration in such fields as cybersecurity, state administration, healthcare, and environmental regulation. With the growth of digital platforms, harmonised data governance is the key to the stable and ethical implementation of AI in the world (Rong et al., 2025).

13.6.2 Joint Innovation Programmes and Research Networks

Another important mechanism on enhancing AI governance is international cooperation in innovation. The AI study is fast growing and demands great amounts of money, computing resources, and skills. The demands cannot be fulfilled by many countries on their own. Through joint innovation, there is the possibility of shared research, technological development, and collaboration between universities, governments, and the private companies. Such programmes also allow knowledge and resources to be pooled to expedite the process of scientific advancement (Liebig et al., 2024). Research networks provide spaces in which scientists and policy makers investigate solutions to common problems including climate change, public health, and sustainable development. The testing of the standards of ethical guidelines and safety standards in real-life situations is also facilitated in collaborative projects. Joint innovation eliminates work redundancy and enables countries to enjoy the fruits of collaborative discoveries. In the case of emerging countries, joining such networks allows them to access superior tools, experience, and the world research community. This is beneficial in closing the gap between technologically developed countries and those that have a weak research capacity (Birkstedt et al., 2023). The global collaboration in the area of innovation promotes cultural exchange as well as the creation of diverse AI solutions that take into account local languages, values, and social behaviour. The collaboration of countries provides AI systems which are diverse and efficient in terms of technological development throughout the whole world (Makridis et al., 2024).

13.6.3 Knowledge Sharing and Capacity Development for Emerging Economies

Most countries, especially in Africa, Asia Pacific, and Latin America, struggle with the adoption of AI because of the weak infrastructure, lack of trained professionals, and inadequate financial resources. Devoid of assistance, they will end up relying on the technologies of other countries or being left behind in AI-driven growth.

Dissemination of knowledge and capacity building are thus important aspects of international collaboration (Rezaei et al., 2025). Capacity development involves educating the government officials to come up with responsible AI policies, enhancing technical abilities among the students and professionals, and developing local ecosystems that assist in innovation. International organisations like the United Nations, OECD, the World Bank, and regional development banks are significant as they provide guidance, technical assistance, and educational programmes. They assist nations with developing national AI plans that are aligned with local interests, including agricultural development, healthcare, or e-governance (Birkstedt et al., 2023).

It is also through knowledge sharing that countries can learn the working practices in other countries. Policy makers and researchers can share information and localise global frameworks to fit the local conditions through workshops, conferences, open research platforms, and regional centres of excellence. This collaboration assists the emerging economies in coming up with governance systems that are culturally acceptable and economically viable. They have more capacity to be involved in the global policy discussions and strike agreements that cater to their interests (Yang & Turi, 2025).

13.7 Challenges and Limitations of International AI Governance

13.7.1 Power Asymmetries and Representation Gaps

The technological advanced nations have been centralised into a few countries that lead AI leadership. The United States, China, and the EU members are leading AI research, cloud computing infrastructure, and international digital platforms. These countries also affect the process of setting standards and governing discourses. Not all developing countries are equal in terms of technical knowhow, financial resources, and political influence to play an equal role. Consequently, international regulations might have biased interests and values of the strongest nations (Png, 2022). There are representation gaps between nations as well as within societies. Governance meetings do not usually include civil society groups, Indigenous populations, and marginalised populations. They leave out information that decisions could fail to consider the difference in culture, access, or harms of vulnerable populations. In situations where the decisions of governance lack the interests of every citizen, AI can strengthen inequality instead of diminishing it (Ishkhanyan, 2025). There is no equal participation and it is hard to come up with truly global and fair governance. There must be more powerful structures of representation in which each region is represented in a serious way.

13.7.2 Conflicting National Interests and Geopolitics

The nations are not always unanimous about the way AI is to be regulated. There are governments with a focus on innovation and global competitions and others have more focus on ethics, public safety, or human rights. These conflicting interests slug the negotiation process and mostly create compromises that are not as efficient as required (Li, 2025). The competition in geopolitics complicates cooperation even more. The AI technologies are regarded as the strategic tools that could make economic power and military power grow. Countries might reduce technological sharing due to the need to preserve national security or such that can give them a competitive advantage. Indicatively, export quotas and online trade restrictions limit the possibility of cross nation cooperation. Due to the increase in competition, the countries can make regional partnerships where they have varying governance philosophies resulting in fragmented standards globally (Roberts et al., 2024).

Regulatory attitudes are also affected by the political systems. Democratic countries are normally endorsing transparency, freedom of expression, and independent control. On the contrary, authoritarian governments can apply AI to mass surveillance, censorship, and social control. Such conflicting values complicate the creation of universal principles regarding such matters as facial recognition or algorithmic surveillance. The issue of national sovereignty is also one of the reasons why some nations oppose international regulations which they perceive as limitations to domestic powers. Such political frictions undermine the capability of global institutions to establish shared systems of governance fast (Emery-Xu et al., 2025).

13.7.3 Limited Enforcement Mechanisms

Enforcement is also a significant constraint even in cases where there are agreements. AI governance systems in other countries do not always consist of binding legislation, but they usually suggest recommendations. Most of the principles are voluntary and depend on self-regulations by governance and companies. This imbalances implementation since certain actors can go unpunished to breach the rules (Roberts et al., 2024). It is also hard to enforce as AI regulations demand technical skills to check non-compliance. Proprietary algorithms, datasets, and internal audits may not be available to regulators. This transparency is not easy to monitor and be accountable for. Businesses might present themselves as being ethically committed on the one hand, but on the other hand, they may not behave in a morally responsible manner (Birkstedt et al., 2023).

Inter-country problems like cyberattacks, misinformation, election interference, are additional enforcement problems. The legal reactions are delayed and complex when the damaging actions are not within the limitations of a country. The international mechanisms to probe or punish the perpetrators of such violations are few (Söderlund & Larsson, 2024). The harm caused through AI is not necessarily obvious. The negative outcomes may be caused by developers, providers of the platform, and users, and it is hard to hold people responsible. In the absence of explicit liability structures, victims are likely to be denied justice and malpractices might persist (Attard-Frost & Lyons, 2025).

13.8 Conclusion

The international organisations are in the centre of the coordinated and human-centred AI governance. As AI systems have more and more influence on transnational societies, national regulations will not be sufficient to deal with international risk of privacy, security, discrimination, and economic disparity. Bodies like the United Nations, OECD, and UNESCO offer forums on which countries can come up with common principles, ethics, and technical standards. Their activities contribute to the alignment in the spheres of data governance, protection of human rights, and public and private application of AI in a transparent way. The role of regional organisations and consortia of industries can also help by development of standards, facilitation, and responsible innovation. Nevertheless, global governance continues to be challenged and some of these challenges are power imbalances, geopolitical tensions, and poor enforcement mechanisms. To solve these problems, it is necessary to include all regions in this work, engage civil society in a meaningful way, and increase the accountability system. International cooperation is needed, although it is limited to making sure that AI can help humanity but not cause harm in the most possible way. The harmonised global governance can help ensure safe technological advancement, ensure communities that are at risk, and build a just and long-term digital future.

References

Afzal, J. (2024). *Implementation of Digital Law as a Legal Tool in the Current Digital Era*. Springer. https://doi.org/10.1007/978-981-97-7106-6.

Agarwal, A. and Nene, M.J. (2025). A five-layer framework for AI governance: Integrating regulation, standards, and certification. *Transforming Government: People, Process, and Policy*. https://doi.org/10.1108/TG-03-2025-0065.

Attard-Frost, B. and Lyons, K. (2025). AI governance systems: A multi-scale analysis framework, empirical findings, and future directions. *AI and Ethics*, *5*(3), 2557–2604. https://doi.org/10.1007/s43681-024-00569-5.

Bean, E., Burleigh, C., Haskell, C., Burris-Melville, T., Payne, J. and Pathak, B. (2025). Eavesdropping on UNESCO AI Policy, Leadership, and Ethics. *Journal of Leadership Studies*, *18*(4), 98–110. https://doi.org/10.1002/jls.70007.

Birkstedt, T., Minkkinen, M., Tandon, A. and Mäntymäki, M. (2023). AI governance: Themes, knowledge gaps, and future agendas. *Internet Research*, *33*(7), 133–167. https://doi.org/10.1108/INTR-01-2022-0042.

Bjola, C. and Manor, I. (2025). Digital diplomacy in the age of technological acceleration: Three impact scenarios of generative artificial intelligence. *Place Branding and Public Diplomacy*, *21*(3), 303–308. https://doi.org/10.1057/s41254-023-00323-4.

Brandão, A.P. (2024). The European Union narrative on artificial intelligence: The path to international leadership. In: *Artificial Intelligence in Production Engineering and Management* (pp. 145–191). Woodhead Publishing. https://doi.org/10.1016/B978-0-12-819471-3.00009-4.

Calderaro, A. (2025). Human rights and cybersecurity: Contentious communities in cyber diplomacy practice. In: *The Palgrave Handbook on Cyber Diplomacy* (pp. 211–230). Cham: Springer Nature Switzerland. https://doi.org/10.1007/978-3-031-93385-1_10.

Camilleri, M.A. (2024). Artificial intelligence governance: Ethical considerations and implications for social responsibility. *Expert Systems*, *41*(7), e13406. https://doi.org/10.1111/exsy.13406.

Cantero Gamito, M. (2024). The Role of ETSI in the EU's Regulation and Governance of Artificial Intelligence. *Innovation: The European Journal of Social Science Research*, *37*(5), 1425–1440. https://doi.org/10.1080/13511610.2024.2349627.

Cantero Gamito, M. and Marsden, C.T. (2024). Artificial intelligence co-regulation? The role of standards in the EU AI Act. *International Journal of Law and Information Technology*, *32*, eaae011. https://doi.org/10.1093/ijlit/eaae011.

Corrêa, N.K., Galvão, C., Santos, J.W., Del Pino, C., Pinto, E.P., Barbosa, C., ... & de Oliveira, N. (2023). Worldwide AI ethics: A review of 200 guidelines and recommendations for AI governance. *Patterns*, *4*(10). https://doi.org/10.1016/j.patter.2023.100857.

David, P., Choung, H. and Seberger, J.S. (2024). Who is responsible? US Public perceptions of AI governance through the lenses of trust and ethics. *Public Understanding of Science*, *33*(5), 654–672. https://doi.org/10.1177/09636625231224592.

Effoduh, J.O., Akpudo, U.E. and Kong, J.D. (2024). Toward a trustworthy and inclusive data governance policy for the use of artificial intelligence in Africa. *Data & Policy*, *6*, e34. https://doi.org/10.1017/dap.2024.26.

Emery-Xu, N., Jordan, R. and Trager, R. (2025). International governance of advancing artificial intelligence. *AI & Society*, *40*(4), 3019–3044. https://doi.org/10.1007/s00146-024-02050-7.

Erkkilä, T. (2023). Global indicators and AI policy: Metrics, policy scripts, and narratives. *Review of Policy Research*, *40*(5), 811–839. https://doi.org/10.1111/ropr.12556.

Gill, A.S. and Germann, S. (2022). Conceptual and normative approaches to AI governance for a global digital ecosystem supportive of the UN Sustainable Development Goals (SDGs). *AI and Ethics*, *2*(2), 293–301. https://doi.org/10.1007/s43681-021-00058-z.

Girasa, R. (2025). AI as a disruptive technology. In: *Artificial Intelligence as a Disruptive Technology: Economic Transformation and Government Regulation* (pp. 3–38). Cham: Springer Nature Switzerland. https://doi.org/10.1007/978-3-032-02827-3_1.

Gohr, C., Rodríguez, G., Belomestnykh, S., Berg-Moelleken, D., Chauhan, N., Engler, J.O., ... & von Wehrden, H. (2025). Artificial intelligence in sustainable development research. *Nature Sustainability*, *8*(8), 970–978. https://doi.org/10.1038/s41893-025-01598-6.

Huang, K., Joshi, A., Dun, S. and Hamilton, N. (2024). AI regulations. In: *Generative AI Security: Theories and Practices* (pp. 61–98). Cham: Springer Nature Switzerland. https://doi.org/10.1007/978-3-031-54252-7_3.

Huang, Z.A. (2025). Terminology, AI bias, and the risks of current digital public diplomacy practices. *Place Branding and Public Diplomacy*, *21*(3), 327–333. https://doi.org/10.1057/s41254-024-00324-x.

Ishkhanyan, A. (2025). Governing AI across borders: Corporate power, state sovereignty, and global regulation. *Digital Policy, Regulation, and Governance*. https://doi.org/10.1108/DPRG-03-2025-0057.

Justo-Hanani, R. (2022). The politics of Artificial Intelligence regulation and governance reform in the European Union. *Policy Sciences*, *55*(1), 137–159. https://doi.org/10.1007/s11077-022-09452-8.

Keith, A.J. (2024). Governance of artificial intelligence in Southeast Asia. *Global Policy*, *15*(5), 937–954. https://doi.org/10.1111/1758-5899.13458.

Kong, J.D., Fevrier, K., Effoduh, J.O. and Bragazzi, N.L. (2023). Artificial intelligence, law, and vulnerabilities. In: *AI and Society* (pp. 179–196). Chapman and Hall/CRC.

Küçükuncular, A. (2026). Addressing Ethical Challenges in Cyberspace Governance: Recommendations for the Digital Sovereignty Era. *Digital Society*, *5*(1), 3. https://doi.org/10.1007/s44206-025-00241-3.

Kulkov, I., Kulkova, J., Rohrbeck, R., Menvielle, L., Kaartemo, V. and Makkonen, H. (2024). Artificial intelligence-driven sustainable development: Examining organizational, technical, and processing approaches to achieving global goals. *Sustainable Development*, *32*(3), 2253–2267. https://doi.org/10.1002/sd.2773.

Kuzio, J., Ahmadi, M., Kim, K.C., Migaud, M.R., Wang, Y.F. and Bullock, J. (2022). Building better global data governance. *Data & Policy*, *4*, e25. https://doi.org/10.1017/dap.2022.17.

Lane, L. (2023). Artificial intelligence and human rights: Corporate responsibility in AI governance initiatives. *Nordic Journal of Human Rights*, *41*(3), 304–325. https://doi.org/10.1080/18918131.2022.2137288.

Li, J. (2025). Governing High-Risk Technologies in a Fragmented World: Geopolitical Tensions, Regulatory Gaps, and Institutional Barriers to Global Cooperation. *Fudan Journal of the Humanities and Social Sciences*, 1–25. https://doi.org/10.1007/s40647-025-00445-4.

Liebig, L., Güttel, L., Jobin, A. and Katzenbach, C. (2024). Subnational AI policy: Shaping AI in a multi-level governance system. *AI & Society*, *39*(3), 1477–1490. https://doi.org/10.1007/s00146-022-01561-5.

Madavarapu, J.B., Kasula, B.Y., Whig, P. and Kautish, S. (2024). AI-powered solutions advancing UN sustainable development goals: A case study in tackling humanity's challenges. In: *Digital Technologies to Implement the UN Sustainable Development Goals* (pp. 47–67). Cham: Springer Nature Switzerland. https://doi.org/10.1007/978-3-031-68427-2_3.

Makridis, C.A., Borkowski, A.A. and Alterovitz, G. (2024). Perspectives on advancing innovation and human flourishing through a network of AI institutes. *Science and Public Policy*, *51*(3), 557–562. https://doi.org/10.1093/scipol/scad088.

Marcucci, S., Alarcón, N.G., Verhulst, S.G. and Wüllhorst, E. (2023). Informing the global data future: Benchmarking data governance frameworks. *Data & Policy*, *5*, e30. https://doi.org/10.1017/dap.2023.24.

Marwala, T. (2023). Artificial Intelligence in politics. In: *Artificial Intelligence, Game Theory and Mechanism Design in Politics* (pp. 41–58). Singapore: Springer Nature Singapore. https://doi.org/10.1007/978-981-99-5103-1_4.

Misuraca, G., Rossel, P. and Sibal, P. (2024). Mastering AI governance in the public sector. In: *The Routledge International Handbook of Public Administration and Digital Governance* (pp. 338–353). Routledge.

Natorski, M. (2024). Compromise in multilateral negotiations and the global regulation of artificial intelligence. *Democratization*, *31*(5), 1091–1116. https://doi.org/10.1080/13510347.2024.2351583.

Natorski, M. (2025). Multilateralism in the Global Governance of Artificial Intelligence. *arXiv preprint arXiv:2508.15397*. https://doi.org/10.48550/arXiv.2508.15397.

Nuño-Santana, F.E. (2024). International Cooperation, Multilateralism, and Civil Society in the Face of the Technological Revolution 4.0. In: *International Relations and Technological Revolution 4.0: World Order, Power, and New International Society* (pp. 173–187). Cham: Springer Nature Switzerland. https://doi.org/10.1007/978-3-031-66750-3_11.

Olugbade, O. (2025). In search of a global governance mechanism for artificial intelligence (AI): A collective action perspective. *Global Public Policy and Governance* (pp. 1–23). https://doi.org/10.1007/s43508-025-00113-z.

Oviedo, J., Rodriguez, M., Trenta, A., Cannas, D., Natale, D. and Piattini, M. (2024). ISO/IEC quality standards for AI engineering. *Computer Science Review*, *54*, 100681. https://doi.org/10.1016/j.cosrev.2024.100681.

Png, M.T. (2022, June). At the tensions of south and north: Critical roles of global south stakeholders in AI governance. In: *Proceedings of the 2022 ACM Conference on Fairness, Accountability, and Transparency* (pp. 1434–1445). https://doi.org/10.1145/3531146.3533200.

Radanliev, P. (2025). Cyber diplomacy: Defining the opportunities for cybersecurity and risks from Artificial Intelligence, IoT, Blockchains, and Quantum Computing. *Journal of Cyber Security Technology*, *9*(1), 28–78. https://doi.org/10.1080/23742917.2024.2312671.

Rezaei, M., Pironti, M. and Quaglia, R. (2025). AI in knowledge sharing, which ethical challenges are raised in decision-making processes for organisations? *Management Decision*, *63*(10), 3369–3388. https://doi.org/10.1108/MD-10-2023-2023.

Roberts, H., Hine, E. and Floridi, L. (2023). Digital sovereignty, digital expansionism, and the prospects for global AI Governance. In: *Quo Vadis, Sovereignty? New Conceptual and Regulatory Boundaries in the Age of Digital China* (pp. 51–75). Cham: Springer Nature Switzerland. https://doi.org/10.1007/978-3-031-41566-1_4.

Roberts, H., Hine, E., Taddeo, M. and Floridi, L. (2024). Global AI governance: Barriers and pathways forward. *International Affairs*, *100*(3), 1275–1286. https://doi.org/10.1093/ia/iiae073.

Rong, K., Ling, Y., Yang, T. and Huang, C. (2025). Cross-border data transfer: Patterns and discrepancies. *Journal of International Business Policy*, *8*(1), 10–32. https://doi.org/10.1057/s42214-025-00209-7.

Roumate, F. (2022). Artificial Intelligence and Digital Diplomacy. *Artificial Intelligence To Strengthen or to Replace Traditional Diplomacy*. https://doi.org/10.1007/978-3-030-68647-5.

Sayles, J. (2024). Aligning AI Governance with Other Internal Governance Models for Trustworthy AI: "The Convergence of Governance Frameworks". In: *Principles of AI Governance and Model Risk Management: Master the Techniques for Ethical and Transparent AI Systems* (pp. 113–172). Berkeley, CA: Apress. https://doi.org/10.1007/979-8-8688-0983-5_5.

Sepasspour, R. (2023). A reality check and a way forward for the global governance of artificial intelligence. *Bulletin of the Atomic Scientists*, *79*(5), 304–315. https://doi.org/10.1080/00963402.2023.2245249.

Söderlund, K. and Larsson, S. (2024). Enforcement design patterns in EU law: An analysis of the AI Act. *Digital Society*, *3*(2), 41. https://doi.org/10.1007/s44206-024-00129-8.

Strange, M. and Tucker, J. (2024). Global governance and the normalization of artificial intelligence as 'good' for human health. *AI & Society*, *39*(6), 2667–2676. https://doi.org/10.1007/s00146-023-01774-2.

Tampubolon, M. and Tampubolon, M.J.P. (2025). Cybercrime, Human Rights, and Digital Privacy: Navigating the Complex Landscape of Protection and Freedom. In: *Integrating Artificial Intelligence, Security for Environmental and Business Sustainability* (Vol. 2, pp. 75–85). Cham: Springer Nature Switzerland. https://doi.org/10.1007/978-3-031-96641-5_7.

Taylor, R.D. (2025). Saving global human rights: A "Global South+ AI" strategy. *The Information Society*, *41*(2), 123–138. https://doi.org/10.1080/01972243.2024.2442916.

Van Norren, D.E. (2023). The ethics of artificial intelligence: UNESCO and the African Ubuntu perspective. *Journal of Information, Communication, and Ethics in Society*, *21*(1), 112–128. https://doi.org/10.1108/JICES-04-2022-0037.

von Ingersleben-Seip, N. (2023). Competition and cooperation in artificial intelligence standard setting: Explaining emergent patterns. *Review of Policy Research*, *40*(5), 781–810. https://doi.org/10.1111/ropr.12538.

Walter, Y. (2024). Managing the race to the moon: Global policy and governance in Artificial Intelligence regulation: A contemporary overview and an analysis of socioeconomic consequences. *Discover Artificial Intelligence*, *4*(1), 14. https://doi.org/10.1007/s44163-024-00109-4.

Wirtz, B.W., Weyerer, J.C. and Kehl, I. (2022). Governance of artificial intelligence: A risk and guideline-based integrative framework. *Government Information Quarterly*, *39*(4), 101685. https://doi.org/10.1016/j.giq.2022.101685.

Yang, L. (2023). Recommendations for metaverse governance based on technical standards. *Humanities and Social Sciences Communications*, *10*(1), 1–10. https://doi.org/10.1057/s41599-023-01750-7.

Yang, X. and Turi, A.N. (2025). The Impact of AI on Economic Growth: A Take for Emerging Economies. In: *Tech Transformation and AI Readiness: Pioneering Paths for the Global*

South (pp. 31–38). Cham: Springer Nature Switzerland. https://doi.org/10.1007/978-3-031-73639-1_2.

Yilma, K. (2025). *The Global Governance of AI: The Role of the United Nations.* Routledge. https://doi.org/10.4324/9781003607366.

Zambrano, R. and Sanchez-Torres, J.M. (2021, October). AI Public Policies in Latin America: Disruption or more of the same? In: *Proceedings of the 14th International Conference on Theory and Practice of Electronic Governance* (pp. 25–33). https://doi.org/10.1145/3494193.3494294.

14 Designing Inclusive and Participatory AI Governance Frameworks

Participatory and inclusive AI governance is necessary to have all members of the society reflected in the Artificial Intelligence systems in their needs, rights, and values. Top-down traditional regulation methods usually dismiss the views of marginalised groups, the civil society, and stakeholders in the communities. This chapter examines methods for designing governance structures that enhance equity, openness, and participation by the people. It examines options, like stakeholder consultations, co-design processes, citizen assemblies, and community-based oversight. Accessibility, representation, and cultural sensitivity to the formulation of equitable AI policies are also emphasised in the chapter. In making it more participative and inclusive, AI governance will be more democratic and trusted as well as responsive to various social contexts.

14.1 Introduction

AI is rapidly influencing the contemporary society functioning in the digital world. Nowadays AI technologies affect the decision making in healthcare, education, finance, public services and personal digital interactions (Alshahrani et al., 2024). An opportunity to be efficient and innovative is also generated by these technologies, also of concern is fairness, accountability, and social impact. When the AI systems are found to be integrated in the provision of key services, care should take precedence to ensure that the systems run in a manner that does not infringe on the human rights, and ensure that the interest of the populace is not endangered (Dunleavy & Margetts, 2025). Regulatory systems are aimed at regulating safe and responsible AI usage. Nevertheless, the conventional methods of governance have been largely top down in which the policymakers, states, and the technical professionals formulate regulations without consulting a significant population. Such a solution is not comprehensive enough to satisfy varying needs and lives of different communities. The numerous victims of the algorithmic decisions lack a voice in the manner the systems are made, executed, or are being monitored (Huang et al., 2024).

Inclusive and participatory AI governance will be used to alter this trend and engage various stakeholders in making a decision. The stakeholders refer to the government agencies, corporations, educational professionals, civil society groups, and the general population. All groups provide varied information regarding risks, benefits, and ethical factors. The use of additional voices assists in outlining the possible harms not only apparent to technical specialists (Moon, 2023). Unless

DOI: 10.1201/9781003776659-14

the data or experiences of marginalised communities are taken into account, then the algorithmic bias can exhibit a disproportionate impact on them. There are also problems of accessibility in cases where digital systems lack solutions to persons with disabilities, rural communities, or of the language minority. Engagement facilitates the designing of technologies to suit the requirements of the varied users and enhances creation of socially conscious and culturally relevant systems (Shafik, 2025).

Participation enhances trust in AI-based systems as well. Having the ability to communicate and challenge the way some decisions are made, people will become more susceptible to believe that technology is utilised in a fair way. Trust is particularly vital where there is a high risk as in policing, welfare examination, and diagnosing health care. Participatory governance promotes transparency by opening up communication channels, dialogue and providing avenues of access to publicity (Afroogh et al., 2024). Inclusive governance is favourable to the on-going improvement, as AI systems change over time and need to be monitored constantly as opposed to adherence to fixed policies. It also facilitates innovation to the advantage of a greater population. By listening to the communities, governments, and companies can develop a solution that incorporates the actual human needs and contributes to the social development (Walter, 2024).

This move to participation is in line with democratic principles, which allow citizens the right to shape systems that concern them. It embodies the perception that AI governance must not be in the hands of limited and strong actors but it should embrace the wisdom of the army of people. With the growing scope of AI efficiency in all spheres where citizens live, participatory governance is one of the avenues to more ethical, fair, and trusted technological advancement (Rasoulzadeh Aghdam et al., 2025).

14.2 Principles of Inclusive AI Governance

14.2.1 Equity, Fairness, and Non-Discrimination

Inclusive AI governance is based on equity and fairness. AI systems are not supposed to treat individuals differently, but rather not promote discrimination. Nonetheless, numerous artificial intelligence (AI) applications are based on past data which is socially biased. Algorithms might give biased results when biased data is relied upon without significant analysis. As an illustration, recruitment algorithms can be discriminating in favour of individuals with a particular background. Systems of health care can ignore underrepresented groups in the medical records. Such consequences may enhance pre-existing inequalities (Akhtar et al., 2024). The AI governance should consequently take care of bias throughout the development process. Inclusive design involves a variety of data inference, equal consideration to the model, and frequent review of decisions. It is also worth participation of affected populations. Their participation assists in detecting some undetected risks that the professionals might not be aware of (Giovanola & Tiribelli, 2023).

Equal consideration must be made as well through equity so that the benefits of AI can be made reachable to other categories. When access to high quality digital services is only provided to the rich or urban population, then the digital divide is increased. When everyone has equal access to the AI innovations, fairness is attained (Lütz, 2024).

14.2.2 Transparency, Accessibility, and Public Accountability

The other major principle of inclusive governance is transparency. AI systems are frequently used as black boxes where they cannot visualise the way decisions are made. This causes distrust and hinders individuals to defy detrimental consequences. Clear information regarding the manner in which AI tools operate, the information which they utilise and the method of making a decision is essential to transparent governance. This does not imply that the trade secrets are being revealed, but just that it has to be explainable. Individuals must know the reason why they could not get a loan, could not get a job, or were caught by a surveillance unit (Olsen et al., 2024). The availability makes information on AI easy to comprehend by other users. There may be the use of technical language that locks out the non-experts. Opportunities to engage in the system of AI governance as informed participants are provided by accessible communication. It is also connected with the creation of technologies that might be employed with the disabled, non-dominant language speakers, and digitally deficient individuals (Akhtar et al., 2024).

The notion of public accountability implies the necessity of those who create and implement AI systems to be accountable. There ought to be a system of checking the algorithms, complaints, and errors in the institutions. Once harms are incurred, then individuals must be allowed to find redress. Responsibility is also necessitated by independent oversight institutions that will impose the rule of the law and ethical considerations. It is impossible to have fairness and transparency without accountability (Hosseini Tabaghdehi & Ayaz, 2025).

14.2.3 Human Rights and Social Justice Foundations

The inclusive AI governance is based on human rights. The privacy, dignity, freedom of expression, and equal opportunity must be honoured using AI systems. They must not endorse mass surveillance and censorship, and discriminating against certain groups of people. According to many global systems, technology should be used in human interest. Nevertheless, the exceptionally perceived speed of AI development poses difficulties in the consistency of the application of such principles. Rights infringements could be followed in case AI systems gather personal information without any consent or in case decisions are made by AI and are not analysed by humans (Gentelet & Mizrahi, 2024).

Social justice is aimed at eliminating power disparities. Employment of AI has the potential of reinforcing existing systems of inequality provided it is not regulated. As an illustration, predictive policing tools can be used to focus on some neighbourhoods more. The automated welfare systems can punish the people who have less computer access. Inclusive governance gives the marginalised individuals not only security, but also power. Policies and technologies have to impact them and their knowledge has to aid in shaping them (Buccella, 2023). Significant participation is also endorsed on human rights principles. Individuals are entitled to participate in making decisions in their lives. The inclusion of the affected communities enhances greater fairness, empower legitimacy, and design more responsible technological development. Rights-based governance points out that technology is created on behalf of people and not to dominate or exploit a person (Robles & Mallinson, 2025).

14.3 Stakeholder Participation Models

14.3.1 Government, Industry, and Public Sector Roles

Governments play a major role in AI governance. They develop legislations, policies, and regulatory models to inform how AI should be used safely. AI allows improving the work of the public agencies, but at the same time, they should guarantee transparency and safeguard the rights of citizens. The involvement of governments will aid in making sure that AI should adhere to social ideals and not only to businesses (Choi & Park, 2023). AI technologies are largely developed and deployed by industry. The number of innovations promoted by the work of private companies is large: they invest in research, collections, and uptake in the market. Since companies have a direct role in designing and using AI products, they have to adhere to the principles of ethical behaviours. Industry ought to participate in decision-making by collaborating with regulators and the civil society. It must make use of responsible innovation, internal auditing, and accountability systems to keep it out of abuse (Alshahrani et al., 2024).

The government is a consumer and a controller of AI. The government departments have welfare delivery, policing, transportation, and health services systems. The way they make decisions determines the trust of the people in AI. Thus, the government has to establish high transparency, equity, and data security standards. The government and industry should work in such a way that technological advantages are beneficial to the people and not the sole motive of making profits (Chen et al., 2023).

14.3.2 Civil Society and Community Representation

The civil society organisations play critical roles in communicating missions of different communities. Such groups are human rights groups, advocacy networks, labour associations, community groups, and non-profit institutions. They assist in the detection of risks and disparities that can be found with the help of AI. Civil society supervises the notion that governance systems deny vulnerable groups the right to discrimination, exclusion, and exploitation (LePere-Schloop &

Zook, 2023). The communities who will be directly impacted by the AI choices should also be given a chance to voice their experiences. Individuals receiving social welfare, gig workers, and minorities are examples of those who are usually affected by automated decision-making most. Their involvement makes sure that the policymakers are aware of the practical problems, in particular, the problems associated with algorithmic bias and unfair treatment. The feedback on the community also assists in changing the AI systems to accommodate the local cultures, languages and social requirements (Moon, 2023). Civil society can help through creating awareness and informing the people on AI. They offer digital literacy and an active role in policymaking. The high participation of a civil society enhances democratic accountability and helps to make a decision that is more inclusive (Sieber et al., 2025).

14.3.3 Academia and Expert Participation

Scientific understanding and technical expertise needed in responsible AI governance are offered by academia and experts. Researchers contribute to understanding the risks, system performance, and ethics issues in algorithms development. Their autonomy enables them to criticize practices in the industry and give alternative solutions which are in tandem with societal values (Birkstedt et al., 2023). It is particularly imperative to have a multidisciplinary expertise. AI governance needs not only computer scientists, but legal, psychological, sociological, ethical, and economical scholars as well. The specialists can help in policy making by demonstrating the impact of AI in various facets of society. Transparency is also promoted through academic institutions through research that describes the impacts of technologies in simple and understandable terms (Ter-Minassian, 2025). Experts are important in his or her role in coming up with standards, benchmarks, and assessment frameworks. They assist governments not only in complex technical matters but also in future outcomes. The global partnerships between universities would also be instrumental in dispensation of knowledge to the rest of the world and assist developing economies with a small research force (Yang, 2023).

14.3.4 Citizen Assemblies and Deliberative Engagement

Democratic legitimacy of AI governance by citizens is enhanced. A common citizen has a right of voicing his opinions on technologies that affect their day to day activities. Citizen assemblies enable the groups of various people to deliberate on AI policies and give recommendations to the decision-makers. These groups promote discussion, contemplation and wise decision-making (Buhmann & Fieseler, 2023). Public consultations and town hall meetings can also allow the citizens to use such avenues and air their concerns. Digital platforms promote greater involvement as they permit online surveys and feedback tools and open forums. Such mechanisms are particularly useful to individuals that are unable to meet physically because of distance, disability and other barriers (Duberry, 2022).

Deliberative participation enhances trust as it mitigates the fact that there is a distance between the policymakers and the members of the general population. It makes sure that technological savvy and big companies do not overrule the decisions of governance. As citizens get involved, the AI policies are more representative and correspond to societal values. Such interaction also makes people know how AI functions, which facilitates responsible use and increased collaboration with governance practices (Jain & Dienel, 2024).

14.4 Governance Tools and Mechanisms for Inclusion

14.4.1 Participatory Policy Design Platforms

Policy design platforms that involve participation of stakeholders enable policy makers to participate in the AI governance directly. These networks establish organised forums through which individuals are able to air their views and offer experiences and suggestions on policy areas. Such platforms are often used by governments when writing AI plans, data protection laws, or digital transformation plans. These tools aid in involving individuals early enough such that the policies are tailored prior to implementation (Ter-Minassian, 2025). The participatory platforms aid in minimising power imbalance. They provide civil society bodies, industrial bodies, researchers, and citizens with a chance to make comments regarding laws that are relevant to them. This is done to promote transparency since policy drafts and deliberations are exposed to the people. Involvement also enhances the quality of decisions. The policymakers get to understand practical challenges to various communities. Such a form of group decision-making establishes some policies that are not solely determined by professional considerations (Parthasarathy et al., 2024).

Digital platforms increase reach because of the elimination of geographical boundaries. Individuals that are unable to move to government offices can also get involved online. Such inclusiveness is significant to rural populations, people with disabilities, and individuals with limited time or functionality. The key to effective participatory design would involve effective communication, the use of simple language, and reach as many people as possible so that it becomes clear how to participate (Moon, 2023).

14.4.2 Community Based Data Governance Models

The data governance models that are community based make local communities central in the process of making decisions about the collection, storage, and otherwise use of data. These models acknowledge that data are social and cultural resources, but not only the technical ones. People should thus be a part of the decision-making process of how their data are processed, particularly when such data are sensitive or are employed in risky AI uses (Micheli et al., 2022). In this model, communities will be capable of establishing their own data sharing policies. They can determine the possible use of data, the persons that can be able to access the data, and the security that is required. Indigenous and migrant populations and minority communities that had historically been abused with their data, especially require community governance. These models can prevent exploitation and encourage useful data work ethics by making communities have control over them (Bui, 2025).

Trust is also facilitated by community-based governance. Individuals feel more at ease engaging in the digital systems when they are aware that data practices are visible as well as equitable. Such a solution is also able to produce local data commons, where communities gather and share common datasets to social advantage. These data sets can be used to conduct health related, environmental, urban planning, or education programmes. Engagement in the community will make AI technologies based on such data mirror the local priorities and be culturally considerate (Cooper et al., 2023).

14.4.3 Ethical Review Boards and Oversight Committees

Ethical review panels are a significant tool in analysing the risks and benefits of AI systems. These boards have members of government, academia, civil society, and occasionally the masses. They evaluate AI projects prior to their implementation to ascertain that they comply with ethical and legal provisions. Issues that are reviewed by the ethics boards include fairness, prejudice, privacy, consent, and probable harm to vulnerable populations (Sharma, 2024). Constant monitoring is done by oversight committees. They guarantee adherence to laws and address issues that are raised by the citizens. Monitoring organisations assist in determining issues at an initial stage, including algorithmic bias or automated decision-making that is unsafe. It is possible, they can ask audits, insist on updating systems, or stop working on the ones that do not follow ethical principles. Good committees should be independent so as to avoid conflict of interest. They ought to be open and public in decision making (Hadley et al., 2025). Examples of high risk applications that need ethical review and oversight systems are policing technology, biometric applications, algorithm hiring systems, and technology in government welfare initiatives. They are also known to facilitate accountability as they make it impossible to evade responsibility for bad outcomes by the organizations (Schuett et al., 2025).

14.4.4 Digital Tools for Public Dialogue and Feedback

The digital participation tools facilitate ease of the involvement of the populace in AI governance. These are online surveys, open consultations, public comment portals, interactive forums, and mobile applications that can enable one to report their concerns. They enable the governments and institutions to receive feedback from a large number of people. Transparency is also aided by digital tools whereby the information on AI systems is published to the public (Pislaru et al., 2024). The tools are useful in collecting various perspectives particularly those of a population whose opinions might not be included in the official decision-making procedures. They also promote interaction to the extent of constant contact as opposed to rare consultations. The digital platform can help institutions notify the population about the changes in the policies, describe the functioning of AI systems, and address the concerns as they are raised (Wilson, 2022).

The online engagement should be friendly, safe, and readily available. It ought to embrace several languages and formats in order to shun out non-technical users. Good tools form better relations between humans and institutions creating greater trust in AI governance (Schmank & Buchkremer, 2024). Table 4.1 indicates important governance instruments that contribute to more populace and inclusion in AI decision-making in various communities.

Table 4.1 Key Governance Tools for Inclusive AI Participation.

Governance Tool	*Purpose*	*Contribution to Inclusion*
Participatory Policy Platforms	Collect public input on laws and policies	Ensures diverse voices shape decision-making
Community Based Data Governance	Local control of data collection and use	Protects vulnerable communities and builds trust
Ethical Review Boards	Assess ethical risks in AI deployment	Promotes fairness, safety, and accountability
Digital Dialogue Tools	Enable online consultation and feedback	Expands participation across different populations

14.5 Challenges in Implementing Inclusive Governance

14.5.1 Power Asymmetries and Under Representation

The imbalances of powers are reflected in the development and regulation of AI technologies. Innovation and policy in AI are controlled by giant technology and strong governments. They manipulate data resources, research funds, infrastructure, and technical expertise. Consequently, they are more powerful in terms of governance, decision-making and standards. Less resourceful communities like Indigenous communities, the rural areas, or those in the poorer nations have fewer avenues to present their needs and issues (Panarese et al., 2025). This is a power imbalance when it comes to representation in formal governance. The consultations with stakeholders can include experts, business leaders, and policymakers, as well as leave the common citizens out who are direct users of the results of AI. Women, disabled people, minorities of other languages, and groups that are socially marginalised are often ignored. Their experiences matter since they might be more at risk of being discriminated against, being surveilled, and becoming victims of algorithmic bias (Correa Lucero & Martens, 2025).

There is also power asymmetry in knowledge. AI systems can be more authoritative to those who comprehend the systems compared to other people who lack technical understanding. This creates an unequal situation of participation between different groups of people even where they are physically present. Significant inclusion would demand that there should be adjustments in the decision-making process which lead to reallocation of power in favour of the people to be most affected by the use of the AI systems (Hughes et al., 2025).

14.5.2 Digital Access and Literacy Barriers

One of the approaches used to engage the populace in AI governance is digital participation. The online platform is becoming a valid avenue that governments and organisations utilise to collect comments, provide information, and hold consultations. Nevertheless, not all people have access to digital infrastructure. Most of the citizens do not have stable internet access, particularly in rural and remote communities. There are others who lack digital devices or simply cannot afford the data services (Djatmiko et al., 2025). Another issue is digital literacy. AI governance can only be properly perceived through internet access and understanding of the technical terms of technology and navigation of online tools as well as critical analysis of complicated data. Individuals having low education and exposure to technologies or those with disabilities might not be successful at participating. This is also true of the older generation who might not be comfortable with digital interfaces (Allmann & Radu, 2023).

The cost of participation is also accompanied by barriers to accessibility whereby places of participation are unfamiliar with local languages, or assistive technology, or varying levels of literacy. In the case where digital participation is based on written responses, less literate people will be unable to communicate and take full advantage of it. In their failure to be designed in a way that is inclusive, platforms recreate social inequalities rather than decrease them (AbdulKareem & Oladimeji, 2024). Hence, digital inclusion needs to be enhanced. Governance initiatives cannot be described as participatory in the absence of equal access to digital spaces.

14.5.3 Cultural, Linguistic, and Social Differences

AI governance is usually associated with the values of prevailing cultural groups. Though, societies are not uniform and different communities can share certain ethical perceptions, privacy anticipations, and worries over technology. The governance frameworks that fail to respect the differences in culture may risk the establishment of rules that do not apply in every setting (Roche et al., 2023). Another participant obstacle is language. A great number of informal debates on AI are conducted in international languages including English. Individuals with local or oral language background might not be able to decipher technical text or policy materials. They can also get excluded during the conversation that fails to address their cultural expressions or styles of communication (Walter, 2024).

The influence of social norms is that they influence those who are comfortable to raise opinions. Certain societies do not encourage speaking in front of the people in authority. Otherwise, gender roles can limit the availability of participation to women or non-binary people. Moreover, those who have been discriminated against can be wary of the institutions and not engage at all (Sartori & Theodorou, 2022). Participation tools should thus be made to fit various cultures. The participation must be able to honour the local cultures and offer secure platforms to discuss. The discussions may be inclusive and sensitive to the culture and that can be supported by multilingual platforms and community mediators (Koniakou, 2023).

14.5.4 Resource and Institutional Capacity Constraints

Inclusive governance involves the financial resources, competent personnel, and institutional frameworks. A good number of organisations and governments do not have these necessities. Consultations, training of the facilitators and participation platforms require time and money. The poor nations might find it difficult to have such initiatives at the expense of dealing with more pressing issues including medical care, education, or joblessness (Roberts et al., 2024). Most areas also have limited institutional capacity. This governance of AI needs people, technology, ethics, and social scientists. In the event of lack of trained personnel, there is ability to assess algorithmic systems or monitor adherence. The smaller organisations might lack committed staff with knowledge of the risks and public participation strategies regarding complex AI (Papagiannidis et al., 2023). Bureaucratic barriers might also haunt some institutions thus slackening down the decision-making process. In the absence of effective procedures, the contribution of the people to the policy might not be immediate enough to motivate them to participate. International alliances can assist in closing such gaps as they would offer experience and resources. Nonetheless, sustainable governance must be supported through the establishment of the capacity at the local level and not by external assistance alone. The engagement should be supported with a long term investment and no single program ones (Olugbade, 2025).

14.6 Strategies for Strengthening Participatory Governance

14.6.1 Trust Building, Transparency, and Responsible Communication

Inclusive governance requires the establishment of trust. The lack of trust can cause citizens not to participate in it or grant them unwillingness to provide personal information. The issue of trust can be achieved when governments and organisations apply transparency in the way AI systems work and make decisions. Such transparency enables people to know what is being targeted, risks, and answers of the adoption of AI (Visave, 2025). The importance of responsible communication is that AI can be unintelligible in many instances. People can be confused in technical terms and complicated explanations. Effective communication contributes to sound involvement. When making explanations on how AI policies and projects will work, governments should use plain language and graphic illustrations. They are also supposed to be proactive in terms of information sharing of key decisions and not wait until issues crop up (Mądra-Sawicka et al., 2025). There is also the need to disclose sources of data, system restrictions, and possible biases which would maintain the transparency. It is the right of the user to know why decisions are being made to them, influencing them particularly in sensitive fields like healthcare or work. This makes developers and decision makers accountable (Blom et al., 2025).

Trust building involves a two way communication. Individuals will be required to have the ability to raise questions, report issues, and get their concerns met in a prompt manner. This connection can be achieved with the help of public consultations, systems of grievance redress, and online communication channels. The trust also grows when the citizens feel that they are respected and that their contribution is evident in the process of making policies (Al Chami, 2025). Transparency also covers responsibility with independent audits and control mechanisms. When such systems exist and are operational, the general attitude of the population towards the use of AI becomes more trusting. Relationships of trust build over time and need constant effort on the part of all the stakeholders (Park & Yoon, 2024).

14.6.2 Capacity Building for Marginalized and Under Represented Groups

A good number of the population will be unable to actively engage in the governance of AI due to a lack of knowledge, skill, or resources. These groups should be engaged in capacity-building activities. Training on digital literacy, rights awareness, and participatory decision-making should be given by governments, academic and civil society organisations (Mutambara, 2025). Capacity-building programmes may be provided in schools, in the community, and online. In these programmes, the mechanisms of collecting data, decision-making, as well as the impact of AI systems on everyday life should be explained. Communities will be able to recognise risks and propose better solutions to the system when they learn more about them (Nanni & Napolitano, 2024). Special attention is needed for the marginalised groups. Assistive technologies could be required by people with disabilities. The speakers of non-dominant languages might demand the assistance of the translators. The rural populations might require enhanced connectivity and access to digital tools. Equal representation will also be necessary, hence involvement in genders (Roberts et al., 2024).

Capacity building is not all about technical knowledge. It involves empowerment of communities to take their own case. Peer networks, workshops, and leadership development programs assist individuals in airing their opinions without fear. Engagement of local leaders also enhances its participation through trust creation in the local communities (Wasi, 2025).

The second activity is the knowledge sharing between scholars and the society. Communities will be exposed to technical knowledge and the experts can learn on community experience. This threefold association gives the two parties a chance to make their contributions to governance (Sayles, 2024). International collaboration can also aid development in the developing countries in terms of capacity building. Collaborations with international organizations may offer resources in training and funding along with policy advice. Nevertheless, it takes long-term successes with local ownership and support structures. The capacity building should assist in the ability of the communities to participate not just once but endlessly as AI changes (Khan et al., 2024).

14.6.3 Integrating Local Knowledge and Adaptive Policymaking

AI governance should be diverse concerning social settings. The relevant sources of knowledge are the local values, local culture as well as the community experiences. By implementing this local knowledge in AI governance, the decisions should be timely and approved. Cultures are more familiar with their surrounding environments than the external authorities and are able to detect hazards which are not evident during any formal evaluations (Yigitcanlar et al., 2024). Ethical perceptions are curbed by local knowledge as well. As an example the expectation of privacy can vary according to regions. The cultural norms define how individuals perceive fairness or harm. These differences can be effectively addressed by the adaptive governance models which must have the local perspectives (Liebig et al., 2024).

Focus group and participation research programmes along with community-based consultations can enhance the collection of local knowledge. These issues ought to be recorded and incorporated into legislation by policymakers. Oversight committees and policy making groups should have local experts as well to ensure that it is constantly representative of the views of the community (Chakravarty & Gattupalli, 2024). Adaptive policymaking acknowledges the fact that AI technologies are evolving at a fast rate. The government will need to adapt. The given fixed rules can be outlived when algorithms undergo changes and when new threats are created. Policies using adaptive models can be updated by the regular review, monitoring and consultation (Sahu & Mallick, 2025).

Adaptive governance heavily depends on feedback loops. Such loops assist institutions to monitor the effects of real worlds and amend decisions when need be. There should be a way to report issues by the citizens and the authorities should react to it in an open and quick manner. This is a dynamic process which enhances fairness and safety (Santos & Carvalho, 2025). Incorporation of local knowledge also helps in innovation. In cases when AI systems are developed with consideration of cultural and linguistic diversity, they will be more helpful and reachable to various populations. This will minimise inequality as systems will not dominate other systems that are meant only to address a small percentage of the population (AbdulKareem & Oladimeji, 2024).

14.7 Conclusion

AI governance should be inclusive and participatory in the establishment of technology that helps humanity to thrive socially and in wellness. The unfolding of AI into everyday reality requires the system to be driven by a set of values that put into perspective the rights and needs of everybody. Participation offers perspective of the rich views of governments, industries, civil society, experts, and citizens. Such different opinions facilitate the occurrence of risk identification, avoidance of discrimination as well as fostering fairness. Inclusive governance also enhances trust and transparency which are required to make the AI systems acceptable to the population. Nonetheless, to succeed in the participation, it is necessary to cope with the challenges of power disparities, digital disparities, and weak institutional capacity. There must be powerful governorial instruments and techniques that will make sure that all groups are given the platform to express themselves. It involves establishing health and trust by means of responsible communication, enabling underrepresented communities via capacity building, and incorporating the local knowledge in flexible policies. The collaboration, mutual respect, and constant interaction are the foundations of AI governance. In situations where individuals are consulted in making decisions that determine technology, AI will be more democratic and close to social values. An action-oriented strategy will guarantee that no one will be left behind based on the progress of AI and make it a fairer, more equal, and inclusive society.

References

AbdulKareem, A.K. and Oladimeji, K.A. (2024). Cultivating the digital citizen: Trust, digital literacy, and e-government adoption. *Transforming Government: People, Process and Policy*, *18*(2), 270–286. https://doi.org/10.1108/TG-11-2023-0196.

Afroogh, S., Akbari, A., Malone, E., Kargar, M. and Alambeigi, H. (2024). Trust in AI: Progress, challenges, and future directions. *Humanities and Social Sciences Communications*, *11*(1), 1–30. https://doi.org/10.1057/s41599-024-04044-8.

Akhtar, M.A.K., Kumar, M. and Nayyar, A. (2024). Ensuring Fairness and Non-discrimination in Explainable AI. In: *Towards Ethical and Socially Responsible Explainable AI: Challenges and Opportunities* (pp. 165–192). Cham: Springer Nature Switzerland. https://doi.org/10.1007/978-3-031-66489-2_6.

Al Chami, R. (2025). From talk to trust: Cultural dynamics of AI-driven social responsibility in negotiations for strategic communication. *International Communication of Chinese Culture*, 1–20. https://doi.org/10.1007/s40636-025-00331-4.

Allmann, K. and Radu, R. (2023). Digital footprints as barriers to accessing e-government services. *Global Policy*, *14*(1), 84–94. https://doi.org/10.1111/1758-5899.13140.

Alshahrani, A., Griva, A., Dennehy, D. and Mäntymäki, M. (2024). Artificial intelligence and decision-making in government functions: Opportunities, challenges, and future research. *Transforming Government: People, Process, and Policy*, *18*(4), 678–698. https://doi.org/10.1108/TG-06-2024-0131.

Birkstedt, T., Minkkinen, M., Tandon, A. and Mäntymäki, M. (2023). AI governance: Themes, knowledge gaps and future agendas. *Internet Research*, *33*(7), 133–167. https://doi.org/10.1108/INTR-01-2022-0042.

Blom, J.M., Rivi, V., Tascedda, F. and Pani, L. (2025). Building trust in clinical research: A systems approach to ethical engagement and sustainable outcomes. *Frontiers in Pharmacology*, *16*, 1570899. https://doi.org/10.3389/fphar.2025.1570899.

Buccella, A. (2023). "AI for all" is a matter of social justice. *AI and Ethics*, *3*(4), 1143–1152. https://doi.org/10.1007/s43681-022-00222-z.

Buhmann, A. and Fieseler, C. (2023). Deep learning meets deep democracy: Deliberative governance and responsible innovation in artificial intelligence. *Business Ethics Quarterly*, *33*(1), 146–179. https://doi.org/10.1017/beq.2021.42

Bui, M. (2025). Toward a community-driven approach to urban data-driven governance. *International Communication Gazette*, *87*(1), 34–47. https://doi.org/10.1177/17480485241261572.

Chakravarty, P. and Gattupalli, S. (2024). Integration of indigenous traditional knowledge and AI in hurricane resilience and adaptation. In: *Advances In Hurricane Risk in a Changing Climate* (pp. 125–158). Cham: Springer Nature Switzerland. https://doi.org/10.1007/978-3-031-63186-3_6.

Chen, Y.C., Ahn, M.J. and Wang, Y.F. (2023). Artificial intelligence and public values: Value impacts and governance in the public sector. *Sustainability*, *15*(6), 4796. https://doi.org/10.3390/su15064796.

Choi, H. and Park, M.J. (2023). To govern or be governed: A|n integrated framework for AI governance in the public sector. *Science and Public Policy*, *50*(6), 1059–1072. https://doi.org/10.1093/scipol/scad045.

Cooper, C., Martin, V., Wilson, O. and Rasmussen, L. (2023). Equitable data governance models for the participatory sciences. *Community Science*, *2*(2), e2022CSJ000025. https://doi.org/10.1029/2022CSJ000025.

Correa Lucero, H. and Martens, C. (2025). Colonial structures in AI: A Latin American decolonial literature review of structural implications for marginalised communities in the Global South. *AI & Society*, 1–17. https://doi.org/10.1007/s00146-025-02547-9.

Djatmiko, G.H., Sinaga, O. and Pawirosumarto, S. (2025). Digital transformation and social inclusion in public services: A qualitative analysis of e-government adoption for marginalised e communities in sustainable governance. *Sustainability*, *17*(7), 2908. https://doi.org/10.3390/su17072908.

Duberry, J. (2022). Artificial intelligence and democracy: Risks and promises of AI-mediated citizen–government relations. In: *Artificial Intelligence and Democracy*. Edward Elgar Publishing. https://doi.org/10.4337/9781788977319.

Dunleavy, P. and Margetts, H. (2025). Data science, artificial intelligence, and the third wave of digital era governance. *Public Policy and Administration*, *40*(2), 185–214. https://doi.org/10.1177/09520767231198737.

Gentelet, K. and Mizrahi, S.K. (2024). A Human-Centered Approach to AI Governance: Operationalizing Human Rights through Citizen Participation. In: *Human-Centered AI* (pp. 215–230). Chapman and Hall/CRC.

Giovanola, B. and Tiribelli, S. (2023). Beyond bias and discrimination: Redefining the AI ethics principle of fairness in healthcare machine-learning algorithms. *AI & Society*, *38*(2), 549–563. https://doi.org/10.1007/s00146-022-01455-6.

Hadley, E., Blatecky, A. and Comfort, M. (2025). Investigating algorithm review boards for organizational responsible artificial intelligence governance. *AI and Ethics*, *5*(3), 2485–2495. https://doi.org/10.1007/s43681-024-00574-8.

Hosseini Tabaghdehi, S.A. and Ayaz, Ö. (2025). AI ethics in action: A circular model for transparency, accountability, and inclusivity. *Journal of Managerial Psychology*. https://doi.org/10.1108/JMP-03-2024-0177.

Huang, K., Joshi, A., Dun, S. and Hamilton, N. (2024). AI regulations. In: *Generative AI Security: Theories and Practices* (pp. 61–98). Cham: Springer Nature Switzerland. https://doi.org/10.1007/978-3-031-54252-7_3.

Hughes, K.D., Konnikov, A., Denier, N. and Hu, Y. (2025). Problematizing the role of artificial intelligence in hiring and organizational inequalities: A multidisciplinary review. *Human Relations*, 00187267251403902. https://doi.org/10.1177/00187267251403902.

Jain, A. and Dienel, H.L. (2024). Deliberative democracy in times of crisis: The capability of citizens' assemblies to overcome societal polarization. *Innovation: The European Journal of Social Science Research*, *37*(3), 681–686. https://doi.org/10.1080/13511610.2024.2381958.

Khan, M.S., Umer, H. and Faruqe, F. (2024). Artificial intelligence for low income countries. *Humanities and Social Sciences Communications*, *11*(1), 1–13. https://doi.org/10.1057/s41599-024-03947-w.

Koniakou, V. (2023). From the "rush to ethics" to the "race for governance" in Artificial Intelligence. *Information Systems Frontiers*, *25*(1), 71–102. https://doi.org/10.1007/s10796-022-10300-6.

LePere-Schloop, M. and Zook, S. (2023). AI governance and civil society: The need for critical engagement. In: *Handbook of Critical Studies of Artificial Intelligence* (pp. 878–889). Edward Elgar Publishing. https://doi.org/10.4337/9781803928562.00087.

Liebig, L., Güttel, L., Jobin, A. and Katzenbach, C. (2024). Subnational AI policy: Shaping AI in a multi-level governance system. *AI & Society*, *39*(3), 1477–1490. https://doi.org/10.1007/s00146-022-01561-5.

Lütz, F. (2024, March). The AI Act, gender equality, and non-discrimination: What role for the AI office? In: *ERA Forum* (Vol. 25, No. 1, pp. 79–95). Berlin/Heidelberg: Springer Berlin Heidelberg. https://doi.org/10.1007/s12027-024-00785-w.

Mądra-Sawicka, M., Gołuchowski, J. and Paliszkiewicz, J. (2025) Trust-Building in the Generative AI–Future Perspectives and Emerging Trends. *Building Trust in the Generative Artificial Intelligence Era* (pp. 3–21). Routledge.

Micheli, M., Gevaert, C.M., Carman, M., Craglia, M., Daemen, E., Ibrahim, R.E., ... & Vespe, M. (2022). AI ethics and data governance in the geospatial domain of Digital Earth. *Big Data & Society*, *9*(2), 20539517221138767. https://doi.org/10.1177/20539517221138767.

Moon, M.J. (2023). Searching for inclusive artificial intelligence for social good: Participatory governance and policy recommendations for making AI more inclusive and benign for society. *Public Administration Review*, *83*(6), 1496–1505. https://doi.org/10.1111/puar.13648.

Mutambara, P.D.E. (2025). Strategic Framework for AI Deployment. In: *Deploying Artificial Intelligence to Achieve the UN Sustainable Development Goals: Enablers, Drivers, and Strategic Framework* (pp. 245–267). Cham: Springer Nature Switzerland. https://doi.org/10.1007/978-3-031-88423-8_11.

Nanni, R. and Napolitano, M. (2024). Dataspaces, public administration, and collective rationality: Opportunities and limits for data-driven policy-making. *Public Money & Management*, *44*(6), 484–490. https://doi.org/10.1080/09540962.2023.2298260.

Olsen, H.P., Hildebrandt, T.T., Wiesener, C., Larsen, M.S. and Flügge, A.W.A. (2024). The right to transparency in public governance: Freedom of information and the use of artificial intelligence by public agencies. *Digital Government: Research and Practice*, *5*(1), 1–15. https://doi.org/10.1145/3632753.

Olugbade, O. (2025). In search of a global governance mechanism for artificial intelligence (AI): A collective action perspective. *Global Public Policy and Governance*, 1–23. https://doi.org/10.1007/s43508-025-00113-z.

Panarese, P., Grasso, M.M. and Solinas, C. (2025). Algorithmic bias, fairness, and inclusivity: A multilevel framework for justice-oriented AI. *AI & Society*, 1–23. https://doi.org/10.1007/s00146-025-02451-2.

Papagiannidis, E., Enholm, I.M., Dremel, C., Mikalef, P. and Krogstie, J. (2023). Toward AI governance: Identifying best practices, and potential barriers and outcomes. *Information Systems Frontiers*, *25*(1), 123–141. https://doi.org/10.1007/s10796-022-10251-y.

Park, K. and Yoon, H.Y. (2024). Beyond the code: The impact of AI algorithm transparency signalling on user trust and relational satisfaction. *Public Relations Review*, *50*(5), 102507. https://doi.org/10.1016/j.pubrev.2024.102507.

Parthasarathy, A., Phalnikar, A., Jauhar, A., Somayajula, D., Krishnan, G.S. and Ravindran, B. (2024). Participatory Approaches in AI Development and Governance: A Principled Approach. *arXiv preprint arXiv:2407.13100*. https://doi.org/10.48550/arXiv.2407.13100.

Pislaru, M., Vlad, C.S., Ivascu, L. and Mircea, I.I. (2024). Citizen-centric governance: Enhancing citizen engagement through artificial intelligence tools. *Sustainability*, *16*(7), 2686. https://doi.org/10.3390/su16072686.

Rasoulzadeh Aghdam, S., Bababei Morad, B., Ghasemzadeh, B., Irani, M. and Huovila, A. (2025). Social smart city research: interconnections between participatory governance, data privacy, artificial intelligence, and ethical sustainable development. *Frontiers in Sustainable Cities*, *6*, 1514040. https://doi.org/10.3389/frsc.2024.1514040.

Roberts, H., Hine, E., Taddeo, M. and Floridi, L. (2024). Global AI governance: Barriers and pathways forward. *International Affairs*, *100*(3), 1275–1286. https://doi.org/10.1093/ia/iiae073.

Robles, P. and Mallinson, D.J. (2025). Artificial intelligence technology, public trust, and effective governance. *Review of Policy Research*, *42*(1), 11–28. https://doi.org/10.1111/ropr.12555.

Roche, C., Wall, P.J. and Lewis, D. (2023). Ethics and diversity in artificial intelligence policies, strategies, and initiatives. *AI and Ethics*, *3*(4), 1095–1115. https://doi.org/10.1007/s43681-022-00218-9.

Sahu, S. and Mallick, N. (2025). Enhancing Governance through Fuzzy Logic: A Framework for Adaptable and Inclusive Policymaking. In: *Fuzzy Logic in Smart Sustainable Cities* (pp. 309–354). Jenny Stanford Publishing.

Santos, M.R. and Carvalho, L.C. (2025). AI-driven participatory environmental management: Innovations, applications, and future prospects. *Journal of Environmental Management*, *373*, 123864. https://doi.org/10.1016/j.jenvman.2024.123864.

Sartori, L. and Theodorou, A. (2022). A sociotechnical perspective for the future of AI: Narratives, inequalities, and human control. *Ethics and Information Technology*, *24*(1), 4. https://doi.org/10.1007/s10676-022-09624-3.

Sayles, J. (2024). Capacity Building for AI Actors. In: *Principles of AI Governance and Model Risk Management: Master the Techniques for Ethical and Transparent AI Systems* (pp. 321–331). Berkeley, CA: Apress. https://doi.org/10.1007/979-8-8688-0983-5_16.

Schmank, J. and Buchkremer, R. (2024). Navigating the Digital Public Sphere: An AI-Driven Analysis of Interaction Dynamics across Societal Domains. *Societies*, *14*(10), 195. https://doi.org/10.3390/soc14100195.

Schuett, J., Reuel, A.K. and Carlier, A. (2025). How to design an AI ethics board. *AI and Ethics*, *5*(2), 863–881. https://doi.org/10.1007/s43681-023-00409-y.

Shafik, W. (2025). The Intersection of Technology and Inclusion for People with Disabilities and Marginalized Communities. In: *Global Sustainable Transition with Inclusion: A Focus on the People with Disabilities and the Marginalized* (pp. 185–212). Singapore: Springer Nature Singapore. https://doi.org/10.1007/978-981-96-6557-0_7.

Sharma, R. (2024). Governance and Oversight of AI Systems. In: *AI and the Boardroom: Insights into Governance, Strategy, and the Responsible Adoption of AI* (pp. 353–370). Berkeley, CA: Apress. https://doi.org/10.1007/979-8-8688-0796-1_28.

Sieber, R., Brandusescu, A., Sangiambut, S. and Adu-Daako, A. (2025). What is civic participation in artificial intelligence? *Environment and Planning B: Urban Analytics and City Science*, *52*(6), 1388–1406. https://doi.org/10.1177/23998083241296200.

Ter-Minassian, L. (2025). Democratizing AI Governance: Balancing Expertise and Public Participation. *arXiv preprint arXiv:2502.08651*. https://doi.org/10.48550/arXiv.2502.08651.

Visave, J. (2025). Transparency in AI for emergency management: Building trust and accountability. *AI and Ethics*, 1–14. https://doi.org/10.1007/s43681-025-00692-x.

Walter, Y. (2024). Managing the race to the moon: Global policy and governance in Artificial Intelligence regulation: A contemporary overview and an analysis of socioeconomic consequences. *Discover Artificial Intelligence*, *4*(1), 14. https://doi.org/10.1007/s44163-024-00109-4.

Wasi, A.T. (2025, March). AI for Social Good and Public Impact in Marginalized Communities: A Cross-Cultural Framework. In: *International Conference on Social Impact of AI* (pp. 1–12). Cham: Springer Nature Switzerland. https://doi.org/10.1007/978-3-031-98949-0_1.

Wilson, C. (2022). Public engagement and AI: A values analysis of national strategies. *Government Information Quarterly*, *39*(1), 101652. https://doi.org/10.1016/j.giq.2021.101652.

Yang, L. (2023). Developing collaboration between research-oriented and practice-oriented experts in public administration: How does expert participation make a difference in public policy making and governance practice? *Public Policy and Administration*, *38*(1), 58–82. https://doi.org/10.1177/0952076720958468.

Yigitcanlar, T., David, A., Li, W., Fookes, C., Bibri, S.E. and Ye, X. (2024). Unlocking artificial intelligence adoption in local governments: Best practice lessons from real-world implementations. *Smart Cities*, *7*(4), 1576–1625. https://doi.org/10.3390/smartcities7040064.

15 Future Directions in AI Policy and Governance

Artificial Intelligence (AI) is evolving gradually, giving a rise to new opportunities and challenging policy issues. Future AI governance will have to keep up with the new technologies, change in ethical issues, and alteration of geopolitical relations. This chapter discusses potential ways in enhancing AI policy in the near future. It explores such trends as risk-based regulation, international collaboration, human focused regulation, and increased integration of values in society. Another point which is raised in the chapter is the necessity of adaptive legal frameworks, transparency tools, and effective enforcement systems. It focuses on cooperation between governments, industries, researchers, and communities in order to make innovations responsible. By uncovering ways forward, the chapter contributes to establishing the AI governance models that are adaptive, visionary, and democratic and human right oriented.

15.1 Introduction

Artificial Intelligence (AI) is steadily influencing world societies and has taken over key industries like healthcare, finance systems, transportation, governance, and education. The high pace of AI technologies development has offered novel economic and scientific opportunities. It is also associated with complicated policy issues regarding privacy rights, security threats, changes in employment, and equitable treatment of every member of society (Qin et al., 2024). Various nations are creating systems and regulations to inform the use of AI. To achieve responsible innovation and to benefit the broader population, international organisations are making suggestions of shared standards. This development is indicative of the fact that AI governance has become a crucial priority in both national and global policy objectives (Schmitt, 2022).

The situation with governance constantly is that it fluctuates due to fast development of AI technologies. Machine learning is dynamic, and it needs regular control as opposed to a single supervision. The policies should, therefore, be flexible and be able to do away with changes in technology (Zaidan & Ibrahim, 2024). Governance is not on current challenges only but it should be inclined to look into the future challenges and opportunities. Proactive policy enables the governments and institutions to anticipate the long-term implications of AI to every social, political, and economic system. This involves anticipating future human resource changes, new ethical issues and digital infrastructure (Yar et al., 2024).

DOI: 10.1201/9781003776659-15

The relevance of adaptive models of governance is that the common methods of regulation used are slow-moving and inflexible. The technological advancement of AI systems can surpass the human ability to revise legislation. Rigid regulation helps ensure timely intervention in the event of a problem, but at the same time innovative and developing processes are encouraged. It also enables other nations to test new policy strategies as per their societal priorities, economic connections, and cultural values. With increased AI competition across the world, a good governance structure is now a significant element in the national development policies (Holzinger et al., 2025).

Another significant element of AI governance is meaningful cooperation between governments, industries, researchers, and citizens in the future. The AI does not know national borders. The flow of data is between countries, and AI services are conducted on the platform of other countries online (Birkstedt et al., 2023). International collaboration is needed to handle international risks like cybercrime, false information, and online monitoring. The governmental systems should respond to issues of international trade, common data formats, and technologies that ensure individuals are secured irrespective of geographical location (Roberts et al., 2024).

Another factor of significance in the future direction of governance is public confidence. Human beings communicate with AI in various fields of everyday life with or without their awareness. This trust can be developed by institutions speaking straight to the point regarding the usage of AI and the reasons why we make certain choices (Lee et al., 2023). Clear policies are useful in eliminating fear or misunderstanding. Law enforcement and accountability depict the existence of checks and balances where officials are ready to act in case of damages. In case of high trust by the population, AI acceptance will be easier and more advantageous to the society (Choung et al., 2023). The world has changed and AI governance should keep up with the development. The emergence of new technologies will introduce new challenges, to which any specific policy response will have to be thoughtful and collaborative in relation to the research and public inclinations (Zaidan & Ibrahim, 2024).

15.2 Technological Trends Shaping Future Governance

15.2.1 Autonomous Systems and Advanced Robotics

Autonomous systems are developed to do functions with some little or no human involvement. The latter are self-driving cars, drone carriers with deliveries, industrial robots with AI, and sophisticated defence technologies. They also have sensors, machine learning algorithms, and decision-making models that make them operate independently (Chen et al., 2022). Such systems have the ability of enhancing safety, enhancing productivity, and also lowering human labour in hazardous locations. To illustrate, robots are able to reinforce the efforts of disaster response, help in medical operations, and even increase agriculture. Nevertheless, there are also some problems of liability, security, and ethical responsibility in autonomy. In the case when an autonomous vehicle is involved in an accident, it is hard to determine who is to be blamed: the user, the manufacturer, the programmer or the data provider (Yazdanpanah et al., 2023).

Governments have to create explicit policies on safety testing, human oversight policies, and certification protocols. There must always be accountability mechanisms involved in the autonomy of decision-making. There should also be a policy against malicious utilisation like weaponised robots or systems that threaten human rights. The growing autonomy of machines will cause adaptive governance to play a greater role in the future (Azar & Koubaa, 2023).

15.2.2 Generative AI and Information Integrity Challenges

Generative models of AI produce novel content in the form of images, text, video, and audio. Some of these examples are AI chatbots, deepfake systems, and creative design tools. These technologies aid in the media, entertainment, education, and business innovation. Their content creation speed and personalisation is very useful in numerous industries (Taeihagh, 2025). Nevertheless, generative AI also poses great fragilities. Misinformation is the one which can be delivered more rapidly and seems more persuasive. Deepfakes can make people famous and corrupt the elections, or reinforce fraud. The credibility of online materials is more difficult to be checked. The citizens can lose confidence in the news and online communication (Badawy, 2025).

They should be governed to maintain integrity of the information. Transparency, watermarking, and content authentication tools are the policies that should be encouraged. There is a need to have digital literacy programmes to make the population aware of manipulated content. Proper licensing to conduct responsible use in prevention of wrong use without hindering positive innovation is possible. Generative AI proves the idea that the future governance should refrain from its technical safety to an adequate extent, but it should also be concerned with the safeguarding of democratic values and truth in the informational space (Wang et al., 2025).

15.2.3 AI for Scientific Discovery and Public Innovation

AI systems are actively implemented in scientific studies and public developmental projects. They have speeded up the discovery related to other fields like medicine, agriculture, climate, and energy. AI models have the capability of processing big data, modelling complex systems, and discovering patterns that might be overlooked by human beings. As an illustration, AI enhances quicker drug development, better disease recognition, and enhanced forecasts of climatic conditions (Bianchini et al., 2022). In urban innovations, AI is used to enhance cities in regard to planning, disaster management, and resource allocation. It assists governments to make superior choices using data. These applications can be used to solve challenges faced by the world and contribute to sustainable development (Agrawal et al., 2024).

Nonetheless, the science of AI should be guided by the principles of ethical conduct and free research. Scientific results should be reproducible and accountable; hence, there is the need to have transparency. The reasons behind the importance of data governance frameworks are to ensure sensitive health, environmental or citizen data is safeguarded. There is also a need to collaborate globally and have equal access resources in innovation. Inclusive policies lead to concentration of scientific AI advantages in affluent regions in the absence of the policies (Wang et al., 2023). AI in science and public innovation demonstrates that governance in the future requirements encourages available knowledge, equity in the dispersion of technology, and prudent utilisation of potent academic instruments (Yu et al., 2025).

15.2.4 Human–AI Collaboration and Workplace Transformation

AI is not the only cause of losing jobs, but it also transforms the way of work. The Human–AI partnership is a joint venture that integrates human creativity and judgement, and machine speed and accuracy. These may take the form of workplace assistants, decision support systems, and collaborative robots in factories. With the help of these tools, the productive work can be enhanced, the number of manual operations minimised, and personalised service advanced (Babashahi et al., 2024). Nonetheless, this change brings other difficulties as well. The automation of some of the tasks will lead to the displacement of jobs in some sectors. The employees will have to acquire new competencies to work and handle AI-driven systems. Inequality on the workers having advanced digital skills and those without may escalate without appropriate support. Fair work conditions and labour rights have to be supported in the sphere of the AI interest decision-making (Tenakwah & Watson, 2025).

Governance should then be concerned with employment practices that are ethical, reskilling, and inclusion of the workforce. The issue of human control is also significant in ensuring AI does not make decisions that disfavour employees or infringe rights. It should mean that the economic positive aspects of AI should be distributed equally and not accumulate in the hands of big companies (Fenwick et al., 2024). The Human–AI partnerships point out that governance is necessary to facilitate innovation without jeopardising employment, human dignity, or the welfare of workers.

15.3 Adaptive and Risk-Based Regulatory Models

15.3.1 Dynamic and Flexible Policy Structures

Adaptable and dynamic policy frameworks assist the regulators in revising the rules as AI progresses. The design of policies can be developed to have a mechanism of constant revision, which keeps the policies pertinent to technological advancements.

This can also enable the policy formulators to experiment on their solutions on a small scale before mass implementation. One of these tools is regulatory sandboxes. They involve controlled conditions under which the developers of AI and similar controls collaborate with regulators in order to discover and enhance safety before a broad release of products (Liebig et al., 2024). Flexibility in policy structures is another form of encouraging inter-government collaboration, research, and company collaboration. With open communication channels, it is easier to deal with any arising problem in a short time. Regulations could change gradually with the experience of the world around. This minimises time wastage in the policymaking process and makes the governance very realistic and efficient. It is not aimed at eliminating rules but to come up with ones that can be easily modified and not through lengthy legal procedures (Zaidan & Ibrahim, 2024).

15.3.2 Risk-Tiering and System Classification

Risk-tiering is used to guarantee AI systems are controlled according to the amount of damages they can inflict on people or society. It acknowledges the fact that AI tools are not homogenous in the purpose or effect. The systems that are less risky such as in the case of entertainment recommendations do not require the same degree of restrictions like systems that utilise high risk like the medical diagnosis or policing (Currie et al., 2025). The governments may categorise AI by such criteria as autonomy, sensitivity of data, the effect on rights, and the extent of implementation. The high risk systems have to adhere strictly to certain standards such as audit trails, safety testing, and human supervision. Moderate risk systems need moderate controls whereas the low-risk systems can be guided through simple directions. This will be a way of not over regulating but having good protections where regulations are required (Edward et al., 2025). Risk classification is not a decision made once. The AI systems can work out or be applied in other contexts that raise the risk level. Classification should thus be re-examined on a regular basis. Clear-cut criteria would assure the population as to why certain AI systems have to be regulated more than others. Risk-based governance can efficiently allocate regulatory effort, as well as devoting resources to those places where harm would be most extreme (Prem, 2025).

15.3.3 Continuous Monitoring, Auditing, and Compliance

The AI systems are dynamic and therefore require around the clock supervision. In the case of any change in the environment or the introduction of a new piece of information forming a bias, their performance can be diminished. Monitoring enhances organisations to monitor precision, equity, and protection in the lifecycle of the system. Reporting, logs, and user feedback aid in the detection of problems early. Systems can be fixed or restricted when there are any concerns to avoid any damage (Naoufal, 2024). Auditing also provides more evaluation of AI behaviour. Technical audits are conducted to look into the strength of algorithms where ethical audits are conducted to look into fairness, discrimination, and accountability. Audits may either be internal or independent. Open auditing assists in providing assurance that the organisations adhere to policy standards at all times. All systems that are not in compliance should be corrected (Minkkinen et al., 2022).

The compliance mechanisms put the blame on developers and system operators. Companies have to keep documents and forward them to government regulators in case of need. In other instances, sanctions can be taken against violations, namely, in instances where the systems that are of high risk lead to injury. The compliance rules prompt organisations to view safety and ethics as processes that have no beginning and no end (Mökander, 2023). Trust is also enhanced by monitoring and compliance. Human beings would like to be more accommodative towards AI once they are informed that there is monitoring of activities after integration and the accountable parties assess the consequences. Constant governance should be used to maintain the relevance of policy to the reality on the ground, and not with the old assumptions (Turksen et al., 2024).

15.4 Strengthening Global Cooperation and Harmonisation

15.4.1 International Standards and Cross-Border Alignment

International standards assist in developing a common language on responsible AI development. Such organisations as ISO, IEC, and IEEE introduce principles of safety, fairness, transparency, and interoperability. Once the countries harmonise their regulation systems with these standards, companies are able to run across boundaries without any hustles. This will ease compliance load and induce innovation (Ishkhanyan, 2025). Shared accountability is also supported by cross border alignment. When a single nation permits negative AI applications, the consequences can be passed to the rest of the world. Standardised norms eliminate regulatory loopholes and save citizens all over the globe. Alignment does not presuppose the same policies, although it promotes some consistency in key sectors such as human rights protection, auditability of the system, and data governance. Standard setting via co-operation makes sure that the governance is based on the global views as opposed to the interest of a few, influential countries (Huang et al., 2024). Mutual recognition agreements also need to be done between governments where each government recognises the other testing, certification, and compliance process. This eliminates redundancy in work and enhances more effective international cooperation (Rong et al., 2025).

15.4.2 Joint Research, Innovation, and Safety Initiatives

The new knowledge that stems out of AI research is useful to all societies, particularly those that deal with important matters like healthcare, climate adaptation, and disaster response. Joint innovation practices enable nations to pool expertise and transfer scientific resources and speed up the discovery. There is the contribution of international academic networks and cross border research centres which make the capacity of problem solving to be enhanced (Wen, 2024). The research on safety is also necessary. Joint initiatives may centre on risk detection, robustness tests, as well as on the creation of secure systems. Broader and fairer testing of AI systems can be performed because of shared datasets and secure testing environments. Combined exercises assist in establishing international levels of ethical experimentation and responsible application (Salhab et al., 2024). Collaboration minimises overlaps in efforts as well as reduces the cost of newness. It further enhances fair access to emerging technologies. Unless there are collaboration programmes, AI benefits can be concentrated in more affluent regions. The cross-border initiatives are therefore contributing in a global development, and they make sure that development is divided more favourably (Buocz et al., 2023).

15.4.3 Inclusive Participation of the Global South and Under-represented Regions

The international collaboration should involve nations that have varying technological and economic potentials. Limited digital infrastructure, AI expertise, and inadequate funding of innovation are some of the problems encountered in many parts of the Global South. When this is not included in the global regulation of governance, there are chances that AI policy may disregard the needs of billions of individuals (Mutambara, 2025). Inclusive participation is a way of ensuring governance structures are inclusive of various cultures, laws, and social realities. It further discourages digital colonialism where technologies created in other regions foster destructive values or biases on the population in the local industries. Equal participation in standard setting, research collaborations as well as capacity-building policies should be facilitated (Nkwo et al., 2025). The underrepresented regions can be encouraged to create their solutions to AI by investing in digital skills, infrastructure, and an open access to tools and data. The regional and South-South collaboration and alliances, e.g., strategies by the African Union AI could be good moves towards collective governance leadership. Inclusion enhances the validity of the global cooperative work and minimises the structural inequalities (Jamba & Marambi, 2024).

15.4.4 Cybersecurity and Responsible Data Governance Norms

AI systems require greater reliance on data and digital infrastructure. Such cybersecurity risks such as hacking, data poisoning, and system manipulation may be extremely detrimental. In the absence of aligned governance, bad players can use the lax security systems in one part to invade systems in other parts. Global actions are required to come up with equal measures on cybersecurity (Camilleri, 2024). Rules of responsible data governance are also required to handle the cross-border data flows. The countries should agree on agreements that strike the right balance between the economic interests, privacy protection and national security. **Common values:** The use of law, consent, and responsibility are some of the principles that help us form trust between the states and the citizens (Gill & Germann, 2022). To avoid the illegal surveillance, safeguard sensitive data sets, and provide transparency to the operations in the world digital arena, governments have to collaborate. The damage related to AI-related cyber attacks can be minimised through cooperation on incident reporting and crisis response (Sarker, 2024). The relationship between large spheres of cooperation that benefit unified global AI governance and contribute to enhancing fairness, safety, and innovation are summarised in Table 15.1.

Table 15.1 Areas of Global Cooperation for AI Governance.

Key Area	*Main Focus*	*Expected Benefit*
International Standards	Interoperable safety and ethics rules	Reduced regulatory fragmentation
Joint Research & Innovation	Shared scientific progress and risk evaluation	Accelerated and fairer innovation
Inclusive Participation	Representation of Global South and under-represented groups	Equitable access to AI benefits
Cybersecurity & Data Governance	Secure infrastructure and trusted data sharing	Protection from cross-border threats

15.5 Ethical Priorities for Future AI Governance

15.5.1 Human Dignity and Rights-Centred Approaches

The key to the governance of AI should be human dignity. AI systems also affect the choices of people in terms of their opportunities, freedoms, and well-being. These systems are potentially harmful in cases where they are operated without considering the dignity of the individual although they may seem efficient or accurate. A rights-based approach can be used to make sure that AI bolsters human autonomy instead of destroying or diminishing it. This involves having people have relevant control over decisions that influence their lives (Hogan & Lasek-Markey, 2024). Basic human rights, including privacy, freedom of expression, and freedom of discrimination, should not be infringed by AI. Police, surveillance, border control, or social welfare systems are particularly in need of intense protection. Rights-based governance needs to have regulations that restrict intrusive data gathering, stop unfair vigilance, and ban damaging profiling actions. Governments should ensure that AI does not enhance surveillance by the state and democratic involvement (Prabhakaran et al., 2022).

An anthropocentric approach would also demand on-site control in high risk environments. However, despite the ability of AI to process information fast, human beings should be in charge of making decisions that have significant ramifications. Monitoring keeps people in check and holds them responsible to save them from mistakes or injustices. The responsibility should be explicitly distributed in such a way that it does not harm the people who might fall victim to the systems that have no transparency or individual human participation (Wong, 2025). Respect towards cultural diversity and moral values are also part of human dignity. AI systems cannot be classical in their views of the world. On the contrary, they need to be representative of social and moral norms of various communities. The rights-based governance extends discussion, involvement of people, and responses of groups that might be at risk due to some special factors or being vulnerable. This will make AI more legitimate and trustworthy to the general population (Thomaidou & Limniotis, 2025).

15.5.2 Fairness, Equality, and Social Benefit

Ethical fairness needs to be a critical AI requirement. AI should not discriminate against them based on race, gender, disability, socioeconomic status, and other identity factors. Nevertheless, most AI systems use historical data that is indicative of forms of inequality. Unless these biases are eliminated, systems may generate unequal results as well as social hierarchies. The governing of the AI needs to demand fairness testing, periodical audits, and prejudice control measures throughout the complete procedure of the system (Camilleri, 2024). Equality is another factor that implies that the benefits of AI should be equally shared. AI is able to enhance healthcare availability, increase education, and promote economic development. Nevertheless, unless there is good governance, such advantages can only be enjoyed by rich areas or those with high technology. Inequality will grow as one of the communities will have access to advanced AI services and the rest are unable to access anything digital. Ethical governance demands bridging this divide by investing in digital infrastructure, inclusive design and equal policy support (Moon, 2023).

With social benefit AI must also serve. The governance systems ought to promote technologies that reinforce the social good, environmental sustainability, and community. Systems that encourage manipulation, exploitation, or commercial practices that are detrimental to ethical practices are discouraged by ethical guidelines. AI cannot be utilised in order to boost unfair working conditions, surveillance capitalism, or environmental degradation (Panarese et al., 2025). Social good and justice must be constantly monitored. The AI systems are developed, and their effects can vary through time. On-going assessment should be supported in the policies in order to make fairness the priority. Problems should be corrected by having mechanisms that can swiftly fix the problem. Fair governance enhances stability in society and advances trust on technology (Qian et al., 2024).

15.5.3 Transparency, Explainability, and Safe Design Principles

The other critical ethical priority is transparency. The processes that AI systems operate on can be complex, and they are hard to comprehend by people. Accountability is weak in the case of opaque decisions. People are not able to question results that are harmful when they are not familiar with the process of decision-making. Transparent design needs documentation, openness, and accessibility in explanations as well as the availability of the limitations of the system (Walter, 2024). Transparency is associated with explainability. It needs to reason the decisions, which impact the rights and opportunities of people, in an understandable way as conducted by AI systems. This is of particular concern in healthcare, credit rating, employment, and law enforcement. There is no reason why explanations have to disclose sensitive intellectual property yet they should provide people with sufficient information to appeal, question, or contest decisions (Chen et al., 2023).

There should be safe design principles that will direct the formation of AI. Safety is not only a technical problem, but it is also an ethical issue. The AI systems are supposed to be configured in a way that results in less harm, prevention of cyberattacks, and stability even in unpredictable situations. Testers have to test systems in realistic conditions to get to know their failures. Data security and protection against unauthorised access should also be addressed in terms of safety (Gianni et al., 2022). Responsible design has mechanisms of human control and fall back. In case of AI failure, human intervention should come in time. Systems must also not deal with falsely designed systems that control users or conceal vital information. Ethical design promotes clarity, control by the user, and responsible communication (Erman & Furendal, 2022). Transparency and safe design will help to build a better trust in the population. With the awareness of the AI systems and their safety oriented approach, people are more prone to technological change and its acceptance. These moral priorities would remain influential in the future in relation to the way governments and institutions approach emerging AI issues (Radanliev, 2025).

15.6 Institutional Capacity and Public Trust

15.6.1 Building Regulatory and Technical Capability

With further development of AI, regulators have to comprehend the functionality of systems, the risks they propose, and their evaluation. The traditional regulatory bodies were intended to control the physical products or fixed software. AI is however dynamic, and can learn through machine learning. This makes it difficult to have the necessary technical expertise of the regulators. Capacity creation would involve recruiting personnel focusing on computer science, data governance and cybersecurity, social sciences, and ethics. There is also the need to create training programmes that should assist the current staff in learning how to behave algorithms, detect bias, and audit techniques. Government units and institutes in charge of AI may contribute to facilitating work and exchanging expertise in different sectors (Agarwal & Nene, 2025).

Infrastructure also matters, such as technical infrastructure. In order to investigate the problem of algorithmic decision-making, regulators should have access to testing environments, secure data-sharing platforms, and analytical tools. It is an absence of such resources that makes oversight a weak component, and detrimental systems can remain unnoticed. Cases of collaboration with learning institutions and global organisations may be used to help in enhancing capability, especially where the resources are minimal (Birkstedt et al., 2023). The capacity to respond swiftly on emerging issues is also part of institutional capacity. Regulators need to be empowered to coordinate in cases where dangerous consequences emerge, revamp the policies, or simply paralyse unsafe systems. Effective governance systems enhance resiliency and make sure that society is safeguarded as technologies keep on changing (Cancela-Outeda, 2024).

15.6.2 Public Engagement and Digital Literacy

A significant role of AI governance is played by public trust. Individuals tend to embrace innovations when they know their operations and they feel that their issues are addressed. Communication with the populace ensures that the citizens voice their opinion about implementation of AI, particularly in places of high consequences like surveillance, law enforcement, or welfare distribution (Polizzi, 2025). The involvement can be done through various methods, such as consultations, workshops, online forums, citizen assemblies. Through these platforms, the policymakers are taught the practical effects and social demands. Transparency is also enhanced as people are able to participate in the decision making process because decision making is not a secret (Wilson, 2022). Engagement has close relation to digital literacy. And there are a lot of people who engage with AI on a daily basis. Misunderstanding may lead to a fear, bafflement, or suspicion. They should empower people to be critical of the systems by conducting education programs that describe AI in straightforward words. Learning about digital rights, data privacy, and processes of these algorithms can be supported in schools, universities and in libraries, and in media platforms (Marmolejo-Ramos et al., 2022).

There should be work towards equalising digital access. Individuals without internet connectivity, devices, or without any technical skills, cannot play on an equal footing. The strategies will have to include the rural communities, some of the elderly, persons with disabilities, and linguistic minorities. Having more citizens who have access to digital skills would enable them to enjoy the optimism of the technology and the participation of anyone making meaningful contributions to the decision-making process in governance (Pislaru et al., 2024). Democratic values are enhanced by society participation. It also makes sure governance is based on the needs of the society, not just the interests of industry or government machinery. The trust is established when communities realise that their feedback does not go to waste when it comes to the policy outcomes and also the authorities address the issues in a timely and respectful way (Sieber et al., 2024).

15.6.3 Accountability Processes to Strengthen Trust

Accountability is required in order to demonstrate that the actions of the AI systems can be attributed to the agencies and developers. Reliable governance has to have systems of review, supervision, redress, and enforcement in place. Accountability would make the usage of AI both legal and ethical and would provide individuals with chances to be compensated in case of negative results (Visave, 2025). Categories should be covered by clear regulations to define the decision-maker in the systems operated by AI This eliminates cases of passing on of accountability or evading since the system is independent. There should be a level of responsibility taken by developers, operators, and organisations of various elements of system performance. Responsibility is aided by audit and reporting requirements. The AI systems must be appraised every now and again to identify bias, errors, and risks. Results on issues should be shared when there is a crisis. Lack of compliance can be checked by independent overseeing bodies and ethics can be ensured by organisations adhering to ethical standards and legal requirements (Lahusen et al., 2024).

Redress is required in order to guard individual rights. The complaint mechanisms and appeals need to be availed to users in case they feel wronged or harmed. These processes need to be accessible, visible, and prompt. They assist in preventing the situation when people are helpless before algorithmic decisions. Trust is strengthened by enforcement mechanisms since they indicate that rules are not considered imaginary. More penalties, fines, or operational limitations can be followed in case organisations do not fulfil their duties or misuse AI technologies. With successful enforcement, citizens are able to witness that systems are also accountable just as humans as well as institutions are (Novelli et al., 2024). There is also accountability that entails communication. It should be known to people how the data is being utilised, what decision-making is being taken, and what are the safety precautions. Fear and uncertainty are minimised through responsible communication. It demonstrates that institutions play a role in ensuring safety to the masses.

15.7 Conclusion

The future of AI governance is to strengthen institutional capacity and develop public trust. As AI is becoming a part of the daily routine, societies should make sure that the institutions established to oversee it possess the necessary skills and resources and structures that will allow them to address the risks that are likely to arise. Tough regulation needs qualified specialists, technical means, and timely decisions. In the absence of this, the governance actions might not save individuals and communities against the negative consequences. The trust of the people is also critical. Individuals should be made to believe that the AI systems are fair, open, and in manners that do not violate their rights. Engagement and digital literacy empower citizens with the knowledge of AI and include them in making decisions that determine its progress. With communities involved, they will support innovation and take new technologies well. Accountability processes strengthen the trust aspect because it makes organisations accountable towards their actions. The ethical principles are being observed because of auditing, oversight, and an available system of redress. These aspects combined control an environment of governance, which is both consistent and receptive. Safe and human-centred AI futures have their basis in institutional capacity and trust among people. By laying money in both fields, the societies are able to steer the advancement in technology towards a path that is of benefit to all.

References

Agarwal, A. and Nene, M.J. (2025). A five-layer framework for AI governance: integrating regulation, standards, and certification. *Transforming Government: People, Process, and Policy*. https://doi.org/10.1108/TG-03-2025-0065.

Agrawal, A., McHale, J. and Oettl, A. (2024). Artificial intelligence and scientific discovery: A model of prioritized search. *Research Policy*, *53*(5), 104989. https://doi.org/10.1016/j.respol.2024.104989.

Azar, A.T. and Koubaa, A. (Eds.). (2023). *Artificial Intelligence for Robotics and Autonomous Systems Applications*. Berlin/Heidelberg, Germany: Springer. https://doi.org/10.1007/978-3-031-28715-2.

Babashahi, L., Barbosa, C.E., Lima, Y., Lyra, A., Salazar, H., Argôlo, M., ... & Souza, J.M.D. (2024). AI in the workplace: A systematic review of skill transformation in the industry. *Administrative Sciences*, *14*(6), 127. https://doi.org/10.3390/admsci14060127.

Badawy, W. (2025). Algorithmic sovereignty and democratic resilience: Rethinking AI governance in the age of generative AI. *AI and Ethics*, 1–8. https://doi.org/10.1007/s43681-025-00739-z.

Bianchini, S., Müller, M. and Pelletier, P. (2022). Artificial intelligence in science: An emerging general method of invention. *Research Policy*, *51*(10), 104604. https://doi.org/10.1016/j.respol.2022.104604.

Birkstedt, T., Minkkinen, M., Tandon, A. and Mäntymäki, M. (2023). AI governance: Themes, knowledge gaps, and future agendas. *Internet Research*, *33*(7), 133–167. https://doi.org/10.1108/INTR-01-2022-0042.

Buocz, T., Pfotenhauer, S. and Eisenberger, I. (2023). Regulatory sandboxes in the AI Act: Reconciling innovation and safety? *Law, Innovation, and Technology*, *15*(2), 357–389. https://doi.org/10.1080/17579961.2023.2245678

Camilleri, M.A. (2024). Artificial intelligence governance: Ethical considerations and implications for social responsibility. *Expert Systems*, *41*(7), e13406. https://doi.org/10.1111/exsy.13406.

Cancela-Outeda, C. (2024). The EU's AI Act: A framework for collaborative governance. *Internet of Things*, *27*, 101291. https://doi.org/10.1016/j.iot.2024.101291.

Chen, J., Sun, J. and Wang, G. (2022). From unmanned systems to autonomous intelligent systems. *Engineering*, *12*, 16–19. https://doi.org/10.1016/j.eng.2021.10.007.

Chen, Y.C., Ahn, M.J. and Wang, Y.F. (2023). Artificial intelligence and public values: Value impacts and governance in the public sector. *Sustainability*, *15*(6), 4796. https://doi.org/10.3390/su15064796.

Choung, H., David, P. and Ross, A. (2023). Trust in AI and its role in the acceptance of AI technologies. *International Journal of Human–Computer Interaction*, *39*(9), 1727–1739. https://doi.org/10.1080/10447318.2022.2050543

Currie, W.L., Leimeister, J.M., Schlagwein, D. and Willcocks, L. (2025). Rethinking technology regulation in the age of AI risks. *Journal of Information Technology*, *40*(3), 236–245. https://doi.org/10.1177/02683962251378815.

Edward, S.G., Bhattacharya, R. and Sinha, V. (2025). Responsible AI and Risk Framework. In: *Enterprise Guide for Implementing Generative AI and Agentic AI: A Practical Guide to Developing, Deploying, and Operationalizing AI-Driven Applications for Enterprise Use* (pp. 337–383). Berkeley, CA: Apress. https://doi.org/10.1007/979-8-8688-1603-1_7.

Erman, E. and Furendal, M. (2022). The global governance of artificial intelligence: Some normative concerns. *Moral Philosophy and Politics*, *9*(2), 267–291. https://doi.org/10.1515/mopp-2020-0046.

Fenwick, A., Molnar, G. and Frangos, P. (2024). Revisiting the role of HR in the age of AI: Bringing humans and machines closer together in the workplace. *Frontiers in Artificial Intelligence*, *6*, 1272823. https://doi.org/10.3389/frai.2023.1272823.

Gianni, R., Lehtinen, S. and Nieminen, M. (2022). Governance of responsible AI: From ethical guidelines to cooperative policies. *Frontiers in Computer Science*, *4*, 873437. https://doi.org/10.3389/fcomp.2022.873437.

Gill, A.S. and Germann, S. (2022). Conceptual and normative approaches to AI governance for a global digital ecosystem supportive of the UN Sustainable Development Goals (SDGs). *AI and Ethics*, *2*(2), 293–301. https://doi.org/10.1007/s43681-021-00058-z.

Hogan, L. and Lasek-Markey, M. (2024). Towards a Human Rights-Based Approach to Ethical AI Governance in Europe. *Philosophies*, *9*(6), 181. https://doi.org/10.3390/philosophies9060181.

Holzinger, A., Zatloukal, K. and Müller, H. (2025). Is human oversight to AI systems still possible? *New Biotechnology*, *85*, 59–62. https://doi.org/10.1016/j.nbt.2024.12.003.

Huang, K., Joshi, A., Dun, S. and Hamilton, N. (2024). AI regulations. In: *Generative AI Security: Theories and Practices* (pp. 61–98). Cham: Springer Nature Switzerland. https://doi.org/10.1007/978-3-031-54252-7_3.

Ishkhanyan, A. (2025). Governing AI across borders: Corporate power, state sovereignty, and global regulation. *Digital Policy, Regulation, and Governance*. https://doi.org/10.1108/DPRG-03-2025-0057.

Jamba, F. and Marambi, S. (2024). Sustainable Use of Artificial Intelligent Technology: What Is It for the Global South in Achieving Inclusive Development Goals? In: *Fostering Long-Term Sustainable Development in Africa: Overcoming Poverty, Inequality, and Unemployment* (pp. 343–374). https://doi.org/10.1007/978-3-031-61321-0_16.

Lahusen, C., Maggetti, M. and Slavkovik, M. (2024). Trust, trustworthiness, and AI governance. *Scientific Reports*, *14*(1), 20752. https://doi.org/10.1038/s41598-024-71761-0.

Lee, S., Lee, M. and Lee, S. (2023). What if artificial intelligence becomes completely ambient in our daily lives? Exploring future human–AI interaction through high fidelity illustrations. *International Journal of Human–Computer Interaction*, *39*(7), 1371–1389. https://doi.org/10.1080/10447318.2022.2080155.

Liebig, L., Güttel, L., Jobin, A. and Katzenbach, C. (2024). Subnational AI policy: Shaping AI in a multi-level governance system. *AI & Society*, *39*(3), 1477–1490. https://doi.org/10.1007/s00146-022-01561-5.

Marmolejo-Ramos, F., Workman, T., Walker, C., Lenihan, D., Moulds, S., Correa, J.C., ... & Sonna, B. (2022). AI-powered narrative building for facilitating public participation and engagement. *Discover Artificial Intelligence*, *2*(1), 7. https://doi.org/10.1007/s44163-022-00023-7.

Minkkinen, M., Laine, J. and Mäntymäki, M. (2022). Continuous auditing of artificial intelligence: A conceptualization and assessment of tools and frameworks. *Digital Society*, *1*(3), 21. https://doi.org/10.1007/s44206-022-00022-2.

Mökander, J. (2023). Auditing of AI: Legal, ethical, and technical approaches. *Digital Society, 2*(3), 49. https://doi.org/10.1007/s44206-023-00074-y.

Moon, M.J. (2023). Searching for inclusive artificial intelligence for social good: Participatory governance and policy recommendations for making AI more inclusive and benign for society. *Public Administration Review, 83*(6), 1496–1505. https://doi.org/10.1111/puar.13648.

Mutambara, A.G. (2025). *Artificial Intelligence: A Driver of Inclusive Development and Shared Prosperity for the Global South*. CRC Press. DOI: 10.1201/9781003511014.

Naoufal, G. (2024). Continuous auditing/continuous monitoring. In: *Continuous Auditing with AI in the Public Sector* (pp. 143–162). CRC Press.

Nkwo, M., Ikwunne, T., Adejoro, C. and Anuyah, O. (2025). Exploring Usability of AI Systems in the Global South: Toward Responsible Human-Centered AI for Sustainable Cities and Communities. In: *Usability for the World: Building Better Cities and Communities* (pp. 125–165). Cham: Springer Nature Switzerland. https://doi.org/10.1007/978-3-031-88326-2_5.

Novelli, C., Taddeo, M. and Floridi, L. (2024). Accountability in artificial intelligence: What it is and how it works. *AI & Society, 39*(4), 1871–1882. https://doi.org/10.1007/s00146-023-01635-y.

Panarese, P., Grasso, M.M. and Solinas, C. (2025). Algorithmic bias, fairness, and inclusivity: A multilevel framework for justice-oriented AI. *AI & Society*, 1–23. https://doi.org/10.1007/s00146-025-02451-2.

Pislaru, M., Vlad, C.S., Ivascu, L. and Mircea, I.I. (2024). Citizen-centric governance: Enhancing citizen engagement through artificial intelligence tools. *Sustainability, 16*(7), 2686. https://doi.org/10.3390/su16072686.

Polizzi, G. (2025). Digital literacy and strategic (dis) engagement: Examining how functional and critical digital literacy shapes participation. *Information, Communication and Society*, 1–20. https://doi.org/10.1080/1369118X.2025.2452282.

Prabhakaran, V., Mitchell, M., Gebru, T. and Gabriel, I. (2022). A human rights-based approach to responsible AI. *arXiv preprint arXiv:2210.02667*. https://doi.org/10.48550/arXiv.2210.02667.

Prem, E. (2025). Managing Entrepreneurial AI Ethics Risks. In: *Artificial Intelligence, Entrepreneurship and Risk: Reflections and Positions at the Crossroads between Philosophy and Management* (pp. 453–475). Wiesbaden: Springer Fachmedien Wiesbaden. https://doi.org/10.1007/978-3-658-45544-6_23.

Qian, Y., Siau, K.L. and Nah, F.F. (2024). Societal impacts of artificial intelligence: Ethical, legal, and governance issues. *Societal Impacts, 3*, 100040. https://doi.org/10.1016/j.socimp.2024.100040.

Qin, Y., Xu, Z., Wang, X. and Skare, M. (2024). Artificial intelligence and economic development: An evolutionary investigation and systematic review. *Journal of the Knowledge Economy, 15*(1), 1736–1770. https://doi.org/10.1007/s13132-023-01183-2.

Radanliev, P. (2025). AI ethics: Integrating transparency, fairness, and privacy in AI development. *Applied Artificial Intelligence, 39*(1), 2463722. https://doi.org/10.1080/08839514.2025.2463722.

Roberts, H., Hine, E., Taddeo, M. and Floridi, L. (2024). Global AI governance: Barriers and pathways forward. *International Affairs, 100*(3), 1275–1286. https://doi.org/10.1093/ia/iiae073.

Rong, K., Ling, Y., Yang, T. and Huang, C. (2025). Cross-border data transfer: Patterns and discrepancies. *Journal of International Business Policy, 8*(1), 10–32. https://doi.org/10.1057/s42214-025-00209-7.

Salhab, W., Ameyed, D., Jaafar, F. and Mcheick, H. (2024). A systematic literature review on AI safety: Identifying trends, challenges, and future directions. *IEEE Access*. https://doi.org/10.1109/ACCESS.2024.3440647.

Sarker, I.H. (2024). CyberAI: a comprehensive summary of AI variants, explainable and responsible AI for cybersecurity. In: *AI-Driven Cybersecurity and Threat Intelligence: Cyber Automation, Intelligent Decision-making and Explainability* (pp. 173–200). Cham: Springer Nature Switzerland. https://doi.org/10.1007/978-3-031-54497-2_10.

Schmitt, L. (2022). Mapping global AI governance: A nascent regime in a fragmented landscape. *AI and Ethics*, *2*(2), 303–314. https://doi.org/10.1007/s43681-021-00083-y.

Sieber, R., Brandusescu, A., Adu-Daako, A. and Sangiambut, S. (2024). Who are the publics engaging in AI? *Public Understanding of Science*, *33*(5), 634–653. https://doi.org/10.1177/09636625231219853.

Taeihagh, A. (2025). Governance of generative AI. *Policy and Society*, *44*(1), 1–22. https://doi.org/10.1093/polsoc/puaf001.

Tenakwah, E.S. and Watson, C. (2025). Embracing the AI/automation age: Preparing your workforce for humans and machines working together. *Strategy & Leadership*, *53*(1), 32–48. https://doi.org/10.1108/SL-05-2024-0040.

Thomaidou, A. and Limniotis, K. (2025). Navigating Through Human Rights in AI: Exploring the Interplay Between GDPR and Fundamental Rights Impact Assessment. *Journal of Cybersecurity and Privacy*, *5*(1), 7. https://doi.org/10.3390/jcp5010007.

Turksen, U., Benson, V. and Adamyk, B. (2024). Legal implications of automated suspicious transaction monitoring: Enhancing integrity of AI. *Journal of Banking Regulation*, *25*(4), 359–377. https://doi.org/10.1057/s41261-024-00233-2.

Visave, J. (2025). Transparency in AI for emergency management: Building trust and accountability. *AI and Ethics*, 1–14. https://doi.org/10.1007/s43681-025-00692-x.

Walter, Y. (2024). Managing the race to the moon: Global policy and governance in Artificial Intelligence regulation: A contemporary overview and an analysis of socioeconomic consequences. *Discover Artificial Intelligence*, *4*(1), 14. https://doi.org/10.1007/s44163-024-00109-4.

Wang, H., Fu, T., Du, Y., Gao, W., Huang, K., Liu, Z., ... & Zitnik, M. (2023). Scientific discovery in the age of artificial intelligence. *Nature*, *620*(7972), 47–60. https://doi.org/10.1038/s41586-023-06221-2.

Wang, X., Liu, B. and Bao, L. (2025). Generative artificial intelligence policies: Information governance. *Management Decision*. https://doi.org/10.1108/MD-06-2024-1422.

Wen, H. (2024). Human-AI collaboration for enhanced safety. In: *Methods in Chemical Process Safety* (Vol. 8, pp. 51–80). Elsevier. https://doi.org/10.1016/bs.mcps.2024.07.001.

Wilson, C. (2022). Public engagement and AI: A values analysis of national strategies. *Government Information Quarterly*, *39*(1), 101652. https://doi.org/10.1016/j.giq.2021.101652.

Wong, P. H. (2025). Global Governance of AI, Cultural Values, and Human Rights. In: *A Companion to Applied Philosophy of AI*, 359–371. https://doi.org/10.1002/9781394238651.ch25.

Yar, M.A., Hamdan, M., Anshari, M., Fitriyani, N.L. and Syafrudin, M. (2024). Governing with intelligence: The impact of artificial intelligence on policy development. *Information*, *15*(9), 556. https://doi.org/10.3390/info15090556.

Yazdanpanah, V., Gerding, E.H., Stein, S., Dastani, M., Jonker, C.M., Norman, T.J. and Ramchurn, S.D. (2023). Reasoning about responsibility in autonomous systems: Challenges and opportunities. *AI & Society*, *38*(4), 1453–1464. https://doi.org/10.1007/s00146-022-01607-8.

Yu, H., Liu, S., Yang, H., Yan, Y., Qu, M. and Jin, Y. (2025). Unlocking the potential of AI researchers in scientific discovery: What is missing? *arXiv preprint arXiv:2503.05822*. https://doi.org/10.48550/arXiv.2503.05822.

Zaidan, E. and Ibrahim, I.A. (2024). AI governance in a complex and rapidly changing regulatory landscape: A global perspective. *Humanities and Social Sciences Communications*, *11*(1). https://doi.org/10.1057/s41599-024-03560-x.

Index

About the Author

Dr. Azamat Ali is an Associate Professor in the School of Liberal and Creative Arts (Journalism and Mass Communication) at Lovely Professional University, Punjab, India. He obtained a PhD from the Central University of Gujarat, Gandhinagar, and a M.Sc. in Science Communication from Devi Ahilya Vishwavidyalaya, Indore. His research interests span emerging technologies, development communication, public policy, and health and science communication. Dr. Ali research is directed toward bridging the divide between scientific innovation and societal application, with a particular focus on harnessing the transformative potential of emerging technologies to drive innovation, address developmental challenges, and enhance societal well-being.

For Product Safety Concerns and Information please contact our EU representative GPSR@taylorandfrancis.com
Taylor & Francis Verlag GmbH, Kaufingerstraße 24, 80331 München, Germany

www.ingramcontent.com/pod-product-compliance
Ingram Content Group UK Ltd.
Pitfield, Milton Keynes, MK11 3LW, UK
UKHW022223190926
475702UK00003B/482
9781041308966

ROUTLEDGE LIBRARY EDITIONS:
MONETARY ECONOMICS

Volume 3

MONETARY POLICY AND PUBLIC FINANCE

MONETARY POLICY AND PUBLIC FINANCE

G. C. HOCKLEY

Routledge
Taylor & Francis Group
LONDON AND NEW YORK

First published in 1970 by Routledge & Kegan Paul Ltd

Published in 2017 by Routledge
4 Park Square, Milton Park, Abingdon, Oxon OX14 4RN
605 Third Avenue, New York, NY 10017

Routledge is an imprint of the Taylor & Francis Group, an informa business

British Library Cataloguing in Publication Data
A catalogue record for this book is available from the British Library

ISBN: 978-1-138-73264-3 (Set)
ISBN: 978-1-315-16457-1 (Set) (ebk)
ISBN: 978-1-138-70479-4 (Volume 3) (hbk)
ISBN: 978-1-315-20245-7 (Volume 3) (ebk)

Publisher's Note
The publisher has gone to great lengths to ensure the quality of this reprint but points out that some imperfections in the original copies may be apparent.

Disclaimer
The publisher has made every effort to trace copyright holders and would welcome correspondence from those they have been unable to trace.

Monetary Policy and Public Finance

G. C. Hockley

London Routledge & Kegan Paul

First published 1970
by Routledge & Kegan Paul Ltd
Broadway House, 68-74 Carter Lane
London, E.C.4
Printed in Great Britain by
Northumberland Press Limited
Gateshead

SBN 7100 6691 0

To my Parents

Contents

Acknowledgments

I wish to record my great indebtedness to Professor B. Tew of Nottingham University for comments on 'The Monetary System' Part I of this manuscript, and Mr J. Bates for comments on Parts II and III. Also Professor J. Perrin of Lancaster University and my colleagues Mr J. H. Loosemore, Mr B. L. Jones and Mr J. F. Mackeson for comments on Chapters 12 and 13. Professor Brinley Thomas, Professor Gethin Davies and Mr J. D. Pole have been particularly helpful with advice and encouragement. I received invaluable assistance from the late Professor H. D. Dickinson, who read the whole of the draft manuscript and made many improvements in style and content. Shortcomings and omissions remaining are, of course, my responsibility.

I am indebted to the editors of the *British Tax Review* for permission to use material from my articles 'Taxation and the Employment of Married Women', May/June, 1967, and 'Capital Gains and Inflation', Jan./Feb., 1968 and *The Banker* for 'Incentives under a Value-Added Tax', March, 1968, and to the following for permission to quote from the works listed:

George Allen & Unwin for
  D. R. Denman, *Origins of Ownership*, 1958 and
  R. M. Titmus, *Income Distribution and Social Change*, 1962.
The Bank of England for several issues of the
  Bank of England Quarterly Bulletin.
The *Economic Journal* for
  A. Rubner, 'The Irrelevancy of the British Differential Profits Tax', June, 1964 and
  G. L. S. Shackle, 'Recent Theories concerning the Nature and Role of Interest', June, 1961.
Longmans Green & Co. for
  A. J. Merritt, *Executive Remuneration in the U.K.*, 1968.
Oxford University Press for
  A. T. Peacock and Jack Wiseman, *The Growth of Public Expenditure in the United Kingdom*, 1961.

Prentice-Hall Inc. for
W. J. Schultz and C. L. Harriss, *American Public Finance*, 1965.
C. A. Watts & Co. for
Joan Robinson, *Economic Philosophy*, Pelican, 1962.

As a recent writer on public finance, I must record a general debt to R. A. Musgrave for the stimulation of *The Theory of Public Finance*, McGraw-Hill, 1959.

Finally, as is proper, the last word goes to a woman—my wife—whose help and forbearance greatly eased my task.

University College, Cardiff GRAHAM C. HOCKLEY

Terminology

Since the publication of the *Report of the Committee on the Working of the Monetary System* in 1959, Cmnd. 827 (hereafter referred to as the *Radcliffe Report*, after its Chairman) the following terminology has been widely adopted and will be followed in this book:

Monetary sector is taken to include the Bank of England, the commercial banks, the discount houses, savings banks and the central government.

Monetary authorities are the dominant part of the monetary sector, and comprise the Bank of England and the central government.

The public: all individuals and institutions outside the monetary sector.

Long-term bonds: bonds which have five years or more to run to maturity or are undated.

Short-term bonds: less than five years to run to maturity.

Introduction

This book is intended as an introduction to a university course in public finance and for use of students of professional examinations. Also, I hope, it will be intelligible, and of interest, to the general reader. Taxation and poverty have been two of the most-discussed questions in recent years. In these matters most of us judge from a purely personal standpoint: a good tax is a tax that is paid by somebody else; wise government spending is spending that benefits oneself; correct monetary policy is regulation that protects one's own interests. The multitude of voices raised on almost every aspect of public finance, each claiming right on their side, but frequently each seeking their own ends, tends to drown out general considerations.

Essentially a study of public finance is an attempt to break away from this Babel, to see through arguments based on the interests of this or that group, and attempt to establish rational principles on which policy can be based.

The scope of a public finance course is ill-defined. Government spending and revenue are central to it, but there is considerable overlap with monetary policy. The government can, after all, merely create money to pay for the goods and services it requires, or it can borrow from its citizens as well as taxing them. This book takes the view that it is impossible to have a very realistic understanding of public finance matters without some understanding of the operation of the monetary system.

Part I is therefore devoted to the monetary system. Chapter 1 discusses the nature and attributes of money and then goes on to discuss the value of money—a section that can be omitted at first reading by anyone new to the subject. The following chapters deal respectively with the Bank of England, the discount market and the commercial banks. These institutions have a unique and long-established relationship with each other. Following this is a description of other financial institutions which in recent years have transformed much of the financial scene. Our concern is not so much with the detailed working of these institutions, but with obtaining an understanding of their interrelationships and how they form the monetary system. Chapter 6 draws the previous discussion together in looking at the implications for monetary policy of a Budget surplus or deficit. This chapter therefore provides many of the links between the sphere of public finance and that of money, which will be taken up and developed later in the book.

A description of the monetary system, it will be clear, is a description not of a static framework, but of an evolving structure. The rapidity with which change can take place is indeed one of the remarkable things about the collection of institutions labelled the 'British Monetary System'. As with many rapidly changing things, the spice of controversy is never far away.

Part II introduces the public finance section with four chapters which briefly outline how government expenditure and revenue have changed in this century. This background forms an essential part to understanding the system as it exists today. In this context policy can be discussed from two angles: one approach is to look at reasons for government expenditure and its change over time; the other approach is to concentrate on ways of ensuring that expenditures, given that the decision to spend has been made, are wisely and not wastefully applied. This book has a number of things to say which are relevant to this latter, important question, particularly on simplification of the system of tax and benefits, which could lead to large savings. But the detailed Parliamentary and administrative procedures, and statistical techniques, that attempt to ensure efficiency in this narrow sense have been considered outside the scope of this volume.

Changes up to April, 1969 have been incorporated. Thus the selective employment tax, capital gains tax, land tax, corporation tax, changes in investment allowances and grants, the special charge on investment income, and benefit allowances to individuals are detailed. In addition, a chapter is devoted to looking at a value-added tax, which Britain will have to adopt if she enters the Common Market.

Chapter 11 is a key chapter, setting out the accretion principle of income. This concept is used thereafter as a yardstick to evaluate the current system of taxes and benefits which are detailed in the following chapters. The National Debt raises complex monetary and fiscal issues, and it was decided to include this in Chapter 17, after the monetary and fiscal details have been given. Chapter 18 gathers together previous threads and looks at ways the system can evolve.

Part III, on Policy, does not attempt a detailed assessment of the use of policy in the post-war period: this has been well covered in recent publications; but it outlines the problems of using monetary and fiscal policy to control the economy. The difficulties in control have important fiscal implications which are developed in the final chapter.

Current objectives in society include equity, the full employment of resources, stability of the value of money, a satisfactory balance of payments, and the steady growth of the economy. The heading of 'Growth' covers the effects of monetary and fiscal policy on savings, consumption, investment, prices, output and work effort. All of these aspects are important, but the author is firmly of the opinion that the need for equity in the whole system of taxation and government spending has been very much underplayed, with serious consequences for growth and other objectives.

In a superficial sense, all taxes may be said to have unfavourable effects on growth. The issue is unrealistic. Governments need revenue, and by their investment and other spending policies can make a substantial contribution to growth. The real point at issue is whether an equitable tax and benefit system contributes more to growth and other objectives than an inequitable one. The volume of comment that occurs, almost daily, in the Press and elsewhere on the alleged drawbacks of the current fiscal system is evidence of the concern for this issue. The present system leaves a high-income-earner about 10% of his earned income, 70% of his long-term capital gains, a major part of his gambling winnings and usually all of the sums he receives by way of gifts. This can be put another way. Because of the way income is defined, the majority of employees are taxed on the whole of their spending power, since for most income only comes to them via earnings. They are overtaxed relative to taxpayers with mixed incomes. They are taxed at source, and most of the expenses of earning that income are not allowed to be deducted for tax purposes. It will be argued in Chapter 11 that this is the major flaw in the tax system, all the items mentioned represent purchasing power and a case can be made for taxing them at the same progressive rate. Whether the top rate should be nearer the 30% level of capital gains or the 90% level of surtax then becomes the real question for the community to debate and decide. On the benefit side of the fiscal system even more serious distortions appear: it can almost be described as a system that helps most the richest members of society. Given this situation, the wonder is not that an incomes and prices policy, on which successive governments have pinned so much of their hopes for improvements in the economy, has had so little success, but that it has had any success at all.

Part III also points out that, given the existing state of knowledge, fiscal and monetary changes have only limited ability to achieve the other objectives of society. Excessive concentration on particular taxes or benefits to achieve these ends can distort the impact of the fiscal system as a whole, with serious consequences of the kind mentioned above. A look at the fiscal system as a whole, both from the tax and benefit sides is overdue.

The issue before society is not the stark choice of either/or: of achieving either growth or equity, for example. Inevitable conflicts between objectives will occur and a balance will have to be struck. However, a wide variety of measures are possible, and if equity should be the prime concern of the fiscal system, as is argued here, it is possible that the harmful effects on other objectives can be compensated for in a way that does not seriously distort equity.

To argue for equity is not, it must be stressed, to argue for equality. The concept of equity is treated more fully in Chapter 11. It is composed of two strands: that people in equal positions should be treated equally, and that people in unequal positions should stand in a correct relationship with each other, with regard to the taxes they pay and the benefits they receive. The consensus of opinion in contemporary society seems to be, at its simplest, that a poor person should pay less in tax and receive more in benefits than a rich person. The exact amount of less or more is a matter of choice for the community concerned.

Although no serious commentator on the fiscal system claims that it is an equitable one, opinions differ on the need for, and the urgency of, rectification. Policy since the war has been primarily concerned with 'quantity'. The size of the national income and its rate of growth has been elevated to a prime economic desideratum. Concern for 'quality' and for the distribution of resources has tended to be pushed to one side.

Economists and politicians cannot complain if cynical policies meet with cynical responses. Tax policies that have the effect of helping most those least in need are hardly conducive to the acceptance of an incomes policy. Small taxes on income from gambling and capital gains and zero taxation on gifts, compared with highly progressive taxes on work income, is hardly an inducement to work harder. The pretence that we have a savage rate of estate duty, while it may comfort the wealthy, is likely to exacerbate the feelings of other members.

Better living standards of a community are multi-dimensional. The growth of national product (the amount of resources available) is one dimension; others are the way in which these resources are used (e.g. hospitals or motor-cars) and the way in which these resources are shared amongst the community. Our present fiscal system is inherited from different periods in the past, with many pieces added to patch up this or that particular deficiency. The end-result is less than satisfactory. The adoption of the accretion principle, which is set out in Chapter 11, is important because it helps to turn attention away from special pleading on behalf of interested parties towards more fundamental issues. When income is so defined, it makes sense to discuss the required degree of progression of taxation and benefits.

The belief in the need for growth in the economy is so widely held that it seems necessary to justify the treatment accorded here to equity in rather more detail.

Persuasive arguments are put forward that growth is more important than abstract notions of equity, which can, in any case, never be achieved in practice. Growth, it is argued, provides the means whereby everybody can be better off. This is a comfortable doctrine held, consciously or unconsciously, by many people. Is it possible that by being mesmerized by the concept of growth we have neglected deep-seated currents of human emotion?

In the international field it is generally recognized that the growing disparity between the developed nations and the less-developed nations creates dangerous conflicts and is a serious problem. It is not so much that the less-developed nations are becoming worse off, although in some countries this may be so, as that the developed nations are improving their living standards very much faster than the less-developed. Poverty and wealth are relative concepts. It is curious how little, at the present time, this trend of thought is carried over to standards of living of different sections within a country

Growth, as an aim of society, is seldom made explicit. Growth of what? The measuring-rod of real national product per head is frequently used: it is a crude measure. National product will increase by the same amount if £1,000,000 is spent on hydrogen bombs or if it is spent on hospitals, cars, schools or anything else. There is at least likely to be complete agreement, in that nobody would give equal weight to this collection of things. The further question of how this growth is to be translated into 'better living standards for all' is seldom mentioned. The record is pretty dismal. Britain's national income in real terms has increased considerably since the war: this is not much consolation to the old, the chronic sick, the disabled and the large families who in many cases show little or no improvement. Perhaps the sociologist can explain why the richest nations on earth are so obsessed with getting richer and so little concerned with what it is that is increased, or what happens to it when it has been produced? In any case, this comforting doctrine, that growth will solve the problems of distribution, has received a sharp, bitter shock. Few can doubt that one of the main causes of the rioting, looting, burning and murder which have scarred recent American summers is economic underprivilege of the non-white population. It is irrelevant to the situation that the poor in America may be well off compared to the poor in many other lands. A man compares himself to those around him. Slight improvements in the standard of the underprivileged may exacerbate feelings if this enables them to see more clearly the gap that separates them from the privileged and the nature of the barriers, some of them fiscal, that foster this divide. This is the error of those who define an increase in welfare as a situation where somebody can be made better off without making anyone worse off. Such a situation worsens relative positions, and relative disparities of position can be built up into explosive situations. The desire for fairness, or equity, is a powerful human emotion, but unfortunately, since the desire cannot be measured, it tends to be left out of account.

The idea of growth embodies the important concept that more can be done with a greater output than with a lesser output. Taken as a statement, at this moment of time, this is true, but trite. It does not necessarily follow that a nation, having achieved an increase in national product, will find it any easier to provide more hospitals or more schools. National product is an accounting concept: it shows, in money terms, what was produced in a particular year. If the increase in national product has been achieved by building more hospitals or by making more cars, that is that: the product is not then available for something else. We cannot, as some people would have us believe, have it both ways. Concentrating on growth in the abstract by, for example, suitable fiscal and monetary measures gives an increase of products and services that constitutes the growth. This increase, if it takes the form of consumption goods, will be distributed amongst the community in some way, but it is not then available again to achieve any other social objectives. The point is elementary, but frequently confused.

Growth, then, means more output, which can be planned output of particular things, or growth as dictated by the market-place and distributed by market processes, or some compromise between social and private goods.

The existing fiscal system has therefore grown up piecemeal. Additions and alterations have been made in the past with little thought given to its overall impact on different sectors of the community. Growth, since it is currently fashionable, tends to be the measure by which changes in a fiscal system are now judged. Equity considerations take second place. Lack of facts concerning the impact of the fiscal system might in the past have served as an excuse: this is no longer adequate. The known impact of the fiscal system, on both the tax and expenditure side, for single persons and married persons with and without children is set out in Chapter 18. Paradoxically, it has been pointed out that concentration on growth, to the virtual exclusion of equity, may defeat its own ends by building up resentment in sections of the community. This has probably been at least a contributory cause of the singular lack of success of a prices and incomes policy in the post-war period. The author is sufficient of an optimist to believe that people will work harder to improve a system they believe to be basically fair than they will to continue a system they believe to be basically unfair.

Part I
The monetary system

1
The nature of money

But it is pretty to see what money will do.
SAMUEL PEPYS, March 21st, 1667.

Essential properties of money

To make a comprehensive list of all the items which have been used as money at various times and in various places would be tedious. What have the following items used as money in common: cattle, rice, bark-cloth, women, gold, iron, stone and cigarettes?

These and all items used as money have the common intangible property of *general acceptability*. Within the community concerned, money is accepted because it is confidently believed that it in turn can be passed on for goods and services. The item serving as money in many communities is often scarce, and therefore valuable in its own right, but this is by no means necessary. A look at a £1 note will make this clear. It says: 'Bank of England. I promise to pay the Bearer on Demand the sum of One Pound. Chief Cashier.' It is of itself just a piece of printed paper. If you do demand £1, you can have another £1 note with a different number on it, or two pieces of paper each marked 'ten shillings', or a handful of coins whose intrinsic value—the cost of the metal—is only a few pence. The note is worth having, not because the paper on which it is printed is valuable or because the printing on the note has intrinsic worth, but because it is generally acceptable in Great Britain. That is, whatever goods or services are desired can be obtained by the exchange of a sufficient number of notes. The 'Promise to pay' engraved on the note is a reminder of the origin of banknotes; at one time they were receipts for precious metals deposited with goldsmiths, and it was expected at any time that the note or receipts could be returned and the metal repossessed. It is only in this century that 'backing' for notes, in the form of gold or silver, has been effectively done away with for purposes of transactions internal to a country. Banknotes and coins are not the only form of money in a modern society, for example, the majority of transactions are carried out by means of drawings on current accounts with the commercial banks. More will be said later on the types of assets which should be considered as money, and on the factors which determine the quantity of money in the economy.

Money has been described so far in terms of its function as a *medium of exchange*. The reason why all but the most primitive of societies need a medium of exchange should be self-evident, and is summed up in the phrase, 'the sheer inconvenience of double coincidence of wants'. That is, the need to find a seller of the item you require who at the same time needs what you have to offer.

Money, by its nature, also acts in some degree as a *store of value*. If money were like a day-return ticket on a railway, valueless after the day had ended, nobody would keep it. It is because money is expected to have general acceptability and more or less the same purchasing power the day after, and the day after that, that money is held, and this function is described as a store of value. It is unfortunate that the phrase *store of value* is often taken to mean that the value is constant. What determines the 'value of money'—that is, the amount of goods and services for which it can be exchanged and the problem of its value over time—will be taken up again in this chapter.

Money usually also acts as a *unit of account* and as a *standard of deferred payments*. The unit of account refers to the fact that instead of valuing each and every article and service in terms of all others, it is valued in terms of a common denominator, the medium of exchange. In a similar manner, contracts for future payments are usually made in terms of the medium of exchange, but they can be made in terms of the value of gold, or a foreign currency, or a quantity of goods. It is usual for money to act in both these ways, but is by no means necessary; the guinea today sometimes acts as a unit of account, but it does not circulate as a medium of exchange.

Definitions of money: liquid assets, primary and secondary money

It was a deliberate choice not to start off with a definition of money in our society. This seemingly simple question does not admit of a simple answer. A commonly quoted definition tells us that money is 'anything generally accepted in exchange for goods and services and for settlement of a debt'. This definition, while it is useful, needs further clarification.

The following distinctions will be found useful and can be given empirical content. The first, between *money* and *liquid assets*, is based on the function performed by the asset in question. Money on this definition is used for assets that act both as a medium of exchange and as a store of value, while liquid assets are used for securities which, while acting as a store of value, do not circulate in exchange. Money is liabilities of the Bank of England—that is, coin and notes and bankers' deposits (i.e. deposits of commercial banks at the Bank of England), together with deposits by the public at commercial banks. Liquid assets are such items as deposits at the Post Office Savings Bank, trustee savings banks, building societies, local government and hire purchase companies. These differ from money when the moment for payment arises; they must first be turned into money, rather than exchanged directly for commodities. It should be clear from this distinction that what is money at any particular time is a matter of law and of custom. Deposits at the Post Office Savings Bank could be made transferable by cheque, and these deposits would then fall into the category of money, rather than liquid assets.[1]

There is no hard-and-fast line that can be drawn that enables us to classify an asset into one category or another. For some purposes, it may be desirable to draw the line more widely than has been done above, for other purposes more narrowly. It is important to realize that the presence of a variety of assets with the characteristics of liquidity will affect the demand for money. The determining characteristics of 'liquidity' will be discussed.

Money itself, as defined above, can be split into primary and secondary money. *Primary money* consists of coin, notes and bankers' deposits—often simply referred to as 'cash'. Deposits at commercial banks on both current and deposit accounts are, in this country, what constitutes *secondary money*.

Money should not be confused with legal tender. Only notes, 'silver' coin up to £2, and copper coins up to 1s. are legal tender. In spite of this, the value of payments by cheque are many times the value of payments by cash and notes. The risk of default by banks in Great Britain and most other developed countries is nowadays considered so small, i.e. confidence is so great that transfer of deposits to third persons will be honoured, that deposits are included with notes in the definition of money. In Great Britain also no distinction is usually drawn between current and deposit accounts, because deposit accounts can usually be drawn on with almost as much ease as can current accounts.

[1] After a great deal of procrastination, a decision to set up a giro system was made (*Post Office Giro*, 1965). It started operation in October, 1968. A giro is a means whereby the payer can pay cash into the Post Office (or have his special account debited), and the sum credited or paid to the payee. Facilities for transfer between giro and savings bank accounts are provided. Post Office accounts are therefore now even more close to the money end of the spectrum of assets.

Current accounts, sometimes called 'demand deposits', are subject to cheque and withdrawal on demand. Deposit accounts, often called 'time deposits', formally require seven days' notice before withdrawal, but in practice a cheque would not be dishonoured if it were covered by a balance in a deposit account. An added reason for not distinguishing between these two accounts is that British banks, unlike, for example, American banks, do not have to observe different reserve ratios for each type of account.

Quantity of money and liquid assets

In 1967, in approximate figures, notes and coins outstanding in the economy amounted to £3,250 million, while deposits at commercial banks were three times as large at some £10,000 million. Post Office securities (Savings Certificates, Premium Bonds, Defence Bonds, Post Office and Trustee Savings accounts) amounted to nearly £8,500 million, Treasury bills to nearly £4,000 million. Short-term deposits with local government authorities amounted to over £1,500 million and shares and deposits with building societies to about £7,000 million.

The list of liquid assets is not intended to be a complete one, e.g. for some purposes, deposits with finance houses, accumulated funds in insurance companies, and others may be included. It can be seen that notes and coin are small in relation to bank deposits, and in their turn liquid assets are bigger than bank deposits.

Liquid assets perform some of the functions of money. They act as a store of value and, while they cannot be used directly as a medium of exchange, they affect the demand for money. Coin and notes, together with current account deposits at banks, do not earn interest, deposit accounts earn a small rate of interest, liquid assets, as a rule, rather more. So a change in interest rates may cause the public to switch some money from bank deposits to liquid assets. Alternatively, the public can switch from liquid assets to money by, for example, demanding repayment of some of their Post Office securities. The amount of money in the economy is thus not necessarily a good guide to the spending power of the public. This latter point was very much the concern of the Radcliffe Committee.

Liquidity

The concept of liquidity has unfortunately been used in a number of ways, and come to mean different things to different people. In this book we shall regard it as: *the speed and certainty with which an asset can be turned into money without loss, or into a known amount of money in relation to its face value.* Shares in quoted companies, gilt-edged securities and Treasury bills can all be turned quickly into money: just pick up the telephone and call a stockbroker. Equity shares and gilt-edged would not, however, be classified as liquid assets, for the amount of money obtainable by sale on the market is not known in advance, whereas Treasury bills are highly liquid, for they have only to be held to maturity, at most three months, to be paid face value; or, alternatively, they can be discounted straight away at a rate which is known in relation to Bank Rate. If Bank Rate doubled overnight, a most unlikely occurrence, it will still only inflict a very small capital loss on having to discount a bill, whereas it would severely depress gilt-edged prices.

A second distinction between these assets is that equity shares are the liability of various companies, and therefore there is a possibility of default, whereas government securities are, in most countries, deemed to have a negligible risk of default. In a financial panic, it is better to be holding liquid government assets than liquid private assets.

It is evident that assets can be arranged on a scale: at one end completely liquid, i.e. money; at the other end, illiquid—say, an IOU from me to you or a piece of real property. If liquidity, the ability to exchange an asset quickly for a known sum of money, was the only consideration governing the holding of assets, we should expect to find that the yield on securities would increase as the asset became more illiquid, the better yield being necessary to induce the public to hold the more illiquid securities. It is found that securities do, as a rule, follow roughly this pattern, although a number of other things have to be taken into account. Money, unless it is held in the form of a deposit account at a bank, does not earn interest, while the yield on short-term government securities will normally be lower than the yield on long-term securities. Business fixed-interest securities will normally yield rather more than government securities because of a higher risk of default. Equity shares, since they offer both the attraction of sharing in business profits and the risk of getting nothing, are likely to be more volatile as to yield, depending on the market assessment of their worth.

In the previous paragraph, the terms 'yield' and 'interest' have been used. A fixed-interest security is issued at a particular price and at a particular rate of interest. Say it is issued at £100 at 4%. This means that each year the holder will receive £4 until such time, if the security has a redemption date, it is repaid at £100. The yield on this security is the market price of the security divided into the rate of interest paid. Thus, if the security in our example is sold on the market for £50 the yield is $\frac{100}{50} \times 4$, or 8%. It it fetched £75 the yield would be $\frac{75}{100} \times 4$, or $5\frac{1}{3}\%$. The yield on an equity is calculated in the same way, by dividing the market price into the face value of the security and multiplying by the dividend. It is important to grasp this inverse relationship between the price of a security and its yield. If the price of securities goes up, the yield must go down; if the price of securities falls, the yield must increase—in both cases on the assumption that the rate of interest or dividend paid on the security remains unaltered. The stock of liquid assets (stock = assets in existence) is large; in particular, it is large in relation to the flow of new liquid assets. Also the stock of company securities is large in relation to new securities coming on to the market. For this reason a change in the price of existing securities (as we have seen, we are also saying by definition that yields have changed) is likely to affect the terms on which new securities will be taken up by the market. Many of the matters touched on in this section will be taken up later in more detail.

The value of money

This section is more difficult, and can be left until later by those who wish. It has already been established that when we talk about money performing as a 'store of value', this should not be taken to mean that the value of money is constant. In general, we mean by value of money, the amount of goods and services that money will buy, compared to what it would buy, say, last year. The value of money is thus the inverse of the price level. When it is said that the price level has gone up, the same idea could be expressed by saying that the value of money has fallen. In the words of J. Hicks, 'If we have equiproportional changes in all prices, all commodities can be considered as a single composite commodity with price p, where p = the absolute price level.' Putting the matter in this stark form brings out the difficulties of using the terms 'price level' or 'value of money'. If prices do not change in an equiproportional manner, we have no unambiguous measure of the value of money. Everyday habits of talking about the 'cost of living' or 'fall in the value of the £1' may hide, but they do not solve, this problem. They get round it by a more or less arbitrary system of selecting the components to go in the index, and by more or less arbitrary weighting of the components, once these have been selected.

We are faced with a number of variables that interact with one another; we need a general equilibrium system to solve for any variable. A change in the amount of money in the economy is likely to change output and prices in the economy. However, changes in output and prices can occur independently of changes in the amount of money, but they will nevertheless affect the value of money. Talking of a change in the amount of money in the economy, as we have just done, without specifying how the amount of money comes into the economy, can also hide important differences. If the public desire to hold more money, this can come about, for example, by their exchanging some assets for money. If the assets exchanged are Post Office securities, no great effects may be apparent. The net effect is that the government has issued more notes and fewer securities. If the public attempt to obtain the money by selling securities on the market, this does not (unless the monetary authorities themselves buy the securities) increase the amount of money in the economy; the public will be exchanging the same quantity of money and securities amongst themselves, it has the effect of driving down the price of securities, i.e. increasing the yields. The initiative for the increase in money may come from the monetary authorities who buy government securities in the market. If the public's desire for money has not changed, then this increase in money will be spent on securities or goods with probable effects on prices, interest rates and output. When the desire for increased money holdings comes from the public, we should not expect a direct effect on output and prices, the money we have postulated is required by the public to hold, not to spend. When the increase is brought about by the monetary authorities, we may expect direct effects on spending. Increased spending in times of unemployment is likely to result more in increased output than increased prices, while in times of full employment by definition output cannot be increased without changing techniques of production.

The quantity theory of money

There are a number of concepts in economics that, like land-mines, seem to exist for the purpose of trapping the unwary. The quantity theory of money is one of them. In the hands of skilful practitioners, the theory is a useful one in explaining the role of money; in less careful hands it degenerates into a mechanical formula that conceals rather than reveals the truth. The theory is set out very briefly below.

Money has been defined as coin, notes and bank deposits: this (as with any other definition of money) is a *stock* concept. That is, at any particular time there is a certain amount in existence; it has a definite magnitude. Now, money can change hands many times in the course of a year, and we can measure the money value of the annual flow of final purchases of goods and services—the gross national product (G.N.P.). By dividing G.N.P. by the amount of money in existence, we find out the average number of times money turns over in the period, i.e. its velocity of circulation.

In the example above, money was divided into G.N.P. to arrive at the income velocity of money. This concept relates money to final purchases on goods and services. If money is divided into the value of all transactions in the economy, the transactions' velocity of money is arrived at. The latter relates to all purchases in the economy and includes intermediate purchases by firms of raw materials and fabricated parts, whereas the former relates only to finished goods.

Money times its transactions' velocity of circulation or MV can be equated with the total flow of the things that are purchased for money, i.e. the volume of trade, T, multiplied by the price level, P.

So we get $PT \equiv MV$ or $P \equiv \frac{MV}{T}$. This is an identity. That is, the statement is true by definition. The number of transactions times the price level must be equal to the quantity of money times its turnover.

An alternative way of expressing this is the so-called cash balance equation $M \equiv kPT$. Here k is the reciprocal of V and expresses that fraction of the period's expenditure on goods and services, which on average is held in the form of money. If V is 10 in a period, then average money holding is $\frac{1}{10}$th.

These identities can be misleading if figures are substituted and conclusions drawn. Working with $P \equiv \frac{MV}{T}$, it is not legitimate to draw the conclusion that it is always the case that the price level varies proportionally with the quantity of money and its velocity of circulation, and indirectly with the volume of transactions. The reason for this is that we cannot assume that M, V, P and T, are independent of each other. For example, it may be that, as has already been pointed out, as M is increased V decreases because people wish to hold more money. Or the increase in money could go to the company sector, which in depressed times may not want to use it. Or during a depression the increase in M may lead not to higher prices, but to more output and sales, i.e. an increase in T. It has also been pointed out that prices can increase independently of a change in the money supply or a change in the velocity of circulation.

Summary

The inconvenience of barter has led to nearly all societies using money. Money has taken the form of a very wide variety of items at different times and in different places, having only one thing in common—the intangible property of common acceptability within the community concerned.

The term 'money' is used for assets that act both as a medium of exchange and as a store of value. The term 'liquid' is the name given to assets which, while acting as a store of value, do not circulate in exchange and in addition have the property that they can be turned into money without loss, or into a known amount of money in relation to face value. Examples of liquid assets are Treasury bills and deposits at the Post Office Savings Bank. The distinction between money and liquid assets is not a rigid one, but will depend on law and custom in the society concerned.

In Great Britain the term 'primary money' is used for coin, notes and bankers' deposits at the Bank of England. Secondary money consists of deposits at banks on both current and deposit account. Once again what constitutes secondary money will depend on prevailing law and custom in society.

All economists are agreed in rejecting the crude quantity theory of money that a change in the quantity of money of x% will necessarily lead to a like change in prices of x%. The effect of changes in the quantity of money on prices is not direct and proportional; there is, in the words of J. M. Keynes, 'many a slip 'twixt the cup and the lip'.

The manner in which a change in the quantity of money may influence prices is a complicated one, which is likely to vary at different levels of employment, according to how the increase comes about, according to the division of the increase between people with different income and wealth, and many other complicating interactions and relationships.

The above remarks are particularly relevant to the short-run, which is our main concern. The long-run relationship between money and prices may have some simpler relationship; Keynes regarded this as a question for historical generalization, rather than pure theory (Keynes, J. M., 1936, 306).[2] Keynes saw the tendency for the long-run course of prices to be nearly always upward as due to the fact that when money is relatively abundant wages rise; and when money is relatively scarce some means is found to increase the effective quantity of money. The latter point has a very Radcliffe ring about it, which we shall be examining.

[2] The custom will be followed of giving an abbreviated reference within the text. A full list of works cited, arranged alphabetically, will be found on pp. 283-6. Books and articles are indexed under the author's name, and anonymous articles and reports under the first substantive word of the title.

2
The Bank of England

A catalogue of changes and developments in the position and character of the Bank of England, over, say, the last forty years, looks impressive; but it cannot conceal the fact that all too often, if not indeed typically, they have failed to match the pace of change in the external situation which they were supposed to meet. . . .

ARTIS, M. J. (1965), *Foundations of British Monetary Policy.*

Today the Bank of England (referred to as the Bank) is one of the partners of the sector termed the 'monetary authorities'.

Starting out as a joint-stock business venture of rather dubious quality in 1694, the Bank soon developed into the Bank of the government and achieved a position of importance in monetary affairs. Since relations between the government and the Bank have grown up as a result of long association, an explanation of these relations is not to be found by examination of legislation. This 'club-like' atmosphere is typical of the British monetary system; rules are obeyed, not because of laws, but because of conventions. It can form a source of strength. Modifications can come about gradually without the need for changes in statutes which may confer on the change a dramatic character it does not warrant. The converse of this is that opportunities for the legislature to have full-scale debates on the institutions are removed.

The organization of the Bank of England

The effective managing body of the Bank now consists of the Governor, the Deputy Governor, and four full-time executive directors. There are a further twelve part-time directors. The Governor and the Deputy Governor are appointed for five years, the directors for four years. All can be reappointed.

The part-time directors are appointed for their expertise in industry, commerce, banking or trade-union affairs, and may be called upon by the Governors for advice on any problem in which they have qualifications. In addition, they attend a weekly meeting—the 'Court', as it is called.

The main work of the Bank is done through committees, of which the principal one is the Committee of Treasury. This committee is the policy-making body of the Bank and receives the reports of all other committees before they are submitted to Court: membership consists of the Governor, his Deputy and five other directors.

No mention has been made of the Bank of England Act, 1946, whereby the State acquired the whole of the capital stock of the bank and brought it into public ownership. Formal powers are written into the Act, whereby the Treasury may from time to time give such directions to the Bank as, after consultation with the Governor of the Bank, they think necessary in the public interest. This provision has not essentially changed the working of the system, which is one based on persuasion and discussion, and one in which the use of coercive powers is considered foreign. The Bank was, under this Act, also endowed with statutory powers to direct the affairs of the commercial banks. Again compulsion is relegated to the background: directives are issued only after consultation with the commercial banks.

Functions of the Bank of England

A look at a simplified statement of the Bank shows up many of its functions.

Bank of England Statement as at December, 1967

Figures in £ million

	Issue Department		
1. Notes in circulation	3,160	6. Government securities	3,199
Notes in banking department	40		
	3,200		3,199
	Banking Department		
2. Bankers' deposits	259	6. Government securities	454
3. Special accounts	213	7. Discounts and Advances	97
4. Public deposits	12	Other	29
5. Other accounts	118	Notes and Coin	41
	602		621

Source: *Bank of England Quarterly Bulletin*, September, 1968, Table 5.

The division between the issue and banking departments is historical. The number of notes in circulation is, as we shall see, whatever the public demands at any time. Notes are *not* issued to finance government expenditure. This matter will be taken up in more detail later. We note here the function of the Bank to maintain a sufficient supply of notes to meet whatever is the demand for them.

The function of the Bank, as banker, is brought out by items 2, 4 and 5 in the statement. The relative smallness of the sums appearing under these items should not mislead one into under-estimating the importance of this function. The Bank is providing for its customers a wide range of services, analogous to those offered by commercial banks to their customers, with the difference that the main customers of the Bank are the government, other banks, both home and foreign, some of the financial intermediaries and international organizations.

Bankers' deposits refer to the accounts of the commercial banks. They form, together with the till money of the commercial banks, their cash reserve. Inter-bank indebtedness will be settled by drawing on bankers' deposits and more important transactions between the commercial banking sector (and their customers) and the government will be reflected in withdrawals or replenishing of these deposits.[1] The cash reserve of the joint-stock banks is kept at a figure of 8% of deposits, so that the figure of bankers' deposits will not show great variation; a surplus of cash is loaned to the discount houses at 'call or short notice', and likewise a deficit is met by calling in some of these loans. This should not be allowed to obscure the importance of bankers' deposits, and the function of the Bank to exercise monetary control over the banks and other financial institutions.

'Public' has been used to denote all individuals and institutions outside the monetary sector. The term 'public deposits', item 4 in the statement, has, however, the meaning of government deposit. Once again the smallness of the account should not be allowed to mislead. The account is deliberately kept to a working balance. The government does not, as a rule, borrow from the Bank, with the minor exception that small sums may be borrowed overnight by way of 'Ways and Means Advances', to meet residual requirements. A deficit will be made up by the issue of government securities, either Treasury bills or bonds, and likewise a surplus will be used to buy securities, i.e. fewer securities will be offered on the market. The Bank itself

[1] For example, if Smith pays the Inland Revenue a £100 cheque for tax owed, the joint-stock bank will debit Smith's account, and the joint-stock bank, in turn, will have its bankers' deposits account, at the Bank of England, debited in favour of the Exchequer.

manages the sale or purchases of these securities on behalf of the government.

Special deposits (item 3) are also deposits by the joint-stock banks, but in this case they are not allowed to treat these deposits as cash or as liquid assets. This is a recent form of monetary control which will be dealt with more fully later on.

Other accounts (item 5) covers the accounts of discount and acceptance houses, of overseas central banks and of such bodies as the International Monetary Fund. In addition, the Bank keeps accounts for a few individuals, amongst them its staff, and for a few private and public companies—a legacy from the days when the Bank was active in general banking.

Item 7, discounts and advances, points the way to one of the Bank's crucial functions, that of lender of last resort. This means that any institution with the privilege of access to the Discount Office of the Bank with 'eligible paper' (e.g. Treasury bills) knows that the Bank will re-discount them. Bank Rate is the rate at which the Bank normally lends at last resort; it is announced by the Court of Directors, customarily on Thursday mornings, after the Governor has consulted with the Treasury and the Chancellor of the Exchequer. Bank Rate is a key rate among short-term rates, because it exercises a powerful influence on other rates. It will be shown that the rate on Treasury bills moves in sympathy with Bank Rate; commercial banks' rates are geared by convention to it. With these important rates changed as a result of a change in Bank Rate, market influences spread the impact through to other rates. In practice, rates given by local authorities on short-term borrowing change overnight, and financial institutions and intermediaries change their rates with different time-lags, as the effect of higher rates to be obtained in the markets mentioned draws funds away from them.[2]

Although Bank Rate is the usual rate at which the Bank will lend at last resort, this is at the discretion of the Bank. In recent years, on occasions, the discount houses have been charged more than Bank Rate, and they can always be assisted by the Bank buying bills in the market—so called 'open-market operations'.

Interest rates are also influenced by the activities of the government broker—one of the discount houses, which acts under instructions from the Bank. 'The prices he [the government broker] bids in response to an offer are therefore seen as the expression of the Bank's current policy, and are closely watched by the jobbers for any sign

[2] In Chapter 6 we shall look at a proposal that commercial banks should drop the convention whereby they maintain fixed differentials with respect to Bank Rate, and instead leave themselves free to compete with each other, and with other institutions for deposits.

of a change of emphasis in the policy, such as might lead the market to expect new movements in prices' ('Official Transactions in the Gilt-edged Market', June, 1966).

The Bank also acts as an agent for the government in administering exchange control; it manages the Exchange Equalization Account—which holds the reserves of gold and foreign exchange; and acts as registrar of government stocks, stocks of nationalized industries and of some local authorities, public boards and Commonwealth governments.

The final function of the Bank is one that is not apparent from the statement: that of financial adviser to the government. Its leading position in the financial structure of Great Britain and activities and contacts abroad means that the Bank is in an unrivalled position to tender advice.

Relations between the Bank of England and the government

The relation between a central bank and the executive is always a tricky one. Checks and counterchecks are needed to ensure, on the one hand, that the government does not resort to the printing of notes to solve its fiscal problems, and, on the other, that the management of the monetary side of the economy, in so far as it is within the control of the central bank, shall be in accordance with the wishes of the government. The personalities of the Governor of the Bank, together with that of his opposite number in the Treasury and the Chancellor of the Exchequer, is probably as good a guide as any to their influence at any one time.

Enough has been said to make it clear that the relations between the Bank and the government are subject to change. One recent example to illustrate what has been said will be given. In the words of a former Governor, the Bank has 'the unique right to offer advice and to press such advice even to the point of nagging; but always, of course, subject to the supreme authority of the government'.

What is not as yet clear is whether this right to offer advice should be confined within the circle of discussion of the monetary authorities, or whether the Bank should be free to make its disagreements known. The American practice in these respects is to have much fuller public discussion and to publish dissenting views. There is less search for a viewpoint on which all can agree.[3]

Britain seems to get the worst of both worlds, in that the few times the Bank is moved to make their disagreements public may help to make the situation (it is usually one of confidence in the £1) worse,

[3] Contrast the *Radcliffe Report* and the *American Report of the Commission on Money and Credit.*

and in addition has all the appearance of trying to coerce the government to its point of view. Either the adoption of the convention that disagreements are fought out in private or much fuller publication of information and views would seem to be a better solution. The Bank, until the publication since December, 1960, of its *Quarterly Bulletin*, was notorious for the secrecy with which it conducted its operations. The *Bulletin* has done much to enable an informed discussion of monetary issues to take place.

This section deals with contentious matters that largely lie outside the scope of this volume. It has been stressed in this chapter that the monetary system, and within it the Bank, is not subject to formal regulations. It has changed a great deal over the last forty years. Inevitably it has not changed, as the quotation that heads this chapter indicates, as fast or in as radical a manner as some of its critics would like.

Summary

The effective management of the Bank is in the hands of a small group: the Governor and his Deputy, who are appointed for five years, and four full-time directors appointed for four years. They are assisted by twelve part-time directors.

The Bank manages the note issue, acts as banker to the government, other banks and many financial intermediaries and international organizations. It exercises monetary control as agreed by the monetary authorities, of which the Bank itself forms an important part. One of its crucial functions is that of lender of last resort to the discount houses, which gives the Bank influence over short-term interest rates. The Bank manages the Exchange Equalization Account and acts as registrar of government, nationalized industries and a number of public authority stock issues.

Finally, the Bank, because of its leading position in the financial structure of Great Britain and activities and contacts abroad, tenders advice to the government on economic matters.

3
The discount market

Because that is the way the market has always been, going back a long way.
Verbal evidence of the London Discount Market Association to the Radcliffe Committee.

It is easy to imagine the despair of people when they attempt to understand the English monetary system. Because it has grown up over so many years, it appears haphazard, full of illogicalities. If the system were being constructed afresh, the monetary system would probably appear simpler and more tidy. For example, the functions performed by the discount houses could be performed in other ways; it was, however, the considered opinion of the *Radcliffe Report* that they performed effectively and efficiently, and it seemed unlikely that savings in cost or manpower would result from a change. With these preliminaries in mind, we will consider the organization and functions of the discount houses.

Structure of the London discount market

The London discount market now consists of twelve major discount houses. They stand as an intermediary between the government and the Bank of England in the sense that we have seen that the government borrows (other than overnight), not from the Bank, but by issuing securities which are chiefly channelled through the discount houses. In a similar manner, the discount houses stand as an intermediary between the Bank of England and the commercial banks; funds required by the latter are channelled through the discount market rather than by the commercial banks borrowing directly from the Bank.

The discount houses are commercial bodies and, like banks, they aim to make a profit by borrowing money more cheaply than they lend it. They operate for the most part in the short end of the market, and operate almost entirely on money which is borrowed on even shorter terms than they lend. They are able to do this in safety because the discount houses enjoy access to the Bank as lender of last resort.

Source of funds

Normally the cheapest source of funds for the discount houses is provided by borrowing 'money at call and short notice' from the commercial banks. This money, as the name implies, can be recalled by the banks either immediately or at very short notice. The cost of this money to the discount houses is related to Bank Rate and will be, at best, 1⅝% below the existing level of Bank Rate.[1] We can now see how the commercial banks are able to maintain a rigid cash ratio of 8% in spite of differences, day to day, in the calls for cash. Any cash above the 8% level can be loaned overnight to the discount houses; a shortfall can be met by recalling funds. A surplus, or deficit, which continued for any length of time will call for more fundamental action by the commercial banks, but temporary departures from the 8% ratio are taken care of by the buffer provided by the discount houses.

The money at call and short notice is the cheapest source of borrowed capital of the discount houses. They also borrow at slightly higher rates of interest from acceptance houses and foreign banks with surplus funds in London, and minor amounts from other sources. They also, as we have noted, have access to the Bank of England; funds borrowed from the Bank will normally be charged at the same rate as Bank Rate, which, as we shall see, is a penal rate for the discount houses. However, if the Bank wishes to influence the money market in a particular way, the Bank can accommodate the discount houses at less than Bank Rate, and in recent years has on occasion charged more than Bank Rate.

Functions of the London discount market

The discount houses, for their part, undertake to 'cover the tender' of Treasury bills issued weekly by the government. This means that, however many Treasury bills the government decides to issue, they can be sure that, failing other buyers offering better terms, the discount houses will take them up. In turn, the discount houses sell the bills to commercial banks in suitable maturities and to the Bank and other holders. The discount houses are able to give this undertaking

[1] Part, so termed 'regular money' is borrowed at the rate 1⅝% below Bank Rate. Other call money is loaned at rates which vary from day to day, but will approximate to the less favourable rates the discount houses have to pay from other sources.

to cover the tender only because they know that, if they are unable to borrow funds from other sources, they can borrow from the Bank. The discount houses do not normally keep the bills they buy until they mature, but sell them, chiefly to the commercial banks, as and when the banks require them. The commercial banks could tender directly for bills, but prefer to keep to the custom whereby they buy from the discount houses the bills in the quantities and maturities that suit them best.

The discount houses, as well as channelling finance to the government, provide finance to the private sector by discounting bills of exchange. They also act as jobbers in short-term government bonds. Historically, commercial bills should be mentioned first, because the discount houses grew up to provide discount for them. It was not until the 1880s that the Treasury bill came into existence and much later before it came into widespread use.

The bill of exchange is an old device whereby the seller of goods draws on the purchaser of the goods an order for the sum of money involved to be paid on demand or at a fixed time in the future. Once the purchaser 'accepts' the bill by signing on the face of it, the seller is able, if the acceptor is sufficiently well known, to rediscount the bill through the money market. The purchaser doesn't have to pay for the goods before receipt, and the seller, for a small discount, can obtain his money as soon as the goods are sold. The convenience of this in times past, when delivery of goods, particularly between countries, took months, is obvious. Hence also the growth of acceptance houses, who specialized in accepting bills—that is, adding their names to a bill and so making themselves liable to pay the bill if the original acceptor defaulted. Once a bill had been accepted by a reputable house it became an easily negotiable instrument.

So convenient a device has been widely adopted by governments by means of Treasury bills. These have no counterpart in the dispatch of goods, but otherwise are similar to bills of exchange, being promises to pay a stated amount, usually ninety-one days from the time of issue. In amount the Treasury bill outweighs the commercial bill in importance. The amount of the former outstanding at any one time can rise to £500 million or more. Paradoxically, the commercial bill becomes important during a credit squeeze. An obvious source of funds to certain traders if they are denied bank credit is to make more use of bills of exchange; that this is done shows clearly in the figures of amounts of bills outstanding. Recently directives to the joint-stock banks on restricting credit have also included bills of exchange.

The Treasury bill market

It remains to outline briefly the market structure for Treasury bills. These are issued weekly. Tenders (minimum sum £10,000) are invited every Friday for the bills to be issued in the following week. In general, the highest tenders, i.e. those offering the nearest to the face value of the bills, will receive the bills. The difference between the tender price and the face value of the bill represents the rate of interest the government pays for borrowing money. The quantity coming on to the market depends on two factors: the requirements of government finance, which will be considered later, and the amount of surplus funds held by government departments. These surplus funds are used for Treasury bills—the so-called 'tap issue'—and the remaining bills are offered on tender.

The discount houses submit a 'syndicated bid'—that is, they submit a common tender price between them. This 'price' or discount at which they will take bills is fixed somewhere between the cost of their cheapest and dearest source of borrowed funds. That is somewhere between the cost of funds borrowed from the commercial banks and the cost of borrowing from the Bank of England at penal rate. Since the cost of borrowing from commercial banks is at best 1⅝% below Bank Rate, the discount houses' bid will normally be below Bank Rate by a slightly smaller percentage, to cover the cost of dearer money and allow for a small turn of profit. Other tenderers must normally submit better terms than this to secure an allocation of bills.

The structure of interest rates

The Bank, because of its key position as issuer of the securities and as lender on its own terms, can normally get the bill rate to the level it requires. Important implications follow from this. The cost of funds to the discount houses moves in the same way as Bank Rate. The commercial banks automatically change the rates at which they lend so as to maintain the customary differentials with Bank Rate, and rates from other sources are likely to move in the same direction as Bank Rate. Thus, the rate (or discount) on Treasury bills will move with Bank Rate. In practice, if the discount houses have correctly judged the state of the market, the change in the rate on Treasury bills will precede the change in Bank Rate. Thus, if the rate on Treasury bills is increased slightly for a number of weeks, this is an indication that the discount houses expect an increase in Bank Rate, and vice versa. This is because the discount houses try to anticipate the course of Bank Rate (and hence the cost of funds to them) over the life of the Treasury bills for which they are tendering.

The following picture thus emerges: because Treasury bills overshadow in quantity any other kind of short-term paper, the rate on Treasury bills is of key importance in influencing the structure of interest rates throughout the short end of the market. And the rate on longer-term securities will also tend to move in sympathy with short-term rates. Thus, the level of interest rates in the economy is under the control of the monetary authorities in the sense that changes in Bank Rate will influence most other rates. The monetary authorities can also, as we have seen, reinforce their influence on the key Treasury bill rate by lending money to the discount houses above Bank Rate (if they wish to keep interest rates up), or below Bank Rate in the reverse situation. The monetary authorities can also, in a way to be explained, ensure that the discount houses are forced to borrow from the Bank; that in the terminology 'money is tight'.

The reservation above that, 'the level of interest rates in the economy is under the control of the monetary authorities *in the sense that* changes in Bank Rate will influence most other rates', must not be taken to imply that Bank Rate can be manipulated at will by the monetary authorities. There are a number of constraints which the monetary authorities have to consider when setting the level of rates. The most important of these is the level of interest rates abroad and the state of the home economy. The much-quoted reason that the cost to the Exchequer of servicing the National Debt must also be taken into account is, as we shall see in the public finance section, important, but of less significance. Also, we must not prejudge the significance of high- or low-interest rates in affecting the economy.

It will be seen from the above account that the discount houses operate on an extremely narrow margin between the cost of the funds they borrow and the return on the funds they lend by buying securities. It may also be noticed that they are in a 'monopolistic' type of position where, because they bid collectively, they could manipulate the market to their own advantage. The narrow margin on dealing in bills is taken care of by the huge volume of bills that are dealt in. The second point can be met by saying that there seems to be sufficient counter-checks in the system to ensure that the market is not so manipulated. The commercial banks can vary the terms on which they lend and so can the Bank of England. The discount houses' position is thus very dependent on the goodwill of the other partners. Para. 590 of the *Radcliffe Report* does complain about the practice at one time of the 'syndicated bid' being jumped up and down in order to discourage outside tenderers. The 'frown' on the face of the monetary authorities seems to have been sufficient to stop this practice.

Summary

The discount houses were originally set up to discount commercial bills. Today Treasury bills form the major part of their business. There are now twelve major discount houses enjoying access to the Bank as lender of last resort. This access enables them to act as an intermediary between the government and the Bank in the sense that the government normally borrows not directly from the Bank, but by the issue of securities which are channelled through the discount market. The discount houses also stand as an intermediary between the commercial banks and the Bank. The commercial banks replenish cash not by borrowing from the Bank, but by calling in their loans to the discount houses.

The discount houses operate almost entirely on money borrowed at call and short notice. Their cheapest source of funds will normally be the commercial banks and the rates at which they borrow will be linked to Bank Rate. The discount houses try to anticipate changes in Bank Rate, so that movements in the Treasury bill rate will normally anticipate a change in Bank Rate.

Because of the volume of Treasury bills, the rate on these is important in influencing other short-term rates: since the rate on Treasury bills is linked to (though it may anticipate) changes in Bank Rate, we can say that the level of short-term interest rates is under the control of the monetary authorities, although this must not be taken to imply that Bank Rate can be manipulated at will by them. The most important constraint on the monetary authorities is the need to take account of the level of interest rates abroad.

4
The commercial banks

> We consider that the banks can in fact successfully take such initiatives (to stem this decline in their relative importance) and that the contrary view implicitly rests upon an assumption that the volume of bank deposits is arbitrarily determined at some level by the monetary authorities. It is, of course, true that the actions of the monetary authorities play a crucial role in determining the volume of bank deposits, but they do so in the context provided by the preferences of the public (including financial institutions) about the kinds of assets it wishes to hold and the ways in which it wishes to borrow. The actions taken by the monetary authorities —for example, in buying and selling bonds or in making calls for, or releases from, special deposits—will be taken with the ultimate aim of securing the stability of the economy, and are directed at such variables as the level (and pattern) of interest rates, the flow of lending and the general state of liquidity. This being so, it seems to us that the volume of bank deposits can be greater—consistent with the monetary authorities realizing their aims—the more attractive are bank deposits and the less inclined is the public to shift funds into other liquid claims.
>
> *Bank Charges* (1967), Report No. 34,
> National Board for Prices and Incomes.

This chapter is concerned with the domestic banks, known as the London clearing banks. The term 'clearing banks' comes from the mechanism that has been developed for settlement of inter-bank indebtedness.[1] Merchant banks or accepting houses, and overseas banks, are important and will be looked at in the next chapter. The clearing banks will hereafter be referred to as commercial banks.

[1] Strictly, an account of domestic banks should give a separate account of the Scottish banks, as there are minor differences between them and the clearing banks. For example, they have limited power to issue notes and slightly different reserve requirements. In practice, the Scottish banks are not sufficiently large enough, or different in operation, to distort the picture, and most of what is said about the clearing banks applies to the Scottish banks. For details of the Scottish banks, see *Radcliffe Report*, paras. 149-61.

Structure of the commercial banks

The structure of British banking had been stable, apart from regrouping amongst some of the smaller banks, since the 1930s: a system of eleven clearing banks, dominated by the 'Big Five'—Barclays, Midlands, Lloyds, Westminster and National Provincial—with Martins Bank coming next in size of total deposits. This stability was broken early in 1968 when a merger was announced between the Westminster and National Provincial, the smaller two of the 'Big Five', which would put them at, or near, the top in size. Shortly afterwards Barclays, Lloyds and Martins announced their intention to merge.[2] The merger would have made, ranked by deposits, the second biggest bank in the world, exceeded only by the San Francisco's Bank of America. This triple merger was referred to the Monopolies Commission and advised against by a majority of six to four.

In spite of this decision, a period of change in the structure of the commercial banks is likely for several reasons. One is the success of other types of financial intermediary and foreign banks in attracting deposits. Another is the possibility of economies in staff at headquarters and the possibility of some reduction in the number of branches where these duplicate each other. If branch reductions on a sufficient scale turn out to be possible, considerable capital could be realized from the sale of sites and premises. Of more immediate importance are the greater financial resources, which would enable the groups to meet the needs, at home and abroad, of the largest industrial organizations. Also, the banks are at present engaged in expensive installations of computing equipment, and financial economies could be expected from this source.

On the wider issue, of whether these mergers would result in better service to the public, the answer depends so much on the way the proposed groups would operate. The reader will be in a better position to judge this issue for himself after he has read this section of the book and taken in the criticisms that have been made of the current structure of banking.

Commercial bank operations

The clearing banks are profit-making institutions, drawing their revenue from the difference in rates which they pay for borrowed money (nil in the case of demand deposits) and the return they obtain by lending or investing in financial securities of various kinds. The

[2] Two Scottish banks, the Royal Bank of Scotland and the National Commercial Bank of Scotland, also announced their intention to merge at this time.

commercial banks maintain an interest-rate structure geared to Bank Rate. Loan and overdraft rates vary with the class of borrowing, but follow a set pattern. The rate for most industrial, commercial and private customers is usually 1% above Bank Rate, with a minimum rate of 4½% or 5%. Local authorities, building societies, insurance companies and other first-class industrial and commercial borrowers pay ½% below Bank Rate. Nationalized industries are normally charged Bank Rate. Rates paid on deposit accounts are 2% below Bank Rate. Corresponding levels are maintained on such other rates as loans at call and short notice. The result is that the commercial banks do not compete with each other by means of rate differentials, and, a more important point, they do not compete with other institutions who adopt flexible interest-rate policies.[3] In Chapter 1 it has already been explained that deposits both in current and deposit accounts are counted as money.

Banks are not confined to lending out only the money which is deposited with them; they can 'create money' by creating claims on themselves, e.g. allowing a customer to overdraw his account. A clear knowledge of the process by which banks create credit, the limits to this process, the influence and limitations of the monetary authorities in controlling it, and the similarities and differences of other financial intermediaries in creating credit are essential and form our chief concern in this and the next two chapters.

Creation of credit

In order to make this process clear, we start with a very simplified system. When this is understood, it is relatively easy to bring in real-life complications. Let us assume an economy with only one bank, where any money lent by the bank is redeposited back in the bank. Further, it is assumed that this bank has found from experience that it need only keep 20% of whatever sum is deposited with it as a reserve, in case cash is demanded back by its customers. (20% has been chosen to make it quite clear that our system is not intended to be a replica of the current banking system.)

Stage 1 starts, we will assume, with the deposit of £1,000 in the bank. Of this the bank needs to keep only £200 (20%) as a reserve.

Stage 2 is the process whereby the bank lends out the remaining £800, or, what amounts to the same thing, purchases securities for this amount. (Our assumption is that the whole of this £800 is

[3] Except indirectly in the sense that commercial banks have set up a number of subsidiary or affiliated companies who are chiefly concerned with hire-purchase financing. These companies do compete for deposits. For details refer to 'How the Banks compete for Deposits' (July, 1967) 582-7.

redeposited back in the bank.) If we assume that Holder A obtained an overdraft of £800 and paid this to Holder B by cheque, then the bank makes a simple book entry. Holder A is indebted to the bank for this sum, his liability has not decreased, while the deposit account of Holder B has increased by £800.

Stage 3 is a repetition of Stage 2, with the bank free to lend or buy securities to the value of £640, keeping the remaining £160 as a reserve, and so on. The ultimate value of the credit created is given by the formula:

$$\text{Total deposits created} = \frac{\text{new reserves}}{\text{percentage reserve ratio}}$$

which in our example is $\frac{1{,}000 \times 100}{20} = £5{,}000$. An initial deposit of £1,000 has led to a 'multiplier' process, whereby total deposits have increased by £5,000.

Table 1 sets out the process in detail.

Table 1

Hypothetical example of the creation of bank credit

Stage	Loans and Investments made £	Total £	Deposits created £	Total £	Reserves required for Deposits created £	Total £
1.	—	—	1,000	1,000	200	200
2.	800	800	800	1,800	160	360
3.	640	1,440	640	2,440	128	488
4.	512	1,952	512	2,952	$62\frac{2}{5}$	$550\frac{2}{5}$
Final	—	4,000	—	5,000	—	1,000

From Table 1 we see that Stage 1 is the deposit of £1,000, of which the bank needs only £200 as a deposit. Stage 2 records that a loan or investment is made by the bank of the remaining £800. This results in a return of the £800 to the bank as a deposit by another party. The bank needs to keep £160 of this as a reserve and can therefore in Stage 3 make loans or investments of £640. The final result of this process is recorded in the bottom line, where we see that total loans and investments made by the bank come to £4,000; so deposits are up by £5,000, £1,000 of which must be kept as a reserve.

The assumption of our model, that there is only one bank, does not alter our argument in any essential way. A number of banks must make sure that they keep in step in their credit-creation, otherwise one bank would lose deposits to another.

The fact that the banking system is not a completely closed system of payments leads, as we shall see, to an ability to create credit which is much below that indicated by this simple model. Before examining this point, the reserve ratios of the commercial banks are described.

Cash and liquid asset ratios

It was mentioned in the beginning that commercial banks are profit-making institutions, but they must conduct their activities so as to maintain the confidence of the public. The history of banking is a long and fascinating one that we cannot go into. It is sufficient for our purpose to know that the banks now maintain a cash ratio equal to 8% of deposits. As we have seen, 'cash' consists of money in the tills of the banks and their deposits with the Bank of England, and this ratio can be strictly maintained at 8%, because the banks are able to call in money they have lent to the discount market to meet a shortfall, and likewise to lend any surplus funds to the discount houses. This ratio is also buttressed by keeping a quantity of liquid assets. It is now the rule that joint-stock banks must keep liquid assets equal to at least 28% of deposits. The Bank of England lays down what constitutes the assets which the banks are allowed to count in their liquid-asset ratio. Cash itself will form 8% of them; Treasury bills and commercial bills the bulk of the remainder. Commercial bills which have been accepted by a British bank or by an acceptance house, if it has one other British name on it, are eligible paper. In addition a number of miscellaneous items may be included. For example, in order to encourage banks to make certain loans to help exporters, these loans in the last eighteen months before maturity were declared eligible paper.

In terms of the simple model set up in the beginning of this chapter, we could arrive at two versions of the credit multiplier. One would be the reciprocal of the cash ratio—that is, 12½ times the increase in deposits. The other would be the reciprocal of the liquid-asset ratio, or 3·9 times. Which ratio would depend on whether the monetary authorities control the cash or the liquid assets of the banks. It will be argued that this attempt to decide the ability of the banks to create credit by some mechanical formula relating to the reserve ratios of the banks is a misleading one. Expansion of deposits is in most circumstances not likely to exceed two times the initial sum. Contraction of deposits, for reasons which will be outlined, is even more circumscribed. The advantage of setting out the credit multiplier, as we have done, is so that the process whereby credit is created in the economy may be clearly understood, it should not be used to derive a ratio. A better understanding is obtained by an analysis of leakages in the flow of money in the banking system, to which we now turn.[4]

The limits to the process of creating credit

In the simplified example used, the multiplier, or limit to credit creation, is simply determined by the formula:

$$\frac{\text{new reserves}}{\text{\%age reserve ratio}}$$

The higher the reserve ratio the lower will be the amount of credit that can be created. The actual reserve ratios kept by the joint-stock banks will give us the upper limit of the bank's power to create credit. This limit is of theoretical interest only for the assumption of our simplified model—namely, that any money lent by the bank is redeposited back in the system—must be subject to important qualifications. The circular flow of money from bank to A, A to B and B back to the bank which we envisaged in our simple model is subject to 'leakages'.

Given below are some important leakages:

Firstly, some receivers of bank money will require cash; for them a deposit at a commercial bank is not an acceptable means of payment. The bank has no option but to 'pay for' the asset in cash—that is, to run down its deposit with the central bank. From an aggregate viewpoint, the more cash the public wish to hold the less will be the amount of bank deposits.

Secondly, and more importantly, transactions between banks or members of the public (using their bank accounts) and the government result in equal and opposite movements of bankers' deposits. This is so, as indicated earlier, because the government do not bank with the commercial banks. Thus the purchase of bonds from the government by banks or purchases from the government by the public reduce bankers' deposits. Purchases of bonds from the banks or the public by the government increase bankers' deposits. In a

[4] The economic journals have for some years contained a recondite debate over the cash and liquid-asset ratios of the banks. For example, Newlyn, W. T. (June, 1964), Crouch, R. L. (December, 1964 and August, 1965). A criticism of points of view expressed in these articles is given by Cramp, A. B. (June, 1966 and October, 1967). For a discussion of the value of the multiplier see Cramp, A. B. (February, 1963).

similar manner, all payments to the government—for example, tax payments—reduce bankers' deposits, and payments by the government to the public increase them.

Thirdly, we have so far been implicitly talking about a closed system. As soon as we admit the possibility of payments to foreigners we get another leakage, as these holders are unlikely to bank with the commercial banks.

Fourthly, there are a large number of foreign banks with branches in Britain. Sums that find their way to these banks represent a leakage from the commercial banking system. From a monetary viewpoint, this transfer of assets to foreign branch banks is, however, merely a transfer of the power to create credit from the commercial banks to these foreign banks. This important difference will be taken up in the next chapter.

As a simple illustration of the difference between flows of money between the banks and the public and flows between banks and the government, let us take the balance-sheet entries for the banks: firstly, when they extend a loan to a customer of £100, and, secondly, when they purchase £100 worth of securities from the government:

Result of commercial banks making a loan of £100 to a customer

Liabilities		*Assets*	
Deposits (i.e. credit balances of customers represent a liability to pay by the bank)	+£100	Loans (liability on the customer to repay, i.e. an asset of the bank)	+£100

Deposits created for the public are not lost to the banking system as a whole, since members of the public bank with the commercial banks. A, who has the added deposit originally writes a cheque to B. This is from the bank's point a transfer of ownership, deposits and loans still remain at +£100, and the bank can extend further credit, subject to the need for sufficient reserves and no leakages.

Results of commercial banks acquiring assets from the government

Liabilities	*Assets*	
No change	Cash (i.e. bankers' deposits at Bank of England)	−£100
	Securities	+£100

London Clearing Banks: averages of monthly figures

Year	Total Gross Deposits £ million	Of which Advances £ million	Assets as a percentage of total Deposits			
			Liquid Assets	Special Deposits	Investments	Advances to Customers
1958	6,636	1,923	34	—	32	29
1959	6,935	2,522	33	—	27	36
1960	7,236	3,123	32	1·0	20	43
1961	7,395	3,357	33	2·4	15	45
1962	7,611	3,408	33	2·1	16	45
1963	7,971	3,880	32	—	16	49
1964	8,550	4,328	30	—	14	51
1965	8,989	4,653	31	1·0	12	52
1966	9,376	4,732	31	1·5	12	51
1967	9,772	4,725	31	2·0	14	48

Composition of liquid assets *£ million*

	Cash	Money at Call	Treasury Bills	U.K. and Other Bills	Investments
1958	543	435	1,167	110	2,149
1959	565	489	1,089	135	1,836
1960	588	562	1,007	142	1,407
1961	607	606	992	233	1,122
1962	623	718	933	272	1,194
1963	647	748	842	297	1,244
1964	696	738	790	365	1,220
1965	739	910	653	461	1,087
1966	767	1,006	689	446	1,137
1967	798	1,136	564	492	1,340

Source: *Financial Statistics*, No. 61, Table 37, May, 1967, and No. 76, Table 35, August, 1968.

The purchase of a security from the government results in no change in bank liabilities, but a rearrangement of assets. Cash is down while there is a corresponding increase in securities.

When a member of the public purchases securities from the government with a cheque drawn on his account, bank liabilities are down by this amount with no corresponding increase in assets of the bank, a process described earlier as a leakage.

The conclusion of this section is that an initial increase in deposits of the commercial banks as a whole sets in motion an expansion of the credit structure. The banks know from experience that the bulk of this increase can be used to purchase financial instruments (investments or advances) giving a positive yield. It is not possible to deduce the size of the ultimate increase in credit by a look at either the cash or the liquid-asset ratios of the banks. The expansion is limited in a number of ways, in particular by the whole complex of operations between the government, the banks and the public sector. Chapter 6 takes up the story at this point.

Reversibility of bank expansion

So far the analysis has been conducted in terms of an expansion of bank deposits. Similar reasoning applies to a contraction of deposits.

Table 2 shows the composition of commercial banks' assets from 1958 to 1967. In spite of this period being one of 'stop-go', with a variety of credit squeezes in force, total deposits and advances which form part of total deposits show an upward trend. This trend should not cause too much surprise. It has been indicated that the multiplier in credit-creation is not large, and it will be found that there are several ways in which the commercial banks can resist making a reduction in deposits and advances.

Let us enter the picture with the monetary authorities trying to squeeze the liquid assets of the joint-stock banks (see 'Bank Liquidity in the United Kingdom', December, 1962).

This will normally take the form of attempts, termed 'open-market operations', to increase the amount of government debt held outside the banking system. This pressure can be applied, as we have seen, by trying to induce the non-bank public to take up Treasury bills or, better still, long-term debt. Or the authorities can try to increase the public's holding of non-marketable debt by, for example, offering a better return on National Savings. Such sales reduce bankers' deposits, as they are transferred to the government's account. As the cash ratio must be maintained, this will initially cause a reduction in liquid assets and the liquidity ratio. The reactions of the banks firstly in the short run and then in the longer run to this reduction in their liquidity is outlined below.

THE SHORT RUN

The commercial banks do not borrow directly from the Bank of England. If they wish to replenish cash, they will first of all recall some of the money at call and short notice from the discount houses.

The discount houses, provided that they cannot get the money from elsewhere, e.g. from foreign banks with funds in London, will go to the Bank of England. The Treasury bill rate is, as we have seen always below Bank Rate and the commercial banks provide the cheapest source of funds for the discount houses. The effect of this borrowing from the Bank on the discount houses is therefore to reduce their profits.

The discount houses can wriggle out of this in two ways: borrowing more from outside the banking system by offering better rates or raising their rate on Treasury bills so that more will go to outside tenderers. The result is the same: a tendency for the Treasury bill rate to increase and for other short-term rates to follow, by the market mechanism of funds seeking, other things being equal, the highest return.

If the monetary authorities do not wish market rates to rise, they can stop the process right at the start by accommodating the discount houses at market rate. The 'Special Buyer' (one of the discount houses acting for the Bank of England) will be instructed to buy Treasury bills on the market and so release cash into the system.

The implications should be quite clear: the monetary authorities can operate on either the rate of interest or the quantity of money. Only fortuitous circumstances will enable both to be achieved at the same time. The authorities' policy has been to seek to establish the rate structure they would like.

The above account details the short-term reactions of the commercial banks and the discount houses to a squeeze. Below are detailed the longer-term reactions.

THE LONG TERM

A look at Table 2 will show ways in which the banks reacted in the years 1958-67. The simplest method is, if their liquid assets are above the minimum level, merely to acquiesce in the reduction of their liquid assets. Thus from the table it will be seen that while liquid assets comprised 34% of total deposits in 1958, this figure was down to 31% in 1967, and in 1964 it was 30%.

Another method open to the banks is to try to replenish their liquid assets by running down their other investments. This process is also in evidence during this period. Table 2 shows investments accounted for 32% of deposits in 1958, but only 12% in 1966; they had increased slightly to 14% in 1967.

Attempts by the monetary authorities to reduce the number of Treasury bills (a policy successfully undertaken in this period) can be overcome by the banks if they are able to substitute alternative liquid assets. Table 2 shows that a drop in the banks' holding of Treasury bills of £603 million was partly compensated for by an increase in 'U.K. and other bills' of £382 million.[5]

The above account is far removed from a mechanical formula which can be applied to give us the final adjustment which a bank has to make in order to compensate for a change in deposits. The process described above whereby the banks can compensate by running down their other investments is a complicated process which can have different results in different circumstances. In order to understand this, it must be borne in mind that these portfolios are largely gilt-edged holdings in short-dated stocks with less than five years to run to maturity. These stocks can normally be realized without substantial loss. The simplest, but slowest, way to reduce these portfolios is for the banks not to renew the securities as they come up for redemption. The effect of actual sale of the stocks before maturity will vary with the identity of the other parties to the transactions:

1. If the banks' sales are taken up by the monetary authorities (they may not wish to see the established pattern of interest rates disturbed), such sales will increase the banks' liquid assets by the proceeds of the sale, leaving deposits unchanged, but, of course, the banks more liquid.

2. The sales may be made to the discount market. The discount market can finance these holdings either by selling Treasury bills to the banks or by borrowing more call money. The effect is the same as before. There is, however, a limit to the amount of stock that the discount houses are able, or willing, to hold.

3. Lastly, the banks may sell to the general public. This reduces bank deposits and leaves liquid assets unchanged and so improves the liquid-asset ratio. From the banks' point of view (but not from the point of view of monetary control), it is a less satisfactory method

[5] The increase in commercial bills is due to a number of factors: the replacement of the *ad valorem* duty of 1s.% by a flat duty of 2*d*. per bill in 1961, the increase in international trade, the growing use of bills to finance hire-purchase transactions, and the resort to bill finance by firms during a time of restrictions on bank-lending. For greater detail see 'London Money Market' (May, 1966).

than the other two ways. Even so, however, if the public finances its purchases of stock from the banks by holding less Treasury bills or non-marketable government debt, its deposits will be unchanged, and the final effect will be the same as if the banks had sold the stock direct to the authorities.

The fact that banks in recent years have run down their liquid assets nearer to the minimum levels, and also have greatly reduced their investment portfolios, means that these methods of replenishing their liquid assets in future are more circumscribed.

The conclusion to this section is that attempts to control the cash and liquid assets of the banks is subject to important qualifications. It depends in particular on the attitude of the public to holding cash and government debt, the willingness of the banks to substitute assets, and the fiscal policy being pursued by the government. Many of the factors noted that tend to offset monetary control may only operate at certain times and be of limited duration. But time is often the essence of the problem in monetary matters. It is not surprising that other methods of control have been devised to supplement control over cash and liquid assets. To these we now turn.

Other methods of bank control

BANK RATE

The use of Bank Rate was for a long time considered as the proper means of controlling the banks. An increase was supposed to deter borrowing from the banks since their rates are, by convention, tied to Bank Rate. Similarly, a decrease was supposed to encourage borrowing.[6]

The effects of changes in interest rates will be examined in more detail in the section on policy. It is sufficient to say now that at least in the circumstances of mild inflation which have prevailed since the war, this effect seems so weak in most sectors of the economy as not to be an effective constraint. It has always been recognized in Keynesian literature that low rates, while helpful, were not sufficient to generate business confidence in a depression. It also seems that high rates, by themselves, may not be sufficient to deter expansion in inflationary conditions—at least, within the acceptable range of movements of Bank Rate. The above remarks apply to the dearness

[6] It is worth noting that since the commercial banks do not pay interest on current accounts, an increase in Bank Rate, and therefore an increase in rates at which they lend, means greater profit for the banks. The term 'endowment' has been coined by the report on *Bank Charges* (1967) to cover this element in bank profit.

of money, not to its scarcity—a point which is frequently confused. If borrowing can be made more difficult, the effects are immediate. However, the act of changing Bank Rate has little effect on the scarcity of money. The classical theory of the monetary system tacitly identified dearness of money with scarcity. It assumed that high-interest rates automatically reduced the supply of money. This effect could come about if high-interest rates caused depositors to switch from bank deposits to government securities, an effect which has not been very much in evidence in the post-war period. The only other way in which changing Bank Rate can affect the scarcity of money is if there is a 'liquidity effect'. This effect refers to the fact that banks and other institutions may be deterred from selling securities by an increase in Bank Rate, which, if it affects other rates, will move security prices down. It is argued that the fear of having book losses will deter, in particular, banks from realizing investments and so recouping their liquid assets. From Table 2 we have seen that there is no indication that this has happened in recent years. Banks have dramatically run down their investments in spite of historically high levels of Bank Rate. This is not surprising, as we have seen, because banks' investments are in securities with less than five years to run to maturity, and in any case banks are allowed (rather controversially) to present balance sheets which obscure the detailed working of their operations.

SPECIAL DEPOSITS

Special deposits came into being on the recommendation of the Radcliffe Committee. If the monetary authorities call for special deposits, the banks are required to place a proportion of deposits at the Bank. These, unlike ordinary bankers' deposits, do not count towards either the cash or liquid-asset ratios of the banks. These deposits earn interest $\frac{1}{16}$th nearest to the average Treasury bill rate.[7] Thus, if banks are unduly liquid and the monetary authorities wish to limit credit, they can call for special deposits. As with pressure on the liquid-asset ratio by open-market operations, the banks may be able to overcome the effect of this type of squeeze in exactly the same way—namely, selling securities or substituting other assets. Like other pressures on the banks, it gives them a lever, if they wish to use it, to politely refuse advances.

Special deposits have been used only in a half-hearted manner, although it has been announced that they will be used more flexibly

[7] In May, 1969 the Bank announced that the rate of interest would be halved on these deposits until such time as the banks had conformed to the Request that lending should not exceed 98% of the November 1967 level.

in the future. The arguments used by the Radcliffe Committee to justify special deposits are not very convincing. The adoption of a variable liquidity ratio, as in some countries, whereby the authorities would announce from time to time the level of liquid assets the banks should hold, would seem to be a better device.

DIRECTIVES, REQUESTS OR EAR-STROKING

During the war and until 1951 the banks were obliged to hold Treasury deposit receipts. This at one stage amounted to 40% of their deposits and were a method by which the assets of the banks could be maintained in a manner desired by the monetary authorities. A process of 'forced funding' has been used on one occasion in 1951. For details refer to the *Radcliffe Report*, para. 406. In effect, the banks had to exchange £500 million of Treasury bills for the equivalent of short-term bonds.

Control of the banks by requiring them to hold specific assets, as outlined above, is regarded as an exceptional measure: the process is disliked by both the central and commercial banks. Instead, a process has grown up whereby the Bank of England makes requests to the banks. The procedure is sometimes called issuing directives or, more familiarly, 'ear-stroking'. These 'requests', as they will be called, are conventions which the banks observe even though they have not the force of law. The legal powers which were given to the Bank of England under the Nationalization Act could be used for the same purpose, but the use of such powers is not the way the system is operated. The Bank of England has said that if it had to use force to coerce the commercial banks it would regard this as a breakdown of the monetary system. For our purpose, the distinction is a fine one that need not trouble us; what matters is that requests are carried out.

These requests must take a general form, such as 'Do not lend more than last year' or 'Do not lend more to hire-purchase companies'. They cannot take the form of specific requests not to lend to a particular person or company. The banks are given guidance on the amount of lending: within this constraint they are free to select the happy or unhappy customers who get or do not get the loans.

Summary

The structure in Great Britain of commercial banking—eleven banks dominated by the 'Big Five'—was stable for many years, but is currently undergoing reappraisal. The need for this has been partly brought about by the success of other types of financial intermediaries and foreign banks in attracting deposits, partly by the introduction of a Post Office Giro system, and partly because of the wish to make internal economies and rationalization, both in the number of branches and use of expensive computing and other equipment.

Banks as a whole are able to create credit because, when they relend money that has been deposited with them, a portion of this money finds its way back into the banking system and can in its turn be used to make new investments or advances. The credit-multiplier is not large; it depends in particular on the whole complex of operations between the government, the banks and the public.

It has been shown that there are a variety of methods by which the monetary authorities influence the commercial banks. These are open-market operations, special deposits and requests. Bank Rate is no longer regarded as a direct method of control, although it may be used as a signal by the authorities to indicate their wish for tighter or easier money. The ease with which money control can be exercised depends intimately on the whole fiscal framework, and we pursue this point in Chapter 6.

Commercial banks form only a part of the monetary system, so that control of the banks may not mean control over the monetary system as a whole. In the next chapter we describe other financial institutions that form part of the monetary system and look at some of the implications for monetary policy.

5

Other financial institutions and financial intermediaries

Above all, the maintenance in the primary market generally and by the clearing banks of long-established arrangements on interest rates, following a rigid pattern, left wide-open opportunities which the new markets, with their uninhibited flexibility, were not slow to fill.

Midland Bank Review, August, 1966.

In this chapter financial institutions other than the commercial banks discussed in the previous chapter are dealt with. Firstly, we look at local authority borrowing, because it is their debt which is often held by the other institutions discussed in this chapter. Next we look at acceptance houses and overseas banks. The important growth in these institutions has largely taken place since the *Radcliffe Report*. It coincided with the granting of convertibility to external holders of currently earned sterling in 1958, and has benefited from the general relaxation of monetary restrictions which has taken place since. Then we look at a group of institutions performing various functions which usually go under the title of 'financial intermediaries'. After a brief description of these intermediaries, their implications for monetary policy are taken up, their impact on liquidity and finally their influence on financial markets.

Local authorities

Local authorities have not been included as financial intermediaries, although a case can be made out for doing so. Local authorities are large borrowers on the market, especially on short-term, and in considering financial flows they rank large in the picture. To the extent that local authorities relend for house-purchase and house-improvements, they act in a similar way to other financial intermediaries, but their borrowing is linked to their own needs for finance and not directly to their lending activities, and they are best treated separately.

Until 1955 local authorities had to meet their needs for borrowing by going to the Public Works Loan Board (P.W.L.B.). In 1955, a change of government policy occurred and local authorities were required to meet their needs in the market if they could. Access to government funds through P.W.L.B. was to be available only if funds could not be raised from the market. They were so successful in this policy that at times they embarrassed the monetary authorities, who found that their efforts to reduce liquidity in the economy were being nullified by the increase in short-term borrowing by the local authorities. In recent years this policy has been eased and local authorities now have easier access to the P.W.L.B.

Table 1

Growth of Local Authority temporary borrowing

(£ million)

Year	Up to 7 Days	7 Days to 3 Months	3 Months to 12 Months	Total[1]
1955	—	—	—	169
1961	558	229	146	933
1962	711	359	167	1,237
1963	693	284	291	1,268
1964	878	289	351	1,518
1965	1,239	315	293	1,847
1966	1,188	329	211	1,728
1967	1,238	229	253	1,720
1968	1,545	311	217	2,073

Source: *Financial Statistics*, Table 26, No. 61, May, 1967, and No. 76, August, 1968.

Table 1 shows the growth of local-authority temporary borrowing. From a figure of £169 million in 1955, it has grown to £2,073 million in 1968. The bulk of this money was recallable by the lender within seven days, as the breakdown for the years 1961-8 shows. These funds were drawn from a wide market, including the commercial banks, acceptance houses, overseas banks, other financial intermediaries, individuals and overseas. A detailed analysis of holders for the years 1955 and 1958 is given by Revell, J. R. S. and Hockley, G. C. (July and December, 1960). From 1961 refer to *Financial Statistics* (monthly publication).

In addition to temporary borrowing, local authorities also borrow on a smaller scale by way of mortgages for periods of one or more

[1] Total includes inter-authority borrowing. In 1968 this amounted to £66 million.

years, by the issue of stocks, and more recently by the issue of one- or two-year bonds.

The period since 1955 has therefore seen the rapid growth of a local-authority short-term money market. Local authorities have to pay rates marginally higher than the government for equivalent dated securities. They also pay ½% more than nationalized industries (with Treasury guarantee) for bank loans.

The fact that local authorities have to pay rather more when borrowing on their own account has long been a matter of dispute between them and the government. The Radcliffe Committee gave this and the difficulties it created for monetary control as the chief reasons why the local authorities should be given freer access to the P.W.L.B. The National Board for Prices and Incomes in *Bank Charges* (1967), paras. 90-2, has come out in substantial agreement with the Radcliffe recommendations. As an alternative suggestion, they put up the idea that a new co-operative financial institution, guaranteed by the Treasury, be set up for local-authority borrowing. Our interest is rather that a sophisticated short-term money market has grown up. Since local authority borrowing is secured on the local rateable value of property, their debt has almost the same market standing as government debt, and rates obtainable in this market will exercise a powerful effect on the rates which financial intermediaries need to give in order to attract deposits.

Acceptance houses and overseas banks in the United Kingdom

Acceptance houses and overseas banks are treated together because both are concerned with deposits of British and of foreign residents. First, an outline is given of the functions performed by these two sectors. This section draws on the *Radcliffe Report*, paras. 185-9 and 197-201, and 'Overseas and Foreign Banks in London' (September, 1961, and June, 1968) to which the reader is referred for greater detail.

ACCEPTANCE HOUSES

A wide variety of city institutions are known as 'merchant banks'. This name reflects their origin in the trading of goods. Today they undertake a wide variety of financial services. Eighteen of them belong to the Accepting Houses Committee: to these the term 'acceptance house' can properly be applied. They have always had close associations with the Bank of England, and at one time a merchant-banking background was necessary to obtain a Governorship at the Bank of England. The acceptance of bills of exchange (at a discount plus an acceptance commission) is an important part of their business.

A bill of exchange by a British bank or by one of the eighteen accepting houses is, if it has one other British name on it, 'eligible paper' at the Bank of England, and has therefore the highest degree of liquidity, shared only by Treasury Bills and short-dated Government bonds. Having this maximum of liquidity and the complete assurance of payment (on which of course the liquidity depends), it commands the lowest rate of discount available for any non-Government paper. An acceptance house thus, when accepting a bill, confers on the drawer of the bill (and on anyone who discounts it for him) the certainty of being able to get sterling in exchange for it from a bank or discount house in London, at the least possible sacrifice in discount (*Radcliffe Report*, para. 186).

Besides acceptances, these houses carry out a wide range of other services; in raising loans, dealing in foreign exchange, financial advice (which includes advice to firms contemplating take-over bids, or are themselves the subject of take-over offers) and a wide range of other activities.

OVERSEAS BANKS IN THE UNITED KINGDOM

Statistics of overseas banks now cover over 100 institutions are collected under four headings. These are:

- British overseas and Commonwealth banks.
- American banks.
- Foreign banks and affiliates.
- Other banks. These are distinguished because they were not included in the statistics until 1962.

It will be seen from this list that the category 'overseas banks' covers diverse institutions. Some are head offices of British banking concerns overseas, while others are branches of banks whose head offices are abroad.

These banks:

- operate as exchange dealers, particularly on the Euro-dollar market;
- finance the movement of goods between countries which will include acceptance credits giving rise to bills of exchange which can be negotiated in the discount market;
- accept and deploy funds moving to London from abroad.

Regarding their activities in the United Kingdom, the Radcliffe Committee were able to say:

This domestic business is negligible in comparison with the activity of the clearing banks. It is as holders of Government bonds and as operators in the discount market that the overseas banks have their main relevance to the liquidity structure of the economy (para. 201).

Since the publication of the *Radcliffe Report*, this situation has been transformed. While still important in the fields quoted, these banks have greatly extended 'domestic business'.

While the total gross deposits of the commercial banks have increased from £6,636 million in 1958 to £9,772 million in 1967 (see p. 31), the corresponding figures for acceptance houses and overseas banks have increased from £1,085 million to £9,300 million (see Table 2), an increase of 47% in the former case and of 757% in the latter case. Allowing for the fact that this slightly overstates the position because

Table 2

Acceptance houses and overseas banks in U.K.: Deposits at Dec.

£ million

Year	U.K. Banks	*Other U.K. Residents* Sterling Balances	Other Currency Balances	*Overseas Residents* Sterling Balances	Other Currency Balances	Certificates of Deposits[2]	Total Deposits
1958	—	—	—	—	—	—	1,085
1959	—	—	—	—	—	—	1,327
1960	—	—	—	—	—	—	1,891
1961	—	—	—	—	—	—	2,013
1962	460	431	76	1,096	959	—	3,022[3]
1963	622	655	83	1,208	1,166	—	3,734
1964	760	815	79	1,283	1,752	—	4,689
1965	1,050	1,046	90	1,356	2,042	—	5,584
1966	1,403	1,158	121	1,250	2,793	81	6,807
1967	2,245	1,399	211	1,167	4,030	248	9,300[4]

Source: *Financial Statistics*, No. 76, August, 1968, and *Bank of England Quarterly*, September, 1964.

[2] These certificates, minimum amount £25,000, are in effect deposits mostly for terms up to one year, but since they are negotiable instruments they are more liquid than fixed term deposits and earn only slightly less in interest.

[3] Figures before 1962 exclude 'Other overseas banks' as data are not available. These banks in 1962 account for total deposits of £409 million.

[4] In 1967 a further £298 million can be added to total deposits in respect of institutions included for the first time. These new institutions have not been included in any of the figures shown.

the figures for 1958 excluded a number of overseas banks which were not included until 1962 and the fact that about one-quarter of deposits represents inter-bank balances (mostly with each other) there must still be an impressive increase in the deposits of this sector compared to the commercial banks.

Taking the period from 1962 to 1967, gross deposits of the commercial banks increased from £7,611 million to £9,772 million, or 28%. Acceptance houses and overseas banks increased their deposits from £3,022 million to £9,300 million, or 207%. Of this increase United Kingdom residents, other than banks, increased their sterling holdings by 225%, while overseas residents increased their balances in other currencies by 320%.

Our concern at the moment is with the sterling holdings of the acceptance houses and overseas banks. Overseas holdings will be taken up in the next chapter. It is clear that in this period they were able to compete very successfully with the commercial banks for deposits. First, the reasons for this will be examined and then the implications for monetary policy looked at.

The acceptance houses and overseas banks are subject to some of the restraints that affect commercial banks. They are, for example, now subject to Requests from the Bank of England on their domestic business, but in general they are freer from restrictions. In particular, in much of this period they were not subject to the cash or liquid-asset requirements of the commercial banks, nor do they follow the interest-rate structure of the commercial banks.

The effect of not being subject to a cash ratio is that:

> Their individual cash positions can vary substantially day by day, from the nature of their business, and it is to their advantage to employ to the utmost channels in which they can earn interest on money that is recallable within twenty-four hours. The existence of the discount market, through which they can smooth out the irregularities of their cash position while maximizing their earning capacity, is a great advantage to such banks, and is indeed one of the attractions which have brought many overseas and foreign banks to London and keep them there (*Radcliffe Report*, para. 177).

One explanation of the faster growth of acceptance houses and overseas banks is thus that they have greater freedom to manipulate their funds *vis-à-vis* the commercial banks.

The second reason referred to, their freedom on interest rates, is probably of more importance in explaining their rise in domestic deposits. They are able to offer, in particular to the institution or business with large funds at its disposal, more attractive rates of interest on deposits than the commercial banks. The commercial banks have reacted recently by setting up special subsidiaries offering higher rates for deposits.

The implications for monetary policy of the growth of acceptance houses and overseas banks is that control of the commercial banks is not sufficient to ensure control of the monetary system. The evidence points to the fact that commercial banks have been unduly penalized (or have penalized themselves) by efforts at monetary control. Restrictions on commercial banks are at least partly overcome by expansion on the part of acceptance houses and overseas banks.

Financial intermediaries

One characteristic of a developed economy is the presence of a wide variety of financial intermediaries. This is in contrast to many underdeveloped countries, where an individual who does not wish to spend the whole of his income has little choice but to hold currency or precious metals, deposit the money in a bank, or lend the money directly to an individual or to a business. A developed country has a great variety of institutions interposed between the owner of funds

Table 3

Main financial intermediaries

(*£ million*)

	Stock of Assets *at the end of* 1963	Assets *acquired in* 1963
Insurance Co's: life funds	7,425	577
non-life funds	972	3
Pension and superannuation funds	4,652	362
Building societies	4,359	518
Investment trusts	2,848	68
H.P. finance houses	796	71
Trustee Savings Banks (Special Investment Depts)	755	133
Unit trusts	350	54
Special finance agencies	215	23
	22,372	1,809

Source: *Bank of England Quarterly*, June, 1965.

and the user of funds. Lending can still take place directly, but usually it takes place by means of the intermediaries. The intermediaries receive money from a variety of sources and employ or invest it in a variety of ways.

Financial intermediaries should be clearly distinguished from brokers, who merely act on behalf of their client to arrange a transaction and then drop out of the picture. Financial intermediaries accept claims on other people, and in exchange offer their liabilities, i.e. claims against themselves. If their claims were widely accepted in payment of debts, as bank deposits are, they would be on the same basis as banks. They are inferior in this respect, e.g. a deposit with a building society must first be turned into money to pay off a debt, whereas a bank deposit can be transferred directly. However, these claims do act as a store of value (which can economize in the use of money) and the intermediaries are a source of credit.

Table 3 lists the main financial intermediaries in order of size of their assets at the end of 1963. (This is not necessarily the same as their economic importance.) The figures are a mixture of market, book and nominal values, and so should be treated with caution.

These intermediaries differ widely from each other. In particular, insurance company life funds, pension and superannuation funds and the special finance agencies are on a different footing from the other intermediaries listed. Special finance agencies will be looked at below. Insurance and pension companies, because of the size of their assets and the annual flow of funds to them, have important repercussions on financial markets in a way which will be outlined at the end of this chapter. In general, however, their liabilities to the public are less liquid than those of the other financial intermediaries. Funds in pension and superannuation schemes are not usually available to the beneficiary before retirement. Insurance life policies are in an intermediate category from a holder's viewpoint: encashment before the policy matures usually involves financial loss, particularly in the early years of the policy. However, a policy can frequently be used as collateral for a loan from the insurance company concerned, a bank or other lender.

Deposits in building societies, hire purchase companies and trustee savings banks are liquid, since deposits can usually be withdrawn on demand or at short notice with no capital loss. Investment trusts and unit trusts differ in that the capital subscribed is usually by way of taking up shares or units in the trust. The funds so subscribed are in turn invested by the trusts in company shares and other assets. The value of these assets will in turn determine the market value of the shares or units of the investment or unit trust. These assets are therefore less liquid than deposits, since their capital value is uncertain.

The special finance agencies include four institutions: the Agricultural Mortgage Corporation, the Finance Corporation for Industry, the Industrial and Commercial Finance Corporation and the Commonwealth Development Finance Company. In general, the capital of these institutions comes from the Bank of England and the commercial banks, with, in the case of C.D.F.C., some being subscribed by a number of Commonwealth central banks. These agencies are government-inspired to meet the needs of agriculture and business for medium- and long-term funds, and in particular to meet legitimate needs where the enterprises find difficulty in raising funds from the normal market sources.

The presence of a host of financial intermediaries raises a number of points.

Power to create credit

From a monetary management point of view, one of the major questions is: supposing the banks are controlled, will the presence of financial intermediaries thwart their attempts at credit control?

If the section on how a bank creates credit has been understood it is easy to see that financial intermediaries differ only in degree in their ability to create credit. A bank can create credit because people deposit notes and coin at a bank in the belief that they can always reclaim deposits in notes and coin. In practice banks find that claims on money are accepted in lieu of notes and coin, i.e. most of the payments in the economy take the form, not of exchange of notes and coin (primary money), but of bank deposits (secondary money). This means a large part of initial deposits can be reloaned, subject only to the need to keep adequate reserves. There was a theoretical stalemate at this point for about 100 years *on whether banks created credit or just loaned out part of existing deposits*. This has been sorted out by considering the flow of income. So long as deposits do not leave the banking system, the process of lending by the banks or of the banks buying securities can repeat itself many times. The process comes to an end because of the need to keep a proportion in reserve at each 'round' of lending and because of leakages from the banking system.

An analogous picture can be drawn for financial intermediaries. A building society will be used as an example. It will find that a certain proportion of money that it lends out will be redeposited with it. This money can be relent, subject only to the need to keep a reserve for that proportion of depositors who demand the return of their money. If we postulate the same sort of closed system of circulation of money, as was done for the banking system, e.g. a house-builder who receives the sum of money loaned by the society deposits this sum back in the building society, then it is clear that the building society can reloan this money, less a proportion to build up its reserves.

The difference between banks and financial intermediaries is thus only one of degree, not of difference in kind. Because financial intermediaries' liabilities are not counted as money, they are likely to have to keep a greater proportion of money as a reserve, or, what amounts to the same thing, see that they secure an adequate flow of new deposits. Also the flow of funds back to the building society is likely to be much less than the flow of funds back to the banking system.

As was the case when considering the banking system, it is necessary to distinguish between a single financial intermediary and financial intermediaries considered as a whole. Although lending by, say, a building society may not lead to very much money being deposited back in the building society, collectively financial intermediaries may be taking in each other's loans, and so be able to expand collectively in a way analogous to the banking system considered as a whole.

Credit creation need not be at the expense of the banking system

It is important to realize that the ability of the financial intermediaries to create credit does not necessarily affect the commercial banks, unlike, for example, the purchase of government securities.

Let us take the case where £1,000 is withdrawn from a bank and is deposited in a building society. From the point of view of the banking system, all that has happened at this stage is that an individual's account is debited by £1,000, while the building society's account is credited by a corresponding amount. The total of bank deposits is unchanged, but the total of financial claims has increased by £1,000 the increase in the deposit at the building society (i.e. a liability of the building society to repay this sum).

Whether, and to what extent, the banks are affected at the next stage depends on the use to which the building society and subsequent holders put this money. Let us assume for simplicity that the whole of this £1,000 is lent by the building society to a borrower, who pays it over to a builder for a house. If the builder deposits the money back in the banking system, once again all that has happened from the banks' point of view is that the ownership of deposits has changed once more. It is clear that the banks will only be affected if there is a 'leakage' in the flow of income: from *their* point of view, a cheque drawn in favour of a financial intermediary is no different from a cheque drawn in favour of an individual. This is so because financial intermediaries bank with the banking system. Commercial banks are affected, as we saw, if the money is deposited with an acceptance house or overseas bank.

Implications for monetary policy

From the point of view of the monetary authorities, a transaction as outlined above is not neutral. The transfer of £1,000 to a building society did not alter the total of bank deposits; it did, however, enable the building society to lend more. We see why the presence of financial intermediaries is so essential to a developed economy and at the same time poses problems for monetary management. The financial intermediaries provide a channel for finance to get to ultimate borrowers. Individuals are not likely to lend substantial sums directly for house-purchase, but are likely to lend to a building society, which in turn lends for house-purchase. This aspect will be taken up in the next section. The problem comes if the monetary authorities are trying to control the amount of credit in the economy by limiting the banks' power to lend. If deposits flow to the financial intermediaries (merely a change of ownership of deposits from the banks' point of view), the financial intermediaries can extend the credit instead of the banking system.

The *Radcliffe Report* went to some length to spell out the implications touched on in this section. It might be supposed that in the circumstances the logic of the situation would dictate that controls over the financial intermediaries be recommended and discussed in some detail, to correspond to existing control over the banking system. In fact, this was not the case, and the position was left rather ambiguous:

> Since we envisage the use of monetary measures as not in ordinary times playing other than a subordinate part in guiding the development of the economy, we do not consider such an elaborate extension of compulsory powers to be justified in the conditions immediately before us. In times of emergency we believe that the rough justice of the blunter measures we propose in paragraphs 524 and 528 would be appropriate.[5]
>
> But it is not impossible that there may be longer periods, not amounting to emergencies, in which excessive liquidity persistently embarrasses the authorities in their conduct of economy policy. In such circumstances an extension of direct control over credit-giving to cover other groups of financial institutions besides the banks would reinforce the efficiency of the restraints imposed on the banks, as well as having the appeal of equity,

[5] The measures recommended were a combination of controls of capital issues, bank advances and consumer credit, aimed to contain private borrowing, and so spending, coupled with a critical review of government spending.

and it might therefore be necessary to accept the degree of interference with business, and to overcome the practical difficulties which such a wide-ranging scheme of registration and direction would entail (para. 511).[6]

In practice, informal control, or Requests, by the Bank of England have been extended from the commercial banks to many of the financial intermediaries. Thus on February 1st, 1965, the Bank wrote to the Chairman of the Committee of London Clearing Bankers requesting that bank advances to the private sector should not increase at an annual rate of more than 5%, and that the banks should apply a similar limitation to both their provision of acceptance facilities and their purchase of commercial bills.

The Governor also wrote to the Accepting Houses Committee and to the organizations of overseas banks in London asking that these banks should similarly limit their sterling advances, acceptances and commercial bill holdings. The London Discount Market Association and the leading associations of hire-purchase finance houses were asked to observe a comparable degree of restraint: and members of the British Insurance Association, the National Association of Pension Funds and the Building Societies Association were also requested to co-operate in maintaining restraint—in particular in relation to the finance of building and property development, other than housing for the owner-occupier (*Commentary*, March, 1966, 3).

In 1968 the Bank announced that a 'new, and to some extent experimental' form of control had been agreed with overseas and foreign banks, to be known as the Cash Deposits Scheme. See 'Control of Bank Lending: the Cash Deposits Scheme' (June, 1968), on which this section draws.

The diversity of these banks precluded bringing them within the system of special deposits. Instead, these banks may be required to make cash deposits with the Bank, calculated as a percentage of certain of their deposit liabilities in sterling. The scheme is not intended to affect the banks' business in foreign currencies. The percentage called will normally be the same for all banks, although the right is reserved, in exceptional circumstances, to treat banks individually. The Bank will pay a Treasury bill rate of interest on the cash deposits, but reserve the right to pay a lower rate than this. The Treasury bill rate will often be less than the banks would otherwise have earned.

The Bank has therefore two methods of control over overseas and foreign banks: strict quantitative controls brought about by

[6] This paragraph has the signs of being the result of compromise between different opinions in pursuit of the British passion for unanimous reports. Would it not be better to have stronger majority recommendations with dissenting opinions?

Requests and the less rigid form of control in the new system of cash deposits.

Thus since the time of publication of the *Radcliffe Report* informal control has been extended to embrace the financial intermediaries. We have not yet been told very much about how the Bank's directives are made known to the financial institutions concerned, to what extent they are effective, and, if so, how they are made effective. It is likely that further evolution will take place. It is now clear that in the absence of restraint the financial intermediaries can, at least in some circumstances, frustrate or partially frustrate a credit squeeze, so that control by informal or formal means is essential if credit restriction is to be successful.

Increase in liquidity

In the previous section we dealt with the ability of the financial intermediaries to create credit. Another aspect of a well-developed sector of this kind was touched on: the increase in liquid assets which they bring about. In general, the financial intermediaries enable long- and medium-term investment to be financed, although the securities which they issue in exchange for deposits are often liquid, i.e. quickly convertible into a known amount of cash. One result of this is that medium- and long-term interest rates are lower than they would otherwise be.[7] This is one of the reasons why interest rates are likely to be higher in underdeveloped countries.

The ability to lend money for a longer period of time than the funds borrowed is an important function in a modern economy. Banks have, of course, long cultivated this art. At the root of this process lies the confidence which must be built up between the depositor and the institution accepting the deposit. The early history of banking, and the bank failures that have occurred in some countries in recent times, are evidence of this. The problem of a country trying to establish a financial sector is not merely that of duplicating the institutions of a developed economy, but of engendering confidence in them once they have been set up. In Britain confidence in the financial sector and the financial intermediaries in particular is

[7] It is sometimes asserted that the movement of funds into institutional hands means that they, as opposed to individuals, are less inclined to invest in newer and riskier projects. The special finance agencies must be exempted from this conjecture, as they were set up expressly to provide finance in this field. A counter-argument is used: that we might expect institutions to exercise their responsibilities of share-ownership more effectively. Either of these conjectures could be important, but there is little satisfactory evidence on either side and it is easy to exaggerate both points of view.

achieved in numerous ways. The various parts are linked together in many ways as a result of formal and informal ties, many of the institutions are subject to legal restrictions governing their reserves and other matters, and most are subject to regulation from their own professional associations.

As an illustration of lending longer than borrowing, we can continue with our example of building societies. It might be questioned how, if building societies lend money for from twenty to twenty-five years on the purchase of houses, they can afford to let depositors have their money back on demand or at short notice. The fundamental point has already been made that because there is general confidence in the way societies are run withdrawals are not likely to be panic measures of a kind that would force any financial institution to close its doors. The building societies, like banks, keep reserves to meet normal withdrawal demands, but, apart from this, their lending is not as long as it seems.

Most mortgages are being repaid over the course of the loan, so that a continual flow of capital is coming into the building society's hands: together with early redemptions, this results in a fairly liquid position.

Building societies are also, to some extent, able to influence the flow of deposits into and out of their accounts by changing the rate of interest they are offering. Here we are not considering the general level of interest rates prevailing in the economy, which will be taken up in a later chapter, but the differential effect of particular interest rates. It is well known that building societies do not follow Bank Rate up or down immediately, unlike, for example, the commercial banks. However, if Bank Rate changes for a considerable length of time, they are forced to follow suit. In the case of an increase in Bank Rate, they find funds flowing from them to institutions who have raised rates, e.g. local authorities and finance companies, and existing deposits may be withdrawn for the same purpose. In this circumstance, building societies are forced to increase their rates in order to protect themselves. In a similar way, societies reduce their rates after a decrease in Bank Rate, when their reserves are sufficiently built up.[8]

The argument in this sector is that financial intermediaries increase liquidity, and that this is an important function in a modern economy.

[8] This example of how an institution is able to make loans for periods in excess of twenty years, and yet let its depositors have their money at call or short notice, illustrates the weakness of the case of the commercial banks, who frequently protest that making long-term loans would endanger their financial security. For a critical look at commercial bank practices see *Bank Charges* (1957).

In essence, financial intermediaries lend or invest long while frequently borrowing short. Long-term lending is more hazardous than short-term lending, and they remove much of this uncertainty for the investor *vis-à-vis* his position had he lent direct to the final borrower.

Impact on financial markets

The final aspect of financial intermediaries that we wish to stress is their impact on financial markets. This impact can come about in two ways. Firstly, from the existing flow of funds and, secondly, from switching of existing assets. From Table 3 it will be seen, for example, that insurance company life funds acquired assets of £577 million during 1963. Of this sum 23% went into gilt-edged or local authority stocks, 29% in company fixed-interest stocks and 21% in ordinary company shares, 16% was used for loans and mortgages and the remaining 10% for land property and ground rents.

The size of the financial intermediaries and the size of the flow of funds to them make these institutions of prime importance. We do not know at present how much of this money is channelled into buying old assets and how much into new assets, but the impact on both markets is likely to be very considerable. The Bank of England estimates that the institutional share of turnover in United Kingdom equities in 1963 was about a quarter of the whole, and that they accounted for rather more than three-fifths of the turnover in fixed-interest stocks.

It is clear that if the authorities can keep these institutional investors happy these financial markets are likely to be orderly.

Summary

The commercial banks form an important part of the monetary system, but in recent years acceptance houses, overseas banks and financial intermediaries have been growing much faster. They are important, not only because, like commercial banks, they can create credit, but because they increase liquidity and have a marked impact on financial markets. The fact that the Bank of England now includes these institutions in its Requests and has initiated the cash deposits scheme for other banks indicates that monetary control, to be effective, must take these institutions into account. There are no clear indications that Requests to these institutions will meet with the same success as Requests to the commercial banks. Developments could take place by more formal means of control, or the commercial banks might be encouraged to compete more actively with these institutions. Either of these developments pose difficult problems and raise far-reaching questions of monetary management, which will be developed in the next chapter.

6
Monetary expansion and contraction

We conclude that the proper spirit of approach to control of the money supply is a decent humility in the face of a highly complex task. Both old-orthodox and new-orthodox arguments are inadequate. The only policy for influencing the money supply on which practical reliance could be placed would be based on control, not of bank cash or of liquid assets, but of security sales to the non-bank public. If the authorities are to be criticized it is because of their timidity in experimenting with methods of controlling the gilt-edged market.

CRAMP, A. B. (June, 1966), 'Control of the Money Supply', *Economic Journal.*

The previous chapters have outlined briefly the financial sector of the British economy. A picture of the Bank of England and its relations with the government, the commercial banks, the discount market, other financial institutions and financial intermediaries has been built up. Also some of the interrelations of these institutions with each other have been indicated.

We now turn to the question: What determines the amount of money and liquidity in the economy? This will be tackled by looking first at what determines the amount of primary money and secondary money, and then considering broader issues which are introduced when acceptance houses, overseas banks and financial intermediaries are brought into the picture.

We should not make a common mistake and forget that money has a *demand* as well as a *supply* aspect. Thus the question, 'What is the potential power of the commercial banks to create money?' may not be the same as 'How much do they actually create?' The former question takes us over the whole field of government policy; the latter question brings in bankers' prudence and aspects which they take into account before granting loans and overdrafts. Again the monetary authorities can attempt to diminish the supply of money or they may be able to achieve the same ends by strengthening the demand for money or for government securities.

In looking at these questions, it will be found that the net flows of money to or from the Exchequer *vis-à-vis* the rest of the economy are the crucial factors, together with the ways in which the authorities and the commercial banks are able to deal with these flows. Much of this chapter is taken up in detailing these matters. One section is taken up with a discussion of how a government deficit in a particular year is financed. The next question goes into more detail of the factors affecting the size of a government deficit or surplus in a year. This is followed by a brief look at how the market is managed day to day. These factors are then drawn together to see how they influence the amount of money and liquidity in the economy.

Amount of primary and secondary money

Primary money has been defined to be coin, notes and bankers' deposits at the Bank of England.

Coin and notes need not detain us long. In Britain they are issued by the Bank subject to the formal consent of Parliament. They are kept at the level demanded by the public, so that issues reach a peak just before summer holidays start and before Christmas. For details of the mechanism of the note issued, the reader is referred to 'Note Circulation' (March, 1965).

The practical effect of an increase in the note issue is to lessen the Exchequer's need to borrow on other forms of debt. However, this is merely a by-product of the issue of a token currency. The government *does not* make an issue of notes to finance its expenditure: it does so because there is a demand for notes. Coin and bank-notes are, in a *Radcliffe* phrase, 'the small change of the monetary system'. We should expect to find in normal times that coin and notes bear a relatively stable relationship to national income, or to consumers' disposable income, after allowance has been made for seasonal factors referred to above.

So bankers' deposits at the Bank of England is the main item we should have in mind when we think of primary money. Transactions between the government and the rest of the economy will (except for sums that take place in coin and notes and in addition are not paid into the banking system) be reflected initially in a change in bankers' deposits. For example, to make a payment to the government, an individual will write a cheque on his account in favour of the Inland Revenue or appropriate department. The end-result is that, besides the individual's account being debited, bankers' deposits at the Bank will be debited and the government's account credited.

We know that commercial bankers maintain their cash reserves (bankers' deposits and till money) at 8% of deposits. Thus when implying that bankers' deposits are increased or decreased above this level, we are implying that commercial bankers alter their structure of assets and liabilities so as to maintain the desired ratio of 8% in a manner which has been outlined in Chapter 3.

Payments from the government that take place by way of cheques reverse the process: as well as an individual's account being credited, bankers' deposits at the Bank are increased, while the government's account is decreased.

What is relevant in this situation is the net flow of payments between the government and the rest of the economy and the way in which this flow is financed. To this we now turn.

The financing of a government deficit

Let us suppose that the Budget in a particular year, taking both above- and below-the-line items,[1] shows a deficit—that is, the government will be spending more than it receives, assuming no tax changes are made. The issue of notes and direct borrowing from the Bank of England have both been ruled out as a means of financing the deficit. *It will be met by the issue of securities: it makes a considerable difference whether these are long-term or short-term securities and to whom they are sold.*

We have two streams of payments to consider: on the one hand, payments from the government to the non-government sector in excess of payments the other way, so that individual and company accounts at commercial banks will be increased and, as we have seen, a consequence of this is that bankers' deposits will be increased. On the other hand, we have the consequences following on from the issue of securities. The first effect is a potential increase in purchasing power, while the second may be, but does not have to be, a potential decrease in purchasing power.

Let us first consider that the government attempts to finance the deficit by the issue of long- or medium-term securities (here a decision has to be made on what rate of interest they will be offered to the market, a point that will not be pursued at this stage). This issue may be taken up by:

(a) the public,
(b) the commercial banks.

[1] The distinction between above- and below-the-line items is historical. Items above the line were intended to cover expenditures met out of taxation and revenue derived from taxation; below-the-line items, expenditures and revenue derived from borrowing. The distinction has little economic merit. For a discussion of alternative ways to present Exchequer accounts see Peacock, A. T. (January, 1964).

(a) It is clear that if the public take up the whole of the issue they will draw cheques in favour of the government and bankers' deposits will be reduced. The increase in deposits brought about by the Budget deficit has been matched by a decrease because the public have been induced to exchange cash for bonds.

(b) Sales to the banks have similar effects to sales to the public. The increase in deposits brought about by the government deficit is matched by the banks' transfer of funds to the government in exchange for securities.[2]

Failure to sell long- or medium-term debt will result in the need to issue short-term securities—that is, Treasury bills. In the chapter on the discount market it was seen that the discount houses undertake to cover the tender. They can do this because they can always get accommodation at the Bank of England. In so far as the discount houses take up the securities, there is no offset to the government deficit. Sales to outside tenderers will reduce bankers' deposits by a like amount and reduce their liquid-asset ratio. However, Treasury bills present a potential spending power, since they are very liquid and their holders will, in any case, have money in three months.

We can summarize so far and say that notes and coin come into circulation because the public desire more or less notes. They are not of operational significance. Bankers' deposits and the amount of secondary money depend on the acquisition of debts by the commercial banks and the public, and is the result of the whole fiscal and budgetary process—that is, it depends on the stream of payments to and from the government and public and the method of financing any deficit.

Determinants of the government's annual surplus or deficit

The preceding section presented a static picture of how a deficit could be financed. We now examine more closely the factors that in any one year will determine the size of the government's surplus or deficit, and then go on to examine day-to-day management.

Table 1 presents a fuller picture of changes that occur in a year. The top part of the table presents the items that require financing in a year; the lower section shows how the finance was provided. The bottom is the inverse of the top. Thus net balance is either a deficit, and a figure will appear in the top half showing the amount that requires financing or a surplus, in which case a figure will appear in the bottom half showing the amount of finance provided.

[2] It is unrealistic to postulate the sale of long-term bonds to the commercial banks in current conditions as bonds with five years or less to maturity are preferred. See *Radcliffe Report*, para. 406.

Table 1

Exchequer Financing

(£ million)

Items requiring Finance	1963-4	1964-5	Year 1965-6	1966-7	1967-8
1. Net balance or overall deficit	376	313	499	740	1,331
2. Increase in Exchange Equalization Account	—	—	128	—	—
3. Decrease in overseas holdings of British Debt	—	—	—	62	—
4. Reduction in the note issue and coin	—	—	—	—	—
5. Withdrawal of National Savings	—	—	118	197	5
6. Reduction in Tax Certificates	59	41	59	—	—
7. Reduction in Treasury bills	—	544	—	488	42
8. Reduction in government stocks	8	138	72	—	96
9. Reduction in net indebtedness to Bank of England	—	1	—	—	131
	443	1,037	876	1,487	1,605
Items providing Finance					
1. Net balance or overall surplus	—	—	—	—	—
2. Decrease in Exchange Equalization Account	55	118	—	112	234
3. Increase in overseas holdings of British Debt	13	611	85	—	1,228
4. Increase in the note issue and coin	205	123	212	123	123
5. Increase of National Savings	156	185	—	—	—
6. Increase in Tax Certificates	—	—	—	98	20
7. Increase in Treasury bills	—	—	396	—	—
8. Increase in government stocks	—	—	—	1,130	—
9. Increase in net indebtedness to Bank of England	14	—	183[3]	24	—
	443	1,037	876	1,487	1,605

Source: *Bank of England Quarterly Bulletins*, Table 1.

[3] Includes changes in the Banking Department's holding of government debt resulting from a special swap with the U.S. authorities and its repayment.

Item 1 thus shows the overall deficit in the year. This was the only item considered in the previous section.

Item 2. It may seem strange that an increase in the Exchange Equalization Account (E.E.A.) appears under the heading of items requiring finance and that a fall provides finance. The explanation is simple. When the E.E.A. increases its holdings of gold or foreign currencies (i.e. foreigners exchange their currencies for pounds) the E.E.A. draws on its reserves to provide these pounds. These reserves are mainly held in the form of tap Treasury bills, so that the Exchequer is obliged to replace these bills by borrowing from another source.

Likewise a fall in reserves (foreigners exchanging pounds for gold or other currencies) means that the E.E.A. has more of its assets in pounds. These as we have seen are held mainly in the form of Treasury bills.

Item 3. The change in overseas holdings refers to changes in amounts of government securities held by foreigners. Many of these changes will be accompanied by opposite changes in E.E.A. For example, when foreign currencies are converted into sterling with the E.E.A. (with the result we saw under item 2 of increasing the Exchequer requirements) and then invested in government debt, the Exchequer requirements will be unaffected; E.E.A. will hold less debt, foreigners more. In the same way, government borrowing from abroad usually results in opposite changes in E.E.A., so that it has no effect on the amount of Exchequer financing.

In addition to these movements, balances held in sterling may be put into, or taken out of, government securities with no attempts made to change into other currencies.[4] These movements will affect Exchequer requirements because of the need to replace the foreign holder by some other.

Items 4-6 are straightforward. A reduction in the public's holding of any of these items has to be financed in some other way. These items are 'passive' savings, in the sense that the government are

[4] These balances could, for example, be invested in local authority securities, in equities, or left on deposit with commercial banks. A full analysis would try to take into account the secondary effects of foreign funds being invested in one type of security rather than another. The most important of these would be the effects on the commercial banks, interest rates and on the lending, borrowing and spending of the private sector. For further details see 'Inflows and Outflows of Foreign Funds' (June, 1962). The tentative conclusion reached by this article was: '. . . It may be said that, in a period of restrictive credit policy, such as 1960 and 1961, a substantial part of an inflow or outflow is likely to occur in ways that directly cause no change in bank deposits and domestic spending. Nevertheless, some parts are likely to be in forms that do cause changes in the liquidity of banks and other credit-giving institutions' (p. 102).

always ready to issue Tax Reserve Certificates, Savings Certificates, Premium Bonds and the like on demand. The more of these that people are willing to take up the less need there is to sell other securities and vice versa.

From time to time these issues are made more attractive, but this is usually when the interest on them has fallen behind other rates.

Items 7 and 8. Again a reduction in the public's holding of these requires to be financed. The contrast between Treasury bills and stocks compared with National Savings is that the monetary authorities may actively be trying to alter the composition of the former. In particular, they may be trying to fund—that is sell long-term securities instead of Treasury bills.

Item 9. This item is not important in this context. It has already been explained that the indebtedness of the government to the Bank of England is minimal. The large sum appearing in 1965-6 is the result of a special swap with the United States authorities and its repayment.

From Table 1 and its depiction of actual changes that took place in the economy during the years in question, it is evident that the question of what determines the amount of money and liquidity in the system cannot be separated from consideration of the whole economic system. In particular, it is possible to imagine adverse circumstances for the authorities. Suppose the aim is to reduce the amount of money and liquidity in the economy. Adverse circumstances would be:

1. A budget deficit, i.e. a stream of expenditure being injected into the economy, and the need to increase debt as a result.
2. Inability to fund because of unwillingness of the public and the banks to buy bonds.
3. A large amount of government debt maturing which, because of 1 and 2, will mean short-term debt must be issued to replace it.
4. An inflow of gold or foreign exchange into the Exchange Equalization Account.

The embarrassment of an inflow of gold or foreign exchange may not seem a very realistic worry in present-day conditions. (This is not saying a gold inflow is bad; merely that this results in the Exchequer having to find alternative holders for the Treasury bills that the Exchange Equalization Account formerly possessed.) However, in the post-war period the adverse circumstances numbered 1, 2 and 3 have been present and have coloured a great deal of monetary policy. This being a period in general of overall deficits, of large amounts of debt-maturing, and of the cult of the equity share rather than fixed-interest stock.

The authorities had little choice but to increase short-term debt to provide the necessary finance. In these circumstances it is not surprising that the monetary authorities should feel that control of the banking system—of secondary money—by the traditional means of controlling primary money and liquid assets left something to be desired and sought to supplement control by other means.

Day-to-day management of money

So far we have seen that imbalance in the flow of payments out of, and receipts into, the Exchequer in a particular year results in a change in the amount of securities. Within the context of a deficit or surplus expected in a year, the flow of payments from day to day, which may be distinctly uneven, and from one time of the year to another, has to be evened out. The Bank, working closely with the Treasury, has the job of ensuring, if a deficit on the day is forecast, that finance is available; alternatively, if a surplus is forecast, that these surpluses are used to buy back Treasury bills from the market and so minimize the net cost of the National Debt.

From our point of view, the second connected task—that of managing the London money market—is more important. A new flow of payments to the government has the effect of reducing bankers' deposits. The banks are likely, as a result, to be drawing upon money lent at call to the discount market.

> . . . The discount houses find themselves short of funds in consequence, and unless the Bank take steps to relieve the shortage—usually by buying Treasury bills either from them (the so-called 'direct' method of giving help) or from the banks (the 'indirect' method)—they may be forced to borrow from the Bank at Bank Rate or over. The enforcement of such borrowing increases the average cost of the houses' total borrowings and is one of the main ways (short of a change in Bank Rate) in which the Bank of England exerts an influence on short-term interest rates and particularly on the rate at which the discount houses may be expected to bid for Treasury bills at the following Friday's tender. ('Management of Money Day by Day', March, 1963, pp. 15, 16. This article gives a detailed account of the management of money day by day.)

The monetary authorities are thus faced with a choice either of maintaining the existing structure of short-term rates, with the consequence that they relieve the shortage of money, or of maintaining the shortage and allowing short-term rates to rise. In practice the authorities normally try to create a shortage, to give themselves this option, by issuing Treasury bills slightly in excess of the Exchequer's estimated needs. At this point the issues become more controversial. See Cramp, A. B. (June, 1966) and references therein.

In considering how effective control by means of a money-shortage can be the controversy turns on whether or not the discount houses are able to escape from the penal rate imposed by borrowing at the Bank, either by reducing their share of Treasury bills or borrowing elsewhere. Either way of escape is unlikely to be effective in current conditions, because the discount houses undertake to 'cover the tender' and because the sources of outside finance are limited.

The reasoning of this section leads to the likely conclusion that the authorities would find it very difficult to control the commercial banks by controlling their cash base. Since the authorities are concerned with the level of short-term rates, they are prevented from provoking a severe and long-lasting shortage of money because of the effect this would have on short-term (and eventually long-term) interest rates. The authorities have to be concerned with the level of short-term rates for a number of reasons. A powerful one is the need to keep rates in line with foreign monetary centres so as to avoid undesirable flows of 'hot' money. Related to this is the effects of servicing the debt and the effects on the balance of payments if the debt is held abroad. Domestically they may also wish to keep interest rates from rising for a number of social and economic reasons.

The previous assertion that the amount of secondary money in the economy depends in a complex way on a number of factors, in particular on the fiscal and budgetary policy of the government, the public's attitude to government debt, and the reactions of the commercial banks, has now been justified and spelt out at some length.

Other financial institutions and financial intermediaries

The presence of a large financial sector, apart from the commercial banks, means that wider issues of credit and liquidity have to be considered. It has been argued that a number of factors have to be taken into account in considering the operations of the banks, and it is clear that these factors will also apply to these other financial institutions—for example, the public's choice between holding deposits with the commercial banks or holding them with the acceptance houses, overseas banks or building societies. The monetary authorities have also to take the amount and composition of government paper into account, not only because it affects the commercial banks, but because it is also important to these other institutions.

It was suggested at the end of the previous chapter that control by means of Requests of these other financial institutions may be less easy than control of the commercial banks. If this is so, one way of establishing more effective control would be to subject these other financial institutions to more formal arrangements as to their reserve ratios, of the kind already imposed on the commercial banks. The situation has altered a great deal since the Radcliffe Committee considered, and largely rejected, proposals on these lines. An alternative proposal (or it could be a supplement to control on the lines suggested above) is that commercial banks should compete more actively amongst themselves and with other financial institutions. Although this proposal is not novel, the first 'official' statement on these lines came, not from a monetary body, but the National Board for Prices and Incomes.[5] The major recommendation of the Board was that the convention by which the banks agree between themselves on the rate of interest to be paid or not to be paid on deposits with them should be abandoned:[6]

> We consider that this agreement has led to a loss in their power to attract deposits, to a loss therefore in their power to extend and diversify their lending activities, to an inability to secure to a larger extent the economies of scale which could follow on such an extension—in short, to a loss in their relative place in the entire financial system. A recovery of place for the banks requires in our view a greater degree of competition between the banks themselves for deposits and therefore between the banks as a whole and other financial institutions . . . (*Bank Charges* (1967), para. 182).

In earlier paragraphs the Board considered the implications for monetary policy. They rejected the idea that freeing rates would weaken monetary control and went on to suggest that it might strengthen the hands of the monetary authority. The present immediate link between changes in Bank Rate and clearing-bank rates while other rates lag behind would be likely to give way to a more evenly spread effect throughout the entire financial system. The Board indicated that this could be coupled with liquidity reserve requirements imposed upon non-bank financial institutions and perhaps also with the imposition of a reserve power over the maximum deposit

[5] *Bank Charges* (1967). This was so in spite of the fact that the reference of bank charges to the Board stated explicitly: 'It is not intended that the Board should concern itself with questions of monetary policy, such as Bank Rate and the general level of interest rates.' The Board interpreted this to mean: 'In so far, however, as we recommend changes in the system of bank charges, such changes are likely to have considerable implications for the techniques of monetary control. We have accordingly thought it consistent with our terms of reference to indicate what these implications might be and what possibilities by way of offsetting action might be open to the authorities' (para. 3).

[6] Other recommendations were abandonment of their agreement on rates to be charged for advances, complete disclosure of profits and reserves, the publication of a scale of charges for work done and the allowances made for credit balances, and more flexible opening hours.

rates offered for specific types of deposit.

The Board briefly considered the effect of freer rates on the level of interest rates and considered 'that our suggestions would have greater implications for the relative rates of different intermediaries than for the general level of lending rates'.

Summary

This chapter sets out to examine the forces that determine the amount of money (in the narrow sense of coin, notes and bank deposits) and the amount of liquidity in the economy, and whether the amount of money and liquidity is under the control of the monetary authorities. Not surprisingly, no simple answer emerges. Monetary control is never likely to be a precise instrument, since it depends on so many things—in particular, the whole fiscal and budgetary process and the attitudes of the public to saving and holding government debt. What emerges from this analysis is that while the monetary authorities can control the commercial banks, more or less, according to their wishes, control over other financial intermediaries is much looser.

Recent developments have included the extension of Requests to many of these intermediaries and the introduction of the cash deposits scheme for other banks. It has also been suggested that control would be more successful if the commercial banks competed more actively amongst themselves and with other financial institutions.

Part II
Public finance

7
Introduction to public finance

We cannot therefore settle on abstract grounds, but must handle on its merits in detail what Burke termed 'one of the finest problems in legislation, namely, to determine what the State ought to take upon itself to direct by the public wisdom, and what it ought to leave, with as little interference as possible, to individual exertion'.

KEYNES, J. M., *The End of Laissez-faire.*

The economic welfare of an individual is his command over goods and services. This command comes from a number of sources. It is derived from work, from accumulated wealth, from inheritance and gifts, and from government provision and legislation.

This book will not be concerned with the return from work as such. It is sufficient for our purpose to note that returns from different kinds of work are altered by society in various ways. For example, the beginning of this century saw the start of minimum-wage legislation. Today we see efforts to have a more extensive incomes policy. Of more practical importance has been the extension of the provision of education out of general taxation, so that entry to work requiring formal training is no longer confined to those able to afford the training. Within the existing framework of the returns from work, this section of the book examines how the individual and the corporation are influenced by taxation of income, wealth, inheritance and gifts and the effects of government provision and legislation.

Public finance is about the revenue, expenditure and debt operations of the government and the impact of these measures. The need for government spending (and therefore to raise revenue or debt) is argued on a number of grounds. A start can be made by considering the imperfections of the competitive pricing system.

Imperfections of competitive market prices

The model of a perfectly competitive pricing system has often been held up as an ideal: prices act as a guide-post to producers as to the things and quantities that they should produce and, assuming certain assumptions are met, output will be optimized. The usefulness of prices in this respect, in invisibly (but not costlessly) planning the immensely complex assortment of goods and services found in a modern developed economy, should not be underestimated. It is, however, the imperfections of the pricing system which give much of the interest to a study of public finance.

One drawback of a pricing system in allocating goods is that it only takes account of effective demand (that is, demand backed by money). If income and wealth is unevenly spread, deficiencies in allocation will occur. These deficiencies in allocation provide one reason for State intervention, either to redistribute income and/or wealth to some extent, or to ensure in other ways some standard for its citizens. This point will be developed later in this chapter.

Another important modification to the optimality of the competitive pricing system has long been recognized: it is usually discussed under the headings of 'collective goods', 'externalities' or 'neighbourhood effects'. These terms are used to draw attention to the fact that some goods confer large benefits, not only on the potential purchaser, but on other people. The opposite may also be true; disadvantages may be imposed on other people, e.g. noise, dirt and pollution. In the former case, where benefits are apparent this may result in the demand for this type of good being lower than the optimum level, as persons hope to benefit from the provision made by other people without providing any themselves. Minimum provision for sewerage disposal can be left to the individual in a sparsely populated area: concentration of population in towns makes it essential to ensure that sewage-disposal is adequate. It is no accident that serious plagues have been eliminated from developed countries. Services of this type usually result in 'natural' monopolies. The waste in having more than one company digging up the same street to lay sewage pipes is obvious. The principle applies to other services, such as gas, electricity, water-supply, telephones, and so on. This conclusion leaves open the question of whether in cases such as this the government should itself undertake the provision of the service and, if so, how the cost shall be met. Or whether the government should merely supervise, and, if it is needed, subsidize the private provision of the service. Where a good imposes a cost on the community (usually termed a 'social cost') there are likewise alternatives. The government may just forbid the nuisance—say, the disposal of waste in rivers—and thereby leave the cost of alternative means of disposal on those causing it (or on their customers), it may assist those concerned financially to make other arrangements, or the government itself may make the alternative arrangements and decide how the cost shall be met.

In extreme cases provision of a service at all means provision for everybody. These services are indivisible. Defence against external aggression and police protection are obvious examples. These are sometimes called 'pure public goods'. In cases such as this the pricing system cannot be operated. Provision of these services, if left in private hands, is likely to result in zero supply.[1] Finally the competitive sector may, if left unregulated, be subject to systematic periods of boom and slump.

The government sector

The above account of the inadequacies of the private pricing system helps to put a discussion of the public sector in perspective. Three questions are frequently posed:

1. How big should the government sector be?
2. How to determine how much to produce when the price system is inoperative, either by necessity or through deliberate choice to meet the cost out of general taxation.
3. How to ensure that expenditures are efficiently, and not wastefully, applied.

1. On the first question the writer believes that the economist, as economist, has no unique answer. The question indeed incorrectly implies that a level of activity can be specified which will be valid over time, valid under varying conditions, and which admits of a unique solution. 'Public goods' where externalities are large are not constant over time. The growth, and particularly the concentration, of population means that problems of health, such amenities as open spaces, clean air, water-supply, communications and so on have more externalities. Again, if size is measured by the amount of government expenditure, it is worth emphasizing that different decisions on the way to achieve a particular object will involve different levels of government expenditure. For example, a decision to maintain employment in the shipbuilding sector of the economy

[1] 'There is a still more fundamental bias in our economy in favour of products and services for which it is easy to collect payments. Goods that can be sold in packets to individual customers, or services that can be charged for at so much per head, provide a field for profitable enterprise. Investments in, say, the layout of cities, cannot be enjoyed except collectively and are not easy to make money out of; while negative goods, such as dirt and noise, can be dispensed without any compensation being required.

'When you come to think of it, what can easily be charged for and what cannot is just a technical accident' (Robinson, J., 1962, p. 124).

can be achieved by subsidies to shipbuilders, or by providing cheap loans to purchasers, which will raise expenditure, or by tariffs which will not. The conclusion to which this sector tends is that the level of government activity at any one time is, in a democracy, essentially decided by political means.

2. The question of how much to produce, say, of defence or public health, where the price system is inoperative is one that admits of no easy solution. The principle of achieving equal marginal benefits from various expenditures needs to be borne in mind. It may avoid crude waste of expenditure. For example, the argument is sometimes heard: 'If only one life is saved the expenditure [on say, a road modification or a particular safety device] is worthwhile.' If the objective is to save life, the question that should be considered is: 'In what way can this particular sum of money be spent so as to save the most lives?' However, as a practical guide to day-to-day decision-making—whether £1 million spent on hospitals would yield more benefit than £1 million spent on defence, or roads, it yields little practical help. This principle is likely to be more fruitful in allocating expenditure within a particular field, e.g. whether to spend £1 million on operating theatres in hospitals or on the provision of more hospital beds.

One possible way out of the difficulty of weighing up expenditure in disparate activities is to set up minimum standards of service that it is desired to obtain[2]—say a policeman for every 2,000 of the population, the elimination of serious epidemics, maximum size of school classes of twenty-five, maximum permitted levels of pollution, and so on. Provided these standards are based on the cost and benefits that flow from reaching these standards, these should aid decision-making. The standards will not be obtainable overnight, but the act of quantification of the costs and benefits and listing of the non-quantification advantages and disadvantages should enable more rational decision-making.

On the question of deciding how much of a particular good should be produced in the absence of price-guide-lines, no economist would claim that, with existing knowledge and techniques, he can do more than assist in decision-making. Intuition, judgment and flair have their part—perhaps the major part—to play.

3. The question of ensuring economy in public affairs in the sense that, after expenditure decisions have been made, the money is used efficiently and not wastefully is important. However, the process

[2] Suggested by Drees, W. Jr. (1967). This issue is devoted to the *Papers and Proceedings of the Twenty-second Session of the International Institute of Public Finance*. Many of the ideas touched on in this chapter are dealt with more fully in this volume.

whereby the government attempts to secure economy in this sense, the weaknesses of present methods and hopes for improvement by new statistical and other techniques must be considered outside the scope of this book.

It may be noted in passing that 'extravagance' may be an indication of too little rather than too much administrative expenditure, in the sense that the misallocation of resources might have been avoided wholly or in part if there had been more, or better trained, government officials. Aircraft development costs since the end of the Second World War seem an apt illustration.

The minimum level of government activity

The above outline enables us to discuss the minimum level of government activity—the level on which all reasonable people can agree.

Nearly all societies give some help to those who are incapable of helping themselves (mainly the young, the old, the sick and the disabled) and who have no one on whom they can depend.

Collective goods, such as the administration of justice and defence of the realm, will form part of the government activity for the reasons given. (There may be deep divisions of opinion about the nature and extent of defence, about whether it is necessary at all, but if the need is granted nobody seriously suggests that private armies be formed.)

Again, it is generally agreed that where an operation must, by its nature, be monopolistic in order to be efficient, e.g. sewerage and the supply of electricity, then the State should either control, or itself run, the service at the central or local government level.

General agreement obtains that where there are strong externalities government action is needed. Difficulties occur over those goods which have both a benefit to the individual and externalities: education is an example. Elementary education is recognized as having strong externalities; our present society would be impossible without a certain level of education of the population. Not everybody agrees that, as yet, higher education has sufficiently strong externalities to justify meeting the cost out of general taxation.

This is, then, the minimum scope of State activity: some form of aid for the unfortunate, justice, defence, the regulation of natural monopolies, and goods which have strong externalities. Public opinion in most societies would recognize this as the lowest common denominator of government action. Even at this level disagreements can creep in. If government action is admitted as necessary in a certain area—say, education—it leaves open the question of whether the government should itself undertake the provision of the service or merely supervise and, if it is needed, subsidize the private provision of the service.

Government activity, even at this minimum level, involves some redistribution of resources from the 'better off' to the 'worse off'. The questions raised by redistribution will now be tackled.

Redistribution of income and wealth

Redistribution in a community can take place by provision of services above the minimum levels just discussed, provided these are met out of taxes paid by the 'better off' or, alternatively, by direct money transfers from the 'better off' to the 'worse off'.

In talking about redistribution of income and/or wealth, three strands of thought are apparent. These will be discussed in turn. One is unavoidable if it is granted that help should be given to the unfortunate. The second strand of thought aims at deliberate redistribution above the level required to supplement the lowest incomes. The third strand is directed at changing the conditions which help create and foster the inequalities. In practice, these ideas may be interwoven, but conceptually much confusion can be avoided if they are kept separate.

If it is granted that a society should assist those who are incapable of helping themselves, then this implies that society has already made a decision that some redistribution of income and/or wealth is desirable. This conclusion is inescapable. The government cannot in these circumstances be neutral in its attitude to the redistribution of income and/or wealth, since a decision to help a needy section of the population entails redistribution from a 'better-off' to a 'worse-off' section.

Leaving to one side humanitarian arguments, the core of the case of those who advocate government provision or, alternatively, argue for some redistribution of income and/or wealth above the minimum level just discussed, is that, as we have seen, needs are not satisfied equally if income is unequally spread. That is, that economic welfare can be increased by government provision or redistribution. This case was well put by Dalton, H. (1959), 10:

> Income consists of the means of economic welfare, and great inequality in incomes in any community implies great inequality in the economic welfare attained by different individuals. But this is not all. For it implies also considerable waste of potential economic welfare. Put broadly, and in the language of common sense, the case against large inequalities of income is that the less urgent needs of the rich are satisfied, while the more urgent needs of the poor are left unsatisfied. The rich are more than amply fed, while the poor go hungry. This is merely an application of the economists' law of diminishing marginal utility, which states that, other

things being equal, as the quantity of any commodity or, more generally, of purchasing power increases, its total utility increases, but its marginal utility diminishes.

This quotation contains two ideas. One is that the economic welfare of different individuals can be compared. However reasonable such an idea may seem, particularly when we compare extreme positions, such as giving a loaf of bread to a man who already has plenty with giving a loaf to a man who is hungry, there are those who hold that we have no objective measure by which we can compare needs of different individuals. We need not enter into this controversy, because the second idea contained in this quotation is that the community should judge relative needs. Such judgment will not be to any absolute standard, but will change as ethical, political, social, economic and other conditions change in the community. Much of the study of public finance can be taken up with a consideration of how these changes in community standards have affected ideas about government spending and revenue. Chapters 8 and 9 look briefly at the changes in Britain since 1900.

The more fundamental problem is to change the conditions of society which create and foster the inequalities and this paradoxically seems to receive less practical attention. It is perhaps inherent in most of us to regard as 'normal and just' whatever framework of society exists at the time. Even Plato carried forward the conditions of slavery into his *Republic*. We shall examine two important examples of this tendency. One which will be examined at length in Chapter 11 on 'The Concept of Income' is concerned with the extremely narrow definition of income which has grown up for tax purposes. The second is concerned with the general tendency to regard the laws about inheritance and gifts as though they were ordained by the Almighty from the beginning of time. Far from this being the case, it is found that laws and customs about these matters show wide variation between countries, even when these countries have similar democratic institutions and roughly comparable economic development. Changes within the same country over time may be just as great, but come less to the notice of the observer. The substantial freedom of bequest in England is in large measure due to legislative changes in the nineteenth century, but this freedom is hedged about in important ways. When a person dies intestate, the State steps in to administer the estate according to law, and in the event of no surviving relatives the estate goes to the Exchequer. Where a will has been made, it is restricted in that the deceased cannot validly direct that his property should be destroyed, and there are restrictions imposed in the interests of morality and public policy generally. Property cannot be left in perpetuity and dependants have certain rights, even if they are not named in the will, over other beneficiaries. Far from the laws about inheritance being laid down from time immemorial, they are seen to be restricted both to place and time. Dalton, H. (1959), Part IV, Chapter VI, gives an interesting elaboration of these matters. However a great deal of the discussion that takes place is confined to rates at which taxes shall be applied within the current legislative mould. As we shall see in later chapters, questions about the nature of wealth and income are as important in discussing a tax system as the rates which happen to be applied at a particular moment of time.

Summary

By the economic welfare of an individual is meant his command over goods and services. This command comes to the individual from a number of sources. It is derived from work, from wealth, from inheritance and gifts, and from government provision and legislation.

Imperfections in the competitive marketing price system leave a vacuum for the community to fill. These are due to the uneven spread of income and wealth leading to deficiencies in allocation, the presence of goods which have strong externalities, and the natural bias of the private sector of the economy towards goods for which it is easy to collect payment.

It has been suggested that there is no unique solution to the question about what is the correct level of government activity. The level itself is likely to change with time, with changes in population, and in the complexity of society. Also changes in political ideals are likely to change ideas about goods which could be produced by the private sector, but which the State (for economic or other reasons) decides to control.

In deciding the quantities of goods to be produced, where no pricing system acts as a guide, the economist has a useful, if limited, role to play.

Government provision and legislation forms the backdrop of a public finance study. Government provision out of general taxation or transfer payments, such as pensions, are an obvious way of supplementing income deficiencies. Society judges the extent to which redistribution above this level is desirable. The economic justification for such provision is that command over goods and services is unevenly spread, and a democratic society, in no very exact fashion, judges the relative needs of its members and deems that some minimum needs must be met for all—that is, that some redistribution of command over goods and services shall take place.

8
The pattern of government expenditure since 1900

Crying wolf at the drop of an index.

MISHAN, E. J. (1967), *The Costs of Economic Growth.*

Conceptual difficulties

Government spending and taxation affects every individual. It is not therefore surprising to find that in public finance there are perhaps more attempts made by sectional interests to present biased information than in other economic fields. It is not uncommon to find people asserting opposite things, e.g. one will claim that public expenditure has gone up, another that it has gone down. Ignoring deliberate attempts to mislead by, for example, choosing a base period when prices were either particularly high or particularly low, or deliberately picking on the item which 'proves' the point in question and ignoring all the evidence to the contrary, there are still a number of difficulties to be overcome, which we shall look at briefly. After this the evolution of government spending during this century can be tackled.

First, figures of money expenditure, although useful in showing how expenditures on different sub-categories have changed relative to each other, tell us little about the share of government expenditure in relation to total resources. In order to measure the latter, it is necessary to make allowances in some way for changes in the value of money. This can be done by some form of price index which can be used to present the money figures in 'real' terms, i.e. in terms of command over goods and services, or by expressing government expenditure as a percentage of the gross national product. Unfortunately, all ways of allowing for price changes have limitations, which means, not that the results are useless, but that we must use them with care.

Secondly, items should be related to population. The longer the period under consideration the more misleading it can be to ignore this factor of government activity if population has changed significantly in composition or absolute numbers or both.[1]

Thirdly, we need to take account of the nature of government expenditure and draw a clear distinction between transfer payments on the one hand and direct government expenditure on goods and services on the other. Transfer payments are, as the name implies, payments made by the government, such as pensions, family allowances and interests payments on the National Debt.

Transfer payments do not involve the government in direct use of the nation's goods and services. Transfers may be classified in different ways—for example, transfers between persons, as between rich and poor; transfers over time, as the provision of pensions; and transfers to meet such contingencies as sickness or unemployment. Since the government does not work on the principle of earmarked funds the practical implications of transfer payments on these lines are not easy to sort out. The financing of National Insurance, outlined in the Appendix to Chapter 9, comes closest to the idea of a fund, since only 15% of the cost in 1967 came out of general taxation. However, the use of the word 'fund' can be misleading. It does not represent a transfer over time, in the sense that individuals pay now to build up a fund to pay for their future pensions and other benefits. Current payments are used to pay existing benefits. Pensions, for example, are largely a transfer from the working population, because they pay contributions, to the pensionable group. Existing workers in their turn, on the current method of financing, will have their pensions paid by the population working at the time they are retired. Over 73% of the cost of health is met out of general taxation: the transfer here depends much more on the impact of the tax system as a whole on the particular individual, as well as the benefit to the individual. Given this situation, it seems that the most meaningful concept of transfer between persons is obtained by looking at the whole system of taxation and benefits and taking their net impact on the individual. This will be done in Chapter 18.

Finally, a great deal of confusion is caused because different concepts of government are selected. Should government spending include spending by local authorities? Should it include spending by the nationalized industries? Fortunately, there is no need to seek a non-existing 'right' definition. Sometimes one definition, sometimes another is useful; what we must avoid is misleading conclusions from figures drawn up on different bases.

[1] Looked at from a different viewpoint. If the government undertakes exactly the same functions over a time period, it does not follow that expenditure, when allowance is made for price-changes and population-growth, will also be static. Age changes in the population will mean different amounts need to be spent on, for example, education and old age pensions.

Expenditure since 1900

Table 1 shows government expenditure for selected years since 1900. The definition of 'government' adopted will, throughout this book, include local government, but exclude the nationalized industries unless the contrary is stated. Nationalized industries have been excluded because they are not, as a rule, on the same footing as other government activities. Neither the nationalized industries' investment nor their charges form part of the Budget process in quite the same way as other government activities. This will be taken up in the beginning of the next chapter. Table 1 shows expenditures for central and local government separately and a 'Total' column with them combined. The figures are given in £ million, first at current prices—that is, at prices in the year in question—then in 1900 prices after allowance has been made for the growth of population. For the sake of completeness, a price index and population index are given. Attention to the footnote to this table will make it clear that the price index is intended only as a rough guide. In practice, expenditure in the period 1900-55 was broken down into various parts, e.g. capital-formation and goods and services, and appropriate price indexes were applied to each component part. The 'price' index shown gives a rough average of these price indexes. The index after 1955 is that for 'all goods and services sold on the home market' from the *National Income and Expenditure Tables* for 1968—adjusted to the base year, 1900.

The source of these figures, price index and population index up to 1955 is from Peacock, A. T. and Wiseman, J. (1961). No attempt has been made to match the sophistication of Peacock and Wiseman's price index. The adjustment for price and population changes after 1955 is only intended to serve as a rough approximation. For this reason a line has been drawn across the table and figures for the year 1955 appear from both sources.

Table 1 shows very clearly that government expenditure has increased markedly in this century. The rather meaningless comparison in money terms is an increase from £281 million in the year 1900 to £16,749 million in 1967, or a forty-seven-fold increase. However, prices increased nearly seven-fold in this period and population increased by 33%. When allowance is made for these changes, we get more than a six-and-a-half-fold increase in expenditure in real terms per head (either a staggering increase or a revelation of the fantastic underspending in earlier years, according to one's viewpoint!) The changes in expenditure have not occurred at a steady rate, a point which will be considered later. Central government expenditure has increased more rapidly than local government expenditure. As a proportion of the total, local government expenditure decreased from

Table 1

Expenditure of Central and Local Governments on Current and Capital Account at Current and at 1900 Prices per Head of Population. Selected years 1900-67

(£ million at Current Prices)

Year	*Current Prices* C.G.	L.G.	*Total*	%[2]	*Gross National Product*	*Total Spending as % of G.N.P.*
1900	182	99	281	35	1,944	15
1910	142	130	272	48	2,143	13
1920	1,275	317	1,592	20	6,070	26
1928	695	399	1,094	37	4,523	23
1933	676	390	1,066	37	4,141	26
1938	1,056	531	1,587	34	5,294	30
1950	3,479	1,060	4,539	23	11,636	39
1955	4,607	1,536	6,143	25	16,784	37
1955	4,848	1,622	6,470	25	16,974	38
1960	6,744	2,251	8,995	25	22,790	39
1961	7,305	2,578	9,883	26	24,392	41
1962	7,573	2,866	10,439	27	25,550	41
1963	7,882	3,142	11,024	29	27,163	41
1964	8,428	3,639	12,067	30	29,313	41
1965	9,310	4,112	13,422	31	31,310	43
1966	10,097	4,461	14,558	31	32,858	44
1967	11,684	5,065	16,749	30	34,292	49

1900 Prices deflated by Population Growth

Year	*Price[3] Index*	*Pop. Index*	*C.G.*	*L.G.*	*Total*
1900	100	100	182	99	281
1910	103	109	118	123	241
1920	282	106	432	101	533
1928	197	111	316	184	500
1933	173	113	344	201	545
1938	186	115	494	246	740
1950	380	122	765	215	980
1955	469	124	808	248	1,056
1955	469	124	833	279	1,112
1960	537	127	989	330	1,319
1961	553	128	1,032	364	1,396
1962	574	129	1,023	387	1,410
1963	585	130	1,036	413	1,449
1964	601	131	1,070	462	1,532
1965	632	132	1,116	493	1,609
1966	659	133	1,152	509	1,661
1967	675	133	1,301	564	1,865

35% or higher at the beginning of the century to around 25% after 1945, but in recent years it has shown a tendency to increase once more. The effect of two world wars on centralizing expenditure can be seen, expenditure in real terms by local government being lower after the wars than it was before. Part of the explanation of the change in local government expenditure is the transfer after the Second World War of gas and electricity services to national industries.

Table 1 also shows Gross National Product (G.N.P.) in current prices and total government spending in current prices as a percentage of G.N.P. The results, using deflated values for both sets of figures, do not differ very greatly from those using current prices, so the latter only have been shown in the table.

Government spending as a whole rose from 15% of G.N.P. in 1900 to 49% in 1967. In 1900 most of this expenditure was on goods and services and on capital account. By 1965 spending under this head accounted for 32%, spending on transfers and subsidies 17%, making up the indicated total of 49% of G.N.P.

These facts can be expressed rather differently. The money increase in G.N.P. of rather more than seventeen and half times between 1900 and 1967 has the effect, when allowance is made for price and population changes, of almost doubling real G.N.P. per head. Against this doubling of real product per head, in this period of sixty-seven years, government expenditure in real terms has increased six-and-a-half times; however, government spending on goods, services and capital account increased rather less than this at five and a half times, the difference being made up by the bigger increase in spending on transfers and subsidies.

Tables 2-4 use figures at current prices, but this does not matter,

---

[2] Total local government expenditure at current prices as percentage of total government expenditure (i.e. C.G. and L.G.).

[3] 1900 prices for the years 1900-55 were arrived at by breaking down government expenditure into various parts, e.g. capital formation and goods and services and appropriate price indexes were applied to each component part. The 'price' index shown gives a rough average of these price indexes. The index for the years 1955 onwards, shown beneath the line, is that for 'All final goods and services sold on the home market' from *National Income and Expenditure Tables*, 1966 and 1968, Table 16, adjusted to base year 1900.

Source: Source of figures, price index, population index and G.N.P. up to 1955, Peacock and Wiseman, *The Growth of Public Expenditure in the U.K.*, Table A.20, pp. 201-2, and Table A.2, pp. 153-4. 1955 and after: *National Income and Expenditure Tables*, 1966, Tables 1 and 48, and 1968, Tables 1 and 47.

Because of rounding, figures may not add up to the totals shown.

Table 2

Expenditure of Central and Local Governments at Current Prices on Current Account (Goods and Services and Transfers and Subsidies) and on Capital Account. Selected years 1900-67

(£ million at Current Prices)

Year	*Goods and Services*	*Transfers and Subs.*	*Current Account*	*Capital Account*	*Total Expenditure*	*Capital Expenditure as % of Current Account*
	(1)	(2)	(3)=(1)+(2)	(4)	(5)=(3)+(4)	
1900	194·2	36·2	230·4	50·4	281	21·9
1910	171·8	55·1	226·9	45·1	272	19·9
1920	887·7	602·5	1,490·2	101·9	1,592	6·8
1928	451·9	534·1	986·0	108·7	1,094	11·0
1933	438·9	538·6	977·5	88·5	1,066	9·1
1938	822·7	545·6	1,368·3	218·7	1,587	16·0
1950	2,071	2,031	4,102	437	4,539	10·7
1955	3,192	2,333	5,525	618	6,143	11·2
1955	3,171	2,305	5,476	994	6,470	18·2
1960	4,163	3,260	7,423	1,572	8,995	21·2
1961	4,497	3,616	8,113	1,770	9,883	21·8
1962	4,822	3,822	8,644	1,795	10,439	20·8
1963	5,080	4,129	9,209	1,815	11,024	19·7
1964	5,395	4,307	9,702	2,365	12,067	24·4
1965	5,919	4,822	10,741	2,681	13,422	25·0
1966	6,436	5,182	11,618	2,940	14,558	25·3
1967	7,063	5,925	12,988	3,761	16,749	29·0

as we are here interested in how the proportions spent on various services have changed, and deflating by a price index is not likely to alter these in any significant way. Table 2 splits the total figures of Table 1 into expenditure on goods and services and expenditure on transfers and subsidies. The importance of this distinction has already been commented on in the beginning of this chapter. Together these expenditures equal the current account transactions. If to the current-account expenditures we add expenditure on capital account, we reach the figures of total expenditure, which agree with Table 1.

The bottom part of the table expresses these expenditures as a percentage. Taking the current-account transactions, we see that transfers and subsidies run at much higher levels in the later period. Sub-

Expenditure as a Percentage of the Total

Year	*Goods and Services*	*Transfers and Subs.*	*Capital Account*	*Total*
1900	69	13	18	100
1910	63	20	17	100
1920	56	38	6	100
1928	41	49	10	100
1933	41	51	8	100
1938	52	34	14	100
1950	45	45	10	100
1955	52	38	10	100
1955	49	36	15	100
1960	46	36	18	100
1961	45	37	18	100
1962	46	37	17	100
1963	46	37	17	100
1964	45	36	19	100
1965	44	36	20	100
1966	44	36	20	100
1967	42	35	23	100

Sources: 1900-55: Peacock and Wiseman, *The Growth of Public Expenditure in the U.K.*, Table 5, p. 71, and Table 6, p. 78. 1955 and after: *National Income and Expenditure Tables*, 1966, Table 48, and 1968, Table 47.

Because of rounding, figures may not add up to the totals shown.

sidies are mainly to agriculture; transfers either payment of interest on the National Debt or on social services. Variations in social-service payments will also cover very interesting variations, reflecting, for example, high amounts on unemployment pay during the slump of the 1930s, and more on education, health and housing in the later years. Interest payments exhibit interesting variations during this period. Greater detail is available in Tables 3 and 4.

Expenditure on capital account exhibits wide variation. This is not unexpected, since capital expenditures create durable assets. Neither the creation of the original assets nor their replacement is likely to be spread evenly over time. The mistake should not be made of equating capital expenditures with 'useful' expenditures and current expenditures with 'wasteful' expenditures. Both statements may be true, but both may be false. The tendency is all too apparent which regards expenditure on bricks and mortar as somehow 'better' than expenditure on training and pay of the staff to run the schools or hospitals or institutions once they have been built.

Table 3

Expenditure of Central and Local Governments on Current and Capital Account by function. Selected years 1900-67

(£ million at Current Prices)

Year	*Administration and Other*	*National Debt*	*Law and Order*	*Overseas Services*	*Military Defence*	*Social Services*	*Economic and Environmental Services*	*Total*
1900	17	20	10	1	135	51	48	281
1910	22	20	13	1	74	89	53	272
1920	72	325	33	3	520	412	228	1,592
1928	49	305	31	1	125	434	149	1,095
1933	44	228	31	2	112	497	151	1,066
1938	61	213	39	3	473	596	202	1,587
1950	175	507	79	179	836	2,094	669	4,539
1955[4]	182	707	115	80	1,606	2,739	714	6,143
1955	145	770	118	135	1,567	2,970	600	6,305
1960	194	1,025	174	213	1,612	4,122	1,145	8,485
1961	221	1,108	209	236	1,732	4,574	1,270	9,350
1962	250	1,118	224	230	1,853	4,892	1,367	9,934
1963	208	1,200	247	238	1,905	5,348	1,402	10,548
1964	206	1,263	272	281	2,006	5,871	1,580	11,479
1965	228	1,349	295	301	2,131	6,657	1,800	12,761
1966	253	1,475	339	315	2,246	7,108	2,042	13,774
1967	267	1,599	380	326	2,412	8,003	2,702	15,689

Current Prices expressed as % of Total Government Expenditure

1900	6	7	4	0·4	48	18	17	100
1910	8	7	5	0·4	27	33	19	100
1920	5	20	2	0·2	33	26	15	100
1928	5	28	3	0·1	11	40	14	100
1933	4	21	3	0·2	11	47	15	100
1938	4	13	2	0·2	30	38	13	100
1950	4	11	2	4·0	19	46	15	100
1955[4]	3	12	2	1·0	26	45	12	100
1955	2	12	2	2	25	47	10	100
1960	2	12	2	3	19	49	13	100
1961	2	12	2	3	19	49	13	100
1962	3	11	2	2	19	49	14	100
1963	2	12	2	2	18	51	13	100
1964	2	11	2	2	18	51	14	100
1965	2	11	2	2	17	52	14	100
1966	2	11	2	2	16	52	15	100
1967	2	10	2	2	16	51	17	100

[4] The totals after 1955 are less than those shown in Tables 1 and 2 because grants from the Central Government to local authorities, and other transactions in financial assets, are omitted to avoid double counting.

Sources: 1900-55: Peacock and Wiseman, *The Growth of Public Expenditure in the U.K.*, Table A-15, pp. 186-7, and Table A-16, pp. 188-9. 1955 and after: *National Income and Expenditure Tables*, 1966 and 1968, Tables 52 and 53.

Because of rounding, figures may not add up to the totals shown.

Table 4

Expenditure of Central and Local Governments on Current and Capital Account on Social Services at Current Prices and as a Percentage

(*£ million at Current Prices*)

Year	Education	Health	Social Insurance and Assistance	Housing	Food Subsidies	Total
1920	97	49	213	53	—	412
1928	105	66	202	61	—	434
1933	107	75	269	46	—	497
1938	139	99	278	80	—	596
1950	440	478	674	340	162	2,094
1955	675	582	1,015	420	47	2,739
1955	549	619	1,075	489	238	2,970
1960	916	919	1,574	468	245	4,122
1961	1,012	996	1,721	534	311	4,574
1962	1,172	1,046	1,843	503	328	4,892
1963	1,281	1,118	2,093	562	294	5,348
1964	1,417	1,224	2,214	772	244	5,871
1965	1,588	1,375	2,537	920	237	6,657
1966	1,768	1,515	2,719	898	208	7,108
1967	1,963	1,692	3,055	1,045	247	8,002

Expenditure as a Percentage of the Total

1920	24	12	51	13	—	100
1928	24	15	47	14	—	100
1933	22	15	54	9	—	100
1938	23	17	47	13	—	100
1950	21	23	32	16	8	100
1955	25	21	37	15	2	100
1955	19	21	36	16	8	100
1960	22	22	38	12	6	100
1961	22	22	37	12	7	100
1962	24	21	38	10	7	100
1963	24	21	39	11	5	100
1964	24	21	38	13	4	100
1965	24	21	38	14	3	100
1966	25	21	38	13	3	100
1967	25	22	38	13	3	100

Sources: 1900-55: Peacock and Wiseman, *The Growth of Public Expenditure in the U.K.*, Table 10, p. 92. 1955 and after: *National Income and Expenditure Tables*, 1966 and 1968, Table 53.

The period since the 1930s reflects the growth of Keynesian ideas that government spending can be used to take up the unemployment in the economy. In present-day conditions these ideas have been re-examined. The first crude idea of government expenditure acting as a regulator of the economy—expanding when the private sector contracts and vice versa—looks odd when the nature of much government expenditure is considered. Do we really wish to put off spending on roads, education or hospitals until such time as there is a danger of recession?

In the post-war period the authorities have been groping in a new direction. Fiscal and monetary policy is seen as a means whereby the private sector of the economy can be regulated. If the economy is slack, the private sector can be encouraged to undertake more capital investment by, for example, tax incentives, or attempts can be made to influence private expenditure on goods and services by reducing tax or other changes. This can be in addition to, or in place of, changes in government spending. In a like manner, in times of inflation the private sector can be discouraged from trying to undertake so much investment or consumption by tax increases; the full brunt of the adjustment need no longer be borne by the government sector.

There is probably wide agreement on the principle involved in trying to regulate the economy in the way outlined in the preceding paragraph. Disagreements occur on the ability of the government to undertake the regulation, and on the advantages and disadvantages of various monetary and fiscal weapons as the means to achieve the regulation. Value judgments enter when regulatory measures are at variance with equity aspects. These matters will be taken up in Part III.

Table 3 sets out information on government spending in the same two ways. The first part of the table gives figures in £ million. The second part expresses expenditure on each service as a percentage of the whole.

The following brief notes on the headings should make clear the nature of expenditure referred to and the main changes which have occurred:

ADMINISTRATION AND OTHER

A heterogeneous category covering the cost of tax-collection, government buildings and maintenance. While these have, of course, increased in money terms, they have not done so in percentage terms. Not surprisingly, they take a smaller proportion of the Budget.

NATIONAL DEBT

Simply interest paid to other than government sectors—that is, the so-called 'net' debt, which excludes inter-government transactions.

The National Debt interest payments show interesting variations. In the 1920s they amounted to well over a quarter of government expenditure, falling in the 1930s after the conversion operations in 1932 and 1934. The contrast in the proportion of the Budget going in debt payments after the two world wars is very striking, and reflects the very different ideas of paying for these wars held at the respective times. A great deal of the credit must go to the ideas of J. M. Keynes. In particular see Keynes, J. M. (1940). The difference between the two war periods reflects the greater use of taxation in the Second World War compared to the greater use of debt policy in the First World War. The Second World War also introduced a special war-time tax known as post-war credits. Sums paid in this form of taxation remain to the credit of the individual, returnable at the discretion of the government. At present these are paid back to a woman on reaching the age of fifty-five and to a man on reaching the age of sixty. Since 1959 interest at the rate of 2½% has been paid on sums still retained.

LAW AND ORDER: *Police, prisons, law courts, judges' salaries*

In view of the current emphasis on crime, it may seem surprising that a smaller proportion was spent on law and order in 1965 than in 1900. We can put this in another way: while government expenditure in real terms increased, as we saw from Table 1, about six and a half times, on law and order it increased about four times. This relative change in emphasis poses interesting questions which cannot be pursued here. It might be argued that we are spending too little on this service, that, for example, our prison system is largely a relic from the nineteenth century. On the other hand, it may be that increased expenditure on other services has redressed the balance and reduced the relative needs of this sector.

OVERSEAS SERVICES

Expenditure of the Foreign Office, colonial administration, the British Council and overseas broadcasting. From very small absolute and relative amounts prior to the Second World War, overseas services account for 2% of total government expenditure after 1955. Part of the difference is explained by loans to overseas governments and net lending abroad for private industry, etc., which were excluded from the figures above the line, but included in the figures from 1955.

MILITARY DEFENCE

This includes civil defence. Military defence has always occupied a significant slice of expenditure in this period. From around a third of expenditure pre-1914, a significant drop in the 1920s and 1930s to around a quarter of the Budget in the 1950s, the 1960-67 period shows the proportion slightly declining.

SOCIAL SERVICES

Education, child care, health, National Insurance (unemployment, sickness benefits, retirement pensions, etc.), national assistance, housing (subsidies and capital expenditure) and food subsidies. The importance of social service expenditure from the 1930s is evident from the tables, and now accounts for over 50% of expenditure. The figures hide important changes in the nature of the expenditure which will be looked at in Table 4.

ECONOMIC AND ENVIRONMENTAL SERVICES

Services to agriculture, forestry and fishing, and expenditure on industry and commerce (food subsidies appear under the social service heading). Provision of basic services: roads and public lighting, fire, water, sewage, refuse, land-drainage, coast-protection, town-planning, parks. These expenditures were a higher proportion of total expenditure in most of the pre-1939 period: they now account for 17% of the total.

Table 4 presents the main items of social service expenditure. Differences in classification at this more detailed level mean that the proportions shown for the period 1920-55 are not strictly comparable to those after 1955, but the broad trends are evident. While the proportion spent on education has accounted for nearly a quarter of expenditure during this period, expenditure on health has increased from around 12% to 22%. The most important category, social insurance and assistance, shows considerable variation, and the figures do not bring out the different nature of the expenditure in different periods. The high proportion shown for 1933 reflects the high level of unemployment and hence unemployment payments of this period, while the later figures reflect the growth of social insurance. The fluctuations in housing reflect to some extent the different emphasis put on municipal housing by the Conservative and Labour parties. Food subsidies reflect the relative decline in their importance from their Second World War levels.

Summary

Government expenditure has increased since 1900 in money and real terms per head of population. Of this expenditure the central government has increased its importance relative to local government.

Of the broad categories of government spending we selected, the increasing importance of the social services showed up clearly, and within the social services the largest increase in expenditure was on health. Military defence fluctuated, as we would expect, and it still accounts for a sizeable amount of government spending. Finally, the interest payments on the net National Debt showed interesting variations.

The rate of growth of the government's claim on the national product (as measured by expenditure on goods and services) is impressive if somewhat less than the rate of increase in government expenditure as a whole. Put the other way, expenditure on transfers and subsidies has increased faster than expenditure on goods and services.

9
The pattern of government revenue since 1900

It has been maintained—and the assertion is scarcely an exaggeration that the theorems of Euclid would be bitterly controverted if financial or political interests were involved.

FISHER, I., *The Purchasing Power of Money.*

Introduction

This chapter first of all takes a factual look at the pattern of government revenue since 1900. It then goes on to consider the aims of a tax system and principles of taxation.

In looking at the pattern of government expenditure in the previous chapter, it was possible to treat as a whole the expenditures of central and local government on both current and capital account. In presenting figures of revenue, a similar procedure will be adopted, whereby the items of tax revenue of central and local government will be presented. It is not the intention to present a complete balance sheet, and some revenue items, such as trading income and income from rents, interest and dividends, are not included.

The decision to exclude trading income is in line with the general treatment throughout this book. If, however, a government-run service is operated primarily as a tax device, this decision would clearly be incorrect. For example, some countries have a tobacco monoply, so that 'profits' from this service are no different from the large amounts raised in tax from tobacco in Great Britain. In a similar way, services run at a loss represent a subsidy to the users of the service met out of general taxation. In Great Britain lip-service at least is paid to nationalized concerns breaking even taking one year with another. Three industries do not fit very well into this formula. The postal services have for many years made a profit and contributed sums to the Exchequer but, on the other hand, the National Coal Board and railways have made much larger losses. There appears to be growing up, at least in respect of the railways, the idea that some parts of the service will always have to be run at a money loss, the social or neighbourhood effects of these loss services being held to justify the subsidy involved. In the absence of separation in the accounts of nationalized concerns of that part of the service run for social purposes as opposed to that part run on more commercial lines, taking account of the 'tax' or 'subsidy' involved, is bound to be an arbitrary process.[1] Therefore trading profits or losses are omitted. Our concern will be with the items of taxation which are regarded as variable in the Budget to suit the revenue needs of the government.

Revenue since 1900

Table 1 presents the information on revenue, first in current money prices and then in percentage form. Since our interest is in the amount of revenue drawn from various kinds of tax, we can work in current prices without worrying that price and population changes will seriously distort the picture: see the opening remarks in the previous chapter. A warning is needed that in looking at changes in the amounts yielded by different types of taxes the aggregate figures conceal changes in the rates of tax and of the income or goods which are subject to tax. The details of Customs and Excise taxes will be looked at in this chapter; details of the other taxes will be taken up in later chapters.

Income tax has accounted for a quarter or more of total revenue since the 1930s, and in much of the post-war period for around 31%. This tax is subject to almost annual changes, either as to the rates applied or to tax concessions granted. The impression that we have a steeply progressive tax system is frequently obtained because income tax and surtax are progressive taxes. However, together these only account for about a third of total revenue, and when all taxes are taken into account the picture is rather different.

The percentage yield from surtax shows a diminishing trend from a high of 6% before 1939 diminishing to 2% in the post-war period. It cannot be concluded from these figures that high incomes have diminished significantly in this period. Changes in rates and in the level of income subject to surtax, already mentioned, have to be taken into account and also the extent of legal avoidance. Faced with high tax on money incomes, employers and employees have taken advantage of the fact that many tax-free benefits can be given: free meals, generous expenses, top-hat pension schemes and so on. These benefit those concerned to the detriment of the revenue and of other taxpayers whose taxes are correspondingly higher. It may also

[1] The government paper *Railway Policy* (November, 1967), envisages that this —separation of social services from commercial activities—will be made in respect of the railway accounts. See also *Nationalized Industries: a Review of Economic and Financial Objectives* (November, 1967).

be possible to convert income into a capital gain which until recently was untaxed. For example, instead of a salary increase an executive may be offered share options or better pension prospects. Estate duties have also been eroded by avoidance to a much greater extent. Estate duty accounted for 12% of revenue in 1900, about 6% per cent in the 1930s and 3% post-war. Since death duties are now much higher than they were pre-war, amounting to 80% on estates over £1 million as opposed to 40%, it might be supposed that wealth is now more equally distributed. As we shall see, very little of the change in yield can be explained by redistribution effects. Rather, the explanation is to be sought in the fact that death duties are to a great extent a discretionary tax which can be legally avoided.[2]

Stamp duties cover miscellaneous items of revenue, of which the bulk is from *ad valorum* duties on the sale of houses, land and shares. Also included are the fixed duties payable on cheques and other deeds. A not insignificant source of revenue in the early years of the century, these items in the post-war period account for only about 1% of revenue.

Taxes on companies were introduced to gather some of the excess profits which some companies were able to make in wartime. The high percentage figure shown in 1920 for company tax is a reflection of the abnormal conditions still being felt as a result of the First World War. The corporate form of business has been growing in importance throughout this century, and in interpreting these figures this fact must be borne in mind. The yield has remained at about 4% in the post-war period. Whether companies should be taxed as companies, as opposed to taxing only the owners of the companies, together with the structure of tax and allowances, will be discussed in Chapter 13.

National insurance and health contributions show the biggest percentage increase of any tax in the table, and now account for 14% of total revenue. This increase thus mirrors the increase in expenditure on social services that was noted in the previous chapter. These contributions are in the nature of a poll tax, payable in part by the employer and part by the individual. They are therefore by nature regressive taxes, falling more heavily on small incomes. This has been modified

[2] Those who regard this statement as a wild exaggeration might ponder the advertisements in newspapers. For example, the *Financial Times* on December 16th, 1967, carried two advertisements on this theme. The largest, spaced over two columns, read:

'ESTATE DUTY IS ALMOST A VOLUNTARY TAX!'

'If you have an estate-duty problem and love someone more than the Exchequer, we can assist you.

'We have specialized in designing original schemes for Top People for over 20 years.'

Table 1

Sources of United Kingdom Tax Revenue

(£ million)

Year	Income Tax (Land and Property)[3]	Surtax	Estate Duties	Stamp Duties	Profits Tax[4]	National Insurance and Health[5]	Customs and Excise	Motor Vehicles[6]	Rates	Selective Employment Tax	Other	Total
1900	21	—	19	9	—	—	61	—	45	—	3	158
1909	37	—	18	8	—	—	63	—	68	—	4	197
1920	320	42	41	23	290	29	283	—	119	—	297[8]	1,443
1928	251	61	77	27	2	80	251	25	188	—	86	1,048
1933	252	61	77	19	2	88	288	28	165	—	30	1,010
1939	336	63	77	21	22	104[7]	341	36	214	—	23	1,236
1939	346	65	77	19	28	104[7]	382	34	214	—	23	1,292
1950	1,404	114	190	53	277	440	1,583	59	338	—	16	4,474
1955	1,964	132	184	75	223	594	1,990	85	475	—	17	5,739
1960	2,285	178	236	94	262	913	2,366	123	771	—	28	7,256
1961	2,565	196	259	97	317	1,072	2,540	141	831	—	32	8,050
1962	2,846	230	266	95	379	1,197	2,687	164	916	—	33	8,813
1963	2,823	174	308	92	388	1,303	2,721	182	1,013	—	38	9,042
1964	2,942	179	308	83	408	1,444	3,034	194	1,092	—	46	9,730
1965	3,373	184	290	76	466	1,685	3,425	192	1,228	—	71	10,990
1966	4,120	210	315	78	120	1,806	3,617	174	1,358	298	65	12,161
1967	[illegible]	[illegible]	[illegible]	[illegible]	[illegible]	[illegible]	[illegible]	[illegible]	[illegible]	[illegible]	[illegible]	[illegible]

Year	Income Tax (Land and Property)[3]	Surtax	Estate Duties	Stamp Duties	Profits Tax[4]	National Insurance and Health[5]	Customs and Excise	Motor Vehicle	Rates	Selective Employment Tax	Other	Total
1900	13	—	12	6	—	—	39	—	28	—	2	100
1909	19	—	9	4	—	—	32	—	34	—	2	100
1920	22	3	3	2	20	2	20	—	8	—	20	100
1928	24	6	7	3	—	8	24	2	18	—	8	100
1933	25	6	7	2	—	9	28	3	16	—	4	100
1939	27	5	6	2	2	8	28	3	17	—	2	100
1939	27	5	6	1	2	8	29	3	17	—	2	100
1950	31	3	4	1	6	10	36	1	8	—	—	100
1955	34	2	3	1	4	11	35	2	8	—	—	100
1960	31	2	3	1	4	13	33	2	11	—	—	100
1961	32	2	3	1	4	14	32	2	10	—	—	100
1962	32	3	3	1	4	14	31	2	10	—	—	100
1963	31	2	4	1	4	15	30	2	11	—	—	100
1964	31	2	3	1	4	15	31	2	11	—	—	100
1965	31	2	3	1	4	15	31	2	11	—	—	100
1966	34	2	3	1	1	15	30	1	11	3	—	100
1967	28	2	3	1	9	14	28	1	11	3	—	100

[3] Land and assessed taxes were about £2·5 million until 1924 and thereafter declined in amount. Refer to note 3 to explain revenue changes in 1966 and 1967. Net receipts from capital gains tax is estimated to be £1·5 million in 1963-4, £2 million in 1964-5, £2·5 million in 1965-6 and £15·5 million in 1966-7. These sums are included under income tax.

[4] Profits tax, called at various times excess profits tax, corporation profits tax, national defence contributions (profits), etc. Now known as corporation tax; the switch to this tax is the reason for the unevenness of revenue in 1966 and 1967.

[5] From 1965 Redundancy Fund contributions are included.

[6] Prior to 1921 motor licences were included under Excise. From 1965 export rebates were introduced; these have been excluded from the figures.

[7] Refers to year 1937.

[8] Mainly receipts from the sale of war property.

Sources: 1900-39 Financial Accounts of the U.K. and Statistical Abstracts of the U.K. 1939 and after: *National Income and Expenditure Tables*, 1966 and 1968, Tables 41, 42 and 45.

only slightly by the recently introduced graduated contributions for pension and supplements in respect of sickness and unemployment and industrial injuries. The social services at the present time represent a not very happy mixture of services which are intended to be self-financed, some which are intended to be partly met by way of contributions and partly met out of general taxation, and some met solely out of general taxation. In current conditions the idea of earmarked taxes is a polite fiction that bears little relation to government accounting, a fact which has long been recognized in the case of the Road Fund. The adoption of the total accretion principle which will be discussed in Chapter 11 would abolish this fiction entirely. An appendix to this chapter gives more details on the financing of the national insurance and health services.

The broad category of taxes labelled 'Customs and Excise' has always represented a sizeable portion of revenue. Gladstone called them the 'two fair sisters'! They have accounted since the 1930s for roughly the same proportion of revenue as income tax. Table 2 gives the breakdown of Customs and Excise duty in 1967.

Table 2

Customs and Excise Duty in 1967

		(£ million)	%
Alcohol		725	19
Tobacco		1,038	28
Hydrocarbon oils		949	26
Purchase tax		748	20
Rest: protective duties and temporary import charge	189		
Betting	69		
Other	11	269	7
		3,729	100

Source: *National Income and Expenditure, 1968*, Table 41.

From Table 2 it can be seen that the three standbys of the Exchequer are alcohol, tobacco and hydrocarbon oils, which accounted respectively for 19%, 28% and 26% of Customs and Excise revenue in 1967. Purchase tax is spread over a large number of products: the tendency in recent years has been to simplify the structure by reducing the number of rates and increasing the number of products subject to the tax. Further details are given below. The remainder of Customs and Excise revenue comes chiefly from protective duties, with betting contributing a small amount.

PURCHASE TAX

Purchase tax was first imposed in 1940, and is levied on certain goods, whether home-produced or imported. No services are charged in this way. The tax has been as high as 125% of the wholesale value of certain items. In recent years a simplification in the number of rates charged has taken place. Today goods are charged at one of four rates, 13¾%, 22%, 36⅔% or 55% of the wholesale value.[9]

The tax is charged on registered persons: these are normally manufacturers and wholesalers whose sales of goods exceed £500 a year. The effect is to create a tax-free 'ring'. Goods may pass tax-free between registered traders, but tax is charged when the goods pass outside this ring, i.e. normally to a retailer or final buyer. As a rule, the goods are invoiced with the full value of the tax added on.

In general, the lower rate is applied to garments, footwear, gloves and to goods used in the home, such as floor coverings, wallpaper, fabrics, furniture, hardware, table-ware and kitchen-ware. The second rate is levied on confectionery, beverages, ice-cream, and since 1969 prepared pet foods. The third rate of 36⅔% applies to motor-cars and most durable consumer goods and luxury goods, except for those taxed at the top rate. The top rate applies to furs, jewellery, watches and clocks, gramophone records, smokers' requisites and photographic goods, pictorial reproductions, diaries, calendars and greeting cards, fancy and ornamental articles, perfumery and toilet preparations. Foodstuffs, raw materials used in industry and exports are the main goods exempted from the tax.

The revenue shown under motor vehicles covers the annual licence duty, which for private motor-cars was raised to £25 per annum in 1968. Commercial vehicles are charged at a higher rate, and goods vehicles are subject to a rising scale of charges, based on the unladen weight of the vehicle. Cars are also subject to purchase tax and fuel

[9] In 1963 the number of rates had been reduced to three: 10%, 15% or 25%. An increase of 10% was imposed under the Regulator power given to the Chancellor. The Regulator also applies to duties imposed on tobacco, alcohol and hydrocarbon oils. This was consolidated with these old rates in the Budget of 1967. The Chancellor then estimated the yield from this surcharge as in excess of £150 million a year. The Budget of 1968 increased the rates to 12½%, 20% and 33⅓% and introduced a top rate of 50%. The yield from these changes was estimated to be £163 million a year. In November, 1968, an increase of 10% was again imposed, under the Regulator power and consolidated in April, 1969, giving the rates shown in the text. The yield was estimated to be £250 million a year.

is taxed; the receipts for these appear under the heading 'Customs and Excise'.

In view of the annual outcry that is made against rates, it is perhaps surprising to find that rates as a percentage of revenue show a sharp decline from nearly a third of revenue in 1900 to 11% in 1965. Rates are a local authority's only major source of revenue that is independent of the central government. They are levied by local authorities at so much in the pound on the value of premises. One reason for the unpopularity of rates could be laid on the local authorities themselves. Rates are levied in two annual instalments, so that the householder or ratepayer is faced with two payments to make of quite large magnitude, whereas most income tax is deducted by the employer under 'Pay as You Earn' and indirect taxes in the price of the article subject to the tax. Local authorities are now required to allow payment of rates by instalments. One reason for the decline in the share of revenue from rates is due to derating: this is the exemption, whole or in part, from rates for certain kinds of property. These first occurred in the Depression of the 1930s and have continued with modifications ever since. At the present time buildings of charities are 50% derated and agricultural land and buildings are wholly exempt. Manufacturing premises were 50% derated, but were brought back into the rating system in 1963. Legislation in 1966 takes the amount due for rates into account in assessing the needs of applicants for pensions or other assistance.

Comment

The two main sources of revenue, income tax and Customs and Excise, show only a small percentage change in the twenty-eight-year period from 1939 to 1967 in spite of a world war. The changes in this period have been the decrease in the percentages obtained from surtax, death duties and rates and the increase in sums raised by way of national insurance and health contributions.

The tabulation of the existing sources of revenue that has been carried out in this chapter hides a curious feature. This could be brought out more clearly by having many more headings showing nil returns. The majority of taxes shown in the table fall on current income: wealth as such is virtually untouched, apart from the small amounts raised by death duties and a portion of stamp duty that can be attributed to wealth movements. An outsider looking at this tax system might well conclude that our society despised and generally tried to discourage earned income while it looked up to and tried to encourage inherited wealth. A deeper probe of the system to be found in Chapter 11 on the concept of income will reveal that it is only income very narrowly defined which is heavily taxed. Spending power that comes in the form of gambling winnings, capital gains or gifts was virtually untaxed in the period covered by the table.

The table does not bring out important changes that have been made in recent years, as these have as yet made little impact on the revenue received. A capital gains tax of a very restricted kind was introduced in 1962; a more thoroughgoing tax was introduced in 1965. Chapter 12 on 'Personal Income Taxation' gives details. From the point of view of equity between persons, this change is a major breakthrough, but from the revenue side it will be many years before the capital gains tax brings in very much revenue, as it is only gains made since the passing of the Acts (with offset for capital losses) which have been made relevant for tax purposes. Details of recent changes in taxes on betting and gambling and the selective employment tax will be looked at in the next chapter.

Aims and principles of taxation

A fiscal system serves various purposes besides the obvious one of providing revenue. Following Musgrave, R. A. (1959), 5, these will be collected under three headings:

1. *Allocation of resources.* This aspect of taxation is concerned with the allocation of resources between, for example, private and public goods and between investment and consumption goods. It is also concerned with correcting deficiencies in the pricing mechanism due, for example, to monopoly elements, the existence of external economies or diseconomies, and cases where social costs diverge sharply from private costs.

2. *Distribution of resources.* Chapter 7 has already indicated that the distribution of income and wealth depends on a number of factors, including work, educational opportunities, inheritance, gifts, and from government fiscal policy and legislation. The distribution heading is concerned with the adjustments that society decides to make in order to correct for deficiencies in the distribution of income and wealth.

3. *Stabilization of the economy in terms of current objectives.* Current objectives usually include equity, obtaining and maintaining a satisfactory level of growth, maintaining full employment, ensuring stability in the value of money and maintaining a satisfactory balance of payments.

It should be noted that, until recently, only 1, the allocation of resources, has been considered as a part of public finance. After about 1900 the distribution of resources began to be considered.

Stabilization of the economy is due to the ideas of Keynes in the 1930s.

Within the aims selected by society as relevant, persons have been looking for centuries for a general principle that could be used as a guide to apportion taxes in an equitable manner. Two principles have long been canvassed:

The benefit principle and ability to pay

These principles have mainly been discussed in relation to the allocation of resources. When the aims of public finance are drawn more widely to take in the distribution and stabilization aims, neither will be found without fault, but both can contribute to our understanding of the problems involved. A detailed discussion of these principles will be found in Musgrave, R. A. (1959), Chapters 4 and 5.

The benefit approach dictates that taxes are apportioned to individuals according to the benefits they derive from government activity and spending. Taxes are treated as a payment for the goods and services provided by the government. The provision of government goods and services will, like the provision of private goods and services, be dictated by market demand. In a society where the aims of government are conceived in minimum terms of defence against external aggression and the administration of justice, as in eighteenth-century England, this approach is understandable. The existing structure of wealth and income was taken as given, and the economy was conceived as self-regulating. These ideas have given ground on all fronts. It is generally conceded that private provision will seriously underestimate the need for various social services where there are strong neighbourhood effects. Some redistribution of income and wealth is granted as necessary in all developed countries, and stabilization of the economy since the 1930s is now taken for granted. With these wider aims the benefit rule is clearly ruled out as a principle of general application. The more the government did to help the needy, the more the needy would have to pay. The whole transfer process which has been seen taking place, particularly in this century, would be frustrated. Again the allocation of some benefits—for example, defence—would be an arbitrary process. And the aims of stabilization would not necessarily be carried out by following the benefit principle of taxation. The benefit principle, nevertheless, may have application in limited areas where a close relationship between outlay and benefit can be established. Thus where a government undertakes the provision of a service, which could equally well be undertaken privately and there are no strong externalities present, the danger of not charging according to the benefit principle is that demand for that service is likely to be stimulated at the expense of services where costs are allocated to users. This may represent an uneconomic use of the nation's resources. For some services, e.g. health and education, this extension of demand is deliberately aimed for: neighbourhood effects apply. In others, e.g. government provision of some forms of transport or some forms of fuel, failure to charge users with the costs of the service or commodity is likely to have the effect of distorting the use of the nation's resources in an undesirable way. No general solution emerges: it is necessary in each case to weigh the social benefits and costs involved in charging users for the full costs of the service and in meeting these costs out of general taxation, or of some compromise between these two methods.

The ability-to-pay approach is concerned with the equitable distribution of taxes according to the stated taxable capacity, or ability to pay, of an individual or group. It leaves the correct contribution that government provision should make to be decided on political grounds. This rule, in terms of the objectives stated at the beginning of this section, enables the distribution and stabilization objectives to be carried out in an equitable manner. Its disadvantage, that the allocation objective has to be decided by other means, has just been stressed. With the ability-to-pay principle, the criterion on which ability is to be judged must be identified: whether it is to be income, wealth, income and wealth, or spending power. This will form the main concern of Chapter 11. In their usual formulation these criteria do not take into account benefits from government expenditure that accrue to the individual. However, it is possible to define the criteria to include these benefits. This partial synthesis of the two approaches will be developed further in Chapter 18.

Summary

Income tax and Custom and Excise duties each account for about 30% of government revenue, proportions that have changed relatively little since pre-war. In 1967 73% of Customs and Excise duties came from tobacco, hydrocarbon oils and alcohol; purchase tax, charged at one of four rates on a wide range of commodities, accounts for a further 20%. National insurance and health contributions show the largest increase and now account for 14% of total revenue. The proportions raised from surtax, estate duties and rates show a sharp decline. It is not correct to conclude that high incomes, or the distribution of wealth, have diminished significantly in these years.

Recent years have seen the introduction of a number of important taxes: on capital gains, on betting and gambling and a selective employment tax. Wealth continues to be taxed lightly, in spite of nominally high rates of duty, compared to earned income, because of the ease of avoiding the full impact of estate duties.

A fiscal system is aimed at providing revenue and also serves other purposes. These were collected under three headings: allocation of resources, distribution of resources, and stabilization of the economy. Within the aims selected by society as relevant two principles of tax have been put forward: the benefit principle and ability to pay. Neither of these principles, in present-day conditions, is without fault, but an understanding of them is useful in trying to formulate a satisfactory fiscal system.

Appendix
Financing of National Insurance and National Health Services

A list of the major public social services is given below. Finance comes from diverse sources. These vary from contributions from local authority sources, contributions from employed persons and from employers, part-payment from the users of some of the services and contributions from the State out of general taxation.

SOCIAL SECURITY

National insurance: pensions
unemployment and sickness benefit
maternity benefits
industrial injuries

Family allowances

Social security supplementary benefits (old title 'National Assistance') to meet exceptional need.

PUBLIC HEALTH

National Health Service: hospital and general practioner services.

Environmental Health Services: sewerage, home-refuse, water-supply, etc.

EDUCATION

HOUSING

OTHER SERVICES, as: employment exchanges, retraining, town and country planning, highways, administration of justice, child care, parks and the arts.

With the exception of national insurance, these services are financed in the main out of general taxation of the central government with the lesser part being financed from local authority sources. Attention will be confined to discussing the financing of national insurance and the National Health Service. The use of the term 'contribution', in talking of employees' payments to national insurance followed in this appendix, is conventional. Since payment is compulsory the term tax could equally well be used.

The financing of the services covered by these two schemes has differed from the start. The National Health Service is not an insurance scheme; benefits do not depend on the payment of contributions: it is basically a service available to all. The flat-rate contributions paid by employed persons and their employers for National Health covered only 11% of the cost of the service in the year ending March 31st, 1967.

In looking at the National Insurance Scheme, the position is less clear-cut. Whether the term 'insurance' is the correct one to use has been debated since its inception. There are two basic principles of private insurance; the less important one is basing the premium to be paid on an assessment of the risks involved. Thus a thatched house pays a higher premium against fire risk than a similar house with a tiled roof; motor-insurance premiums may vary with the age of the insured, his accident record and occupation, type of car, etc. A person in chronic poor health or over a certain age is unlikely to be accepted at all in a private medical care scheme. In contrast, State insurance was instituted on the principle of collective risk and flat-rate contributions and benefits. Recent departures from this principle will be noted.

The more important principle of private insurance is the actuarial aim that premiums should more than cover the claims paid out. There has been disagreement from the start whether State insurance should operate on similar lines. The idea that the State should build up a fund to meet future contingencies was not contemplated: the issue is between those who wish to see a 'pay as you go' system and those who wish to see the whole, or part, of the expenditures met out of general taxation. Lord Beveridge, whose Report formed the basis of the extension of the National Insurance Scheme after the war envisaged the scheme as being financed on a tripartite basis: from employers, employees and the State (*Social Insurance and Allied Services*, 1942, and Beveridge, W. H., 1944). It was envisaged that employers' and employees' flat-rate contributions would provide the bulk of the necessary revenue. It was foreseen that the State would need to contribute a large amount for many years towards the provision of pensions, since people nearing retiring age at the start of the scheme would not be able to contribute much towards the scheme.

The meaning of a State 'pay as you go' scheme, largely financed by flat-rate contributions, is assessing the rate of contribution at the minimum age of entry to the scheme which, say, a male would have to pay over his working lifetime to ensure the benefits on an actuarial basis. This rate, or some lesser sum if the State is to bear part of the cost of the services, is the flat-rate contribution for all males. In any one year such a scheme will leave the State with a larger, or smaller, contribution to make, depending on many factors, such as the age-structure of the population, the degree of sickness and unemployment.

Many commentators have pointed out the weakness of this idea. Financing the bulk of the service by flat-rate contributions sets a limit to the amount that can be collected without imposing undue hardship on the poorest paid in the community. The amount so raised may bear little relation to the needs of the community. This fact and the general inflation of money which has occurred since the war has eroded to some extent the concept of self-financing outlined. These ideas of self-financing, on the one hand, and of meeting expenditures out of general taxation, on the other, continue to be debated (e.g. Titmus, 1963).

There follow three tables, one giving the weekly contributions paid by employed persons and their employers and two setting out costs and sources of finance.

At present persons are categorized for payment of flat-rate contributions according to whether they are male or female and whether they are over or under eighteen years of age. Different rates are paid by employed persons and self-employed persons, and other categories are separated, e.g. part-time workers and students.

Table 3

Class I employed persons' weekly contributions from May 6th, 1968[10]

	Paid by Employee				*Paid by Employer*				
	N.I.	N.H.S.	I.I.	Total	N.I.	N.H.S.	I.I.	R.F.	Total
	s. d.	*s. d.*	*d.*	*s. d.*	*s. d.*	*d.*	*d.*	*d.*	*s. d.*
Man	12 8	3 2	10	16 8	14 1	8	11	10	16 6
Woman	11 0	2 6	7	14 1	12 3	8	8	5	14 0
Boy	8 8	1 7	5	10 8	9 6	8	5	—	10 7
Girl	7 1	1 7	3	8 11	7 10	8	4	—	8 10

N.I. = National Insurance.
N.H.S. = National Health Service.
I.I. = Industrial Injuries.
R.F. = Redundancy Fund.

[10] These flat-rate contributions are to be increased for employers and employees by 1*s*. a week for men and 11*d*. for women from November, 1969.

Table 3 lists the contributions paid by Class 1 employed persons who have not contracted out of the pension scheme. It covers the most numerous category.

These sums are paid by the employer fixing a stamp of the appropriate value to the employee's card; the employer deducts the employee's contribution from his wage. The stamp must also cover the employer's contribution to the selective employment tax in respect of each worker, but since this tax is not part of the social insurance scheme, this has been omitted from the tabulation.

It will be seen that a man pays 12*s.* 8*d.* a week for National Insurance, or £33 a year, and 3*s.* 2*d.* a week for the National Health Service, or £8 4*s.* 8*d.* a year. The employer pays £36 16*s.* 8*d.* and £1 14*s.* 8*d.* respectively per year for each man employed. Since 1961 an element of graduation was introduced into the pension part of the insurance contribution. This has not been taken into account in the table of weekly contributions above. Employed persons over eighteen who have not contracted out and whose remuneration exceeds £9 a week, together with their employers, each pay an additional contribution of 4¼% of earnings between £9 and £18 a week. These contributions entitle those who pay to an additional graduated benefit in addition to the flat-rate pension. Persons can only contract out of this graduated scheme if the employer has a private scheme at least as good as the provisions provided by the State. The position is therefore that every person covered is entitled to a flat-rate pension. Those whose wage is above the minimum will, in addition, receive an additional benefit from their firm or from their additional graduated contributions, or both. Those with a wage of £18 a week or more will pay at the highest graduated rate, unless contracted out, and will receive the highest graduated pension.

As from October 5th, 1966, a contribution at the rate of ½% of earnings between £9 and £30 is paid by both employer and employee (whether or not contracted out) to meet the cost of earnings-related benefit supplements under the National Insurance Act, 1966. These supplements are in respect of sickness, unemployment and industrial injuries. From November, 1969 these rates are increased to 2¾% for those who earn between £18 and £30 a week, so that a man earning £30 or more a week will pay 7*s.* 7*d.* and women 7*s.* 6*d.* a week. Employers' contributions are increased by the same amount.

Table 4 shows that for the year ending March 31st, 1967, the Exchequer financed directly 73% of expenditure on health. The Exchequer also, through the rate-support grant finances a proportion of local authority health expenditure. National Health Service flat-rate contributions financed 11% and charges on users 4%. Over half of this expenditure was on the hospital service.

Table 4

Health finance for Year ending March 31st, 1967, to nearest £ million

Cost			Sources of Finance		
	£m.	%		£m.	%
Hospitals: current 685			Exchequer	987	73
Capital 80			N.H.S. contributions	147	11
	765	56	Payments by users	55	4
General medical	97	7	Rates and Exchequer grants to L.As.	166	12
Pharmaceutical	142	11	Rest	3	0
General dental	70	5			
Local health authorities	126	9			
Administration	16	1			
Other	142	11			
	1,358	100		1,358	100

Source: *Annual Report of the Ministry of Health, 1967.*

Table 5

National Insurance Funds for Year ending March 31st, 1967, to nearest £ million

Cost			Sources of Finance		
	£m.	%		£m.	%
Retirement pensions	1,272	68	Flat-rate contributions (from employers and insured persons)	1,165	63
Sickness	262	14	Graduated contributions (from employers and insured persons)	346	19
Widow's	141	8	Exchequer contributions	287	15
Unemployment	78	4	Other	65	3
Maternity	37	2			
Administration	62	3			
Other	24	1			
	1,876	100		1,863	100
Excess of payments over receipts	13				

Source: *Annual Report of Ministry of Social Security, 1967.*

Table 5 shows that in the same period flat-rate contributions from employers and insured persons accounted for 63% of finance to the National Insurance Funds. Graduated contributions accounted for 19% and the Exchequer contributed 15%. On the expenditure side, the major part is accounted for by flat-rate benefits, of which retirement pensions constitute the bulk. Graduated retirement pensions, as yet, hardly figure on the expenditure side. In 1966, the last year for which figures were given, they amounted to less than £2 million.

Proposals after 1972

In January, 1969 a White Paper—'National Superannuation and Social Insurance'—was issued which proposed substantial changes in pensions and social insurance.

The basic change envisaged is earnings related payments coupled with earnings related benefits paid in respect of pensions, sickness and unemployment.

The most important part of these proposals concern pensions and the most controversial part the suggestion that these new earnings related pensions be paid only to those who have paid earnings related contributions, so it will be twenty years after the start of the scheme before pensions at the full new scheme rates are paid. Contributors who reach pension age during the twenty-year build-up period will earn pensions at intermediate rates.

Citizens in otherwise equal circumstances will therefore be differentiated according to the number of years contributions they have made. Based on the illustrative figures given in the White Paper, for a single man assumed to earn the national average of £22 a week we find:

						Existing pension
a man aged	70	in 1972 would be	aged	90	in 1992.	£4. 10. 0.[11]
						Proposed pension
"	60	"	"	80	"	£5. 14. 0.
"	55	"	"	75	"	£6. 19. 0.
"	45	"	"	65	"	£9. 7. 0.

[11] Plus a supplement of a few shillings under the existing graduated scheme. The basic pension for a single person will be increased to £5 in November, 1969.

These proposals which differentiate, not according to need but according to the time a person has contributed to the new scheme, can be contrasted with the proposals introduced after the Second World War. Then, as now, it was envisaged that pensions should be on the basis of 'pay as you go' but then it was accepted that to bring those near retiring age into the scheme would entail a contribution out of general taxation for a period of years. The scheme was largely set up on this basis.

The figures used in the illustration above will not, of course, be the actual rates payable in 1992. The White Paper proposes:

'The government will be required by law to undertake a review every two years of the main rates of benefits in payment, both under the present scheme and under the new. The increases made will, as a minimum, compensate for any rise in prices during the two year period. The amounts of increases beyond this will be decided by the government of the day, in the light of the general situation on each occasion' (para. 6).

The proposals to make the review of pension bi-annual can be unreservedly welcomed as an improvement on the present system whereby pensions receive most attention at times of Parliamentary election. However the issue taken up here is not about the level of benefits, but about the degree of differentiation. If the spread of pensions is maintained as shown in the table, £4. 10*s*. 0*d*.—£9. 7*s*. 0*d*., it is not difficult to forecast that for those near retirement age at the present the closer he or she will be to poverty as they get older. The White Paper, paragraph 9, tells us that nearly one-third of the 7,000,000 pensioners in 1965 were eligible for some form of additional assistance, or in other words had inadequate pensions. If levels of national assistance had been £2 a week higher about three-quarters of all pensioners would have been eligible for assistance.

Proposed rates

The new scheme proposes to charge employees up to a level of earnings of about £33 a week, 4¾% of total earnings for superannuation and 2% for social insurance benefits, so that a deduction of 6¾% from earnings is proposed. Employers will be charged 6¾% on their total payroll with no earnings ceiling. Collection of both employers and employees contributions will in most cases be administered through the 'Pay as You Earn' system of tax collection.

Contributions from employees are therefore not progressive but proportional. However, some redistribution of income is provided because the fully mature pension rates will be based for a single person on 60% of earnings up to half the national average earnings, and 25% of the remainder up to the ceiling of £33 a week. From the table below it can be seen that this results in a man earning £33 a week or more paying 3 times as much as a man earning £11 a week whereas his pension is 1·8 times as much. The table on p. 110 lists the proposed new total contributions for pensions and social insurance.

Level of weekly earnings	*Proposed employees total contribution per week*		*Change on present contribu-ution*		*Fully matured new pension rates*[12]		
	s.	d.	s.	d.	£.	s.	d.
£11 (½ national average)	14	10	− 3	0	6	12	0
£16 10s. (¾ national average)	22	3	−	9	8	0	0
£22 (national average)	29	8	+ 5	0	9	7	0
£27 10s. (1¼ national average)	37	1	+11	10	10	15	0
£33 or above (1½ national average)	44	7	+19	2	12	2	0

Women pay the same rates as men under the new scheme.

[12] That is pensions payable after 20 years of earnings-related contributions, assuming April, 1968 earnings levels.

10
Government expenditure and revenue (concluded)

They [politicians and experts] have to say whether it is better to try for a surplus or to acquiesce in a deficit. They both have to consider economic and political consequences. But, so far as taxpayers are concerned, all such questions are subsidiary to the critical issue of distribution. . . . It is usually assumed that other problems may be best resolved by shifting the burdens elsewhere. And there is no lack of ingenuity in providing the necessary rationalizations for the desired results.

EISENSTEIN, L. (1961), *The Ideologies of Taxation.*

To explain adequately the changes in expenditure and revenue would require a full-scale social and economic history of the period. Similar trends to the ones observed in this country can be seen in most developed countries over the same period. In this chapter the main pressures that have helped to mould the system are outlined.

Pressures on government spending

As long ago as the 1880s Adolph Wagner was predicting that public expenditure would increase (at least for a time) at a faster rate than national output. We get a law of 'growing public expenditure'. He based his observations on the results of a study of developed Western countries and on the grounds that State activity would need to increase as a result of social progress. To date Wagner's prediction has proved to be accurate. The extent to which it will continue to hold good in the future is more problematical. The fact of adult male suffrage in 1887 and the start of female suffrage in 1918 is likely to have played a very important (though largely unquantifiable) part. With adult suffrage, Parliament is likely in its spending and revenue to reflect the needs of the community as a whole more closely than before, because Members of Parliament depend on the goodwill of the majority of the community for their seats.

Not always stressed as much as it deserves to be is the pressure on public spending caused by the *growth* of population and the *concentration* of population. Services which can be safely left to the individual in a sparsely populated country have to be undertaken by the community in a more populated country, sewage and water-supply being obvious examples. The process is still at work today. Government spending or regulation on smoke-abatement in large urban areas is beginning to take on the nature of a social necessity, and we can expect expenditures on this head to increase in the future. The motor-car is creating its obvious pressures on the public purse, and so on.

It is sometimes possible to distinguish two trends under this general heading. One which has been referred to under 'externalities' refers to the benefit which the whole community derives from the service. Leaving the provision of such a service to the goodwill of the individual, who is likely to take only his private benefit into account, would result in serious deficiencies, to the general detriment of all. The basic services referred to in the previous paragraph come into this category.

Secondly, we can distinguish cases where technical considerations apply, where, in order to obtain a better use of resources, collective provision is needed. Thus the generation of electricity could be left to the individual, but each building with its own generator is a very inefficient way, at the present time, of obtaining electricity. The State usually steps in at the local or central level to run the service, or to supervise the provision of the service if monopoly powers are granted to a private concern. New processes and inventions change these technical considerations in no very predictable manner. We have already reached the stage where it is technically an extremely inefficient use of resources for each building to supply its own needs for heat and hot water. Centralized provision of hot water to houses and other buildings could yield large economies in the use of fuel, as well as yielding benefits in terms of cleaner air and better living conditions.

In contrast to the neighbourhood and technical effects stressed above, social reasons for public spending—that is, the wish to spread benefits to the community at large—have played an important (but once again hard to determine) part. This is particularly noticeable in the extension of education, health and the social services generally. The desire to spread income and wealth more evenly has also helped to shape the expenditure and the revenue side of public finance. Finally, since the depression of the 1930s most governments accept that they have a positive role to play in keeping the economy in balance, avoiding both the extremes of slump and of severe inflation. This compensatory aspect will lead to a larger rather than a smaller government sector.

Pressures on government revenue

To pick out some of the pressures that have shaped public expenditure is analogous to explaining price by looking at demand and ignoring supply. If we look at public expenditure and revenue over time we find that they are uneven. In particular, we can single out wars as causing large jumps in government expenditure. By itself this is not a surprising feature: what is interesting is that government expenditure does not go back after the war to its former level. This observation is apparent even when allowance is made for price-changes and when war-related expenditures are excluded.

Peacock, A. T. and Wiseman, J. (1961) use the term 'displacement effect' to cover this phenomenon. Once again we find that many strands knit together to cause this effect. Peacock and Wiseman develop the idea that in normal times there is a dichotomy between the desire for public goods and services and the level of taxation which is considered tolerable. A large-scale disturbance, such as a war, may create an upward displacement of the level of taxation considered tolerable, so that new levels of public spending can afterwards be maintained.

In wartime new methods of raising revenue may be accepted; there is some release from the 'bonds of the revenue'. 'Pay as You Earn' is an example introduced in the last war. War also focuses attention on social ills. 'It has taken the catastrophe of war to bring home to those in power that economic progress does not automatically disseminate the benefits of education and health' (Peacock, A. T. and Wiseman, J. (1961), 93). Such a period may also see an acceleration in reorganization of government accounts, statistical information and in Civil Service procedures. Periods of crisis, such as war and the severe slump in the earlier 1930s, thus seem to act as a catalyst. We do not know what would have happened in the absence of these disasters, but in the light of hindsight they appear to break the 'cake of custom'.

Recasting the system of revenue?

The period 1960-7 is a remarkable one in that, without a marked crisis of the kind previously referred to, major changes have been made on the revenue side. These changes have, apart from the selective employment tax, made little impact to receipts of revenue but their potential is great.

The inequalities of income taxation have been tackled indirectly by subjecting some of the spending power which escaped income taxation to other forms of tax. The most notable change has been the capital gains tax. Wealth has received less practical attention. These matters will be taken up in later chapters. In the rest of this chapter an outline is given of two taxes which have been recently introduced, the selective employment tax and the taxes on betting and gambling.

The selective employment tax

The selective employment tax (abbreviated to S.E.T.) was introduced in September, 1966. It is a tax on labour imposed on all civil employers in the private and public sectors. It varies for men, women, boys and girls, and is differentiated according to which industry employs them. At first the tax was 25*s.* a week for every man, 12*s.* 6*d.* for women and boys and 8*s.* for girls. Boys and girls are those under eighteen years of age. Establishments fell into three categories: those who got back after a six months' delay more than the tax, those who just have the tax refunded, and those who get no refund. Amendments were announced in the Budget of 1967 in respect of part-time workers and staff absent overseas: and considerable changes were made in September and November, 1967 and the budgets of 1968 and 1969. These will be outlined shortly.

General establishments classed as manufacturing came into the first category, and received back, in addition to the tax paid, an extra 7*s.* 6*d.* in respect of each male employee, 3*s.* 9*d.* in respect of women and boys, and 2*s.* 6*d.* for girls. Broadly speaking, transport, agriculture, horticulture, shipping, nationalized industries, local government and universities come into Category 2 and receive back the amount of tax paid. Service, distribution and construction come into Category 3 and get no refund.

Two justifications were given in the White Paper, *Selective Employment Tax* (1966), for this tax. The first, and generally agreed, aim was that service and distributive trades should bear a portion of the tax bill. This has the important advantage of allowing the government to restrict consumer-demand without affecting those industries that are already subject to purchase tax and Customs and Excise duties. The second, more controversial, aim was that it would in the longer term encourage the redeployment of labour from the service, distributive and construction trades to industry. The tax also had the effect of acting as a mild stimulus to exports, since wage costs in manufacturing industries were lowered. However rebates are now confined to manufacturing industries in development areas and are due to end there in April, 1970, and S.E.T. unlike a value-added tax cannot be rebated on exports.

If a system of indirect taxes is in operation, the only economic arguments for taxing a small range of goods and services is ease of collection. On social grounds it may be desired to tax goods consumed mainly by the rich, but such goods are not easy to discover. On economic grounds the case for taxing all goods and services, rather than taxing more heavily fewer items, is that consumer prices will reflect more closely their relative costs. In turn this is likely to lead to a more efficient allocation of resources. In the past, relative prices of services and manufactured goods have been distorted because the former were untaxed while the latter were subject to various rates of tax. Under any system of tax, some items, such as alcohol and tobacco, will probably be taxed more heavily for social reasons: but here the deliberate intention, as well as to raise revenue, is to choke off some of the demand for these products.

If it is decided to tax a wide range of goods, the problem then arises as to the best method of collecting the tax. On this point disagreement is sharp. The reason given for this rather clumsy method of taxing all industries and then giving rebates to some, in order to tax the service sector, was that the only machinery readily available was the Ministry of Pensions and National Insurance organization for receiving the national insurance and health contributions. The insurance contributions do not draw any distinction between employees in different industries, and therefore this method was adopted.

The second aim of encouraging redistribution of labour by giving what is in effect a subsidy to manufacturing establishments is more open to criticism. Manufacturing as well as other concerns may be guilty of hoarding labour, and the S.E.T. does nothing to encourage the manufacturing sector to use its labour wisely—rather the reverse.[1]

The tax also came under attack because it discriminates against part-time and disabled workers, who are subject to the same rates of tax. This may have the paradoxical effect of causing a reversal, or a slowing down, in the distributive trades of the trend towards the employment of more part-time workers—in particular, the employment of married women. The 1967 Budget modified the tax, with effect from September, 1967, in respect of part-time workers, but not disabled workers. In establishments not entitled to a refund—that is, in general the service, distribution and construction industries—one-half of the tax payable in respect of adult employees who normally work less than twenty-one hours a week will be refunded. In effect, these industries are charged 12*s.* 6*d.* for every part-time male employee, 25*s.* for full-time male employees and 6*s.* 3*d.* for part-time female employees. Employers with staff who are absent overseas for over three months had a concession whereby their S.E.T.

[1] The element of subsidy to manufaucturing firms is effectively reduced to the extent that the services bought by the manufacturer will be increased in cost.

would be refunded. This was intended to help the construction industry with long-term contracts abroad.

Further changes were later announced in *Development Areas Regional Employment Premium* (1967). These charges came into operation from September, 1967. The tax was now envisaged as a major way of increasing employment in the development areas. Since January, 1966, development areas are defined to include, except for small areas deemed to be sufficiently developed, Scotland, northern England (i.e. the four northernmost counties of England, plus the North Riding of Yorkshire), Wales, Merseyside and the south-western area, which takes in much of Devon and Cornwall. Premiums to manufacturing industries in these areas are to paid out for not less than seven years and then phased out over another two or so years. The premiums are in addition to the refunds already received, and amount to 30*s.* for men, 15*s.* for women and boys, 7*s.* 6*d.* for girls, with part-time employees getting half of the premium in each case. The premiums will be worth about £100 million a year to the development areas.

The aim of these premiums is to reduce the disparity in unemployment levels between the development areas and the rest of Britain; if successful this would have the effect of helping Britain's growth without, it is thought, adding to inflationary pressure or leading to any worsening in the balance of payments, and without the need to increase taxation. These desirable effects will be brought about, it is believed, because any increase in demand for imports will be offset by increased exports, and the competitive loss by maufacturing industry in the rest of the country will offset the extra demand deriving from the higher levels of income and output in development areas. Therefore higher levels of tax will not be required to release resources for the subsidy. The White Paper discounted the idea that the premiums would only result in increases in wages, and that firms would use them to increase profits and not reduce prices. It remains to be seen whether the assumptions which have just been outlined are correct.

In November, 1967 at the time of Britain's devaluation of the £1, it was announced that the rebates (7*s.* 6*d.* in the case of full-time male employees) would be withdrawn from manufacturing industries outside the development areas, but retained within them. This measure goes a little further in favouring the development areas. However it is proposed to stop this premium in April, 1970.

The Budget of 1968 announced that rates of S.E.T. for full-time employees would be increased by 50% from September 1968, and some minor modifications were made. Part-time employees were not subject to the increase. Also workers over sixty-five (about 190,000 in 1968) on whom employers at present pay the full rates will be charged only at the same rate as part-time employees. A minor concession was also announced whereby hotels, inns, boarding-houses, and other small establishments with a minimum of four bedrooms in certain rural parts of development areas would be entitled to a refund of payments.

In July, 1969 the rates of S.E.T. were increased by a further 28% so that the rate is 48*s*. a week for an adult male employee, 24*s*. for women and boys, and 16*s*. for girls.

What emerges from this is that a powerful new fiscal tool has been made. The net yield, that is after allowing for refunds and premiums to manufacturing industry in development areas, is about £600 million a year. The tax as shown by the changes that have already been made, is extremely flexible. It is now used to discriminate between different regions of the country, different sectors of the economy, and by age, sex and time worked. More controversially, it could be developed to discriminate between efficient and inefficient firms.

The real question-mark that hangs over the S.E.T. is whether it should be replaced by a value added tax. This will be considered in Chapter 14.

Betting and gambling

To the future historian the most surprising thing about betting and gambling may well be the length of time that elapsed before they were taxed. This was so in spite of the example, from a number of other countries, that large sums could be raised from this source. The reasons for this immunity have been partly objections on moral grounds and partly difficulties of collection. Winston Churchill's betting levy between 1926 and 1929 was a failure, and may have acted as a deterrent.

A pool betting tax was introduced in 1947. This was a tax virtually confined to football pools, which were taxed at 33⅓% on weekly turnover. At 10% totalisator tax on dog-races was also imposed at the same time.[2] The pools tax was reduced to 25% on weekly turnover when football fixed-odds betting was introduced at 25% in 1964. The totalisator tax on dog races was reduced to 5% at the same time.

It was not until the Finance Act of 1966 that an attempt was made to tax gambling and betting more comprehensively. This Act intro-

[2] In 1963 bookmakers at dog-tracks were required to have an excise licence varying from £6 to £48, according to the number of enclosures. In 1964 the licence fees were halved. The duty was abolished with the Finance Act, 1966.

duced a 2½% tax on the amount staked with a bookmaker or on a totalisator, so that the tax on dog-races was again reduced. The tax on football pools remained at 25%. In addition, gaming was taxed by requiring premises where gaming was carried on to have an annual gaming licence.

The Budget of 1968 increased the betting tax from 2½% to 5%, and raised the pool betting duty to 33⅓%. Fees for gaming licences were also raised.

COLLECTION OF THE BETTING TAX

The betting tax on the amount staked on any bet with a bookmaker on or after October 24th, 1966, is now standardized at the rate of 5%, regardless of the type of event or contingency which is the subject of the bet.

The bookmaker or operator of a totalisator is responsible for payment of the duty, which is due when the bet is made and *not* when the account is settled. The collection of the tax is administratively straightforward. The operator of the totalisator normally pays the tax weekly. The most usual method for a bookmaker is to purchase betting-duty sheets in advance of the duty becoming due, on which summarized details of the bets have to be recorded. The sheets are available in various denominations, from £1 to £500.[3] The alternative method of paying the tax applies only to off-course bookmakers, who may apply to make monthly returns. Approval is subject to the bookmaker's satisfying minimum security arrangements in order to safeguard the revenue. Since 1969 an annual licence for premises used for off-course betting has to be taken out. The cost is three times the rateable value of the premises, or £150 in the case of premises with no rateable value.

INCIDENCE OF THE TAX

Bookmakers have not yet, it appears, settled standardized procedures for passing on the betting tax. Initially some appeared to be bearing the tax themselves while others changed the odds so as to recoup

[3] In respect of betting premises, the value of the sheets purchased must be at least equal to the duty liability incurred in the last week but one during which the bookmaker carried on bookmaking on the premises concerned, less any duty credit or plus any duty debit brought forward from that week. In respect of on-course bookmakers, the value of the sheets are related to the price of admission to the track for horse-racing and to the number of enclosures for dog-races.

themselves. An increasing number either deduct the tax from winnings or charge the tax on the money staked.[4]

GAMING

Gaming was first brought into the tax net in 1966 by requiring premises where gaming was carried on to have an annual gaming licence. The cost of this licence varies with the rateable value of the premises and according to whether bingo only is played or other gambling games. In 1969 the system was changed in respect of places where bingo only is played. These are now subject to a duty of 2½% of the stakes plus one thirty-ninth of any amount by which the value of the prizes exceeds the duty. Premises where other gambling games are played are still subject to duty by an annual licence whose cost varies with the rateable value of the premises as follows:

Rateable value of premises	Duty per annum
Not exceeding £1,000	£750
Between £1,000 and £1,500	£7,500
Between £1,500 and £2,250	£20,000
Between £2,250 and £3,000	£40,000
Exceeding £3,000	£100,000

Also an annual licence is required for a gaming machine (one-armed bandit) in a club. If operated by a coin of 3*d*. or less this now costs £50 for a single machine and £150 for each subsequent machine. If operated by a 6*d*. the cost is £100 for the first machine and £300 for subsequent machines. Machines for gambling with prizes in amusement arcades have since 1969 been taxed at £25 for the first and £150 for subsequent machines if operated by a 6*d*. and at half these rates if operated by a coin of 3*d*. or less.

CONCLUSIONS

So soon after the passing of the Betting and Gambling Act only tentative conclusions can be drawn. The overall impression seems to be that the tax is working well, and revenue has been greater than was estimated.

[4] The procedure is sometimes adopted of deducting 6*d*. on winnings (or stake money as the case may be), up to 10*s*., 1*s*. between 10*s*. and a £1, and pro rata. So that a bookmaker with four 5*s*. bets collects 2*s*. This is almost certainly in excess of his expenses incurred in collecting the tax and his liability to pay 1*s*. in the £1 on the amounts staked, an example, with many previous precedents of a sum greater than the tax being passed on to the consumer.

The idea of taxing some forms of betting at 33⅓% and others at 5% is hard to justify. The rate of 5% looks ridiculous when it is compared with the high marginal rates of income tax and surtax and many indirect taxes. The argument is sometimes put forward that betting and gambling reflects a circular flow of income, with most of the stake-money being returned to the winners and being restaked and so on, and that to tax at higher rates would kill the industry. Since all economic activity can be represented as a circular flow, this argument hardly provides a case for lower taxes on betting and gambling.

The device of taxing gambling by grouping rateable values of the premises in five sizes is obviously an extremely crude procedure. This is not the place to examine alternatives, but examples from a number of foreign countries show that there are feasible and better alternatives.

Summary

Britain, in common with other developed countries, shows a marked increase this century in government expenditure, and hence in tax. Political pressures, growth and concentration of population, the wish of the community to spread income and wealth more evenly can be selected as major forces that have helped to shape expenditure and revenue. From the side of revenue, two world wars, as well as focusing attention on social ills has enabled fiscal innovation to take place and given governments larger tax resources after the war to continue a higher rate of expenditure.

Two recently introduced taxes were examined. Selective employment tax, introduced in 1966, is a powerful new fiscal weapon that is extremely flexible. As well as raising considerable amounts of revenue, it is used to discriminate between different regions of the country, different sections of the economy, and by age, sex, and time worked. The harsh comments on this tax, from many quarters, may be a tribute to the success it is having in achieving some of these objectives, but it is too soon to make any objective judgment. The adoption of a value-added tax (necessary if Britain joins the Common Market) would almost certainly replace S.E.T., and it is difficult to see any future Chancellor of the Exchequer being able to give up such a flexible and lucrative tax as S.E.T. for anything less than a tax on value-added lines.

The Finance Act of 1966 introduced a much more comprehensive tax on betting and introduced a tax on gambling. This area of taxation still exhibits many illogicalities, with different forms of betting taxed at different rates and gambling taxed by the crude method of taxing the rateable value of premises where the activity takes place. It is still the case that a person who has spending power from earning will be likely to pay a great deal more in tax than a person who has the same sum as a result of a bet or by gambling.

11
The criterion of ability to pay

There is still much of sham even in our big redistributional reforms. Our taxation is advertised to be, and is commonly believed to be, steeply progressive, but by various devices the tax laws are permitting the rich to become richer while they live well, in spite of their paying most of their 'incomes' in taxes. In Britain and some other countries, where generous means are provided for avoiding inheritance tax by giving away the wealth in advance of one's death, the situation is almost scandalous, though it is largely concealed from workers and salaried people who are really pressed by taxation and social insurance payments. In Sweden and the United States the tax system is more rigorous, but even there the real incidence of taxation is very different from what it seems to be.

GUNNAR MYRDAL (1960), *Beyond the Welfare State.*

From the discussion in Chapter 9 of the benefit and ability to pay approaches it was clear that, given the current objectives of society, the benefit principle by itself cannot serve as an adequate guide to taxation policy. Some form of criterion based on ability to pay is needed and this is now examined.

Horizontal and vertical equity

The ability-to-pay criterion has to be seen in a broad setting. One of the few principles in public finance that commands wide acceptance is the so-called principle of *horizontal equity*—'that people in equal positions shall be treated equally'. On *vertical equity*—that is, the treatment of people in unequal positions—there is no such agreement. Regressive, proportional and progressive taxes have all been advocated at different times. There is probably widespread agreement today that taxes that fall on the 'better-off' rather than the 'worse-off', and are progressive rather than proportional, are to be preferred. Widely differing views are held on the degree of progressiveness that is desired. The author's opinion is that the economist, as economist, has no special competence to decide this question, which is essentially an ethical one. In democratic societies the decision is decided by political means. The economist can help in pointing out the likely economic consequences of this or that degree of progression, but society as a whole has to decide how much these factors shall count.

In the search for a correct criterion to judge ability to pay, in order to achieve horizontal equity, claims are put forward for income, wealth and expenditure.

By 'wealth' is meant the accumulated assets of a person or institution as opposed to 'income', which are receipts that accrue per period of time. Taxing wealth by itself is unlikely to provide sufficient revenue, and the issue is between those who would like to see wealth taxed separately and those who would like to see the definition of income broadened so as to take in changes in wealth. The latter solution is developed in this book, although reference is made to the alternative of taxing wealth separately.

As an alternative, expenditure has been put forward as the better criterion (see Kaldor, N. (1955)). Any distinction between income and wealth becomes irrelevant with an expenditure tax: both are taxed, not as they accrue, but when they are spent. However, the difference in principle between these concepts is not as wide as it might appear at first glance. The issue is not, it should be stressed, one of progressiveness. It is possible to build into a tax system on either base whatever degree of progressiveness is required. An expenditure-based tax does not have to entail the detailed recording of expenditures. These can be computed as the difference between certain money incomings and outgoings. Forms to compute expenditures in this way would be somewhat more complicated than the current income tax form, but not unduly so. The real difference between taxes on these different bases lies in the exemption from tax of savings under an expenditure tax. In a general way, using consumption (i.e. expenditure) as a base is taxing according to what a person takes out of the common pool; income with what he puts into the common pool.

There are a number of reasons for not developing the idea of an expenditure-based tax here, besides the necessity to keep this book within limits. One is that an expenditure tax has been brilliantly elaborated by Kaldor in his book cited above. Another that has just been noted is that in practice the only major difference between an expenditure tax and the tax on total accretion lines that is developed here lies in the different treatment of savings. Most of the problems that have to be dealt with are common to both. The pros and cons of the argument of whether it is desirable (since savings increase with wealth and income) to exempt savings from tax are discussed by Kaldor. It should be noted that because he is arguing for a progressive tax on expenditures, this mitigates to some extent for not taxing savings. Finally, there is the practical consideration that most countries do not use an expenditure-based system. It is income which is used, and the concept has been elaborated over many years. To this problem we now turn.

Definition of income

One concept of income has gained wide acceptance, and is termed *total accretion*. Income is defined to equal consumption during a given period, plus increase in net worth valued at market prices for the beginning and the end of the period. Income is thus defined to include consumption, savings and changes in wealth. The principle is uncompromising: all accretions to wealth are included, in whatever form they are received or from whatever source they accrue. In practice the principle may have to be modified, but if it is accepted as a principle it gives a basis from which to judge our present tax system and proposed changes. The principle accepts that a change in net worth may be negative—in other words, gains and losses should be allowed for.

The Memorandum of Dissent to the *Royal Commission on the Taxation of Profits and Income Final Report* (June, 1955), sets out very clearly the rationale behind this definition (para. 5):

> In our view the taxable capacity of an individual consists in his power to satisfy his own material needs, i.e. to attain a particular living standard. We know of no alternative definition that is capable of satisfying society's prevailing sense of fairness and equity. Thus the ruling test to be applied in deciding whether any particular receipt should or should not be reckoned as taxable income is whether it contributes or not, or how far it contributes, to an individual's 'spending power' during a period. When set beside this standard, most of the principles that have been applied at one time or another, to determine whether particular types of receipt constitute income (whether the receipts are regularly recurrent or casual, or whether they proceed from a separate and identifiable source, or whether they are payments for services rendered, or whether they constitute profit 'on sound accountancy principles', or whether, in words of the Majority, they fall 'within the limited class of receipts that are identified as income by their own nature') appear to us to be irrelevent. In fact, no concept on income can be really equitable that stops short of the comprehensive definition which embraces all receipts which increase an individual's commands over the use of society's scarce resources—in other words, his 'net accretion of economic power between two points of time'.

It cannot be emphasized too strongly that the consequence of adopting this definition of income would be that current rates of income tax could be reduced without a loss in revenue, or indirect taxes could be reduced, or some downward reduction made in both. In other words, at present income, in the narrow sense, bears a disproportionate share of tax precisely because spending power other than income is taxed less or not at all. For example, capital gains are taxed differently according to whether they are made within twelve months or longer: if realized within twelve months they are taxed at income rates, otherwise if, after offset for losses, they exceed £50 they are taxed at what for a standard-rate-payer will be a lesser rate. Betting and gambling is taxed at flat rates, Earned income is taxed less than unearned income. Inherited wealth is not taxed according to the position of the recipient, but according to the wealth of the donor. Gifts were not taxed at all unless the donor died within five years of making the gift. This was changed to seven years in 1968, so that a gift *inter vivos* remains fully dutiable for four years. In the fifth, sixth and seventh years relief is given of 15%, 30% and 60% respectively. Enough has been said to make it clear that the present system is the result of the haphazard growth of the tax and benefit system over the years.

Is the principle workable?

It is one thing to talk about a principle. Is it workable in practice? As a preliminary we shall deal briefly with the drawbacks of the present system, and then go on to deal with the difficulties of implementing the accretion principle. These difficulties are present in our existing system; some would be emphasized in the system of accretion.

Possibly the main drawback of the present system has already been mentioned. It is curious that it has not received more attention. That is, by the present very narrow definition of income, any receipt unfortunate enough to fall into this category is liable to a steeply progressive tax. Widening the base would give the authorities room to manœuvre: a greater range of small incomes could be exempt from tax, or rates throughout the range could be reduced, or some compromise made between these two.

From this advantage it would follow that there would be no gain in reshuffling assets (from, say, income to capital gains), because both would be income and subject to the same tax. The so-called 'blight' of modern times, the amount of time, money and effort which goes into tax-avoidance, would be lessened. (Avoidance is used here to mean legal means to reduce tax.) Tax-avoidance has always, and probably always will be, a profitable occupation, but the great reductions in taxation that can be achieved under the present system has virtually made it into an industry. It is not the purpose of this book to specify the means of avoidance at length, but the subject is important enough to merit mention. Estate-duty-avoidance is looked at in Chapter 15.

Numerous devices have been thought up to reduce tax on income. Some of the practices mentioned have now been stopped, or modified to limit abuse, but efforts to find new loopholes may be expected to continue unabated, given the present very diverse rates of tax on different receipts. Employers, instead of a salary increase to their top executives, may offer generous non-contributory pensions, a wide range of 'fringe benefits' and lavish entertainment expenses. An old favourite is to turn income into capital gains, which formerly went untaxed and now, if long-term gains, are taxed at a maximum rate of 30% if in excess of £50. Share options to employees and various forms of 'dividend stripping' were the best-known among these devices. It will be pointed out in the chapter on 'Personal Income Tax' (Chapter 12) that advantages may accrue to the person who is able to arrange his affairs under the mantle of company status.

Titmus, R. M. (1962), 72, has pointed out that

> The British system of taxation is almost unique in the world in recognizing a payment voluntarily undertaken by the taxpayer as a charge on his income, provided that payment (*a*) is made under a promise backed by a deed of covenant extending to a period of more than six years; (*b*) is not made in favour of an unmarried infant of the convenantor; (*c*) is not in exchange for value received from (or goods or services rendered by) the recipient.

In a footnote to this section he adds:

> Covenants by men in favour of their mistresses can only be regarded as ineligible for tax relief if the Inland Revenue can establish that they are given 'for services rendered' (see Monroe, J. G., 'Annual and Other Periodical Payments', *British Tax Review*, December, 1956, 289).

Implementation of the total-accretion principle

The total-accretion principle is defined as accretion to wealth, which is equal to consumption plus increase in net worth valued at market price for the beginning and the end of the period. The chief problems are presented by (1) valuation, (2) inflation or deflation, (3) fluctuating income, (4) the tax-paying unit.

VALUATION

As anybody who has had something to do with valuation for purposes of estate duties will know, valuation can cause a great deal of work and involve a great deal of arbitrariness. There is little problem with items which are standardized and traded regularly, such as quoted company shares. Unquoted shares, unique items, such as original paintings, plots of land and so on, are much more difficult to value, short of actual sale in the market-place. On the grounds of practicality, it seems that annual or periodic valuation is ruled out. The item would be brought into the tax-net on sale, or on death of the owner, when valuation has to take place in any case. It is argued against this that such a process discriminates in favour of people who enjoy unrealized accretion. This is true, but it seems to have little weight against the bigger distortions that have been mentioned, caused by not taxing some items at all. Similar considerations apply to the argument that treating as income on sale will interfere with the market process of buying and selling. Once again it is necessary to weigh any loss likely to be caused in this way with the undoubted losses and distortions caused by the present system.

INFLATION OR DEFLATION

Should the valuation of assets and liabilities allow for changes in the value of money—that is, for inflation or deflation? It is argued that a gain of, say, £100 on selling shares is a gain in money terms only, that what should be relevant is the gain in real terms—that is, the gain in command over goods and services. In inflationary conditions this gain will clearly be less than £100 and vice versa.

Most commentators agree that in principle changes due to changes in the value of money should be allowed for all receipts, whether income, capital gains or anything else. That is, in principle, it should be in real terms. However, most also agree that in practical terms money values will have to be used. The difficulties of finding a correct index, or indexes, with which to obtain real values are a serious deterrent to working with deflated values, and allowing for inflation would be administratively complex. Because of these difficulties, it is by no means clear that a system which attempts to take account of inflation and deflation would be more equitable than one that doesn't.

To argue for compensation for changes in the value of money for all receipts is not, however, a good argument for compensation for some of these receipts.

At the moment a money-wage increase which restores the real purchasing power of wages to the level of the previous year nevertheless results in more tax being paid if tax rates are unaltered. The claim that one particular slice of income should be protected from changes in the value of money thus begins to look like special pleading on behalf of interested parties.

If the principle is good for one, it is good for all, but of course, adjustment for all loses much of its point. The government starts out with clear ideas of the amount of revenue it wants from the economy; if adjustments were made on the income side for price changes adjustments would have to be made on the revenue side to tax rates to secure that the tax revenue target was reached. The only change from the present system is that the government obtains more revenue[1] from inflation at the moment if it keeps tax rates the same. If adjustments were made automatically to income, then the present hidden increase in tax revenue would not occur. In other words, if the government wanted more revenue it would have to increase rates rather than rely on the automatic increase brought about by inflation.

A similar argument is used when it is asserted that, since capital gains can accrue over a long period of time, it is unjust to tax them at income rates. The valid point in this argument is that the realization of capital gains will, under a progressive tax structure, raise the tax liability in the year in which the gains are realized, over the liability which would have been incurred if the gain had been realized evenly over time. The remedy for this is some form of averaging of income for tax purposes, a measure which is desirable under any form of progressive tax. This will be touched on in the next section. The assertion that capital gains are different from other income cannot be sustained under the total-accretion concept. This concept seeks the 'taxable capacity' of a person: it is irrelevant whether one person has a higher taxable capacity than another, due to higher earnings, receipt of a legacy, receipt of a capital gain or in some other way. A person who invests money in shares which show a gain in money terms is better off than a person whose shares show no gain or a loss: the degree of inflation or deflation cannot alter this conclusion.

It is also argued that a capital gain is illusory if the proceeds are to be reinvested in a similar asset. Thus in the case of a house purchased for £1,000 and sold for £3,000, it is probable that the whole of the proceeds will be needed to reinvest in a similar type of property. This is easily seen as a case of special pleading: that house-owners should be protected against inflation as opposed to other groups. The person who invests £1,000 in a house in the above example gains over the person who invests the £1,000 in securities and makes the same gain. The latter person will pay tax on his gain and be at a disadvantage in entering the housing market in competition with

[1] Whether the government gets more revenue in real terms with inflation depends on the degree to which its expenditures are affected by the inflation, the people who obtain an increase in income and the degree of progression of tax to which these people are subject.

the former householder. The fact that owner-occupied houses are exempt from capital gains for social and political reasons should not be allowed to obscure the fact that once an owner obtains a house (on the assumption that his property moves in line with the general market trend in house prices) he is largely indifferent to the subsequent trend in house prices. A wedge is driven between those who have houses, who are largely protected from subsequent inflation in house prices, and those who subsequently enter the market.[2]

Although housing was selected as an example, the principles involved apply to any asset; exemption from tax confers benefit on existing owners of the asset *vis-à-vis* the rest of the population. It is not suggested that no case can be made for the exemption of certain assets, but that the nature of the privilege being conferred needs careful examination. No presumptive economic argument can be set up that particular assets merit exemption.

PRO OR CON?

In the mass of words on the subject of inflation and capital gains the assumptions of the protagonists are seldom made explicit.

Those who argue that capital gains should take inflation into account presumably have in mind some concept akin to 'keeping capital intact'. If this is the correct premise, it is clear that taxing a paper gain is unjust.

Those who argue against this view take as their starting-point that what is relevant for taxation and equity purposes 'is the relative income positions of taxpayers'. If this is the correct premise, a person who has a capital gain in money terms is better off than a person who has no such gain or a loss, and should be taxed. On this assumption, not to tax a paper gain is unjust *or*, alternatively, everything should be adjusted for price changes.

This argument seems particularly protracted because the principle of 'keeping capital intact' is both a sound accounting principle and an unsound principle of public finance. The point has been investigated by successive Royal Commissions in relation to depreciation allowances for companies and whether these allowances should be based on historic or replacement cost. Allowances based on the latter would, of course, allow for price changes. Such a change has been decisively rejected. These questions will be discussed in some detail in Chapter 13 on 'Company Taxation'. The viewpoint adopted here is that, however desirable it may be for the individual to maintain

[2] This aspect of protection must also increase the demand for houses, and so be responsible in some degree for the rise in house prices.

his wealth position, it is no part of the fiscal system to do this for him. This aim of the fiscal system is not to maintain the status of those who happen to have wealth or to make gains. On the contrary, at any one time society aims for a certain degree of progression and a certain redistribution of income and wealth. The argument adopted here for the rejection of compensation for inflation is clear: inflationary and deflationary conditions affect all sectors of the community in different degrees; compensation for one sector results in less equity, not more. See Hockley, G. C. (January-February, 1968) and Wheatcroft, G. S. A. (January-February, 1968).

FLUCTUATING INCOME

The difficulty posed by any progressive tax is the inequity between those persons whose income fluctuates from year to year and those who receive their incomes in regular equal amounts. Authors, artists, sportsmen, farmers, fishermen and a number of people in professional occupations who rely on fees are likely to be in the former category.

As an illustration of inequity, an unmarried actor on rates of tax applicable in 1966-7, who receives £10,000 for a film and nothing for the next nine years, will pay about £4,284 in tax and surtax. On the other hand, a single man who receives a salary of £1,000 a year for ten years will pay approximately £186 in tax a year, or £1,860 in tax over ten years.[3]

The only provisions for spreading or averaging income at the moment apply to authors, to patent royalties and, since 1969, to painters and sculptors. The author of a literary, dramatic, musical or artistic work who sells the copyright or an interest in it for a lump-sum payment, or is in receipt of royalties from such a work, can sometimes spread his tax payments. This applies if he was engaged on the making of the work for more than twelve months. He can spread the payment over two years if the period of production does not exceed twenty-four months, and over three years if the period was longer. A person who is chargeable for tax in respect of a capital sum received on the sale of patent rights is entitled to spread the sum in equal amounts over the year of receipt and the five succeeding years. There is a further provision for spreading royalties received as consideration for more than two years' use of a patent. In this case the payment is spread back in equal annual instalments,

[3] The matter is not quite so simple as this example suggests. The actor will pay tax in arrears under Schedule D, while the salary-earner will pay as he earns under Schedule E. Claims for expenses are usually treated more leniently under Schedule D. This point will be taken up in Chapter 12 on 'Personal Income Tax'.

subject to a limiting number of six. The Budget in 1969 enabled painters and sculptors to spread the receipt for a work over the period during which it was made.

It needs to be stressed that the problem of fluctuating incomes occurs under the present tax system. The Royal Commission on the Taxation of Profits and Income in 1955 were of the opinion that 'it was quite impossible to regard as satisfactory the present position of fluctuating incomes' (para. 197). The problem becomes more acute under the accretion principle of income because more income will be volatile. Legacies and gifts are examples of receipts which cannot be expected regularly.

The seemingly straightforward solution of aggregating income over, say, a five-year period or a lifetime falls to the ground because if a person has a drop in income in any year, his tax bill in that year will be based on his average income over the relevant period which may be higher than his current income. The fact that a rising income gives a correspondingly lower tax bill does not compensate for the hardship which is likely to be involved in meeting high tax payments during periods of reduced income.

The usual assumption of averaging is that the total sum of taxes paid over the averaging period should be the same as if the income had been received in equal amounts in each year of the averaging period. With a five-year plan, tax could be computed by finding the average income over this period (that is, total income for the five years divided by five) and reworking the tax liability for each of the past years on the basis of this average. Not surprisingly, the Royal Commission on Tax (1955), para. 189, rejected proposals on these lines 'since the administrative burden of operating it cannot be contemplated'. However the assumption of the Commission that to achieve averaging, tax for past years must be reworked, is not a feature of all schemes of averaging. The Royal Commission on Taxation in Canada (1966) suggested the use of special averaging schedules which would mean that only one computation of tax would be necessary instead of a new computation for each year averaged. An alternative, using the current year's cumulative average income and subtracting from this the amount of taxes already paid for earlier years of the averaging period, is outlined by Vickray, W. (1947), 172-95 and 417-27. The deliberations and recommendations of the Royal Commission (1955) follow.

THE ROYAL COMMISSION ON THE TAXATION OF PROFITS AND INCOME, 1955

The Royal Commission considered a scheme of averaging income over five years. This was rejected on the grounds of an 'enormous volume of additional work that is inherent in averaging' (para. 198), and they came up with more limited proposals.

The 'enormous volume of additional work' came, it seems, from the necessity to ascertain income in virtually every case where there was any income at all. At the period the Commission were considering (1953-4), of the 20 million individuals in the U.K. with incomes above the exemption limit of taxation, 4¼ million were relieved of tax by the operation of allowances, and it was merely necessary to ascertain that such persons are free of liability. It was also stated that 'there would be a formidable task of recomputing the tax payable in each past year of the permitted period' (para. 199). Finally it was noted that this would add to the work of employees, in that their present dispensation from keeping P.A.Y.E. records of certain employees earning under £3 5*s*. a week could hardly be maintained.

On the first point the Report is not clear where the enormous volume of work comes from, since under the present system of tax it is necessary to establish whether a person has enough income to subject him to tax. Averaging does not necessary imply a change in tax allowances, and the number of persons assessed to tax need not be very different in the two cases. The necessity to recalculate past income is a characteristic of a particular scheme of averaging, but is not necessarily a feature of all averaging schemes. On the final point the number of employees below the exemption limits must be small.

At present a great deal of administrative effort goes into providing a large number of benefits. Chapter 18 suggests a possible simplification of these. A scheme of tax on the lines of the accretion principle of income with averaging and simplification of benefits might, after the change had been put through, result in a saving of manpower when both the Inland Revenue and other services are taken into account. Developments since 1955 in the field of computers may also have simplified the administrative task. The more limited proposals for averaging, on which the majority and minority reports of the Royal Commission agreed, was:

> Any taxpayer who can show that his total income for any year was not more than 50% of his total income for the previous year shall be entitled to have his total income for each of those two years assessed as if the aggregate income of the two years had accrued evenly throughout the period (para. 203).

If income again fell below 50% of the preceding year, averaging would occur over three years, and so on. It was recognized that special provisions would be needed when a taxpayer retired from active employment. This scheme was, it was said, 'nothing better than a rough-and-ready means of giving some alleviation to extreme cases of fluctuating income'.

Conclusion. Failure to adopt some form of averaging is unfair to those who have fluctuations in income. Any form of averaging will result in some complication of the tax system compared to a similar system without averaging: but not necessarily compared to a modified tax and benefit system. The amount of difficulty that would result from the introduction of averaging was greatly overstressed by the Royal Commission in 1955, because they worked on the assumption that tax in past years of the averaging period would have to be recalculated.

Even if it was found that an averaging scheme would take some years to work into the system, a simpler compromise could be used in the meantime. One possibility is to implement the suggestion of the Royal Commission. That in cases where a drop in income of 50% over the previous year's income occurs, the taxpayer should have his tax recalculated over the preceding year, and to supplement this with forward spreading of income in cases where income increases by 50% or more over the previous year. These situations would be mutually exclusive. The former situation, where income can be spread over the current and previous year being designed to cover the case where a taxpayer suffers a sharp reduction in earned income. The latter situation, where income can be spread in equal amounts over the year of receipt, and, say, the next two or three years (on the lines of current provisions for spreading a capital sum received on the sale of patent rights) being designed to cover exceptional receipts, such as the receipt of a large gift or legacy or exceptional income earned in one year.

These proposals are still 'rough-and-ready', but they do go some way to achieving equity. The scheme of the Royal Commission involves the greater administrative effort, but was considered feasible at the time. Forward averaging of exceptional receipts is not a great administrative burden. Provision could be made for a taxpayer, if he wished, to pay a provisional sum in tax in the year in which his large income occurred. This would be based on his estimated income in the years over which averaging was to take place. Adjustment would be made in future years if actual income differed from estimated income. The sum payable immediately could be discounted by a suitable rate of interest (since a deferred tax liability enables the capital to be invested and earn interest). The taxpayers concerned could then, if they wished, safeguard themselves against not having funds to meet their future liabilities.

THE TAX-PAYING UNIT

The problem of the tax-paying unit has been described as the most neglected problem in public taxation. If the structure of society is such that the composition of all tax-paying units is the same—say, a husband, wife and two children—we have little difficulty. But tax-payers differ greatly from those who are single with no dependants to look after, to married persons with large families and many dependants.

The Royal Commission on Taxation (1954), reported as follows:

> We have come to the conclusion that the taxation of the combined incomes of husband and wife as one unit is to be preferred to their separate taxation as separate units because the aggregate income provides a unit of taxation that is fairer to those concerned. That is why we do not recommend a departure from the present system. The combined incomes of married persons are sometimes described as a joint purse. We do not think that so wide a generalization can safely be made on such a question of social habit: but it does appear to us, on the one hand, that marriage creates a social unit which is not truly analogous with other associations involving some measure of joint living expenses and that to tax the incomes of two married people living together as if each were equivalent to the income of a single individual would give a less satisfactory distribution than that which results from the present rule. Such a method of taxation would mean that one married couple bore a greater or less burden of tax than another according to what must surely be an irrelevant distinction for this purpose—namely, the proportion in which the combined income was divided between the partners . . . (para. 119).

The Commission were sensitive to the abuses that can arise with separate assessment for husband and wife by the transfer of income from the spouse with the highest income (and therefore under a progressive tax to higher tax) to the partner with the lowest income. This abuse is most likely in the case of unearned income, as it is much more difficult to transfer earned income to another before tax is paid. The exception to this is provided by some private companies where the husband or wife can be paid a director's remuneration although they have little or nothing to do with the running of the business.

On the other hand, aggregation is hard on those married couples who both have high incomes. This point makes itself felt in particular where both spouses can earn high incomes. The extreme is found where the spouses earn equal amounts. For example, as single persons, people can earn up to £5,000 without paying surtax. As a married couple their joint income of £10,000 will attract £894 15*s*. in surtax. In addition, a joint salary of this magnitude will attract

£138 more in income tax, because the earned income allowance by which two-ninths is allowed to be deducted from earned income before tax is payable is diminished to one-ninth on incomes above £4,005, and disappears entirely on incomes above £9,945.

We have reached one of the many conflicts in public finance. To make the unit of taxation the individual may seem unjust to single persons who are not in a position to spread their incomes to a wife. To make the unit of taxation the married couple may seem unjust to the married couple when both can earn high incomes. The argument can be extended to children. Should their income be included in the income of their parents? In other words, why should we draw the line of the tax unit at husband and wife, rather than the family or the household? If the family or the household, how should these be defined?

This problem is one that is inherent with any system of progressive taxation. The moral, if one is to be drawn, is that our current system is likely to be far from perfect, that changes in tax modify the impact on the individual and on the family and, in the absence of any clear criteria for finding an equitable tax unit, would seem to call for periodic examination of the current tax position. Such an examination will be deferred until Chapter 18, where it is broadened out to account not only for taxes paid but also for benefits received by single persons and married persons with and without children.

THE TAXATION MIX

It should be clear from what has already been said that the total-accretion principle is an attempt to achieve horizontal equity. The assumption is made that the source of income is a matter of indifference. Whatever the source, it represents purchasing power, and should therefore be included in income. It should also be clear on reflection that other types of tax do more or less violence to the principle of horizontal equity. Taxes on consumption goods will fall unequally on persons in equal positions if they have different consumption patterns. Most noticeable, if tobacco and alcohol are to retain their present very high rates of tax for social reasons, then two individuals in equal positions, except that one smokes and drinks and the other does not, will pay very different amounts of tax.

In Chapter 9 the benefit principle of tax and the social cost argument were examined. It is clear that the application of either is likely to violate the ability to pay approach of the accretion principle.

The impossibility of laying down a universal principle of tax which will be valid under all conditions is that the extent of government activity varies widely. In a mixed economy the government may be providing services which would not be provided at all, or provided on an insufficient scale, if left in private hands. In such cases as this, the benefit principle is not applicable, and defining ability to pay is essential if equity is to be achieved. At the other extreme the government may be providing goods and services which could equally well be provided by private enterprise (albeit under some form of monopoly regulation). Steel, telephones, railways and power are cases in point. Here failure to charge on the benefit principle is likely to cause a misuse of the nation's resources.

A division on these lines is, in a rough-and-ready manner, apparent in our society. The nationalized industries are expected to pay their way—although at any one time this instruction may fail to be realized. It has already been argued that if these industries are to be expected to pay their way, and this is desirable on allocation grounds, then it is essential that social functions which these services are expected to serve should be clearly separated from their strictly commercial activities. Then the commercial side can be expected to pay its way, and the activities that are continued for social reasons, because the social benefits outweigh the money cost involved, should be subsidized out of general taxation based on ability to pay.

Thus the following conclusions are drawn: many government services either cannot be charged to individuals, such as defence and justice, or should not be charged because of neighbourhood and social effects, e.g. transfer payments, education and health. For these services, taxation according to ability to pay is necessary: the accretion principle has been set out as a method of judging ability to pay. Commercial activities should be charged on the benefit principle.

These conclusions do not still controversy. General agreement is, however, likely over a wide range of services which can be classified unambiguously in one category or the other. Some areas remain controversial, e.g. some people argue that higher education should be financed by loans on a benefit basis rather than grants. Here it is necessary to weigh the advantages and disadvantages that flow from the alternative ways of financing. Charging the beneficiary is likely to deter the use of the good or service, and this needs to be weighed against the social loss involved.

Company taxation is rather more controversial. It can be argued that companies belong to individuals and that company income (both distributed profits and undistributed profits) should be allocated to individuals as part of their income. Imputing undistributed profits to shareholders is not difficult administratively, but is impractical for incentive reasons. A case can be made for taxing companies as well as individuals. This will be further considered in Chapter 13 on 'Company Taxation'.

Whether estate duties should continue is once again a wider issue that a democratic country has to decide through the polls. The accretion principle would, we have seen, include bequests and gifts, along with other additions, as income. The issue is whether estate duties should be imposed as well. On the grounds of the very marked inequality of wealth in Great Britain, a case can be made for additional estate duties in some form.

It is estimated (by Revell, J. R. S., quoted by Meade, J. E. (1964)) that in 1960 the wealthiest 1% of the population owned 42% of personal wealth and the wealthiest 5% owned 75%. In this example the population is taken as individuals over twenty-five years of age in England and Wales. The difficulty in interpreting these figures is to know what degree of concentration of wealth is to be expected. If wealth was accumulated only out of savings, the natural progression would be for a person to have low or negative wealth under, say, thirty-five years of age as family commitments are taken on. Ages fifty on to retirement would see wealth at a peak, with gradually diminished wealth after retirement. Even more important is whether wealth is primarily held by husbands, by wives, or jointly. It is likely that those with very much wealth will adopt some form of sharing in order to minimize the impact of death duties.

Table 1 sets out the home population of England and Wales as given by the 1961 Census of Population, divided into males and females and those below thirty-five years of age and those thirty-five and over.

Table 1

(Thousands)

Age	Total Population	Males	Females
All	46,105	22,304	23,801
Below thirty-five	22,492	11,427	11,065
Thirty-five or over	23,613	10,877	12,736

Source: *Annual Abstract of Statistics, 1967*, Table 8.

On the assumption that wealth is owned by both males and females over thirty-five years of age, this would mean that wealth would be owned by 23,613,000 persons, or 51% of the population. On the extreme assumption that wealth is owned only by males over thirty-five, this would be 10,877,000, or 24% of the population, as potential wealth-owners.[4] The figures above give 5% of the population, or 2,305,250 persons, as owning 75% of the wealth. This represents a marked degree of inequality on any reasonable assumption about the sector of the population that can be expected to hold wealth.

In concluding this brief section on the coexistence of different types of tax, we again come up with the problem that not all the considerations involved are economic ones. In trying to establish horizontal equity between taxpayers, we find that other taxes usually breech this principle. However, principles of taxation are set up as a guide to policy not as inflexible rules. There may well be social and other reasons for deliberately departing from a principle in particular cases. This does not make the principle invalid. On the contrary, it illustrates the use of the concept very well: instead of taxing in the present haphazard way, it enables taxes to be justified; it makes it that much harder for particular groups to indulge in special pleading.

Summary

Horizontal equity—that people in equal positions shall be treated equally—presents few problems of principle. The correct treatment of people in unequal positions, or vertical equity, is more difficult. Even when, as in all developed economies, progressive tax is generally agreed on, the precise degree of progression is an open one that has to be decided by political consensus.

Even in setting aside questions of progression as a political decision, the important point remains as to the criterion on which equal and unequal positions shall be judged—that is, what shall be the taxation base? Two claims have been put forward and generally acknowledged. One is that taxation should be based on expenditure. On this criterion, the source of spending power, whether it comes from income or wealth or exceptional receipts, is irrelevant: taxation accrues as spending takes place, not as accumulation proceeds. The other base broadens the definition of income so as to take in changes in wealth and other receipts. These concepts, at first sight so very different from each other, turn out to have only one major difference in principle: that expenditure as a base exempts savings from taxation while the other does not. The problems posed by valuation, inflation and deflation, fluctuating incomes (or fluctuating expenditures) and the tax-paying unit which are detailed in this chapter are common to both and indeed to any system of taxation.

[4] This assumption is clearly unrealistic for older persons. On average, women live longer than men, and it is known that in the upper age-groups, wealth is concentrated into the ownership of women, particularly widows.

12
Personal income taxation

Albert Einstein once admitted that working out his income tax was beyond him: he had to go to a tax consultant. 'This is too difficult for a mathematician,' said Einstein. 'It takes a philosopher.' *Time.*

In this chapter an outline will be given of the main taxes on personal income. However, as will be shown, it is impossible to treat personal tax entirely separately from tax on businesses. It is necessary to distinguish between the individual, the incorporated business, usually termed a company, which has a separate legal entity, and what will be termed unincorporated businesses. The most common form of unincorporated business is the partnership. Income of the unincorporated business is treated as the income of the persons concerned, but, as we shall see, treatment for tax differs in important respects from the tax treatment of the individual. Incorporated company tax will be treated in the next chapter.

This chapter deals first with income tax. Income tax was introduced by Pitt in 1797 as a temporary tax to help finance the Napoleonic Wars. It ended in 1816. It was reintroduced by Gladstone in 1842 again as a 'temporary measure', and has continued ever since. In the course of looking at income tax, the position of unincorporated businesses will be taken up. Surtax is then considered and an evaluation of income tax and surtax is made. Consideration is then given to the tax on capital gains.

The structure of income tax

Income tax is imposed by a Finance Act introduced every year, which determines the rates of tax and other details which are to apply to the next year beginning April 6th. The tax is chargeable under a number of schedules:

Schedule B applies to woodlands managed on a commercial basis.

Schedule C covers interest on public loans.

Schedule D covers income of a professional and business nature, namely:

Trades, including farms,
Professions and vocations,

and in addition income from a variety of sources, e.g.

Interest not taxed at source, e.g. bank interest.
Foreign securities.
Foreign possessions.
Miscellaneous profits, e.g. from letting.
Furnished accommodation.
Short-term capital gains.
Rents and other receipts from lands and buildings.

Schedule E covers income from employment—that is, wages, salaries, pensions and the like. The tax is collected by the employer under the system known as 'Pay as You Earn', so that the employee receives his remuneration net of tax.

Schedule F covers assessments on companies in respect of tax deducted by them from interest and dividends.

The missing Schedule A used to cover the imputed income from owning land and property before it was abolished in 1964-5. The important schedules for the majority of individuals are Schedules D and E.

The individual is allowed to make certain deductions from his income before tax is charged. The main deductions are:

(1) In the case of earned incomes, including pensions, a deduction of two-ninths is made on the first £4,005; on income between £4,005 and £9,945 one-ninth is deducted. Thus (ignoring other allowances for the moment) a person who has an income of £9,945 or more from investment income will be assessed for tax on the whole amount. Whereas, if the income is wholly earned, the maximum reduction is £1,550, leaving £8,395 to be taxed from an earned income of £9,945. Thus although it is common to regard the marginal rate of tax as the standard rate of tax in force (at present 8*s.* 3*d.* in the £1) this is incorrect for the majority of earned incomes. Relief of two-ninths brings the marginal rate down to 6*s.* 5*d.* in the £1. The marginal rate of tax refers to the amount of tax paid on the last £1 of income.

(2) Since 1969 from the sum arrived at under (1) a married man deducts £375, single persons, including widows and widowers, £255. If a wife is working, she is also, in effect, allowed an allowance equal to that of a single person if her salary or wage is great enough; otherwise she gets a proportion of the allowance.

(3) Further deductions are made in respect of children: £115 for each child under eleven, £140 for each child over eleven but not over sixteen, £165 for each child over sixteen. The latter allowance is subject to the child's receiving full-time educational instruction. Moreover, if a child has income in its own right exceeding £115 the allowance is reduced by the amount of its income in excess of £115.[1]

(4) Deductions are allowed to cover a variety of circumstances: for a widow or widower who has to employ a housekeeper; for dependent relatives; in respect of age and blindness; in respect of life assurance and interest payments on house mortgages. Since the 1969 Budget, interest on bank overdrafts is no longer generally allowed as a deduction.

(5) The Budget in 1967 allowed single women, widows and separated wives who are the sole supports of a dependent relative an increase in allowance from £75 to £110. Also the additional personal allowance of £40 for single people with single-handed responsibility for bringing up children was increased to £75 and increased again to £100 in 1969.

(6) Certain expenses occurred in obtaining the income are deductible before tax is charged.

The allowances outlined in (1) to (5) above apply to all individuals. As we shall see, the treatment of expenses, (6) above, differs according to whether tax is paid under Schedule D or Schedule E. After the appropriate allowances have been deducted, the first £260 of the remaining income is taxed at 6*s.* in the £1, the balance at 8*s.* 3*d.* in the £1. However, the computation of the income which is subject to tax differs for Schedule D and for Schedule E taxpayers.

Schedule D and Schedule E

The most important category falling under Schedule D are shopkeepers, professional persons working on their own account and

[1] These child tax allowances should not be confused with children's allowances, which are paid irrespective of income. These were introduced in 1946 at the rate of 5*s.* a week per child for all children except the first. This was raised to 8*s.* in 1952 and again by 2*s.* per week for third and subsequent children in 1956. From April, 1968, these were increased to 15*s.* for the second and 17*s.* for each younger child, and in October, 1968, these rates were increased by a further 3*s.* Although child allowances are paid irrespective of income, the increased benefit above 8*s.* is confined to small-income families, as tax allowances are changed so as to recoup the increase from income-tax-payers. This supplementation was well below the estimate of Beveridge of the average cost of subsistence of children, and still remains so, with the result that many low-income families have to seek Supplementary Benefit (see Hemming, M. F. W. (August, 1965)).

other unincorporated businesses; wages, salaries and pensions are covered by Schedule E.

In the case of wages, salaries and pensions, the matter is straightforward. Income as defined by current law (not to be confused with the definition of income under the total-accretion principle) is, using standard-tax terminology, called 'gross income'. From this gross income the appropriate personal allowances are deducted in order to arrive at 'taxable income', which is charged under Schedule E through the system known as 'Pay as You Earn'.

In the case of income from trades, farms and professions, it is necessary to ascertain the total statutory income; from this sum adjustments are made to cover the using up of capital involved in the business in order to arrive at the figure of taxable income. If more than one person is involved, the taxable income is allocated to the partners in whatever proportions the partnership has agreed on. This portion of the profits is then the 'gross income' of the person concerned, and after the personal allowances have been deducted we arrive at the taxable income of the individual as before.

First- and second-class citizens?

The growth of unincorporated and incorporated businesses in this century, and the increase in tax rates, brings up some of the most contentious problems in taxation. Incorporated businesses are taxed separately from individuals; the method of tax will be treated in Chapter 11, on 'Company Taxation'. A problem in equity arises if the incorporated company is in effect a 'one-man business' or partnership rather than a company owned by a large number of shareholders. Profits retained in the business do not count as income of the owner and are not therefore subject to progressive rates of personal income. This problem has long been recognized, and provision is made for a closely-controlled company which makes inadequate distributions to be charged income and surtax on the shortfall, except to the extent that it can show that retention of profits is necessary or advisable for the maintenance and development of its business. In the past this provision appears to have been used only rarely, and some income must have been subject to lower tax as a result.

A not dissimilar problem is in achieving equity between taxpayers who receive their income by way of wages and salaries and are therefore subject under Schedule E and those who receive income from unincorporated businesses and pay under Schedule D. The latter are able to deduct for the using up of capital before arriving at a figure of taxable profit,[2] and expenses are dealt with more leniently under Schedule D. Both the majority and minority reports of the Royal Commission on the Taxation of Profits and Income (1955) had much to say on this aspect of tax. The following quotations are from the Minority Report; the paragraph references therein refer to the majority report:

The other main aspect in which the present legal definition of taxable income causes inequality of treatment between classes of taxpayers concerns not receipts, but outlays. As the majority point out one particular source of these differences consists in the allowances given for the wastage of capital. The original theory which ignored the wastage of capital altogether 'has been profoundly modified in the course of time, but not to the same extent or in the same way in respect of all the different sources of income' (para. 38). While incomes derived from trades, vocations or professions 'now received a full allowance out of taxable income to make good money expended in acquiring assets that are used up in the production of the income' (para. 39), no allowances are given with respect to the capital expenditure incurred in vocational and educational training or for the expenditure which a man incurs 'in developing and improving his expert knowledge' (para. 41). . . . Another and, in our view, even more important cause of such inequality arises out of the difference in the legal definition of deductible expenses in respect of income from a trade, profession or vocation assessed under Schedule D, and in respect of income from an office, employment or pension assessed under Schedule E (paras. 19 and 21).

Both the Majority and Minority Reports of the Commission were agreed that it would be impracticable to extend the scheme of capital allowances to expenditure incurred on investment by the individual in the human person. The Minority Report adds: 'we believe therefore that short of withdrawing capital allowances altogether—a course that, on grounds of expediency, we should not favour—the difference in treatment cannot in this respect be avoided and ought therefore to be recognized and compensated for' (p. 361). Compensation could be achieved by taxing individuals at a lower rate or by imposing an annual charge, perhaps graduated to the size of the business, for the privilege of company status, whether of unincorporated or incorporated form.

On the 'even more important' point of deductible expenses no obviously best solution emerges.

[2] The taxable sum may be more or less than the profits shown in the books of the company. For example, if capital items have been charged to revenue this will be disallowed, as will purely personal expenditure of the proprietor. That is, these sums will be added back to arrive at a figure of taxable profit. Certain types of capital investment attract allowances, but the details of these will be left to Chapter 13.

Advertising and entertaining are typical examples of expenses incurred for building up the goodwill of a business, which though fully chargeable against the current year's receipts, are frequently linked with receipts, if at all, only through the enhancement of future rather than current earnings. Nothing similar to this would be a deductible expense under Schedule E. The wage- or salary-earner cannot charge as expenses the cost of entertaining his present or his potential future employers even though the expense might be 'wholly and exclusively' incurred with a view to securing for himself a better job. Nor could he charge the cost of training or education (whether in the form of a capital allowance or as current expenses) or the annual wear and tear to his physical earning powers. For all these reasons 'income' under Schedule E is not analogous to the net profit under Schedule D; it is more analogous to some conception of a 'gross profit' of trade, before the deduction either of depreciation or of all those other expenses which are not directly associated with the current receipts from trading activity (paras. 113 and 114).

The minority report goes on to point out the economic distortion that can result from these expense provisions. It refers to the 'very considerable subsidy from the Exchequer on outlays of doubtful value, which it might not have been worth the trader's while to incur at all in the absence of taxation'. The argument against extending these expense provisions to taxpayers under Schedule E is that these 'outlays of doubtful value' would be extended rather than curtailed. The argument against stopping these provisions is the difficulty of separating legitimate business expenses from other outlays, and the handicap which exporters would face if their overseas competitors continue to receive tax advantages.

Since the Report of the Royal Commission, action has been taken on two fronts. Deductible expenses under Schedule D have been tightened up and a slight relaxation of allowable expenses has occurred under Schedule E. The position, perhaps inevitably, still leaves many loopholes, and further changes are likely in the future.

If a value-added tax is adopted this would provide an opportunity to look afresh at the whole concept of capital allowances and deductible expenses. The agreed system of taxes towards which the Common Market countries are working would mean, if adopted in Britain, that her exporters would not be under a competitive disadvantage *vis-à-vis* European competitors.

Schedule D: other items

The other item under Schedule D which calls for comment is short-term capital gains. These are gains realized within twelve months of purchase. The types of gain which attract this tax will be dealt with in the section on the capital gains tax.

Surtax

Surtax was first introduced in 1909. It is an additional tax payable on incomes exceeding a certain amount. The practical effect of the tax is that since 1961 it is payable on earned income of a single person exceeding £5,000 and earned income of a married couple exceeding £5,120. For unearned incomes the figures are respectively £2,000 and £2,120.[3]

The actual computation of surtax need not concern us, because reliefs are allowed for children, dependent relatives and a housekeeper; the figures given above are the minimum figures at which surtax is payable. Because of these allowances, the figure at which an individual actually pays the tax will vary.

Income above the surtax limit is liable at the following rates:

	s.	*d.*	
On the first £500	2	0	in the £1
„ next £500	2	6	„ „
„ „ £1,000	3	6	„ „
„ „ £1,000	4	6	„ „
„ „ £1,000	5	6	„ „
„ „ £2,000	6	6	„ „
„ „ £2,000	7	6	„ „
„ „ £2,000	8	6	„ „
„ „ £3,000	9	6	„ „
On all beyond £15,000	10	0	„ „

The tax-paying unit

Chapter 11 looked at the problem of the tax-paying unit. In Great Britain the general rule is that income of husbands and wives is aggregated for tax purposes. The position of children's income depends on the source of the income. If the child has earned income in its own right, this is not aggregated with the income of the parent. However, for income, earned or unearned, in excess of £115 (the tax-allowance figure for a child) the parents lose a £1 of allowance for every £1 the child's income exceeds £115. For unearned income the general rule is that if parents settle property on their child the income is nevertheless counted as part of the income of the parents. This rule is an obvious one to reduce tax-avoidance. At the present time

[3] It is by virtue of a rebate on earned income and an additional earnings allowance of £2,000 that the starting-point of surtax for a single person is raised from £2,000 on unearned income to £5,000 on earned income. The corresponding figures for a married couple are £2,120 and £5,120 respectively.

there is a loophole: if the income is accumulated for the benefit of the child until he, or she, reaches twenty-one years of age surtax is not payable. The Chancellor announced in his Budget speech in 1968 that he was intending to alter this provision in 1969.

At the present time, where a grandparent or other person not being the parent makes a settlement of capital on a child (provided the donor receives no material benefit from the gift), the income thus produced can be applied for the child's benefit, e.g. for school fees, and this income is not aggregated with that of the parent. However, as from the tax year of 1969-70 this income will be aggregated with that of the parents. This change is on the lines suggested by the *Report of the Royal Commission on Tax* (1954), 77ff. The Budget in 1969 following the recommendation to reduce the age of majority from 21 years to 18 years also reduced the age for the aggregation of children's unearned income with parents' income to 18 years.

Evaluation of current income tax and surtax

A number of criticisms have been made in previous chapters. The prime one is not about the nature of income and surtax in itself, but the definition of income which is subject to these taxes. In this chapter attention has been drawn to some of the advantages which many individuals can obtain by forming themselves into unincorporated or incorporated companies.

Another criticism can be made: that reliefs given by way of tax concessions do not help the most needy. The present tax system, as we have seen, makes fairly elaborate provision for differences in taxpayers' circumstances. To recapitulate: earned income relief, single person's allowance of £255, married person's allowance of £375, allowances for dependent children, dependent relatives, in respect of age, for blind persons, and for certain interest payments, e.g. house mortgage payments, and life assurance premiums. In addition, the first £260 of taxable income is liable at 6*s*. in the £1, and the balance at 8*s*. 3*d*. in the £1.

Thus, because of earned income relief and a single person's allowance of £220, using the figures that applied up to April, 1969, a single man does not start paying tax until his income is just under £300; the corresponding figure for a married man is nearly £475. Thus the additional reliefs that a person might be entitled to are of no value to a single man whose income is below £300 and a married man whose income is below £475. To take an example, a married man with income below £475 obtains no benefit from the children's allowances even though he has children.

In a similar way, if we take children's allowances into account, a couple with one child do not start paying tax until their income is nearly £600, with two children over £700, with three nearly £900. Because of reduced rates of tax on the first £300 of taxable income, then, these figures become £900, £1,000 and £1,200 respectively before full tax relief is obtainable on further concessions, as, for example, interest or mortgage payments.

The tax system thus has built into it a system which helps those who are relatively well off without assisting the really poor. The surtax-payer gains most from the system of reliefs, the poorest members nothing. This paradox of the tax system is inseparable from the system of giving reliefs via income tax.[4]

It has been suggested that tax concessions should be extended to all citizens. Those citizens, for example, who have children and an income below £475 should receive a supplement equal in value to the allowance for a standard-rate taxpayer. Thus for a child under eleven the allowance against assessable income is £115, which at standard-rate tax of 8*s.* 3*d.* in the £1 is worth £47 8*s.* 9*d.* The present housing mortgage scheme was designed to overcome the drawback discussed above: a person can opt from 1968 either to pay the market rate of interest and claim a deduction from his assessable income or to take a loan at a reduced rate of interest. The basis of the social services and social provision is currently undergoing a reappraisal, and it can be questioned whether the housing scheme does more than partly patch up a system which needs more drastic remodelling. It can be argued, for example, that the need to extend the current tax concessions on life insurance is as great as in the case of mortgage interest. These matters will be extended in Chapter 18.

A look at the tax rates in force and working out a few examples will soon convince the reader that both the average rates of tax (income divided by tax) and the marginal rates of tax (tax paid on the last increment of income) do not impinge on higher and higher income levels in a smooth progression. Income tax is nearly a flat-rate tax, over £5,000 of earned-income surtax leads to progression.

The high rates of tax on very high incomes have frequently been said to act as a disincentive to effort, or to drive high-rate taxpayers

[4] Abel-Smith, B., and Townsend, P. (1965). This survey indicated that in 1960 there were 7·5 million persons, or 14% of the population, who were not living at a higher standard than 140% of the basic National Assistance scales. Poverty, as thus defined, *showed an increase* over a previous survey for the years 1953-4. The immediate causes of poverty were mainly old age and large families. The number of children in these households was estimated at 2¼ millions. They conclude (page 66): 'On the whole the data we have presented contradicts the commonly held view that a trend towards greater equality has accompanied the trend towards greater affluence.' See also Cole, D. and Utting, J. (1962) and *Circumstances of Families* (1967).

to take up residence abroad, although empirical evidence on this matter is largely lacking. Taking the latter point first, it has already been shown that these high rates are to some extent a sham because of the way income is at present defined. If the definition of income is reworked on the lines of the total-accretion principle then it may well be that the degree of progression in the system and the levels reached by the highest rates will have to be looked at anew. The present levels may well be tolerated because people reason that rough justice is being done: high rates on some parts of income being offset by low or no tax on other parts of income. The waste that this causes by the reshuffling of income and assets has already been noted. If income is redrawn on total-accretion lines and comes to form the main source of revenue, then also the problem of jumps in the degree of progression take on a more serious aspect.

A glance at the table on sources of revenue that appears in Chapter 9, on 'Revenue', will reveal a common error. There seems to be an almost universal tendency to take a particular tax in isolation from the rest of the tax system and to make judgments about the regressiveness or unfairness in one way or another of that particular tax. A particularly blatant form of this error is to assume that, because income and surtax, taken together, are highly progressive, we therefore have a highly progressive tax system as a whole. However, as the revenue table shows, income and surtax together account for roughly 33% of government revenue. Some of the other sources of revenue are regressive in their impact—for example, many of the Customs and Excise taxes and National Health contributions.

Capital gains tax

Sufficient has already been said to make it clear that the position before a capital gains tax was introduced was far from satisfactory.

The Finance Act, 1962 (passed by a Conservative government), was the first attempt at taxing capital gains. The importance lies not so much in the Act itself as in introducing the principle of taxing capital gains. The debate that preceded and followed the Act did much to blow fresh air into this corner of taxation, and made the passage of the more throughgoing Act of 1965 much easier. In 1965 the debate was hardly about the principle of taxing capital gains, which was now no longer a matter of party politics. Brief details of these two Acts follow before we attempt an evaluation of how far they succeeded in clearing up the previously unsatisfactory situation.

THE FINANCE ACT, 1962

This Act introduced the taxation of short-term gains. The short-term was defined as six months, except for land and buildings, where the period was three years or less. The tax applied to new transactions only: disposal of an asset acquired before April 10th, 1962, was not subject to the tax.

Assets chargeable to the tax included all forms of property other than those specifically excluded, whether situated inside or outside the United Kingdom. Thus stocks, shares, securities and land were included. The main assets excluded were an individual's main residence, tangible movable property and buildings (factories, shops, etc.) and ancillary land occupied and used solely for the purposes of a trade, profession or vocation, in the case of an acquisition and disposal by a person who occupies and uses them for such purposes.

Capital gains on chargeable assets, after allowance had been made for any capital losses, were treated as unearned income and taxed accordingly. The tax did not apply to gains on property passing at death.

It will be seen that this tax was a discretionary one in the sense that keeping assets other than land for six months and one day, and land for three years and one day gave complete immunity from the tax. Its importance, it has already been suggested, was in introducing the idea of taxing capital gains.

THE FINANCE ACT, 1965

This Act introduced a two-stage tax on capital gains realized by persons on the disposal of assets which occurred after April 6th, 1965 (companies' capital gains are charged to corporation tax). The first stage is a tax on short-term gains realized from the disposal within twelve months of acquisition of assets acquired after April 6th, 1965. These, as we have already seen, will be charged as income. They can thus be taxed at zero rate, or at surtax, or some intermediary rate according to the tax status of the recipient of the gain. The second stage is a long-term capital gains tax, i.e. on gains disposed of twelve months or more from the date of acquisition. These will be taxed at a flat rate of 30% unless it is to the individual's benefits to have the gains taxed on an alternative basis.

The alternative basis is that an individual may elect to settle his liability for tax (on the whole capital gain) by having part of the gain taxed at his marginal rate of income or surtax, as the case may be. The fraction of the gain to be counted as income is: (*a*) one-half where the net gains are less than £5,000, (*b*) where the net gain is more than £5,000, the sum of £2,500 is deducted from the total net gain. This alternative is a substantial concession. Rule (*a*) can be stated as: one-half of the marginal rate of tax is payable on the whole net capital gains where gains are below £5,000. With the standard rate of income tax at 8*s*. 3*d*. in the £, this is equivalent to a tax of 20·6% instead of 30%.

From the tax year 1967-8, long-term capital gains of individuals will be exempt from tax if, after deducting allowable losses, they do not exceed £50 for the year.

THE SHORT-TERM TAX

This tax followed the previous Act in charging short-term gains to income tax, but widened the range of assets and extended the time-period from six to twelve months. The range of assets is the same as that for long-term gains and will be dealt with under that heading. The 1962 time-limit of three years for land was abolished, land being treated in the same way as other assets chargeable under the short-term tax if realized within twelve months, or the long-term tax if over twelve months. However, since the Land Commission Act, 1967, land is now treated separately if it is sold for a new use. Details of this Act are given in Chapter 16. A gain made on the change of ownership of land where no change in the land's existing use occurs is still taxed as a capital gain.

The short-term tax does not, however, apply to capital gains deemed to be realized at death. These gains, even though the assets have been owned for less than twelve months, are chargeable to the long-term tax, i.e. at what in most cases will be a lower rate.

Losses can be offset against short-term capital gains and, if necessary, carried forward; offset is not allowed against long-term capital gains or other income.

THE LONG-TERM TAX

The long-term tax applies to assets sold after April 6th, 1965, which have been held for one year or more. The time of acquisition of the asset is immaterial: it could have been acquired before or after 1965, but the tax is not retrospective. For assets owned on April 6th, 1965, only the proportion of the gain attributable to the period after April 6th, will be taxable. The gain can be ascertained in one of two ways. One is the difference between the amount actually received on sale and its market value on April 6th, 1965. In the case of securities quoted on the Stock Exchange, there is no difficulty in ascertaining market value at this date; in some other cases this may be difficult if a valuation of the asset has not been undertaken. The second method of ascertaining the taxable gain is a straight time-apportionment formula. Thus an asset acquired for £100 one year prior to April 6th, 1965, and sold one year after for £200 would attract tax on half of the gain, i.e. £50. If the asset had been kept for two years after April 6th, 1965, and if it was still sold for a gain of £100, then two-thirds of this sum would attract tax, i.e. £66⅔.

ASSETS CHARGEABLE

The general presumption is that all assets are chargeable to either the short- or long-term tax unless they are exempt. The main exemptions are a principal private residence to the extent that it is occupied as such, Savings Certificates, Premium Bonds, Defence Bonds, and National Development Bonds, normal life-assurance policies on surrender or maturity, tangible movable property (i.e. chattels) disposed of for £1,000 or less and, since March, 1958, tangible movable assets which are wasting assets; important works of art and other objects of national, scientific, historic or artistic interest, provided that they remain in this country and are not sold otherwise than to a national institution, university or local authority, the first £5,000 of net gains (i.e. gains less losses) deemed to be realized at death, gifts of chargeable assets, provided that their value does not in total exceed £100 for each individual donor each year, and private motor vehicles. Since April 1969 government securities, or securities issued by a public corporation and guaranteed by the government, are not chargeable to long-term capital gains tax or, in the case of long-term gains of companies, corporation tax. This budget also excluded from the long-term capital gains tax, gains that do not exceed £50 in any year.

OFFSET FOR CAPITAL LOSSES

Losses can be offset against capital gains in any year, and if gains are not sufficient, net losses can be carried forward without time limit and set against gains of future years. Losses, however, can be offset only against long-term gains, and cannot be offset against short-term gains or other income.

GAINS ON BEQUEATHED PROPERTY

Assets are deemed to be realized on the death of their owner and capital gains are taxed at the long-term rate (even if the assets were acquired within twelve months); however, the first £5,000 of net gains are exempt from the tax.

EXEMPTION FROM THE TAX AND SPECIAL CASES

A number of bodies which are normally treated in special ways for tax purposes are exempt from the tax. These are chiefly charities, approved superannuation funds, friendly societies, registered trade unions and local authorities.

Trustees are in general liable to pay capital gains on assets in the trust, with some provisions to ease the number of times the assets are deemed to be realized. An important clause makes discretionary and other trusts which have no limited interests in possession liable to tax on their accrued gains every ten years.

Evaluation of the capital gains tax

How does the capital gains tax stand up to the standard of the 'total accretion of income'?

The first thing to note is that the revenue from this tax is likely to be quite modest for many years to come. An asset acquired twenty years ago may have appreciated several hundred times in value, but the change in value from April 6th, 1965, is on the valuation basis all that matters for the purpose of the tax. If the asset in question depreciates in value from this date then a loss is available, which can be offset against other gains, in spite of the fact that the asset may have appreciated many times in value over its purchase price. This criticism does not apply if the time-apportionment formula is used. There is a general presumption against retrospective legislation, and in particular retrospective tax legislation. There may be very good grounds for circumscribing a government's power in this direction, but at the same time it must be pointed out that it gives an excellent weapon to vested interests to resist changes that are not in their interest, but could conceivably be in the nation's interest. In view of the sharp rise that has taken place in many capital values since the war, and in view of the general agreement that the old system was inequitable, a case can be made that the tax should have been backdated for a number of years, or at least that where the value of the assets was known at April 6th, 1965, the overall gain should be taken into account before allowing loss offset.

Although the revenue gain is likely to take many years to build up, the tax represents in principle a major breakthrough—one of the few major changes in the fiscal system that has come about in peacetime conditions. Some of the criticisms that can be made of the tax comes from the inevitable conflict that results from putting principles into practice. Of this kind is the exemption from tax of gifts of chargeable assets, provided that their value does not in total exceed £100 for each individual donor each year, and exclusion of chattels disposed of for £1,000 or less. Because of the ease of evasion and the cost of trying to collect tax on small sums, it is almost inevitable that such exemption should be given, and is the reason for the exclusion of the first £50 of gains from the long-term tax since 1967-8. The same reasons of ease of evasion and cost of collection are given for the exclusion of gambling winnings (presumably without offset for gambling losses). It may well be that separate taxation of these winnings is preferable.

It is much more difficult to justify the taxation of long-term gains at a maximum flat rate of 30%. The principle of progressive taxation of 'income' (narrowly defined) has long been accepted, and it seems illogical to charge a flat-rate tax on part of income when this is more widely drawn. It seems little justification to argue, as some commentators have done, that current income tax rates are too high. Income tax rates are to some extent as high as they are because income is so badly defined, and one of the benefits to be expected from widening the scope of income is that tax rates and the progression of the tax can be looked at anew. The conclusion seems inescapable that if it is right to charge short-term gains, arbitrarily drawn at one year, to income tax, it is right to charge long-term in the same way. The fact that short-term gains may result from speculation is, under the total-accretion principle, irrelevant.

The only valid case that it seems possible to make, on total-accretion lines, for the more lenient treatment of capital gains is the present inability to spread fluctuating income over a number of years. In Chapter 11 on 'The Criterion of Ability to Pay', it was argued that some form of averaging was desirable under any form of progressive tax. The argument against taxing that part of the gain which is due to inflation was dismissed on the grounds that there is no case for protecting one section of income from inflation.

Since capital gains on a significant scale are likely to accrue to a very small section of the population, the case for a flat rate appears even more inequitable. A single man with an earned income of £10,000 will pay just over £4,280 in tax and surtax. A capital gain of £10,000 will be liable to a maximum tax of £3,000, regardless of how much or how little income and wealth the owner already possesses. The peculiar ethic that it is only income, narrowly defined, which should be taxed at highly progressive rates has still to be excised from the system.[5]

[5] It may be argued that the man may have less 'real capital' after realizing his gain of £10,000 than when he made the original investment, and that he is paying £3,000 of tax on a non-existent real gain. The pros and cons of this argument were dealt with in the previous chapter at some length. It was there concluded that public finance should be concerned with a person's relative tax position, changes in the value of money affect all sectors of the community in different degrees, compensation for one sector results in less equity, not more.

In view of the very unequal distribution of wealth in this country, which has already been commented on, the exclusion of the first £5,000 of net gains at death seems indefensible in a country where all political parties pay lip-service to the need for some redistribution of wealth. Redistribution at death is the least painful way of achieving this end, and the one likely to cause least economic disturbance.

It was argued in Chapter 11 on the 'The Criterion of Ability to Pay' that the total exclusion of owner-occupied houses from the capital-gains tax confers a benefit on house-owners as compared with those who rent property, and is, in addition, likely to inflate the demand for houses. In America, where capital gains have been taxed for many years,

> Gain on the sale of a residence is taxable as a capital gain but a loss is not deductible. Since 1954, for the federal tax, the capital basis of a residence sold may be transferred to a new one acquired within 18 months if the cost of the new is the same or higher than the sale price of the old, and pro rata if the cost is less, so that capital gains is in effect postponed for such 'paired' transactions. In 1964, Congress allowed additional exemption for gains on homes sold by persons over age 65.
>
> Shultz, W. J. and Harriss, C. L. (1965), 249.

Amendment on these lines would appear to be desirable. Owner-occupied houses would then be liable for capital gains, either when the proceeds were used for other purposes or at death.[6]

[6] The complete exclusion from tax of capital gains in the case of owner-occupied houses serves to further entangle what has been for many years an illogical, absurd and unjust situation. The only people who do not receive a subsidy from public funds are the occupants of privately rented houses. About half of these private tenants are 'subsidized' by their landlords because their premises are subject to rent-control. All tenants, both private and council, pay rents out of taxed income, but most council tenants receive subsidies. A much larger element of subsidy usually accrues to the owner-occupier while he is buying his house, because of tax relief allowed on interest payments. Since the abolition of Schedule A tax, no income is imputed to the owner for the value of the services of his property, so that this tax relief results in a direct reduction in tax.

Always an unpopular tax, we are unlikely for political reasons to see the reintroduction of Schedule A, however desirable this would be on grounds of equity. An alternative way is to allow a private tenant to offset the part of his rent that goes towards interest payment on the capital sum invested in his house against tax, in the same way that an owner can offset his mortgage payments. This proposal, while it would go some way to achieving equity between persons, suffers from administrative complexities and the drawback noted previously that the poorest section of the community derive no benefit from income-tax concessions. More drastic remodelling of the system is required if we are to break out of the present near-tragic situation. For a discussion on this and other aspects of housing, see Hemming, M. F. W. and Duffy, H. (August, 1964), 39-59.

Finally, some word should be added on the cost of administering this tax. The exclusion from the long-term capital gains tax of individuals where, after deducting allowable losses, the gains do not exceed £50 for the year will simplify the administrative task, at a sacrifice of some degree of equity. It should be noted that, in so far as it is now less profitable to switch assets around for a pure tax advantage, in time it could lead to a more productive use of manpower, even though the Inland Revenue staff may have to be increased. The costs of tax-collection do not form a large percentage of the amount of revenue collected, but there is no doubt that the capital gains tax will increase costs for some time to come. In the author's opinion, the serious distortions present in the old system justify this increase in cost. The 'cake of custom' has been broken. It can be hoped that a fruitful period of public discussion can now take place on the kind of modifications still needed.

Summary

Past attempts to allow for differences in individual and family circumstances has resulted in a complex code of personal income taxation which nevertheless fails to help the most needy in the community.

In recent years differences between citizens who obtain their incomes from an employer and those who obtain their income from a business have been accentuated, and has led many who are able to do so to arrange their affairs in this form. The latter are able to deduct for the using up of capital before arriving at a figure for tax, profit retained in the business is not, generally speaking, subject to the progressive rates of tax of personal income, and, finally, they are able to claim more generous expenses. Suggestions have been put forward that individuals should be taxed at a lower rate to compensate for these advantages or that an annual charge should be imposed on businesses for these privileges. Both suggestions are not without their difficulties. If a value-added tax is adopted this would provide an opportunity to look afresh at the whole concept of capital allowances and deductible expenses.

The capital gains tax, in spite of the small amount of revenue received at present, represents a major shift in principle. The distinction between short-term gains, already changed from six to twelve months and taxed as income, and long-term gains taxed at a maximum rate of 30% does not appear to be based on any valid grounds except the present inability to spread fluctuating income over a number of years. If a scheme of income-averaging is adopted, the case for counting all gains as income would be very much strengthened.

13
Company taxation

> This indirect benefit of incorporation [retained profits on which surtax is not payable] cannot fairly be ignored in framing the tax system applicable to corporation profits. It is a fiscal matter and bears upon the proper distribution of the burden of tax upon different kinds of income. The difficulty remains, however, that the saving achieved is achieved on behalf of the shareholders as a whole; the money is in most cases outside the control of any one individual shareholder and is certainly not directly at his disposal as free personal income.
>
> *Royal Commission on the Taxation of Profits and Income* (1955), para. 54.

Company taxation is a complex matter in which the public-finance, accounting and legal aspects twist and interweave. This chapter attempts to give a broad description of company tax, concentrating on important issues. It starts with a factual description of changes in company tax. This leads to a discussion of the principles of company tax and to a discussion of the value or otherwise of tax discrimination against distributed profits. With this necessary background, the tax system before the Finance Act, 1965, can be understood and the important changes introduced by the Act with the introduction of corporation tax. One aspect of this, the taxation of companies trading overseas, is treated at some length. The next section then treats important, and even more controversial, matters relating to the concept of profit which is subject to tax. Finally, it looks at the important system of investment allowances and grants which has grown up since the war.

Company tax in this context is used to cover the ordinary meaning of taxes levied directly on company profits. It will be clear from previous chapters that a number of other taxes affect companies, and may be paid in whole or in part by them. Purchase tax has been previously considered and treated as a tax on consumers. As a general rule this is probably correct, but changes in purchase tax may have sharp repercussions on industry in altering demand for the products concerned. This will be taken up in Part III of this book. Capital gains tax, the selective employment tax and employers' National Health and pension contributions were looked at in previous chapters and will not be developed further.

Changes in company taxation

During the years immediately following the First World War a special tax was levied on the profits of companies to absorb some of the excess profits companies were able to make as a result of the war. In 1937 a national defence contribution was imposed. This continued until 1947, when a profits tax (paid on profits above a certain amount) was levied. This differentiated according to whether the profits were retained in the business or distributed to shareholders. The tabulation below lists the changes made in this tax. This was adapted from Rubner, A. (June, 1964), 347-59. For a comment on this article see Harcourt, G. C., and Whittington, G. (1965), 373-8. An opposing view is given by Feldstein, M. S. (December, 1967), 947-53.

Table 1

	Income Tax	*Net Profits Tax*	
Year		On Undistributed Profits	On Distributed Profits
	%	%	%
1947	45·0	5·4	13·8
1949	45·0	5·4	16·5
1951	47·5	5·2	26·3
1952	47·5	2·5	22·5
1953	45·0	2·5	22·5
April, 1955	42·5	2·5	22·5
November, 1955	42·5	2·5	27·5
1956	42·5	3·0	30·0
1958	42·5	10·0	10·0
1959	38·8	10·0	10·0
1960	38·8	12·5	12·5
1961-6	38·8	15·0	15·0

The column under 'Income Tax' merely reflects the changes in the standard rate of income tax to which taxable profits of the preceding accounting year were subject. The next two columns show the additional profits tax which were levied on profits of the current year if these were above £12,000 with reduced rates for profits between £2,000 and £12,000. Except for the period from 1958 to 1966, a heavier—sometimes a much heavier tax—was levied on that part of profit which was distributed to shareholders than on that part which was retained in the business. The discrimination, which seems to be based on no clear logical principle, was at its highest in 1956, when profits tax was 3% on undistributed profits and 30% on distributed profits.

The principles of company tax

The erratic gyrations of the net profits tax lead to the question of whether or not it is possible to find any principles on which company taxation should be based. On reference back to the section on total accretion of income, it will be found that if we are adhering strictly to this principle and if we are trying to treat people in equal positions equally, then it is the shareholders, as owners of companies, that should be taxed rather than the companies themselves. It is only in the case of profits retained in the business that a problem of reallocation arises.

It is sometimes suggested that company tax should be reduced or abolished and that the whole of company profits should be allocated to the owners. In the case of public companies, shareholders would receive with their dividend warrants a statement of their portion of the profits which the company had decided to retain in the business. The shareholder would be liable for tax on both sums.

This solution has weighty objections. It is usually rejected on the grounds that a person should not be liable for more tax than the sum he receives. This could occur under this scheme, e.g. where a top-rate surtax-payer is a shareholder in a company that retains most of the profit in the business. Even if this argument is accepted in principle, it is one which is likely to carry less weight under the total-accretion principle, since the adoption of this would enable a revision of tax rates to be made. The argument that this would stop the flow of funds to companies, from high-tax-payers, even allowing for the adjustments of tax rates under the accretion principle, is more serious. However just on grounds of equity, it seems unlikely, for this reason, to be a practical proposition.

The adoption of the accretion principle of income would greatly reduce the problem of inequity. Distributed profits would be part of the income of the recipient, as at present. Retained profits, to the extent that they enhance the value of the business, would also be taxed as income when the gains are realized. This solution favours the investor, both because he has a deferred liability for tax and because he has a tax cushion if retained profits do not enhance the value of the business. This degree of inequity may be thought tolerable because of the incentive it is likely to give to investment.

The solution outlined above leaves open the question of whether companies should be taxed as entities in their own right, apart from taxing shareholders. On the one hand are those who hold that the only problem is to achieve a system that will tax shareholders as closely as possible to the position that would be reached if all profits were distributed; on the other hand are those who argue that, in effect, companies can be considered as entities or personalities in their own right and should be taxed accordingly. Before definite answers can be given, it is necessary to know the incidence of company taxation—whether, that is, this ultimately falls on the shareholder, the workers or the consumer. The importance of this question also tends to merge with that of tax incentives to business investment, which is taken up at the end of this chapter.

Does tax discrimination against distributed profits help investment?

Post-war British governments have been concerned with increasing capital investment; the changes in tax on distributed profits, as opposed to undistributed profits, reflects to some extent a conflict on ways of achieving this. The rationale behind sharp discrimination against distributed profits is that this should encourage capital investment by the ploughing back of profits.[1] A number of factors have to be weighed in order to evaluate this. Firstly, it can be said that discrimination against paying dividends, by itself, causes no incentive to material investment, since firms may merely acquire liquid assets. The number of take-over bids that took place after dividend discrimination had been in force for some years is often quoted as evidence that this is so, since in a number of these take-overs the excessive liquid position of the company being taken over was an attraction. As many factors enter into the decision to take over another company, this evidence is hard to quantify.

More serious is the question of how important different sources of finance are to companies. Relying on ploughing back profits limits a company to a growth rate that is compatible with its profits. A company wanting to expand faster than this must seek funds from

[1] It is sometimes suggested that discrimination against distributed profits is in effect discrimination against consumption by shareholders. In view of the facilities for consumption given by capital appreciation in the post-war period, this argument is not very sound.

outside. Borrowing on fixed interest by way of debentures or preference shares has its limitations. Too high a 'gearing'—that is, the level of its fixed-interest payments compared to its ordinary or equity shares—leaves a company very vulnerable if profits should fall. In a bad year equity dividends can be reduced or passed over altogether, but fixed-interest payments must be met or, as a rule, the debenture or preference holders have a right to supersede the management by appointing a receiver or other person to look after their interests. An equity issue means that the market for the shares needs to be a good one, and one of the most important means of ensuring this is to have a liberal dividend policy. We thus come to a direct conflict. If dividends are deliberately discriminated against in order to encourage investment, the effect may be to hamper those companies which want very fast growth and need to go to the equity market in order to do so.

What value should be placed on this argument? There is some evidence that equity finance has been important for many fast-growing companies (see Tew, B., and Henderson, R. F. (1959)), but before we conclude that dividend-discrimination has been bad in this respect, it is necessary to establish that the discrimination has been sufficiently severe to draw funds away from the company sector to some other sector of the economy—that is, that there has been a general shortage of funds for company finance. The evidence does not point in this direction; certain sectors—for example, small companies and new companies—may have had difficulty in getting funds, but this has always been so and has little to do with dividend-restraint. Company dividend policy, in spite of high tax at times on dividends, has nevertheless resulted in an attractive market. If company dividend policy is, for one reason or another, inflexible—and there is some evidence for this (Rubner, A. (June, 1964))—we reach the position that it is possible that Britain, by taxing retained profits less than distributed profits, has nevertheless taxed the shareholder more on balance than those countries who discriminate, on grounds of equity, more heavily against retained profits. This argument depends on the assumption that companies have an inflexible dividend policy, that whatever the level of tax on distributed profits they will try to pay out a fixed proportion of profit. The argument should not be pushed too far!

A further point sometimes made against the discrimination of distributed profits is that such a policy favours the *status quo*. Companies making large profits have the ability to grow, but these may not be dynamic companies. Distributing the profits to shareholders leaves them free to invest in any company. The extent to which dividends are used directly or indirectly to finance new investment is once again a field where little empirical evidence is available.[2]

What emerges from this mass of contradictory opinion? It would appear that many factors influence the real investment of companies. These factors are not likely to be stable over time for one company, nor for companies as a whole to lead at one particular time to a predominant influence of any particular factor. This negative conclusion has policy implications. Simple-minded theories that investment will be increased or decreased by this or that amount of dividend discrimination seem incorrect: such discrimination is unlikely to make any substantial difference one way or the other to investment.

The system of tax before the Finance Act, 1965

A company's taxable profits of the preceding year were liable to tax at the standard rate of income tax, and in addition the taxable profits of the current year, if large enough, were subject to profits tax. From 1961 profits tax was an additional 15% if profits exceeded £12,000 per year. The rate was scaled down for profits between £2,000 and £12,000: below £2,000, profits were only taxed to standard rate of income tax. Under this system it was thus a matter of indifference (from a tax viewpoint) to a company whether it paid out profits in the form of dividends or whether it retained these in the business. The system before 1961 was, as we have seen, one where distributed profits were taxed more heavily than retained profits. (The recipient of the dividend was credited with the standard rate of tax paid by the company, so that he had no more to pay if he was himself a standard-rate income-tax-payer. If he paid at lower or higher rates, he was entitled respectively to a rebate of tax or indebted to the Inland Revenue for the difference.)

One reason why it is very difficult to link changes in tax on companies with changes in their investment behaviour is that both their current-year profits and preceding-year profits were liable to tax because the liability to income tax was lagged by one year. Since companies are under no obligation to keep standard accounting dates for making up their accounts, the time over which tax changes affecting companies was spread amounted to two or more years.

The Finance Act, 1965

The Finance Act of 1965 introduced a corporation tax in place of

[2] This argument is important on 'welfare' grounds. If it is good that capital should be mobile and the rate of return should tend to equality in different use, it would seem desirable to distribute profits and let the recipients reinvest (or consume) them as they think fit.

the two-tier system just described. The corporation tax separates the taxation of companies from that of individuals. Companies are liable to this tax on their taxable profit, including capital gains, but will not be liable to income tax. Payment of interest (e.g. on debenture stock) is treated as a charge against profits, and will not therefore be subject to corporation tax. The initial rate of the tax was 40%, increased to 42½% from April, 1968 and to 45% from April, 1969. However, shareholders will be liable to income tax and, surtax, where appropriate, on dividends and other distributions, and, as a matter of machinery, companies will be required to deduct income tax, at the standard rate, from payments to shareholders and hand the sums over to the Inland Revenue. In essence, companies pay a flat rate of tax of 45% and split dividend payments into two, one part of which they send to the shareholders, the balance to the Inland Revenue.

This is back to the position of effective discrimination against dividends that operated before 1958. It is also back to the questions that were raised in the previous discussion to which no satisfactory answers could be given. If dividend policy is very inflexible, this is saying in effect that it is a matter of indifference to company directors how much they have to split off from their dividend payments to send to the Inland Revenue, so long as the flow of funds to the company sector is not adversely affected. On the other hand, it can be argued that directors will reason that every £1 of profit retained in the business is worth 11*s.* after paying corporation tax at 45%, whereas to the average taxpayer it is worth very much less, because the shareholder will in addition be liable for income tax on this 11*s.* If the result is not to affect dividend policy, then the shareholder is in effect taxed more heavily compared to other taxed income on that part of profits which is distributed to him and less heavily on that part which is retained in the business.

In these circumstances, whether the shareholder gains or loses from the tax compared to the position he would be in if he was credited with the whole of profits and liable to income tax depends on the shareholder's tax position. If, however, the result is to cause companies to retain more profit in the business, as well as the problem of deciding the equity position, we have the more serious problem, in this context, of deciding whether it is to the benefit of the economy as a whole to encourage firms to retain profits.

The corporation tax made other changes with far-reaching results, which will now be considered.

Basis of assessment

The old system of tax was concerned, as has been shown, with two years' profits. The new tax fixes the rate of corporation tax each financial year, and that rate will be applicable to the profits of that financial year. Normally, the tax will be payable nine months after the end of the company's accounting year or, for the majority of existing companies, on January 1st. The financial year referred to above starts on April 1st and ends the following March 31st.

If a company's accounting year coincides with the dates of the financial year, no problem arises as to the rate of tax that is applicable to those profits. If, however, the two do not coincide, then a time-apportionment basis will be used. Thus a company whose accounting year ends on December 31st, 1968, will have one-quarter of its taxable profits charged at the rate fixed for the financial year ending March 31st, 1968, and the remaining three-quarters at the rate for the financial year ending March 31st, 1969. (Obviously, if the tax rate remains unchanged, no problem of time apportionment arises.)

General opinion seems to be that this method of assessment, once the complications of the changeover have been assimilated, is a welcome simplification of the tax structure, companies being subject to an assessment on one year's profits rather than two.

Taxation of company profits earned overseas

The corporation tax has been heavily criticized because of its treatment of companies who earn profits overseas. In order to decide whether this criticism is just or whether the corporation tax merely ended a favoured tax position, it is necessary to go back and establish the procedure in force before the change.

The essence of the problem

The essence of the problem can be quite simply stated: should companies who earn profits overseas and who pay taxes to overseas governments be given any allowance against taxes that they are liable for in their home country?

Over the years a general principle has been established that income so earned should be subject to home taxation, with various concessions. Britain has made agreements with about seventy countries whereby she agrees to forgo the right to tax at full rates, in return for concessions of a like nature. The distinction must now be made between a company that has a subsidiary company which is *located, managed and controlled* abroad and other companies. The general rule is that no United Kingdom tax is payable by subsidiary companies in the first group on profits *retained abroad.* Profits that are remitted to the United Kingdom, and *all profits* of other subsidiary companies are subject to United Kingdom tax, but allowance is given for tax paid abroad.

The allowance takes the form, not of a deduction from gross profits to arrive at taxable profit, but as a direct offset to United Kingdom tax liability. Therefore, if foreign tax is no higher than United Kingdom tax, a company pays no more tax than would be the case if the profits were earned in the United Kingdom.

We now come to the core of the argument. The corporation tax in general continued with the arrangements indicated above, whereby tax paid overseas was offset against home company tax. This was deemed to be corporation tax; no offset was allowed against income tax charged to the individual (but collected by the companies) on dividend payments. As a transitional matter, tax relief is being given to companies which pay overseas tax on income from direct investments which is in excess of corporation tax. The relief, which tapers off after two years, comes to an end after five years. See *Corporation Tax* (1965), on which this section draws.

Before the corporation tax a company's United Kingdom tax-bill, if its profits were more than £12,000, amounted to 53¾% (made up of standard rate tax of 7*s.* 9*d.* in the £1, plus 15% profits tax). Corporation tax at 40% means that companies trading overseas who pay taxes in excess of 40% are worse off. They would in this case not have to pay corporation tax, but whereas before the United Kingdom tax incorporated the shareholders' liability to income tax at the standard rate, now it doesn't. An example should make this clearer.

Assume a company which earns a profit overseas of £20,000, on which it pays £10,000 overseas tax and repatriates the remaining £10,000. The standard rate of income tax is taken at the old rate of 7*s.* 9*d.* in the £1 in each case, and corporation tax at the old rate of 40%.

BEFORE CORPORATION TAX

U.K. tax liability, 53¾%, i.e. £10,750, against which it received a credit of £10,000, leaving £750 to pay. Profits after tax thus £9,250. It could pay, say, £6,000 to shareholders tax free, i.e. pay a net dividend of £6,000, which equals a gross dividend of £9,796 (the difference being tax at 7*s.* 9*d.* in the £1 on the gross dividend of £9,796). The company would have £3,250 to retain in the business.

AFTER CORPORATION TAX

U.K. tax liability, 40%, or £8,000. £10,000 already paid overseas, so no further liability for corporation tax in the U.K. Company now has £10,000 profit. If it still wishes to pay a net dividend of £6,000, it must also pay £3,796 to the Inland Revenue. The company would thus have £10,000, less £9,796, i.e. £204 left in the business, compared to the previous figure of £3,250.

Fair or unfair to companies trading overseas?

In the example given above we saw that under the old system of tax, individuals were credited with tax that had been paid, not to the Inland Revenue, but to some overseas government. One argument put forward for changing the system was that (since U.K. tax rates in this respect were higher than most overseas rates) companies had no incentive to take overseas tax rates into consideration when setting up overseas, since so long as overseas tax was below 53¾%, it was offset against U.K. tax. If the view is taken that a tax on dividends is a tax on individuals, then what companies are really complaining about is the fact that tax on companies is now lower in the United Kingdom than it was! Or, put the other way, that overseas taxes have not been reduced in line with U.K. taxes. We come back once more to the paradox: that we have no clear concept in use to judge the taxation of companies. Should we be thinking in terms of tax on the individual shareholder or tax on the company as an entity in its own right?

The concept of taxable profit

So far in this chapter it has been assumed that the 'taxable profit' of a company is a just and equitable one, and we have been looking at ways of taxing this sum. It is now necessary to look at this assumption and find out how taxable profits are determined. It should be stated at the outset that this question is even more controversial than the matters of company tax just discussed. It is just as fundamental: a correct method of taxing companies would give incorrect results if the tax was applied to an incorrect figure of company profit. The divisions on this subject are sometimes between accountants and economists, but not infrequently there are wide differences within each group. The subject is a complex one, and no more is attempted in this book than an outline of some of the most important features.

Profit and taxable profit

A company incurs costs in making a commodity or in providing a service and receives revenue when the product or service is sold. The difference between costs and revenue (which can be positive or negative) during a specified period of time is profit or loss. Profit or loss, being a residual figure, depends on what the tax authorities allow to be called 'costs', and what they allow to be called 'revenue'.

A convenient division of costs is into *fixed* and *variable*. Fixed refers to items which are necessary to carry on business, but are not completely used up in the process, e.g. buildings and machinery. The problem arises of how the costs of these fixed items are to be apportioned to each year's output. Variable refers to costs which cease if output ceases, e.g. labour and raw material costs. These variable costs are more easily apportioned to annual output, but even here doubts can arise. Should advertising, which is partly aimed at selling current output and partly aimed at building up the long-term goodwill of the firm, be allocated to the one or the other, or both? If both, how is it possible to separate the one kind of expenditure from the other? These, and a large number of other definitional points must be decided. In what follows we shall try and concentrate on the most important aspects. Depreciation will be discussed first. Investment allowances will be treated separately, although perhaps the two should be regarded together. A case can be made for separate treatment on the grounds that depreciation allowances take care of the equity aspect, while investment allowances are primarily concerned to increase the level of real investment; although the practical use of these measures may not accord with this simple division.

Depreciation

It is not generally realized how recent is the relief for the using up of assets in the course of business. To quote from the *Royal Commission on Tax*, 1955:

> The conception of depreciation allowances for fixed assets to which the first Tucker Committee gave their support illustrates how far expert views on the tax system had moved since 1920. In that year the Royal Commission were able to assert that income for purposes of taxation should in general be computed without regard to the amortisation of wasting assets. In contrast, in 1951 the Report of the expert committee accepted as a guiding principle ' . . . the general proposition that the Income Tax system should give relief in respect of the wastage of all assets that are used up or consumed in the course of carrying on a business' (para. 322).

A little later the Commission says:

> One thing must be said in this connection. The practical result of the changes since 1920 has been to afford a scheme of protection to 'material' capital that is not available to 'personal' capital. Our predecessors were apprehensive about this possibility when they wrote of the risk of creating 'grave inequalities between different classes of income'; and we have seen that it was on this ground, amongst others, that they rejected proposals for a general allowance for the amortisation of wasting assets (para. 325).

The precise details of current depreciation allowances is the concern of the accountant rather than ourselves. The broad system is to lay down the method of depreciation, the amount or the percentage of the cost of the asset which can be written off, and the number of years over which it is to be written off. These agreed sums may be deducted from gross profit before tax-liability is calculated. The agreed system of depreciation varies for different assets. The main categories are:

1. Industrial buildings and structures.
2. Plant and machinery.
3. Exploration, development and construction work in connection with mines, oil wells and other mineral sources.
4. Agricultural buildings and works.
5. Patent rights.
6. Expenditure on scientific research.

A business may adopt any system of depreciation that it wishes, but it is only allowed to offset against tax on the agreed scale.

Almost every aspect of the depreciation allowances is subject to some amount of controversy. Does depreciation cover the right items? Should more flexibility be allowed to companies to write off assets against tax as they wish, or should more uniformity be imposed? What is the correct treatment for an asset that is sold before it is fully depreciated? And so on. The reader is referred to the *Royal Commission on the Taxation of Profits and Income* (1955), for a discussion on these matters. Below a brief look is given to the principle of depreciation and depreciation and inflation.

THE PRINCIPLE OF DEPRECIATION

On the question of whether or not depreciation should be deductible from profits before tax, no clear principle seems to emerge. The Majority Report of the Royal Commission fell back on the argument: '. . . Whatever be the right rationalization, it is clear to us that they [capital allowances] have come to stay and they must be taken as an integral part of our system of taxing business profits. We are content to accept them on this basis . . .' (para. 328).

The Minority Report of the Royal Commission was more positive. They granted that an anomalous position was created because allowances are not given in respect of the wastage of human capital, but thought it would be impractical to try to introduce human capital into the system of depreciation allowances. The Minority Report put more weight on the anomaly that 'allowance is given for capital wastage, whilst no charge is imposed on capital gains'.

As the Minority rather than the Majority Report was followed in respect of capital gains, and we now have such a tax, this particular anomaly is taken care of. It seems that the general concensus of opinion now is that depreciation provisions should be allowed, the distortions that would be caused by its omission being greater than that due to the omission of human capital from the provisions.

Depreciation and inflation

The present system of depreciation allowances is based on the historic cost (that is, the original money cost) of the asset. In times of rising prices, the replacement cost of an asset may well be higher, and sometimes considerably higher, than the historic cost. Companies and their accountants frequently urge that allowance should be made for the change in the price-level by basing depreciation on replacement cost, or some alternative measure.

This argument, on which so much has been written, is plausible enough, but in the context of the present tax system represents a case of special pleading. It should be noted in this connection that while replacement costs may increase, so also may the receipts from current output of the capital asset, so that a firm is in a position to protect itself from inflation if it can raise prices. The Royal Commission on Tax quoted with approval the findings of the Tucker Committee on the Taxation of Trading Profits (1951): '. . . one objection common to all schemes, namely that they involve giving preferential treatment to all owners of businesses as against other classes of taxpayers' (para. 330). The Royal Commission on Tax summed up their position as follows:

(1) We do not accept that as a matter of principle a trader's profits in times of inflation must be computed with allowance for the cost of replacement of fixed assets or the fall in the purchasing power of money. (2) We think that for the purposes of taxation a system of computing his profits that does not make allowance for these factors is preferable to one that does (para. 368).

The grounds for the rejection of depreciation based on other than historic cost is thus clear: inflationary and deflationary conditions affect all sectors of the community in different degrees; there is no case in equity for trying to compensate one sector. As will be seen in the section on investment incentives, this has the effect of making investment cheaper and can be considered as making some allowance for inflation. It seems better in principle to regard these allowances, not as attempts to allow for changes in the value of money, but as devices whereby the government can attempt to influence investment. They violate equity between different classes of taxpayers, but are accepted on grounds of investment criteria.

Investment incentives

INITIAL ALLOWANCES

Initial allowances were introduced with effect from April, 1946, as part of a new scheme of taxation designed to encourage re-equipment and modernization in productive industry. The scheme was one of accelerated depreciation. In addition to the allowance for depreciation that could be offset against profit before tax, a further allowance was granted in the year of purchase. However, over the remaining period allowed for depreciation, lower depreciation was given, so that over the whole period the same benefit was received. They can be looked on as a device to defer tax-liability or, the same thing, as a tax-free loan from the government.

The rates at the beginning were 20% for plant and machinery, 10% for industrial buildings and 10% for mining works. In 1949 the rate for plant and machinery was raised to 40%. They were suspended from April, 1952, because it was thought that the heavy calls which the defence programme would make on the engineering industry made it desirable to reduce the pressure of civilian demand for plant and machinery. In 1953 they were restored for the purpose of increasing investment in the assets selected: 20% was given for plant and machinery, 10% for industrial buildings and 40% for mining works. In 1954 they were changed by investment allowances.

As an inducement to invest, the initial allowance made only a small impact. Dow, J. C. R. (1964), 205, has estimated that it was equivalent to 'something like a reduction in the rate of interest by ½%. Its importance lay in providing an internal source of finance for the firm undertaking investment, providing the firm was paying taxes'.

INVESTMENT ALLOWANCES

In 1954 investment allowances were given on a range of assets. Initial allowances were not discontinued for those assets that formally received them and were not given the new allowance. The allowances were given in the year of purchase in a similar manner to the initial allowances, but, unlike them, they were not recouped in later years. Industrial and agricultural buildings and works were given a 10% investment allowance, machinery and plant, mining works, and scientific research assets 20%.

The system of initial and investment allowances continued with several switches and changes until 1966, when they were largely superseded by a system of grants.

ASSESSMENT OF INITIAL AND INVESTMENT ALLOWANCES

The Royal Commission on Taxation in 1955 expressed strongly the opinion that these allowances violate the principle that persons with equal incomes should bear an equal burden of tax. They go on:

> For these reasons we think that instruments of this kind will require to be justified in due course by convincing evidence that they are not only effective in achieving the results anticipated but also worth-while in the value of the results contrasted with the revenue foregone . . . (para. 421).

The evidence in 1966 as given in a White Paper on 'Investment Incentives' is that these measures have largely failed in their objectives:

> The National Plan makes it plain that the overriding need during the next few years is to give priority to those sectors of industry which can make the greatest contribution to strengthening the balance of payments. The benefits of the present system are too widely dispersed to be fully effective. Investment allowances are given for some items which have little or no relation to productive investment. For example, purchases of furniture, curtains and carpets in offices or cutlery in dining-rooms or canteens qualify for investment allowances. Television sets rented by the public do so too, since the purchase of the set by the rental firm qualifies (para. 14).

The White Paper goes on to list other defects; the fact that the allowances take an average eighteen months to be felt, that they are spread over a long period and uncertain because of the uncertainty about future tax rates; also firms with small profits get little benefit.

A more fundamental criticism is mentioned as a result of a survey carried out by the Confederation of British Industry. It appears that a substantial number of firms still do not take tax allowances fully into account in investment decisions. In many cases firms seem to have no rational policy of making investment decisions, but proceed 'by God and by guess'.

The remedy carried out to meet these criticisms was not to stop the incentives or to confine them to firms who could present a reasoned case for the allowances, but to convert them into cash grants. No mention was made in the White Paper of the equity aspects that had troubled the Royal Commission. The whole emphasis was on the need to provide an effective investment incentive.

INVESTMENT GRANTS

From January 17th, 1966, the system of investment allowances was swept away and replaced by a system of grants. Initial allowances continued on some assets.

The system of grants applies in respect of expenditure on new plant and machinery used in manufacturing or extraction industries, but excluding furniture and similar items mentioned above, which were criticized as making no contribution to productive investment. Manufacturing covers all the processes of making articles, including the intermediate stages of processing materials. Extraction covers quarrying, mining and the extraction of natural mineral deposits. Excluded from the grants are service industries and construction industries. Special arrangements were made in respect of ships, hovercraft and computers. In addition, the new legislation swept aside the old development districts (areas of the country that were deemed to need special measures) and introduced 'development areas'.

The development areas cover much wider tracts of country. In these areas investment grants are given on a more generous scale. The table on p. 172 shows the main items qualifying for grants with the rates of grant that applied during 1967 and 1968. The most usual grant was 25% in a non-development area and 45% in a development area. In 1969 these rates reverted back to their previous levels of 20 and 40% respectively.

The Development Areas are, as indicated in Chapter 10, now defined to include, except for small areas deemed to be sufficiently developed, Scotland, Northern England (i.e. the four northernmost counties of England plus the North Riding of Yorkshire), Wales, Merseyside and the South-western area, which takes in much of Devon and Cornwall.

Table 2

Rates of Investment Grants and Initial Allowances applicable to capital expenditure between January 1st, 1967, and December 31st, 1968

	Non-development Areas Grant	Initial Allowances, etc.	*Development Areas* Grant	Initial Allowances, etc.
	%	%	%	%
New plant and machinery for manufacturing, extraction or construction	25	—	45	—
Other plant and machinery, including second-hand and most vehicles	—	30	—	30
Plant and machinery for scientific research relating to qualifying processes	25	100 write-off[1]	45	100 write-off[1]
New buildings and structures				
Industrial	—	15	25 or 35[2]	15
Non-industrial	—	—	25 or 35[2]	—
Computers				
New	25	—	43[3]	—
Second-hand	—	30	—	30
Mining Works	25	—	45	—
Ships[5]	25	Free depreciation[4]	25	Free depreciation[4]
Hovercraft	25	—	25	—
Hotels from April, 1968[6]	20	—	25	—

[1] 100% write-off means that assets may be completely written-off against profits in the first year.

[2] These grants are conditional on an adequate provision of employment. The 35% rate is given to certain new undertakings where the Board of Trade consider that the problems involved justify additional assistance.

[3] A 45% grant is paid in a development area for computers if it is solely or primarily (*a*) for integration with machinery or plant which is or is to be used for carrying on a qualifying industrial process, (*b*) for carrying on qualifying research.

[4] 'Free depreciation' means that the taxpayer can claim depreciation allowance for tax purposes at whatever rate suits him, instead of at the rates prescribed under the ordinary rules.

[5] Except for fishing vessels, which receive separate and normally larger grants.

WHAT DO THESE GRANTS MEAN TO BUSINESSES?

Grants will not be treated as part of the taxable income of a business, but are assumed to reduce the capital cost of the assets to which they relate. Thus an asset costing £1,000 that qualifies for a grant of 45% will be deemed to cost the business £550. Depreciation is allowed on the net cost of £550. Future depreciation allowances against tax will be smaller to this extent, but if the allowances continue unchanged, so also will the effective replacement cost of the asset be reduced.

EVALUATION OF INVESTMENT GRANTS

Since the war the government has been evolving a new fiscal weapon to try to influence real private investment. The current system of grants (and initial allowances) gives a weapon that is free from most of the defects noted in connection with investment allowances. Once the scheme of grants is properly in operation, the grants should be paid within six months of the investment taking place. The grant is not dependent on the amount of profits being made, so that, for example, new businesses which have not yet begun to make profits will benefit. The system could be very flexible: it remains to be seen how flexibly it will be operated. It is flexible in the sense that grants differentiate between different geographical regions and different types of real investment. Finally, cash grants are more easily taken into account by firms when making their investment decisions.

Taken together with the depreciation allowances, there is no doubt that in manufacturing and extractive industries firms have been placed on a favourable footing *vis-à-vis* other firms and individuals. In time the benefits are likely to be fairly widely spread over the community in the form of better goods or goods cheaper than they would have been in the absence of grants, and in a better export performance. In the short run it should not be forgotten that these grants create an opportunity for the owners of these businesses to take most of the gain to themselves by not passing on the benefits to the consumer. Time alone will show which path has been taken.

There are strong arguments for modernizing these sectors of British industry, and the arguments as to whether investment grants are the best way to achieve this will go on for a long while. The Board

[6] From April, 1968, hotels qualify for grants towards the capital cost of new hotels and extensions and improvements. These are conditional on certain requirements being met as to the number of rooms available and to the accommodation not being made solely against advanced bookings. Hotels that satisfy these conditions also qualify for loan assistance.

of Trade has been given certain discretionary powers under the Act, and it may be that in future a case can be made for more rigorous selection amongst firms. The granting of allowances to all firms will undoubtedly help the progressive firm to keep in the forefront of developments; it will also have the effect of propping up the inefficient firm for a period of time. If minimum requirements were drawn up for each industry on criteria to be taken into account when making investment decisions, the receipt of an investment grant could be made conditional on these requirements being met. The working out of these criteria would be likely to stimulate fruitful discussion in the industries concerned as well as spreading existing knowledge, a process that can do little but good.

Summary

The taxation of companies raises many contentious problems and conflicts between the aims of equity and the aims of incentive to investment.

If, on the grounds that it will act as a disincentive to investment, the owners of companies are not to have the whole of business profits attributable to them, the adoption of the total-accretion principle would go a long way to achieving equity between shareholders and other taxpayers without seriously weakening investment in business.

On the general question of tax-discrimination against distributed profits, it was concluded that there is no clear evidence that this is likely to have marked effects on overall investment. While such discrimination is likely to help the company relying on ploughed-back profits for investment capital, it hinders rather than helps the company which relies on raising new equity capital. No simple answer can be given as to whether discrimination is desirable on equity considerations, since this depends both on the dividend policy of the company concerned and the recipient's own tax position.

The evidence of previous Royal Commissions on Tax is unanimous that the granting of depreciation allowances puts companies in a privileged tax position *vis-à-vis* the individual taxpayer. The system of initial allowances and investment grants further substantially favours some companies. These tax privileges are generally accepted as desirable in order to achieve investment and growth in the economy, and it is likely that at least some of the benefits will in time be spread more evenly through the economy in the form of prices lower than they would be in the absence of these privileges.

The most serious criticism of the system of allowances, and in particular of investment grants, is that, in spite of clear evidence that many firms were not using sensible investment criteria, the grants were nevertheless given to any firm which invested in the designated assets. They thus serve to prop up the inefficient firm as well as to help the progressive firm. A highly desirable reform would be the recognition that grants are a tax privilege, to be given only to those firms who have evaluated their investment projects on approved lines. The working out of investment criteria between industries and an appropriate government body—perhaps the Economic Development Council—is likely to do more than polite exhortation to see that rational investment policies are widely and quickly adopted by all firms.

14
Value-added tax

Reactions to new taxes conform to a clear pattern: shock, opposition, understanding, acceptance.

The Times editorial, May 7th, 1966.

Introduction

The merits or otherwise of the value-added tax (abbreviated to V.A.T.) are worth considering, whatever the political future of Great Britain, but they are posed in urgent form by British approaches to join the European Common Market.

The Common Market countries agreed in February, 1967, that a single type of turnover tax based on the French T.V.A. (*taxe sur la valeur ajoutée*) system shall come into effect from 1970. This means the other five countries of the Common Market will have to adjust their turnover taxes to conform to the principles of T.V.A. although the rate of tax can be at different levels. A V.A.T. can take different forms: in what follows attention is mainly concentrated on the Common Market type of tax.

The National Economic Development Council in *Conditions Favourable to Faster Growth* (1963), paras. 165-70, suggested that a V.A.T. might be more conducive to economic growth and that it would have benefits for the balance of payments because the tax could, under the rules of the General Agreement on Tariffs and Trade (G.A.T.T.), be rebated on exports and charged on imports. The *Committee on Turnover Tax* (1964), considered such a tax and advised against a change in 1964. This decision was considered controversial at the time and the government has said that it is being reconsidered in the light of new circumstances.

The French system

Before the tax changes that came into force on January 1st, 1968, between a quarter and a fifth of all tax revenue in France came from turnover and sales taxes, of which T.V.A. provided the bulk. The tax is charged comprehensively on all goods, subject only to defined exceptions. Thus it covers consumer goods, many foodstuffs, industrial materials and intermediate products.

The changes in 1968 extend the tax to wholesale and retail trade and to services. The normal rate of tax has been set at 16·66% of the tax-inclusive value. Certain products will be charged at 20%, services at 13% and basic necessities at 6%.

The tax at the appropriate rate is levied at each stage of production, but is levied only on the value added at that particular stage. This is achieved administratively by allowing each stage to deduct the tax paid by previous stages, *as shown on the invoices of their suppliers*. Since the sum of values added at successive stages is equal to the final wholesale price of the product, the amount of tax paid will be the same as if the tax was charged once on this final value.

An example of a value-added tax

An example taken from the *Committee on Turnover Tax* (1964), para. 17, should make this clear:

Suppose the manufacture of a product which requires materials, fuel, and containers (but nothing else) to be brought in from outside suppliers, and suppose that the making of the product is costed as follows, and that there is a value-added tax at the uniform rate of 20% of tax-inclusive values [i.e. 25% of the tax-exclusive values]:

	Tax-inclusive Invoice Price	Amount of Tax included in Price	Price exclusive of Tax
	£	£	£
Purchases:			
Materials	100	20	80
Fuel	45	9	36
Containers	10	2	8
	155	31	124
Value added by the manufacturer by way of salaries, wages, profit, etc.	100		100
Tax payable by the manufacturer	25	25	
Selling price of product	280	56	224

In this example the manufacturer purchases materials, fuel and containers, which cost him £155, of which £31 is tax. The manufacturer adds £100 to the value (his salaries, wages, profit, etc.) and pays £25 tax on this value. So the final wholesale price of the product is £280, of which £56 is tax.

In France firms must send in returns showing the amount of tax payable within a given number of days of the end of the month, and they then pay tax on purchases of the previous month. Firms paying small amounts of tax are allowed to make quarterly returns.

The V.A.T. is, as the example already given shows, basically a tax on sales less purchases. This figure can be arrived at directly by an inspection of the sales and purchases figures or by adding up the money spent on wages and salaries, depreciation, interest and profit. Problems arise from stocks on hand at the start and finish of a tax period, and from purchases of capital equipment. Stocks present an accounting problem, but no problem of principle. With capital equipment the decision has to be made if this is to be subject to the tax or not. The most usual suggestion, on the grounds that investment should be encouraged, is that net capital expenditure should not be taxed. If this is to be the case a firm would be assessed to tax on value added calculated either

(a) upon the difference between the total of its sales; and the total of its purchases, including purchases of capital equipment;
(*b*) upon the sum of its wages and salaries, depreciation, trading profits and interest payments; minus its purchases of capital equipment.

In both cases exports of products would be excepted and imports taxed so that the tax is one based on final expenditure.[1]

Is a value-added tax an incentive to exports?

Purchase tax is also allowed to be rebated on exports and charged on imports. The significance of the change to a V.A.T. would lie in what other taxes were reduced or abolished. If, for example, employers' National Insurance contributions, which cannot be rebated at present, were lowered as a result of the introduction of a V.A.T., export prices would be lower and import prices higher. There are two advantages: one that follows from this price-change and the incentive this gives to exports; the other follows from the possible

[1] If in (*a*) purchases of capital equipment are excluded and depreciation charges are deducted from sales and in (*b*) capital equipment is excluded and profits taken net of depreciation, the tax becomes one on final expenditure and investment.

advantage to profits if a firm exports. Once again the benefit to profits (since firms are not charged purchase tax on exports) lies in the significance to the firm of the alternative taxes which are rebated.

However, the assumption that the present system, whereby all of the V.A.T. can be imposed on imports and rebated on exports, may be unrealistic. At present a country which imposes taxes on companies for social services, in a form which can not be imposed on imported goods, may complain that it is being discriminated against, since its exports will have to bear the V.A.T. of the country to which it is exporting, part of which is used for social service payments. On the other hand, imports to the country do not bear this social service tax. The question is complicated and one that is likely to lead to international retaliation if international agreement cannot be reached. A United States Congressional Foreign Trade Committee has voiced criticism on these lines and has called for an international review of all non-tariff barriers. And the United States Administration has said it may impose retaliatory 'border taxes' to offset the effect of the European Economic Community's use of the V.A.T.

Is the value-added tax a tax on costs or a tax on the consumer?

It is worth looking briefly at the incidence of a profits tax before the incidence of a V.A.T. is taken up. It is generally accepted that, at least in the short run, a tax on profits does not affect prices. The theoretical case is that if a firm is already charging prices that are maximizing profits, an increase in profits tax will not alter the optimum price and output decisions of the firm. There may be exceptions to this rule if a firm is in a monopolistic or oligopolistic position. If an industry's pricing structure is maintained by a firm, or a small number of firms, acting as a price-leader, or if the firms in an industry act together on pricing, and if they look to a level of return on capital *calculated after taxation is taken into account*, then a change in profits tax could be reflected fairly quickly in a change of prices. The consumer is in this case bearing all or part of the tax. In the long run, it is generally accepted that a profits tax is more likely to be passed on to the consumer. For a selection of articles on incidence refer to Musgrave, R. A. and Shoup, C. S. (1959).

Should a V.A.T. be regarded as a tax on consumption which will be paid by consumers or as a tax on business costs which will be paid by firms? The Richardson Committee considered that the former would be the case.

The procedure of invoicing that has been outlined leads to the expectation that the amount of tax will be carried through each stage of processing to the retail level, in the same way that purchase tax is invoiced through to the retailer and thence to the consumer. The question then arises whether or not firms will reduce the price of commodities in line with any tax-reductions that may come about with the introduction of a V.A.T. On the assumptions that both the V.A.T. and the cost savings that result from other tax reductions are passed on to the consumer, differential effects on retail prices can be expected. These are likely because the change in taxation, even if it is designed to bring in the same aggregate tax revenue, will have a different impact on different firms.[2]

On these assumptions the V.A.T. is primarily a tax on consumption, although it can be conceded that some firms faced with an elastic demand for their products may be forced to bear part of the cost themselves.

Is the value-added tax an incentive to efficiency?

If the V.A.T. is, by and large, a tax on consumers, can it at the same time be claimed that it is a spur to business efficiency? The grounds for arguing that this can be the case run on the following lines: A firm will find that its tax bill will be higher than its competitors if its costs are higher than theirs. Attempts to pass on this tax in excess of the amount the most efficient firm in the industry passes on will therefore result in loss of sales, and act as a direct incentive to the firm to reduce its costs by increasing its efficiency. This argument will now be examined.

The tax position in the competitive case

Let us take two firms producing for a competitive market, so that

	Firm A	Firm B
	£	£
Wages and salaries	400,000	500,000
Depreciation	200,000	200,000
Materials	100,000	100,000
Interest	100,000	100,000
Trading profit	200,000	100,000
Total sales	1,000,000	1,000,000

[2] For example, if government services are to be subject to the V.A.T. it makes a good deal of difference whether corporation tax or employers' Insurance and Health Contributions are remitted. In general, government services do not make profits, so that they would not benefit from a reduction in corporation tax.

the pricing policy of the firms is the same. Firm A is assumed to be the more efficient, its labour costs are lower and trading profits higher than firm B and other costs are assumed to be the same.

In this situation, with no capital expenditure, firm A pays more tax under corporation tax, since its trading profit is higher than firm B. However, despite the fact that firm B has lower profit, each would pay the same amount of V.A.T. (other taxes are ignored for the moment). The amount of V.A.T. can be calculated either as: sales, less purchases (£1,000,000, less £100,000), or as the sum of its wages and salaries, depreciation, interest and trading profit. In both cases, for both firms, this leaves £900,000 as the sum subject to the V.A.T. It is not necessarily correct to say therefore that because firm A has lower costs than firm B it will pay less tax. This is so because the tax base given here includes not only costs, but also trading profit, since profit forms part of the value added by the firm. The case where profits are excluded from the base is considered further below.

The 'incentive' to investment comes about firstly because firm B will have the same amount of V.A.T. to pay as firm A. In the competitive situation outlined firm B cannot increase its prices to improve its profits; it needs to reduce costs, or it may find itself insolvent. The direct incentive to investment comes about as a consequence of allowing capital purchases to be deducted from total sales. If firm B invests £500,000 in capital equipment to bring it up to the efficiency of firm A, its tax liability, in the year in which it undertakes the investment, will be reduced by £500,000. This provision does not reward the existing efficient firm, but gives an inducement to the less efficient firm to invest.

It is sometimes suggested that trading profit be excluded from the tax so that it would be calculated as sales, less purchases and profits or as the sum of its wages and salaries, depreciation and interest. In this case firm A would be liable to V.A.T. on £700,000; firm B on £800,000. This form of the tax obviously favours the efficient firm more than the previous example. *However, in both cases, this is looking only at the firms liability for V.A.T.* without taking into account liability for other taxes. The critical consideration is what other taxes will firms have to pay. The combinations of possible reductions in other taxes are endless, and the taxes to be paid have to be specified before it can be known how favourable or unfavourable the whole tax position is to one company or the other.

The imperfectly competitive situation

If the case is now taken where the firms are working in a market which is less than perfect, the situation changes a little. If firm B is able to maintain its profits by charging a higher price, the following situation emerges:

	Firm A	Firm B
	£	£
Wages and salaries	400,000	500,000
Depreciation	200,000	200,000
Materials	100,000	100,000
Interest	100,000	100,000
Trading profit	200,000	200,000
Total sales	1,000,000	1,100,000

Firm B's sales are higher because its final prices are higher. Taking the case where profits are included in the tax base, firm B will pay tax on £1,000,000 as opposed to firm A on £900,000. If firm B passes the tax on to the consumer, its prices and tax bill will diverge even further from firm A. The inducement to firm B to reduce its costs thus depends on two things. Firstly, the amount of tax paid on the difference in cost and profit between itself and the most efficient firm in the industry. Secondly, on the degree of monopoly power it can exercise. While the tax, in these circumstances, is an inducement to reduce prices and improve efficiency, it seems easy to overstate the benefits that can be expected from it. As in the previous example, the main inducement still lies in the tax-reduction that comes about in the year in which capital investment is undertaken.

As in the previous example, if profits are excluded from the base, the situation becomes more favourable, so far as V.A.T. is concerned, to the more efficient firm. Firm A would then be liable to tax on £700,000; firm B on £800,000. The previous reservations about other taxes that firms may be liable for still applies.

A value-added tax and equity

Speaking generally, it is very difficult to devise a tax which is borne by a company. The reason for this is that companies are often in a position to alter their price and output policies and shift all or part of the tax on to the consumer.[3]

Adopting the position that a V.A.T. is a tax on consumers collected by companies, an equity problem arises. It is concerned with the regressive nature of indirect tax. Although (assuming a comprehensive

[3] Part of the tax may, in effect, be shifted on to the employees if the employer is able to use the tax as a counter to resist wage-claims.

tax) the actual amount of tax paid will increase with the amount of expenditure, the tax is regressive because as a rule consumption expenditure represents a decreasing proportion of income, as income levels rise, e.g. with a V.A.T. at 10% a person earning £10 a week will probably have to spend the whole of his income; in this case he will pay £1 in tax or 10% of his income. If a man earning £40 a week can save £10, he will pay £3 tax on his purchases of £30, or 7½% of his income.[4] This question will be taken up in Chapter 18.

Summary

Britain will have to adopt a V.A.T. if she enters the Common Market. In any case, the tax has advantages in its own right. At present the price system is distorted because some goods are subject to purchase tax and other goods and all services are not. (The S.E.T., which was dealt with in a previous chapter, was seen to be a very imperfect way of subjecting service industries to tax.)

V.A.T. could raise large sums in revenue, and the important question is which taxes will be abolished or reduced as a result of bringing in a V.A.T. Speculation as to which taxes should be reduced has been avoided. A 10% V.A.T. would, it has been estimated, bring in something like £2,000 million. If purchase taxes and S.E.T. were abolished, this will still leave a substantial sum, which could be applied to tax-reductions elsewhere.

The claim that a V.A.T. will encourage exports may be true under certain circumstances, but it is subject to important reservations about the reactions of other countries. A clarification of existing international agreements on tax rebates on exports and levies on imports is posed in urgent form by this tax if international retaliation is to be avoided.

If net capital formation is to be excluded from the scope of the tax, it forms a strong incentive to undertake capital investment.

A V.A.T. is a regressive tax. The problem this poses for equity will be considered in Chapter 18.

[4] Some of these expenditures are likely to be ways that do not attract the tax, such as the payment of rates; this does not alter the principle.

15
Wealth

Having regard to all the evidence presented here, it seems fair to conclude that there was no very marked change in the relative importance of inheritance in the creation of the personal fortunes of the top wealth-leavers of the generations of the mid-twenties and the mid-fifties of this century. For either, the chance of leaving an estate valued at over £100,000 or even £50,000 was outstandingly enhanced if one's father had been at least moderately well off.

HARBURY, C. D., 'Inheritance in the Distribution of Personal Wealth', *Economic Journal*, December, 1962.

Anybody that's got money can hire somebody who's smart to make them money. It's a son of a bitch that hasn't got any money that has to be smart.

HIBBARD, R., a self-made multi-millionaire, quoted by Bainbridge, J., *The Super-Americans*.

Apart from minor stamp duties, which may fall on wealth-transfers, the only continuing tax on wealth in Great Britain is that brought about by estate duties. There were legacy and successive duties until they were abolished in 1949. These duties were not important quantitatively, but important in principle, as an example of what is possible. They will be looked at briefly before details of estate duty are given. Estate duty is, then, related to the accretion principle of income. This section continues with a look at the special investment charge in the year 1967-8, and concludes with a brief look at some of the changes that have been proposed from time to time in taxing wealth.

Legacy and successive duties

Legacy and successive duties were minor duties, complementary to estate duties. The rate at which duties were charged was determined solely by the relationship of the beneficiary to the donor. They varied according to whether:

(1) The beneficiary was the husband, wife or lineal issue or ancestor of the donor.
(2) The beneficiary was a brother or sister or a descendant of a brother or sister.
(3) All other cases.

The lowest duty was payable in case (1); the highest in case (3).

The duties were based on the idea that a person who comes into an inheritance may justly be asked for a special contribution to the needs of the State, and that, if the inheritance has in it something of the nature of a windfall, the contribution should on that account be at a higher rate. These duties were abolished in 1949, when estate duty was increased.

Outline of existing estate duties

Estate or death duties were introduced in 1894, although since that time there have been many changes in detail and in the rates which have been applied. The current rates of tax are given in Table 1, and were introduced in 1969 when the size of estates on which duty is payable was raised from £5,000 to £10,000. The system prior to this had been to subject the whole of an estate to duty at a rate which progressed in 24 steps from 1% on an estate between £5,000 and £6,000 to 80% on an estate exceeding £1,000,000. The current system is that the rates of duty quoted are payable only on the appropriate tranche, or slice, of the estate. Thus from Table 1, an estate worth £30,000 will pay tax at 30% on £12,500 (£30,000 less £17,500) and 25% on the lower tranche of £7,500, the first £10,000 of the estate being free of duty. This was not primarily a revenue change, the

Table 1

Rates of estate duty in Great Britain applying 1969

Tranche of net capital value		
Exceeding	*Not Exceeding*	*Rate*
£	£	%
10,000	17,500	25
17,500	30,000	30
30,000	40,000	45
80,000	150,000	65
150,000	300,000	70
300,000	500,000	75
500,000	750,000	80
over 750,000		85*

* with a ceiling of 80% overall

estimated loss of revenue of £8 million a year is mainly due to raising the limit at which duty becomes payable. The adoption of the tranche system avoids the difficulty under the old scale of an estate which just came into a higher category of duty which needed 'marginal relief' so as not to be penalized compared to an estate which was slightly smaller. The change results in some sizes of estate paying a little more duty than under the old system and some a little less but the difference is not very great in either case.

These rates, if they were effective, might be considered unduly harsh. As Chapter 8 pointed out, the yield from this source is comparatively small, accounting for about 3% of government revenue. A system of high but ineffective rates has been described by Simons, H. (1938), 11 as:

> . . . a subtle kind of moral and intellectual dishonesty . . . a grand scheme of deception, whereby enormous surtaxes are voted in exchange for promises that they will not be made effective. Thus, the politicians may point with pride to the rates, while quietly reminding their wealthy constituents of the loopholes.

That the rates quoted in Table 1 are nominal, rather than effective rates, is due to two main causes: one, the extensive concessions that the legislature has granted, and two, the ease of avoidance.

Duty is charged on property passing on death of the individual, less various estate liabilities, which in general are limited to debts created for value. The meaning of debts created for value is to ensure that an estate is not reduced in value by the deceased having created IOU's for which he had not received full value in money or money's worth. We need not enter here into legal niceties of what constitutes property passing at death, except to note that the device of the trust, particularly the discretionary trust, has become increasingly important as a means of avoidance. (A discretionary trust enables the trustee to distribute income or capital to a specified list of beneficiaries. When a beneficiary dies, no property is deemed to pass, so long as at least two beneficiaries are left. An estate may, in favourable circumstances, be isolated from the revenue for up to 100 years, and duty can be minimized at the close of the trust by suitable distributions.[1]) The net value of the property is then usually aggregated to form one value, on which estate duty is levied at the appropriate rate. To this rule of aggregation there are exceptions, which can substantially reduce the amount of tax.

The general rule is that property in which the deceased never had an interest is treated as a separate estate. This is an easy and

[1] In 1969 this loophole was partly closed by a provision that there should be a charge on the capital of such a trust on the death of a beneficiary.

popular way to lessen estate duties. It could be achieved, for example, by taking out an insurance policy vested absolutely and irrevocably, from the start of the policy, in another person—for example, policies by a man in favour of his wife under the Married Women's Property Act, 1882. This loophole was closed in March, 1968.

Aggregation is also not carried out between 'settled' and 'unsettled' property when the 'unsettled' property of the deceased does not exceed £10,000. In lay terms, unsettled property covers the assets of the deceased, while settled property covers property in which the deceased had a limited or life interest only. Thus, if a deceased's estate was worth £6,000 and he was life tenant of a fund worth £25,000, each would be treated as a separate estate. However, if in the above example, the deceased's estate was worth £10,000 or more, the two would be aggregated for estate duty purposes.

Rapid succession relief is available to reduce estate duty if it becomes liable to duty for a second time within five years, e.g. in the case of the husband dying, followed by the death of his wife within five years. Duty is reduced by up to one-half, according to the length of time involved between the deaths.

A significant and curious provision is the relief granted to agricultural land and appropriate property thereon. Relief was first granted in 1925, and since 1949 it has taken the form of abatement of duty of 45%. A minor provision is that timber is not taken into account until the timber is sold. These provisions take no account of when the property was acquired, so that a death-bed purchase qualifies for relief; the distortion which this introduces into land prices is likely to be significant.

This legislation was further extended in 1954 to industrial premises, plant and machinery used by the deceased or by a company under his control where there is no Stock Exchange quotation. In general, valuation of these assets takes place and a reduction of 45% in duty is made. This class of business may well be faced with special difficulties on the death of an individual, but this form of exemption seems an inequitable way to deal with the problem. It encourages more individuals to arrange their affairs under the protection of this form of ownership, to the detriment of the revenue and of individuals who cannot so arrange their affairs in this form.

In Britain the simplest way to avoid estate duty is to give one's wealth away. There is in Britain, unlike many other countries, no gifts tax as such, although gifts within seven years of death are aggregated and taxed with the deceased person's estate. However, even in this case, reduced rates are payable if the donor dies in the last three years of the period. The period for which gifts are caught for estate duties was increased from three to five years in 1946 and from five to seven years in 1968. The reductions allowed are 15% if the donor dies in the fifth year after the gift was made, 30% if he dies in the sixth year, and 60% in the seventh year.

In the words of Grundy, J. M. (1956), 7, 'as far as estate duty is concerned, the Revenue benefit almost exclusively from the unlucky, the ungenerous and the unwise'.

As illustrations, the unlucky would be those who gave away much of their wealth and died within four years, or those who on their death-bed negotiate to buy a farm or woodland (which has an abatement of duty of 45%) and who die before the transaction can be ratified; the ungenerous, those who refuse to part with any of their wealth before they die or to make other provision; the unwise, those who refuse to pay for competent professional advice in setting up their affairs, particularly in setting up discretionary trusts.

Estate duty and the accretion of income principle

The setting up of the total-accretion principle is an attempt, as we have seen, to tax persons on the increment of spending power that accrues to them per period of time. It is immaterial whether the increment comes in the form of earned or unearned receipts, gifts, bequests, or a change in value of assets held.

The adoption of such an approach to taxation does not change the *existing* pattern of wealth ownership. A person with assets of £1 million, which do not change in value, has had no net accretion of income from capital appreciation (he may, of course, have had an income from these assets, which will be taxed), and he, therefore, will pay no more tax than a person with no wealth but the same income.

However, the *future* pattern of wealth ownership will be changed since any disposal of wealth by way of gift, or bequest at death, will be taxed as the income of the recipient of the gift or bequest.

The community may decide to impose an additional tax on wealth in order to secure more equality in the ownership of wealth. The simplest form of such a wealth tax would be one imposed at death. More complicated will be the imposition of an annual or periodic net wealth tax.

An intrinsic part of any form of wealth tax, whether at death or a periodic tax, is that gifts must also be brought into the tax net, otherwise the wealth tax becomes, at least in part, a discretionary tax, which can be escaped by 'giving away' one's wealth. This is one of the loopholes which makes a mockery of death duties in their present form. The effect of the adoption of gifts as part of the income of the beneficiary with death duties imposed in addition on wealth at death is to give a person the possible option of reducing his tax liability by spreading his gifts out over a number of years and thereby reducing both his own liability for estate duties and the recipient's tax liability. This may not, it itself, be undesirable on social grounds, and averaging of income would greatly reduce the magnitude of the problem.

Special charge on investment income

The Finance Bill in 1968 made a special charge on the investment income of individuals for 1967-8, imposed for one year only. Although this is a charge on income, it can be treated in a chapter on wealth, since when income tax, surtax and the special charge are taken into account the tax will be greater than the income on high investment incomes, and will thus tend to lead to some redistribution of wealth. Disregarding the effect of personal allowances, an individual will surrender more in tax than he receives in investment income when that income has passed £18,580. A sum of approximately £411,000, invested to produce the average yield on *The Times* share index, would produce this sum.

The first £3,000 of investment income, after deduction of personal allowances as allowed for surtax, is exempt from the charge. The remainder is charged at the following rates: between £3,000 and £4,000 2*s*. in the £1 between £4,000 and £5,000 at 3*s*., between £5,000 and £8,000 at 6*s*., and above £8,000 at 9*s*. The yield is estimated at £100 million and about 90,000 people are affected.

This tax was seen at the time as a temporary expedient which would not preclude the introduction of a wealth tax in the future. The problems of taxing wealth are now briefly taken up.

Estate duty or net wealth tax?

The chief difficulty with having an annual wealth tax is the administrative problem of valuation. In contrast, valuation at death normally has to take place in any case. On other grounds, a tax at death comes out well; it is likely to cause less disincentive to effort than most other taxes. Also, the tax has the effect of lessening the inheritance of the beneficiaries, which, because they are unearned by their own efforts, is usually preferred on ethical considerations.

An annual wealth tax, by most of those who propose such a tax, attempts to lessen the problems of valuation by reducing the effectiveness of this tax. They do this by proposing that the tax starts only at high wealth levels, or proposing a very low rate of tax, or limiting the tax to selected assets. These are serious limitations, and because of this in what follows a net wealth tax will not be further elaborated.

Alternatives to a net wealth tax

A frequently advocated alternative is that receipts not subject to income tax and other gifts and bequests should be cumulated over the beneficiaries' lifetime and subject to some form of progressive tax (see Sandford, C. T. (1965) and (April, 1967)). The tax to be paid on a particular bequest would thus depend on the total sum already received. A minor difficulty of such a tax is that the position may arise where the tax due on a gift or bequest is greater (because of past accumulation) than the gift or bequest received. In such cases, the tax could be limited to the sum of the gift or bequest. These proposals can be seen as a way of supplementing death duties or as a substitute for them.

A further complication can be introduced if the proposal to tax gifts and legacies is based on the wealth already possessed by the the recipient, as well as the size of the gift or legacy.

It should be stressed that, in spite of administrative difficulties, taxes on wealth have been introduced in other countries. The Scandinavian countries operate a net wealth tax. Australia, Canada, and the U.S.A. operate gifts taxes of various forms.

Summary

Apart from minor stamp duties which may fall on wealth-transfers, the only tax on wealth in Great Britain is that imposed by estate duties. In their present form, estate duties exhibit most of the disadvantages of a bad tax. Yields are low and administrative costs high. High nominal rates of duty are largely ineffective and lead to the channelling of a good deal of time, money and effort into tax-avoidance.

On the assumption that wealth, as well as income, forms a proper component to tax, a wide variety of suggestions has been made as to the form such a tax should take. The question is not independent of the receipts that are counted as income, and therefore subject to income tax.

The argument adopted in this book is that as much as possible of 'current purchasing power' should be brought into the income tax net. Changes in 'net wealth' due to an inheritance or a gift would therefore be treated as income as well as all capital gains: averaging of income will be necessary to cover the problem of exceptional receipts in any one year, causing an excessive tax burden. The chief benefit to be derived from this change is that an overhaul of the existing tax and surtax rates can be undertaken. Death duties in a modified form should continue with legislative changes to counter the present evasion by way of discretionary trusts and other devices.

As an alternative, it has been suggested that inheritances, gifts and capital gains should be subject to a progressive tax, and that these receipts should be cumulated over a person's lifetime. Such a tax could be extended to lump-sum gratuities and other receipts not subject to income tax.

No attempt has been made to go into the many administrative complexities of taxing wealth more equitably. The problems may appear formidable, but they are not insurmountable if other countries' experience is relevant to Britain.

16
Land

The real property laws of this country, from the period immediately succeeding the Conquest down to the present time, presents a history consistent with itself in one particular, that of a perpetual struggle of rival interests.

C. WREN HOSKYNS (1881), *The Land-laws of England in Systems of Land Tenure in Various Countries.*

Introduction: the meanings attached to 'ownership'

Mankind, even at a primitive stage of development, shows an acute interest in land and territorial rights. Ownership itself is not a simple issue: it presents a highly complex tangle of privileges, rights and duties. By way of illustration, does ownership confer—

- The right of alienation, that is, to sell or give it away?
- The right of bequest?
- The right of franchise?
- The right to mineral wealth below ground?
- The right to hunt and fish?
- The right to erect buildings on it?
- The right to neglect land to the detriment of neighbours and future generations?
- Rights above ground?
- What happens on intestacy?
- Are services or taxes required of the owner?
- Does it accord social status?
- Are improvements made by a tenant the property of the owner, or must the tenant be compensated?
- Are improvements to land by acts of the community chargeable to the owner, and is spoilation compensated, e.g. acts such as sea-defences, drainage, town-expansion, siting of airports, roads, etc.?
- Does the community reserve any public rights, e.g. of access?

Has the community the right to acquire the land for the public good?

'Ownership' is the rag-bag into which all aspects are bundled. The history of land and of the privileges, rights and duties that attach thereto exhibits a rich variety of solutions to be found at different times and in different places. Much history is a record of this changing nexus of privilege and responsibility.

The subject of land abounds in legal subtleties. A short summary or outline is hardly possible, and certainly cannot do justice to the niceties that have developed. In Great Britain the Norman Conquest of 1066 brought great changes. After the Conquest the normal position was for the Crown to *own* land, and others to hold an estate under various forms of tenure, either directly from the Crown or from an intermediate holder, who himself had tenure directly or indirectly from the Crown.[1] Feudal tenure involved the granting of an estate for services. These were in the form of military, spiritual or agricultural obligations. Wills of land were not permitted; descent in the male line predominated.

This situation was gradually changed in a number of ways. Feudal services tended to be commuted into annual money payments or 'rents'. The trust device came to be used to get around the ban on bequeathing land; this right was not legally established until 1540. The freehold, as a freely marketable commodity unencumbered by onerous feudal rights, was achieved by statute in 1660. The system thus established is, speaking very broadly, the one existing until 1947, although there were numerous alterations in the laws affecting land during this time, some of considerable importance. Developments since 1947 will be looked at in more detail later in this chapter.

The economics of land

David Ricardo, an economist of the early nineteenth century, developed the idea that land is in a separate category from other factors of production, since its supply could neither be diminished or reduced. He argued that a tax on land could not reduce the available supply,

[1] 'He who held land as tenant of the royal lord could himself become lord by granting the land to another. The primary rung in the feudal tenurial ladder was the tenant in actual possession of the tenement, the tenant *in dominico*. The ultimate rung was the king, the one man in all the realm who was never tenant. Between the two extremes the rungs were either an ascending series of lordships or a descending series of tenures, according to the view taken. There is no land unowned in all England. Land can be without a tenant where he who is in possession is the king; but land without a lord there cannot be—*nulle terre sans seigneur*' (Denman, D. R. (1958), 80).

and hence could have no adverse effect on production: therefore 'rent' should be treated differently from other factor payments. Fundamentally, the quantity of land is limited in supply. A community with a growing population is likely to experience an increasing demand for the limited amount of land available—for food-growing, dwellings, transport and amenities—which will raise its real value. This 'unearned income' may not accrue to every landowner, but it will accrue to landowners *en masse*. We have here the germ of later ideas developed by 'single-taxers', such as Henry George, that land need be the only item to bear tax, an idea which today, even if acceptable, would not yield the amount of revenue required.

Ricardo's ideas have been modified on two fronts. The supply of services from land can be increased by, for example, better agricultural methods or increasing the height of buildings; it can also be reduced by, for example, soil erosion. Secondly, other factors may be akin to land, in that the supply cannot immediately be changed in response to an increase in demand, and these factors will also enjoy an enhanced price, or 'quasi-rent', for a period.

Land has one other attribute which is sufficient to mark it off from most other assets: that is the degree to which the price of land is affected by socially created values.

There is no novelty in proposals to secure for the community at least a share in the values it has itself created. An Act of 1427 sought to recover increases in the value of property attributable to public expenditure on works for sea-defence, and in the reign of Charles II there was statutory appropriation of a part of landowners' unearned enhancement or 'melioration' assessed upon the benefits of street widening in London (*Land Commission* (1965), para. 2).

With increased government activity today, the scope for great changes in land values which accrue without effort on the landowners' part is very much increased. Proposals to build new towns, the reconstruction of existing towns, new road links, the closing of railway lines, siting of power stations, airports and seaports, the planning regulations which permit or prohibit certain types of development are but a few of the more obvious examples of community decisions, which can greatly increase, and less often decrease, the value of land.

Should land be treated differently from other assets?

From the fiscal viewpoint, it is necessary to decide whether the relative uniqueness of land—that is, its 'fixed quantity' and change in value which can occur through public action—is sufficiently marked to call for special tax treatment. In a country which is sparsely populated, the question may seem an academic one; in a well-populated country like Britain it becomes more acute. The problem, as has been indicated, is made more complex since a wide variety of planning regulations have grown up. The redesignation of land from 'green belt'—that is, land that shall not be built upon—to a housing area can increase the price of land many hundred-fold. In a similar way, the price may be adversely affected by planning permission, which goes the other way.[2]

The authors' opinion is that the factors indicated provide clear evidence that land should be taxed. From the account given below of the period since 1947, it will be seen that the tax on land has taken various forms.

The period 1947-67

Land was considered in the *Report of the Expert Committee on Compensation and Betterment* (1942) under the Chairmanship of Mr Justice Uthwatt. The *Land Commission* (1965) White Paper reported as follows:

> The main recommendations of the Uthwatt Committee were implemented by the Labour government in the Town and Country Planning Act, 1947, which vested in the State all development rights in land. Anyone wishing to develop land had to recover the right to develop by payment of a development charge to the Central Land Board. A capital sum of £300 million was available for payments to those who established claims that the value of their land had depreciated as a result of the Act.
>
> The Central Land Board were also given powers to buy land compulsorily for the purpose of disposing of it for development. The Uthwatt Committee had considered that public acquisition, if need be by compulsion, was the only satisfactory answer to the problem of comprehensive development and of securing betterment. In practice, doubts arose about the validity of the powers given to the Central Land Board and they had not been widely used when the Conservative government changed the situation by abolishing development charges in the Town and Country Planning Act, 1953.
>
> The 1953 Act, a stop-gap measure, was followed by the Town and County Planning Act, 1954, which removed the restrictions on private sales, so that those sales took place at market prices. A two-price system was thereby created: prices paid when land with development value was sold privately were higher than those paid when such land was acquired compulsorily for public purposes. This two-price system was so clearly inequitable that the government was forced to eliminate it, and

[2] It was reported in the *Sunday Times* of July 12th, 1964, that 30 acres of land at Mill Hill bought in 1954 for £3,000 was saleable for £700,000 in 1964.

this they chose to do by the Town and County Planning Act, 1959, which restored market value as the basis for compensation on compulsory purchase.

Since the removal in 1959 of the last restraints on the market in land for development, land with planning permission for development or even with the hope of such planning permission, whether stimulated by a development plan or not, has been fetching ever-increasing prices. These prices, which must be paid by public authorities buying land for their essential purposes, place a heavy burden on their financial resources; they are also a deterrent to people wishing to buy their own homes (paras. 3, 4, 5, 6).

1947, therefore, sees an attempt to implement some of the recommendations of the Uthwatt Committee *Report* and secure for the State the betterment value of land. This attempt fails because of legislative shortcomings, the complexity of the Act and probably also resentment of a 100% tax on betterment values, and lead to the gradual abandonment of the attempt: by 1959 a return to free market pricing had taken place.

This period was one in general of steeply rising prices of land. Gains made in this way were, unless caught by the 1947 Act, untaxed until 1962, unless they were undertaken 'by way of trade' and fell to be taxed under normal company taxation. In 1962 capital gains in land and building were taxed, as we have seen, if realized within three years. The 1965 Act charged all gains either to the short-term or the long-term tax.

Land Commission Act, April, 1967

The Land Commission Act, 1967, is an attempt to re-establish some of the recommendations of the Uthwatt Committee of 1942, but to achieve the aims of the Committee in a different way from the Act of 1947.

The Land Commission has a head office in Newcastle and eleven regional offices, which administer a tax known as the 'betterment levy', and it is invested with wide powers to acquire land compulsorily. Compulsory purchase will be based on current market values (less the betterment levy), so it should be a matter of indifference to a landowner whether he sells to the Land Commission, a public authority or a private purchaser.

The betterment levy is at an initial rate of 40% and the stated intention of the government is to increase the rate progressively to 45% and then to 50% at reasonably short intervals. The question of increasing the rate further is not ruled out. The levy thus presents an important change from the Act of 1947, which sought to obtain the whole of the betterment value. Further, the charge is only on the increase in the value for a new use, less the current value in its old one.

Thus if a piece of agricultural land were originally bought for £300, and is currently worth £1,000 if sold as agricultural land, but worth £3,000 if sold as housing land, no betterment levy is imposed in the case of continuing agricultural use; it is payable on £2,000 if sold as housing land (current value in existing use deducted from current value in new use). Where the betterment levy is charged, the capital gains tax will not apply, but this tax will continue to apply where land is sold for existing use.

The betterment levy is charged on the person who has actually realized the gain. This would normally be the seller. In the above example, the seller would pay the 40% levy on £2,000. If, however, the purchaser defers development and the value of the land rises to £4,000, he will be liable to a betterment levy on the difference of £1,000.

In the case of development of land, the levy may be payable even though no sale takes place, but only *material* development as defined by the Act ranks for levy. Thus a person can rebuild his house and increase its size up to 1,000 square feet, erect a garage, or turn his house into flats without incurring a levy. In a like manner, a factory may be rebuilt and enlarged without incurring a levy, provided neither the floor area or the cubic content is enlarged more than 10%. No levy will be imposed on the development or disposal of land held by local authorities for their social services, including comprehensive development and town development, but it will apply to land held by them for commercial purposes. Similarly, the levy will not be payable by statutory undertakings or endowed charities.

An amendment in 1969 exempted from levy cases where the market value of the land does not exceed £1,500. This was expected to reduce by half the number of cases subject to levy. Provision was also made to deal with hardship in cases where a plot of land has been received as a gift and in which the recipient is building a house for his own occupation.

The financial provisions of the Act probably have the effect of taxing gains on land at a higher rate than for other capital gains, since long-term gains accruing to the individual attract tax at a top rate of 30%. However, this is not necessarily the case. It should be borne in mind in looking at the levy of 40% that this is a charge only on the change between its current value in its new use and the current value in its old use. Any capital appreciation of the land in its existing use is untaxed. When the land is sold, appreciation is only taxed to capital gains if the land retains its present use when sold. There seems little justification for this curious anomaly. The argument that it is difficult to establish the value of land at April 6th, 1965, doesn't deter this date being used for capital gains. As an illustration, we can use the figures given in the example above. If we assume that a piece of agricultural land had a value of £300 on April 6th, 1965, and is now worth £1,000 in its existing use as agricultural land, or £3,000 as housing land, the betterment levy takes the difference between £3,000 and £1,000 as the sum to tax; at 40% this yields £800. If we take the difference in value as £2,700 (the difference between its value in 1965 and now), this effectively reduces the betterment levy to a little below 30%.

Probably of more practical importance than the yield of the tax on land, if the intentions of the Act are carried out, are the powers of compulsory purchase given to the Land Commission. It seems to be envisaged that the Land Commission shall be an active body, not just acquiring land piecemeal as the need arises, but ensuring 'that the right land is made available at the right time'. It is envisaged that the Commission will buy, hold, manage and sell land to developers. These powers are to be gradually given to the Commission.

One by-product of the Act is that the government intends local authorities to benefit from the levy:

> It would, however, be impractical and inequitable to relate this assistance directly to the levy arising on conveyances of land purchased by each local authority, since the benefit could vary between local authorities in an arbitrary fashion. Without prejudice to the discussions which are to take place during the current review of local government finance, it is the intention of the government to ensure that the gain to the Exchequer from the operations of the Land Commission will in one way or another be reflected in the new arrangements under which local authorities will receive financial assistance from government. *Land Commission* (1965), para. 35.

Evaluation of the Land Commission Act, 1967

The Act, as we have seen, has two aims: one to secure the better use of land and, secondly, to tax the increment of betterment value. We shall confine ourselves to consideration of the second point.

Although the Act links these two points together, this is not logically necessary. The Land Commission could continue with its powers for the better use of land while the tax is dealt with separately.

The criticism was made earlier that the long-term capital gains tax is a flat-rate tax, while 'income' is subject to very progressive tax rates. The same criticism applies to the betterment levy. If capital gains were counted as part of personal income, as current short-term gains are, the case for a separate tax on land (with its administrative complexities) could be reconsidered. The case for the community securing at least a large part of socially created values is strong. Whether more revenue would be gained by treating betterment on land as part of a person's income depends on the rate of tax to which a person's income is subject, compared to the rate at which the betterment levy finally comes to rest. The wealthy taxpayer would almost certainly pay more if it is assessed to income, unless the betterment levy is raised to 70% or 80%.

Effect on the price of land

The intention of the 1947 Act was to secure for the government the whole of the increment in the price of land. The 1967 Act subjects this to, at present, a tax of 40%. This difference makes it very difficult to discuss the effects of the tax on land prices. With a tax of 100%, the seller has, at least theoretically, no incentive to hold out for a higher price, since only the revenue will benefit.[3] With a tax at a lower rate, the seller may try to hold out for a higher price, so that his gain after tax has been paid is bigger. The extent to which a seller is able to gain a higher price, and so effectively pass the tax on to the buyer, depends on the strength of demand and supply for the land.

The stated intention to increase the rate to 45% and then to 50% and perhaps higher is a partial inducement not to hold out for too long. However, because the tax is on the difference in the value of the land between its existing use and its new use, too much should not be made of this point. This anomaly, already referred to, whereby land, unlike other capital gains, escapes any tax on the increase in value for existing use when it is sold for a new use may create serious distortions. It is likely to lessen the supply of land coming on to the market, since the effect of higher rates of betterment levy is to some extent mollified. It is also likely to increase the demand for land by those who see a chance to make a capital gain which is partly tax-free. It is true that this advantage will be wiped out if the betterment levy is set at a sufficiently high rate, but there are obvious disadvantages in giving the appearance of high rates without, in practice, taxing at these rates. The rates of the betterment levy are, as shown by the example given in this chapter, not the effective

[3] The intention not to interfere with the market in land clearly failed in the case of the 1947 Act. Land was held back by owners in the hope (subsequently fulfilled) that the levy would be abandoned. Also, land was sold at prices higher than its value in 1947.

rates which will apply. It is possible for the rate of 40% to be a lighter tax than a capital gains tax of 30%, because gains on existing use escape the tax net when land is sold for a different use.

In Chapter 15, on 'Wealth', a more serious distortion is pointed out. Agricultural land and property, even if purchased from the deathbed, is entitled to a 45% rebate of estate duty. While such a tax haven remains open, the demand for agricultural land—and therefore its price—can be expected to be artificially inflated, and this in turn is likely to affect the price of other land.

No very firm conclusions can be drawn, so recently after the passing of the Act, on the effects of the levy on the price of land and the supply coming on to the market. Removal of the levy concession and estate duty rebate would go a long way towards creating a more realistic market in land. Their presence is only likely to inflate the price of land. Of crucial importance is how soon it is intended to increase the levy above the present level of 40% and the level at which it is expected to finally come to rest.

Summary

Land in a developed community is a scarce resource, and can by actions of the community be subject to very wide fluctuations in price.

The Land Commission Act, 1967, set out to secure the better use of land by giving the Land Commission powers to purchase land, if necessary by compulsory purchase, and, secondly, to tax the increase in land values. This tax carries on the tradition of imposing a nominal rate of tax (at present 40%) which is not the effective rate, because gains on the existing use of land escape tax when the land is sold for a different use.

The tax on land in its present form seems a needless complication of the tax structure; the difference in yield if land were taxed to capital gains cannot be very large. As with capital gains, treating gains made on land as income seems to be the equitable solution.

17
The national debt

Although the National Debt, in the sense in which we are using the term, is of such great importance for economic policy, there is in existing publications no adequate statistical analysis of it, nor indeed is there any statement of its size, either in published documents or in any official papers that have been brought to our notice. The great advance in official statistical knowledge of national income has not been matched by any comparable advance in knowledge of national assets and liabilities. We have therefore had to piece together, as best we could, a great deal of scattered information, which has been very substantially increased by figures produced specially for us, both by the authorities and by non-official bodies . . .

(*Radcliffe Committee* (1959), para. 536.)

Meaning of national debt

When the government spends more than it receives, this results in the issue of some sort of security to cover the deficiency. In like manner, a surplus results in a reduction of securities. The aggregate of securities issued over time is called the 'national debt'.

In earlier chapters, when looking at government spending and revenue, it was found necessary to define 'government' carefully in order to avoid misunderstanding. We there included central and local government, but excluded the nationalized industries. Likewise, in order to try to make sense of the figures over time it was necessary to be clear whether the figures were in money terms or deflated for changes in the price-level, and whether account had or had not been taken of changes in population. The National Debt seems to arouse more misunderstanding and emotion than either government spending or revenue, and these reservations are even more necessary. An added reason for caution is, as the quotation to this chapter shows, the lack of adequate data. More information has become available in recent years, but still the quality and quantity leave much to be desired.

The terminology and concepts used will be those adopted by the Radcliffe Committee as modified by the Bank of England. The major modification is the omission from the concept of national debt of debt payable in overseas currency, amounting to £1,822 million in 1967. Used without further qualification, 'national debt' is taken to mean the *net* debt of the public sector. That is to say, the obligations of the public sector, excluding debt held by the public sector itself. The term 'gross' is used to mean all debt, whether held by the public sector itself, termed 'official holdings', or whether it is held outside the public sector. Official holdings would be holdings by the Bank of England, the Exchange Equalization Account, the National Debt Commissioners, and certain government departments.

The public sector is a combination of central government, local authorities, nationalized industries and other public bodies. The inclusion of nationalized industries thus gives wider coverage than that used for spending and revenue. It will be argued later that the debt of the nationalized industries may be on a different footing to other debt, and for this reason the debt of these industries has been distinguished in the figures.

Table 1 presents figures of the gross debt of the public sector by

Table 1

Gross debt of the public sector by origin

(£ million nominal value)

Year	Central Government		Local Authorities in Great Britain		Public Corporations		Total
	Consolidated Fund	Bank-notes and Other Debt	To P.W.L.B.	Other Debt	To Exchequer	Other Debt	
1935	6,760	575	289	1,301	—	161	9,086
1952	23,723	1,961	1,818	1,126	480	2,871	31,978
1955	24,804	2,313	2,828	1,505	776	3,364	35,590
1958	25,069	2,766	3,210	2,390	1,796	3,616	38,848
			Percentages				
1935	81		17		2		100
1952	80		9		11		100
1955	76		12		12		100
1958	72		14		14		100

Source: *Committee on the Working of the Monetary System*, Tables 24, 25.

type of issuing authority. In accordance with the definitions adopted, these figures do not include debt payable in overseas currency. In money terms the debt has increased from £9,086 million in 1935 to £38,848 million in 1958. Prices roughly doubled in this period, the debt increased fourfold, mainly due to the Second World War. In 1935 the central government had issued about 80% of the debt, with local authorities accounting for most of the balance. In 1958 the relative share of the central government had declined to 72%, while local authorities and public corporations have roughly equal responsibility for the remainder. It will be seen from the table that the central government has been a substantial net lender since the war, the increase in its debt being much more than offset by Exchequer advances to public corporations and loans through the Public Works Loan Board to local authorities.

Table 2 shows the composition of the net debt of the public sector —that is, excluding holdings of the public sector held by itself. This will be seen to have increased less rapidly than the gross figures— in other words, the holdings of the public sector of its own debt has increased in this period. One explanation of this has already been noted: the increased lending by the central government to other parts of the public sector. Further holdings will be explained by the development of National Insurance and similar funds. This table also shows that the debt was more liquid post-war. Gilt-edged securities had fallen from 62% of the total to 51%, while notes, Treasury bills and National Savings show big increases. Local authority debt was growing rapidly from 1952, and had important monetary implications, since after 1955 much of it consisted of short-term securities. However, the percentage of local authority debt was still substantially below the pre-war percentage. The line at the bottom of Table 2 is important. It expresses the money values of net debt shown in the table as a percentage of the money national income. It can be seen that, in spite of the large increase in money terms of the debt it has not increased as fast as the national income.

These figures, as most that are published on debt, must be used carefully: they will not bear any but broad conclusions. In particular, it should be noted that the analysis is in terms of nominal values. Nominal values are usually taken as the face value of the security, which is usually the value at which the security is originally sold, although on occasions a security is issued either at a discount or a premium. Long-term gilt-edged securities have for many years stood at a substantial discount on the Stock Exchange on their nominal values, and for many purposes details in market values would provide more meaningful information. In many other respects the figures have to be treated as little more than estimates of the true position;

Table 2

Composition of the net debt of the public sector at 31st March

	£ million nominal value				Percentages			
	1935	1952	1955	1958	1935	1952	1955	1958
Notes and Coin	453	1,545	1,858	2,199	6	6	7	8
Treasury bills	371	2,334	3,024	2,938	4	9	11	10
Gilt-edged securities	5,219	13,048	14,024	14,489	62	52	52	51
National Savings plus accrued interest	1,003	5,786	5,735	5,756	12	23	21	20
Tax reserve certificates	—	368	388	346	—	2	1	1
Northern Ireland government and local authorities	34	43	63	87	0	0	0	0
Local authorities in Great Britain	1,301	1,126	1,505	2,390	16	5	6	8
Borrowing from banks or other funds by public bodies	—	281	196	225	—	1	1	1
Overseas loans payable in sterling	—	361	318	134	—	2	1	1
Total	8,381	24,892	27,111	28,564	100	100	100	100
Total as a percentage of national income	204	195	175	154				

Source: *Committee on the Working of the Monetary System*, Tables 24, 25.

most, for example, contain large residual errors.

Of the figure of £25,069 million shown in Table 1 under Consolidated Fund,[1] together with £3,294 million of nationalized industries' stocks guaranteed by the government, in all a figure of £28,363 million, the Bank of England have estimated holders in 1958 as appears on p. 204.

They found in 1958 that official holdings account for a quarter of the total, the banking sector for 16% and official overseas holdings for 11%. Unfortunately, the value of this analysis is lessened by the figure of 'other' holdings, which, besides concealing the holdings of the company sector and the holdings of individuals, contains a large residual item which the Bank was unable to allocate (see below).

	£m.	%
Official Holdings	7,032	25
Public bodies	179	1
Banking sector	4,629	16
Overseas official	3,094	11
Other	13,429	47
	28,363	100

In their evidence to the Radcliffe Committee, the Treasury estimated the time-structure of that part of the debt which consisted of marketable government and government-guaranteed securities as follows:

Year:	1935	1955	1957
Amount in £m.:	5,508	17,521	18,630
	%	%	%
Up to 5 years	3	20	25
5 to 15 years	12	24	25
15 to 25 years	5	21	19
Over 25 years	19	13	11
Undated	61	22	20
Total	100	100	100

[1] The term 'Consolidated Fund' refers to procedure laid down for payment of moneys to or from the State. It is not of practical significance in this context.

This brings out clearly the sharp change in the time-structure of the debt pre-war and post-war. The figures relate to marketable securities of the government or securities under their guarantee. The data for 1958 are not available. Whereas in 1935 80% of this debt was either undated or had more than twenty-five years to run to maturity, the corresponding figure in 1957 was only 31%. It is not surprising that the monetary authorities in the post-war period were concerned about the liquidity of the economy.

Table 3, still largely in terms of nominal values, analyses the gross debt of the Consolidated Fund and government-guaranteed nationalized industries' stocks for the year 1967 in more detail. The debt is broken down into four categories: Treasury bills, stocks which have between nought and five years to run to maturity, stocks with over five years to maturity or that are undated, and non-marketable securities, such as Post Office savings and certificates. These account respectively for 12%, 20%, 48% and 20% of the total. Treasury bills and short-dated stocks thus account for nearly a third of the total.

The breakdown by holders shows: official holdings (29% of the total), public bodies (1%), the banking sector (6%), overseas banks in the U.K. (2%), accepting houses and the discount market (3%), financial institutions (14%), overseas residents, which includes both official and private holdings (14%), individuals (19%), other holders (2%), residual, much of which is believed to belong to individuals (10%). Even if the whole of the residual column is attributed to individuals, we find that less than 29% of the debt is held by United Kingdom individuals.

Within each category of debt besides official holdings, the important holders of Treasury bills are domestic banks, acceptance houses, the discount market and overseas residents. For short-term stocks, the domestic banks, acceptance houses, the discount market, financial institutions, overseas residents and individuals. For long-term or undated stocks, financial institutions, overseas residents and individuals. For non-marketable stock, overseas residents and individuals.

From the point of view of government finance, the sale of non-marketable debt is no different from the sale of marketable debt, e.g. when the public deposits money with the Post Office Savings Bank and the ordinary departments of the Trustee Savings Banks, and when it holds bank-notes, this is in effect lending to the government. Of the official holdings of £9,278 million nearly two-thirds represents securities held for this purpose. That is to say, a deposit by a member of the public at a Post Office Savings Bank has much the same effect as a purchase from the government of a security for the same amount. In the first case the Savings Bank deposit is credited to the government account and the Savings Bank is issued with a government

Table 3

Estimated distribution of the gross debt of the Consolidated Fund and government-guaranteed nationalized industries' stocks, March 31st, 1967

(£ nominal value)

	Treasury Bills	Stocks		Non-marketable	Total	Total holdings as %age of total debt
		Maturity of 0-5 years	Maturity over 5 years			
Official holdings	2,162	1,650	4,487	929	9,228	29
Public bodies	0	56	137	68 (Public bodies to Accepting houses)	193	1
Domestic banks	425	899	568		1,892	6
Overseas banks in U.K.	43	248	267		558	2
Accepting houses and Discount Mkt.	233	715	73		1,021	3
Financial institutions	9	579	3,985	7	4,580	14
Overseas residents	903	860	1,156	1,563	4,482	14
Individuals	0	427	2,251	3,289	5,967	19
Other holders[2]	2	827 (Other holders and Residual)	2,425 (Other holders and Residual)	138	750	2
Residual[3]	108			432	3,182	10
Total	3,885	6,261	15,349	6,426	31,921[4]	100
Total as %	12	20	48	20	100	

Source: *Bank of England Quarterly Bulletin*, March, 1968.

Nationalized industries' guaranteed stocks account for £1,757 million of the above.
Debt payable in overseas currencies of £1,822 million not included in the table.
0 Negligible or small holdings.
[2] Public Trustee, non-corporate bodies, companies and friendly societies.
[3] Much of this is believed to belong to individuals.
[4] Includes £68 million of non-marketable debt which cannot be allocated.

security as collateral; in the second case the individual receives the security as collateral directly. The remaining one-third of official holdings is divided between various government funds, mainly the National Insurance and Industrial Injuries Funds and the holdings of the Exchange Equalization Account and of the Banking Department of the Bank of England.

Summary of statistical data

The national debt shows a large money increase in the post-war period compared to the pre-war period. However, the net debt expressed as a percentage of national income shows a marked decrease. The composition of the debt has changed from being primarily long-term or undated to being primarily short- or medium-term.

Greater detail is now available for that part of the debt that comes under the Consolidated Fund and government-guaranteed securities of the nationalized industries.[5]

Official holdings have increased in recent years, and in 1967 accounted for 29% of the total, domestic banks show a decline in holdings and now account for about 6%, other financial institutions in the economy hold 13%, 14% is held overseas, while it is estimated that individuals hold between 18% and 29%.

The relevance of the national debt

The total amount of the debt has now been looked at, and it has been shown how much of this is issued by the central government and how much by local authorities and by nationalized industries. The time-structure of the debt has been given and a broad classification shown of the main holders. With this information we are in a position to take up some of the important implications of the national debt.

Can any valid comparisons be drawn between the debt of a nation and the debt of a company? Briefly, the answer is 'yes'; but there are also pitfalls to be avoided.

A company balance-sheet over time will normally show an increase in the liabilities of the company, which will be matched by corresponding increases on the asset side. Before a judgment is made that the increase in liabilities is good or bad, it is necessary to know a great deal more about the changes. For example, it makes a difference if it is the issued capital, reserves or bank overdraft which has increased;

[5] Separate details are also available in the financial statistics on local authority debt by type of holder and structure of the debt.

and also it makes a difference how the assets have changed. Has more been put into plant or is it that unwanted stocks are piling up?

It is also necessary, within limits, to take account of both sides of the national balance-sheet. The debt has been primarily incurred as a result of war expenditure. There are no physical assets corresponding to this expenditure. However, the public sector has tangible assets and the public debt in the post-war period is not quite the same thing as the pre-war debt. In particular, the nationalization of industries has resulted in an increase in debt which has been matched by an increase in assets. Much expenditure of local authorities has been on housing, and once again there are corresponding real assets. A reduction in debt could be achieved by selling these assets to the private sector, but, considered solely as a means of reducing the debt, the exercise achieves little. Since the government undertakes 'commercial' activities, there is a case for separating out debt operations of this kind. It may well happen that full commercial criteria should not be applied to all parts of commercial government activity; that, for example, some branch railway lines should be run even though this entails a loss, but separation at least enables a more realistic appraisal of both the national debt and government commercial activities.

The danger inherent in applying company balance-sheet ideas to the national balance-sheet has been labelled the 'cement and steel' concept. The purpose of business finance is to increase its profits and net worth, but this is not the case for government finance (with the possible modification just noted of government commercial activities). Assets held by the firm are the collateral against the firm's debt, but no such reasoning applies to government assets. Applying commercial ideas to the whole of government debt 'reinforces the ancient prejudice in favour of expenditure on hardware as distinct from services': the type of thinking that enjoins the building of schools and hospitals but jibs at paying those who run them adequate salaries. In particular, it has been alleged in recent years that some underdeveloped countries are prone to prestige development rather than undertaking less glamorous but more productive investment.

We can look at this matter from another viewpoint. It is true that the economy will be worse off if the government increases the national debt (i.e. borrows) and uses the money wastefully. But this argument has nothing to do with increasing the national debt. It would be equally valid if the wasteful spending was out of tax revenue.

The technical problems of debt management

So far it has been established that the size of the debt by itself is not a good guide to its economic significance. It nevertheless remains true that a large debt poses problems of debt-management. These were grouped into five by the Radcliffe Committee:

(*a*) The Treasury has to deal with maturities of marketable debt, and to make new issues to replace these and to finance new requirements, beyond current revenue, of the central government.
(*b*) The markets in outstanding liabilities require 'management', both to facilitate (*a*) and to avert undesirable repercussions on the wider financial structure of the economy. This requirement applies both to the very short-term liabilities (management of 'the money market') and to the longer-term liabilities (management of the gilt-edged section of the Stock Exchange).
(*c*) The net capital requirements of the nationalized industries have to be provided; this involves questions of how the money should be raised (which connects with (*a*) above) and the terms on which it should be made available to the industries.
(*d*) Similarly, the net capital requirements of the local government authorities have to be provided.
(*e*) The methods of raising funds by the sale of non-marketable securities (e.g. Tax Reserve Certificates and the 'small savings' instruments) have to be determined. All of these tasks are related to each other, and decisions on any one of them must have regard to repercussions on others. In carrying out these tasks the Treasury has always to have regard to the fact that a considerable proportion of the National Debt is held overseas (para. 532).

The most important problems in the post-war period, it has already been indicated, occurred under headings (*a*) and (*b*) above. As a result of war-time financing, large blocks of debt became due for repayment. The debt was considerably more liquid and presented a threat of inflationary pressure if the assets, as they matured, were spent on consumer goods rather than reinvested. The period has been labelled one of the 'cult of the equity', in other words the market for fixed interest long-term securities, such as gilt-edged, was not buoyant. Clearly these matters impinge on monetary and fiscal policy and affect rates of interest. A related set of problems was the cost of servicing the debt. In so far as the debt is held by residents of Britain the problem is not so serious: high interest costs mean that taxation must be higher than it would otherwise need to be in order to pay the interest charges. The problem may have important considerations concerning the redistribution of income, but this is not our immediate concern in this section. The problem is more serious for that part of the debt which is held by non-residents of Britain (over £4,482 million in 1967). This implies a payment outflow from this country to the foreign holders, and in so far as they are not content to hold sterling, but require their own currencies, this is a factor operating to depress the price of sterling on world markets.

Management of the debt in relation to the economy

In the words of the Radcliffe Committee:

> The most elementary problem of debt management is one that is necessarily solved in some way or other day by day. The previously existing debt, plus any current Exchequer cash deficit, or minus any current Exchequer cash surplus, has to be and is absorbed. Each day the vast majority of holders of government securities continue to hold those securities at the end of the day, but a fraction of the securities is unloaded during the day: this unloaded fraction, and any currently accruing deficit, must be absorbed either by new holders in the private sector or against release of cash by the monetary authorities. And the same is true of a year's operations: in some way or other the government's needs are met, and the debt existing at the end of the year must be held by someone, even if this result can only be achieved by allowing cash to constitute a greater part of the debt than before. If the achievement of this result threatens to entail growth of cash or other highly liquid liabilities to a degree thought dangerous, because of the repercussions of this growth of liquidity in the private sector, the authorities have in theory three courses open to them:
>
> (1) they can make long-term securities so much more attractive that the threat is averted (i.e. 'funding' succeeds);
> (2) they can increase taxation, so enabling themselves to get the real resources they want without adding so much to, and perhaps even bringing about some reduction of, the National Debt;
> (3) they can cut the use of real resources by the public sector (cutting either government expenditure or investment in the public sector) so reducing the amount of debt to be placed with the private sector in the period.
>
> There have been in the last decade examples of all three methods of adjustment (para. 558).

This quotation brings out clearly one problem: that the management of the debt may result in a growth of unwanted liquidity of the debt in which case a number of alternative (but unpleasant) choices are available. Not brought out quite so clearly is the allied problem that, if the debt is changing in total as well as in maturity structure; this implies a different use of real resources. As an example, consider the case of an Exchequer cash deficit (i.e. a need to increase the debt) in a year in which the economy is fully employed.

Even if in these circumstances the most favourable case is taken where the government is able to make good the deficiency by the sale of long-term securities, it is unlikely that private expenditure will be cut back by the whole amount of the deficiency. Unless additional action is taken on one or more of the ways suggested in (1) to (3) above, inflationary pressure will result.

Similar considerations apply if the economy is not fully employed and the government is running a surplus (i.e. reducing the national debt). It is unlikely that the whole of the proceeds will be spent by the private sector on consumer goods or investment projects, and in the absence of offsetting action the economy will be further run down.

It is now possible to understand the statements of the Radcliffe Committee:

> For the debt ought not to be regarded as a given total, whose structure alone can be manipulated. If all possible courses in manipulating the structure threaten serious disadvantages this can be a reason for aiming at a bigger Exchequer cash surplus (or smaller deficit), so as to lessen the difficulties of management of the debt. . . . The debt is not, that is to say, to be regarded as a residual among the quantities of economy policy. Thus debt management can be regarded neither as something to be, as it were, left to the last and adjusted to all other policy decisions, nor on the other hand as a consideration which should override all other policy decisions; it has to be integrated with a variety of measures in the pursuit of the broad aims of economic policy (para. 535).

To recapitulate, the management of the debt has both monetary implications and implications for the use of the real resources in the economy. Because the propensities to spend of the government and the private sectors will usually differ, the problem in ensuring balance in the economy is not just a simple one of, for example, ensuring that increased government expenditure is equally matched by an increase in taxation or by an increase in debt. In full-employment conditions, a greater sum will normally have to be raised, because private expenditure on goods and services is likely to fall by a smaller magnitude than the changes in revenue brought about by the changes in government spending. Likewise, given a reduction in government spending matched by a cut in taxes, it is unlikely that the whole of this sum will be spent on investment or consumption goods, and it may be necessary for the government to take some action to maintain a balance in the economy.

If we revert back to the three courses of action open to the authorities, we find that restraints are present on each of them. The success of funding depends on the public's willingness to take up government long-term debt; there may be periods during which the public is not willing to do this. It may be possible to induce the public to hold more debt at a higher rate of interest (the Radcliffe Committee express some doubt on this), but even so an increase in interest rates has other implications which must be considered. In particular, rates of interest in Britain that are out of line with other developed countries may result in undesirable flows of money (so called 'hot money') into and out of the country, which are very disturbing to the balance of payments.

Changes in taxation can be aimed primarily either at changing spending in the company sector or at changing the level of personal spending. The latter is likely to reflect on the company sector if the change continues for any length of time. A variety of other methods can also be used to influence behaviour in these two sectors, e.g. changing investment allowances or grants, and altering hire-purchase regulations on down-payment and length of time over which payments can be made. Much use has been made in the post-war period of such policies, designed to influence the private sector. This will be taken up later.

Changes in the use of real resources by the government also has obvious drawbacks. Much of government expenditure is on essential services, such as roads, hospitals and various kinds of educational establishments. Many people are of the opinion that expenditure on these items should be increased, not decreased. In the words of Professor Galbraith, 'Public squalor is contrasted with private affluence'. The interruption of capital plans, particularly the capital spending of local authorities and nationalized industries, has been a feature on several occasions in the post-war period. It is particularly wasteful and expensive to try to alter capital expenditure once a certain stage of work has been reached, and this type of action is a desperate resort. The recasting of long-term plans is a different matter, but it is the case that planning techniques have not developed to the extent that much reliance can be placed on such forecasts, and altering long-term plans is no remedy for a current imbalance.

Burden of the debt

The phrase 'burden of the debt' is unfortunately one that seems to be embedded in any discussion about the national debt. The implication of the word 'burden' is that life would be better if only the burden could be got rid of. Discussion about the debt is thus biased in advance. Confusion is made worse by difference about the meaning of 'burden'.

WHAT DO WE MEAN BY 'BURDEN'?

Burden is sometimes construed to mean the current amount of goods and services which the private sector gives up in order to enable the public sector to consume. This may be nil in the case of an under-employed economy, where the use of resources by the public sector need not be at the expense of private consumption, but can come from increased production out of previously unused resources. With full employment of resources, by definition, increased consumption by one sector is at the expense of another if imported commodities remain unchanged. To make sense of the 'burden' argument in conditions of full employment, it is necessary, somehow, to evaluate the government's use of resources and its worth to individuals as opposed to leaving the resources as they were. It is clear that while this line of argument poses important issues, these have nothing specifically to do with debt-financing. Tax-financing raises exactly similar problems.

Another concept of burden relates to the amount of goods and services forgone by the people currently living during the period of their lifetimes. Given full employment, capital projects which take a long time to fructify will lessen the amount of currently available consumer goods, but increase the amount available, say, ten or twenty years ahead. Again, it is clear that important issues are involved which have nothing specifically to do with the national debt.

The two concepts of burden dealt with approached the question from the side of the use of resources. They can be argued in terms of the money burden on the existing population or in terms of the money burden on the future. Real economic issues underly the discussion in money terms, which will be taken up shortly. Again, these issues are misleading when confined to a discussion of debt-financing, with the implied assumption that financing by other means does not also have similar implications. This will be looked at in Chapter 19.

Yet another concept of burden relates to the estimated effects that the debt has upon incentives to work, to save, to take risks and so on.

What emerges from our discussion of the meaning of the 'debt burden' is that government spending raises very important issues. We mentioned the current use of real resources, the stock of capital we should aim to bequeath to the future, and the effect on incentives. The important point emerges that however the government sector obtains the use of these resources, whether it is by commandeering them, by taxation or by debt, these important issues remain. To look at the so-called burden of the debt in isolation is a misleading exercise; it is necessary to consider the advantages and disadvantages of alternative methods of obtaining these resources.

Internal and external borrowing

An important distinction to be made is between internal and externally held debt—that is, between internal and external borrowing. Internal borrowing is a rearrangement of assets: citizens surrender current purchasing power in return for government securities. No increase of real resources is directly created as a result. External borrowing, on the other hand, permits an import of real resources, either of consumption or capital goods. Likewise, interest and repayment of internal debt is the transfer of current purchasing power back to holders of the debt. Interest and repayment of external borrowing mean, however, a corresponding outflow of goods and services unless the external holders choose for a time to reinvest in securities of the country making the repayment. From the point of view of interest and repayment of external debt, it can be said that this constitutes a 'burden' on future output of goods and services. However, it must not be lost sight of that if the borrowing is used to increase the productive capacity of the economy, this may create the capacity not only to do both of these things, but also to yield a return over and above this. The application of this to underdeveloped countries is obvious. It may at times be necessary to use foreign loans for purposes of increasing imports of consumption goods; but the use to increase productive capacity is to be preferred, if at all possible, as this will help to create the output to repay and service the loan.

Equity aspects of the debt

Probably the most frequently mentioned aspect of the internally held national debt is the concern which is expressed over its effects on the distribution of income and wealth. The debt represents a transfer of income from those who pay taxes to those who own the securities. Since all citizens pay taxes of one sort or another, it is not easy to work out how much transference in fact takes place. If the debt was abolished overnight by decree, the government would be able to forgo collecting £1,599 million or so in revenue which is at present paid in interest. The distributional effects of this would depend on whether it is assumed that income tax is reduced as a result or whether indirect taxes are reduced or abolished. Objections on these lines, that the payment of interest is unfair, as it represents a transfer from the poor (who pay taxes) to the rich (who own the securities), is, as we have seen, dependent on assumptions about which taxes are relieved as a result of not paying interest. The real objection that seems to be at the back of this type of argument is to the very unequal distribution of wealth and income in the community. This is a question which is worth discussion in its own right. Interest payments on the national debt are of only subsidiary importance to the topic.

Future generations

Similar considerations apply to the argument that government financing by debt imposes a burden on future generations who have to repay the debt. What, however, is frequently not pointed out, is that future generations also benefit by the repayment. The debt existing at the present time has, as we have seen, the effect of redistributing income from existing taxpayers to existing holders of securities. In 100 years from now both the holders of the debt and the taxpayers will be different people. If we take a shorter time-span—say, thirty years—the argument can be looked at in terms of inter-generation equity: that sons will be paying for the debts of their fathers. This point has some validity, but doesn't boil down to anything more than the truism that our actions today will affect the future in a number of ways, some of them calculable and some of them not. In particular, the argument that raising funds by taxation today, instead of by debt, imposes no burden on the future is clearly false. If a person's wealth and income is taxed today, while it is true that no 'burden' is left to future generations, it is also true that the assets of the individual to leave to his dependants will be less. Or, in terms of the father-and-son argument, that the father will have less to spend on his son. In order to make sense of the argument that raising money by debt finance is a burden on the future, the stream of consequences stemming from raising finance in this way has to be compared with the stream of consequences stemming from raising finance in alternative ways. The number of alternative ways is innumerable, as they can take the form of various combinations of different taxes. In a trivial sense, however we raise the money imposes a burden on the future, in the sense that this question is usually phrased: that raising money by debt imposes more of a burden on the future than raising it by taxation, the question is not capable of a precise answer. Different assumptions about future behaviour are likely to yield different answers.

In this question we come back once more to a more fundamental question that appears to underlie much argument on this subject. That is the question of the perpetuation of the existing structure of wealth by inheritance; and once more it seems that discussion of this question directly is more fruitful than a roundabout discussion of imprecise 'burdens' caused by this or that method of financing.[6]

[6] The reader interested in pursuing this topic to its metaphysical heights is referred to a collection of recent writings edited by Ferguson, J. M. (1964).

Monetary and fiscal implications of the debt

In looking at the so-called burden of the debt, it was found that merely looking at money transfers obscured rather than illuminated some of the problems. In considering the fiscal and monetary implications, it will also be found useful to bear 'real' implications in mind. The following will serve as a summary of points that have been raised earlier:

COMPOSITION OF THE DEBT

The importance of the composition of the debt has been raised on several occasions. In particular, the authorities are concerned with the liquidity of the debt, with the ratio of short-term to long-term debt. The importance, it will be remembered, is that, although money can be obtained by selling both types of security on the market, only short-term debt has a fairly certain value. The implications of liquidity are twofold: (1) the fear that the private sector will be tempted to convert their assets into spending power, and (2) that the banks and other financial institutions may use the assets as a base on which to expand credit. In both cases what is important is the relationship between the monetary authorities and the private sector. A sale of assets from a private individual to another individual or a sale from a bank to a private individual is merely a rearrangement of assets within the private sector, not of monetary importance except in so far as this implies changes in interest rates. If, however, the monetary authorities buy the securities, then this is directly increasing the purchasing power of the private sector. They may have to buy the securities because these are repayable on demand, such as deposits at the Post Office Savings Bank or short-term deposits with local authorities. They may buy marketable securities because they wish to maintain the level of interest rates. They may be forced into raising more money on such short-term assets as Treasury bills, because the public are unwilling to subscribe to long-term issues.

TOTAL OF THE DEBT

We have seen that the absolute size of the debt does not as a rule form a big constraint on the government. If interest payments form a large proportion of the Budget, it is possible that this will form a constraint on government spending because they fear to put up taxes. Since interest payments are taxed as unearned income, this problem is not likely to arise out of normal peace-time financing.

An increase in the total of the debt is important in so far as it affects the composition of the debt on the lines indicated in the previous section.[7]

INTEREST RATES

The effect of interest rates on the economy will be discussed in Part III. Changes in interest rates do affect the economy in various ways, but these effects are not felt in any simple or direct manner. The monetary authorities must bear in mind the effect on the demand for money by borrowers, on the supply of money, and more directly the effects on the flow of money into or out of the country from overseas.

Bank Rate is a key rate in the economy because, in particular, the commercial bank rates are by convention tied to it, and the Treasury bill rate moves in sympathy. Movements in these rates are likely to cause similar movements in most other short-term market rates, and in time to spread to the longer-term securities. Debt-management policy has obvious implications also for affecting the structure of interest rates. It would be possible for the monetary authorities to set the general level of long-term interest rates by making new issues of securities at the interest rate they had selected and operating in the market day by day to support that rate. If the authorities try to maintain a rate that is clearly out of line with market expectations, undesirable repercussions may follow which will lead them to revise the rate structure they have set. The 'cheap money' policy pursued after 1945 had this pattern. The authorities had the policy of maintaining low interest rates. An investor who expects the rate of interest to

[7] A more diffused effect of the size and composition of the debt may be apparent from its effect on private wealth. An increase in debts among the public itself does not constitute an increase in wealth when aggregation takes place. The assets of some members of the public are matched by corresponding liabilities of other members. To what extent an increase in national debt is regarded by the public as a net increase in wealth is empirically uncertain. An increase in the national debt does two things: it increases the public's ownership of claims against the monetary sector, and at the same time it increases the tax liability of the public to service the debt. The public's reaction can vary considerably. One extreme is considering the increase in claims it holds as an increase in wealth without making any allowance for the tax liability. At the other extreme, if full offset for tax liability is conceded no net increase in wealth is apparent. Put simply, in the latter case there would be no change in aggregate behaviour, due to the wealth effect, if the national debt was halved or changed by some other fraction.

The wealth effect will be considered in the Appendix to Chapter 19. In the context of the present chapter, while it may be true that the wealth effect is important as a long-run determinant of behaviour, it is unlikely to be important as a short-run determinant.

This question is discussed in relation to the Federal Debt of the United States by Tobin, J. (1963).

increase (i.e. a fall in the market value of existing securities), not only does not subscribe to new low coupon issues for fear of making a capital loss when interest rates change, but also tends to sell securities and keep liquid in order to take advantage of the investment opportunities when interest rates do change. In the late 1940s the authorities were having to acquiesce in the increasing liquidity of the public, which resulted in their eventual abandonment of the cheap money policy.

The policy followed in much of the 1950s was use of Bank Rate and other measures to affect short-term rates and thereby indirectly long-term rates, but no deliberate manipulation of long-term rates. In general, the authorities followed rather than led the rates in the long-term sector. In the words of the Radcliffe Committee: 'Until the last year or so [i.e. 1958-9] the authorities have not regarded management of the national debt as an opportunity for working on the structure of interest rates . . .' (para. 429).

The position today is that the authorities are more willing to pursue their aims for interest rates throughout the economy by seeking to influence the behaviour of prices and yields in the gilt-edged market. Also:

> Management of the gilt-edged market, and the outcome in terms both of prices and of the net amounts of stock sold or bought in official dealings, have considerable bearing on credit policy and the liquidity of the banks and others, creating conditions that may help or hinder policy in this field. Neither interest rate policy nor credit policy, however, is the dominant long-term consideration in debt-management; this is rather to ensure so far as possible that suitable finance for the Exchequer is available in the future, so that there be no excessive recourse to short-term borrowing from the banks on Treasury bills and accompanying increase in the money supply ('Official Transactions in the Gilt-edged Market' (June, 1966)).

Summary

Details of the available statistical data on the debt, which are still far from adequate, has been given. Although the debt has increased greatly in money terms, as a percentage of national income it shows a marked decrease since 1935. The debt after 1945 is, however, much more liquid, and this poses problems for the monetary authorities. A particular problem is the need, as well as meeting new borrowing requirements, to replace the debt with fresh borrowing as it comes up for redemption.

The implications of the debt on the use of real resources in the economy are complicated and pose difficult choices.

It is necessary to try to trace the effects caused by the size of the debt, the composition of the debt and the structure of interest rates which are influenced by debt management. These factors affect the liquidity of the economy and the ability of the banks and other financial institutions to create credit, and also have direct effects on individuals and companies. The task is a difficult one, and it is not surprising that differences of opinion exist at many points of the analysis. The conclusion reached is that debt-management should not be considered as an end in itself, but as part of the whole fiscal process.

In discussing the so-called 'burden' of the debt, a distinction should be drawn between debt held internally and debt held by foreigners. The discussion of 'burden' unearthed some important problems: the use of resources by the public sector, the amount of capital investment being undertaken, the effect on incentives, the distribution of wealth and income, and the perpetuation of the existing structure of wealth by inheritance. In all cases it was found that discussion of these problems solely in terms of debt-financing obscured rather than illuminated the issues.

18
Public finance critique

> To restrict our Report completely to an analysis of the revenue-raising side would be equivalent to saying that we think it meaningful to ignore one blade of a pair of scissors. There may be some who would say that our efforts should be directed to spreading more equitably the 'burden' of taxation and that we should not concern ourselves with the results of government expenditure. But in many respects one is essential to the other and it is their joint product that must be our concern. Therefore, while we do not attempt to assess government expenditure programmes, we do not ignore them.
>
> *Report of the Canadian Royal Commission on Taxation* (1966).

Summary of major faults in present system

This section has outlined the main changes in government spending and revenue during this century. Chapter 11, set up the total-accretion principle as a yardstick to evaluate the current system, which was detailed in the following chapters. A summary follows of the major faults found:

1. The complexity of the tax-and-benefit system.
2. The appearance of high rates of tax which are not in many cases effective rates. Particularly is this so with estate duty. It applies to the recently introduced taxes on capital gains and land and also to income, because of earned income relief, up to a level of income of £9,945, and the form in which allowances against tax are given.
3. High rates of tax on earned incomes with alleged disincentive effects on incentives, the diversion of effort into forms of output attracting low rates of tax, the unproductive use of resources specifically for tax avoidance, and the setting up of residence abroad by high-rate taxpayers.
4. Lower flat-rate taxes, or zero taxes, on most other spending power.

5. Many social benefits channelled via tax allowances which do not help the most needy.
6. The lack of any consistent principles for company taxation.

These faults add up to a formidable indictment of the system which is likely to have serious economic and social consequences. This chapter attempts to suggest remedies. First, the problem of incidence in its traditional form is looked at in more detail. This concept is modified on the grounds that the approach is too narrow. There is a need to look at the total incidence of taxes and benefits. This is carried out for the income groups for which information is at present available. Finally, ways in which the system can be improved are investigated.

Incidence

The classical concept of incidence deals with the problem of trying to sort out who really pays a particular tax, and what are the effects of a tax change. In this book the problem has arisen on several occasions. For example, should taxes on companies be considered as being borne by the shareholders, the employees or the customers of the company? Are capital gains paid by the seller on whom the tax is imposed, or the buyer, or in some measure between them?

This concept of incidence refers to the location of the 'ultimate' as opposed to the 'direct' money burden of the tax. The direct location of a tax is the person on whom the legal liability is imposed; the ultimate location the person who finally pays it. 'Shifting' refers to the process by which the direct money burden is pushed along through price adjustments from the point of impact (i.e. where statutory liability is imposed) to the final resting-place. 'Effects' refer to all other changes that the tax may bring about, e.g. inflation, changes in output or incomes and transfer effects.

It should be noted that we cannot in any case make practical measurements of the 'ultimate' burden of a tax. Take, for example, a tax on cigarettes. We can measure the consumption of cigarettes and, on the assumption that the consumer pays the whole of the tax, say that this individual pays so much tobacco tax compared to that one. But we cannot catch by this measuring-rod the 'burden' on the person who has had to reduce or stop smoking because of the tax.

Incidence in this traditional sense is an academic exercise. Different assumptions—for example, about the degree of monopoly power being exercised and about the ratio of elasticities of supply and demand—lead to different answers. The argument used in this book is that it can be highly misleading to talk about the burden of a particular tax in isolation from the rest of the tax system. That is the distortion that is involved, for example, in judging from our progressive system of income tax and surtax that the system as a whole is progressive. As we have seen, this is as misleading as to judge that because we have high rates of estate duty we are thereby rapidly achieving greater equality of wealth.

As a first rough check on the equity of the tax system it is possible to use the figures from Table 1, Chapter 9, showing the sources of U.K. tax revenue. National Insurance and Health contributions, Customs and Excise, and rates can be classified as regressive taxes, falling more heavily on those with low incomes.[1] Profits tax, motor-vehicle tax and the selective employment tax are deducted from the total revenue in 1967 of £13,337 million, to leave a figure of £11,566 million. These taxes are not easily classified as regressive or progressive. The taxes labelled 'regressive' then amount to £7,112 million, or 61% of the total of £11,566. Most of the years shown in the table in Chapter 9 record a figure of near to 60% for these regressive taxes. From the tax revenue side the fiscal system therefore looks to be regressive on low incomes, and not progressive.

However, this is only looking at one side of the picture: the side of income after tax. It is possible that when the expenditure side of the picture is taken into account, it will be found that the addition to income in cash, or money's worth, more than covers the tax paid by lower incomes. What picture emerges when both the costs (i.e. taxes paid) and the benefits are taken into account?

The term 'cost-benefit' has been pre-empted in economics for a rather different idea.[2] So to describe the process when both sides are taken into account the term 'incidence' will be retained and

[1] The recent scheme of rates rebate to those on very low income and the fact that size of house may be correlated with income make rates difficult to classify definitely into one category or the other. In 1967, if rates are included with profits tax, motor-vehicle tax and the selective employment tax as not easily classifiable, we get a total of £10,091 million that can be classified. Regressive taxes amount to 69% of this. If rates are classified as progressive taxes, this leaves a total of £5,637 million as regressive taxation, or 49% of the total of £11,566 million. The point made—that regressive taxes are a large part of tax revenue—holds, whichever of these classifications is judged the best.

[2] Cost-benefit analysis attempts to assess the costs and the benefits of a particular item, such as a new road, or airport, or a Channel tunnel. Costs and benefits are defined in the broadest possible way to embrace, not only direct costs, such as money costs of construction, but indirect costs, such as loss of amenities. Similarly, benefits take in not only direct benefits, such as quicker travelling time for persons using the proposed new route, but indirect benefits, such as quicker travel for persons on old routes because of less congestion. What is included on the cost-and-benefit side and how these are evaluated are obviously of crucial importance.

qualified, as the 'incidence of taxes and benefits'.

The incidence of taxes and benefits in 1966

Incidence is transformed into a study of costs (that is, who pays) and benefits of the whole fiscal system. Criticism of this approach has been made on a number of grounds (see Prest, A. R. (1968), and Peacock, A. T. and Shannon, R. (1968)). The criticisms concern the

Table 1

Average incomes before and after taxes and benefits, 1966

(£ per year)

RANGE OF

		£260–	£315–	£382–	£460–	£559–	£676–	£816–
1 adult								
1.	£	279	348	412	507	624	743	904
2.	£	405	447	448	479	455	561	629
3.	£	+126	+99	+36	−28	−169	−182	−275
4.	%	+41·2	+28·4	+8·7	−5·5	−27·1	−24·5	−30·4
2 adults								
1.	£	287	347	424	510	621	759	901
2.	£	513	583	611	653	607	669	727
3.	£	+226	+236	+187	+143	−14	−90	−174
4.	%	+78·7	+68·0	+44·1	+28·0	−2·3	−12·0	−19·3
2 adults, 1 child								
1.	£	—	—	—	—	—	753	891
2.	£	—	—	—	—	—	668	701
3.	£	—	—	—	—	—	−85	−190
4.	%	—	—	—	—	—	−11·3	−21·3
2 adults, 2 children								
1.	£	—	—	—	—	—	766	903
2.	£	—	—	—	—	—	836	843
3.	£	—	—	—	—	—	+70	−60
4.	%	—	—	—	—	—	+9·1	−6·6
2 adults, 3 children								
1.	£	—	—	—	—	—	—	891
2.	£	—	—	—	—	—	—	987
3.	£	—	—	—	—	—	—	+96
4.	%	—	—	—	—	—	—	+10·8

Source: *Economic Trends*, No. 172, February, 1968.
1. Original income before taxes and benefits.
2. Income after all taxes and benefits: 'effective income'.

general methodology used, assumptions about the incidence of taxes and the need to improve the data. This method is here put forward as the one that approaches most nearly the concept of the standard of living of a person or family. It does so by taking the income of the unit, adding to it a money value of services received where it is sensible to allocate these, and subtracting taxes paid. The fact that the value of nearly half of government expenditure, on such items as defence and roads, cannot be allocated and is ignored as a benefit to the individual or family, while most taxation can be allocated, is, it is suggested, the right approach in this context. Improvements can and should be made to Budget studies, but this does not stop this

ORIGINAL INCOME

£988–	£1,196–	£1,448–	£1,752–	£2,122–	£2,566–£3,104
1,087	1,282	1,570	—	—	—
751	843	1,063	—	—	—
−336	−439	−507	—	—	—
−30·9	−34·2	−32·3	—	—	—
1,091	1,314	1,600	1,912	2,319	3,945
798	923	1,112	1,306	1,571	2,540
−293	−391	−488	−606	−748	−1,405
−26·9	−29·8	−30·5	−31·7	−32·6	−35·6
1,102	1,328	1,598	1,922	2,321	3,550
902	1,018	1,220	1,454	1,796	2,533
−200	−310	−378	−468	−525	−1,017
−18·1	−23·3	−23·7	−24·3	−22·3	−28·6
1,096	1,326	1,596	1,918	2,341	3,744
976	1,142	1,330	1,538	1,934	2,788
−120	−184	−266	−380	−407	−956
−10·9	−13·9	−16·7	−19·8	−17·4	−25·5
1,102	1,310	1,619	1,899	—	—
1,116	1,285	1,521	1,725	—	—
+14	−25	−96	−174	—	—
+1·3	−1·9	−5·9	−9·2	—	—

3. Difference between 1 and 2.
4. Difference as % of original income.

approach being a fruitful one. There is still the problem of deciding who ultimately pays the tax and receives the benefits. Studies must obviously make assumptions about this and what these benefits are worth. However, these problems can be seen in perspective. The importance or otherwise of a particular tax or benefit in relation to the whole can be judged. In particular, with this approach it would be feasible to set up alternative assumptions about the incidence of various taxes and benefits to see what overall difference this makes to the 'burden'.

This type of analysis then sets out to analyse the overall effect of government spending and revenue in its distributional aspect.[3]

For several years the Central Statistical Office has published in *Economic Trends* detailed tax and benefit figures for particular income categories, divided into single persons and married persons with and without children (see 'Incidence of Taxes and Social Service Benefits' (February, 1968)). The information is of necessity in terms of averages. It is obtained from the Ministry of Labour annual survey of expenditure of about 3,000 persons. Each household included in the survey is asked to provide detailed information about all forms of income, including National Insurance and other cash benefits received from the State, payments of income tax and surtax, the type of dwelling occupied, the kind of education which any member of the household is receiving, and so on.

In any exercise of this nature the inclusion or exclusion of particular taxes or benefits may make a big difference to the result. The following outline is intended as a guide:

Direct taxes included are income tax, surtax, and employers' and employees' contributions to National Insurance and Health—that is, the employers' contribution is regarded as part of the employees' income and as a tax borne by him. Death duties and taxes on undistributed profits are not included. Customs and Excise taxes, including purchase and betting tax, are assumed to be fully reflected in the prices paid by consumers when buying commodities subject to indirect tax.

Benefits included are sub-divided into cash benefits and benefits in

[3] Ideally we need also to know the total impact on other variables, such as consumption, investment, prices and growth of the economy. It will be argued in Part III that the problems involved in doing this are formidable. It has also been suggested in the Preface that too much emphasis has been placed on these aspects in recent years. A developed country has the resources to drastically reduce if not solve its social problems now; it is not necessary to wait until this or that particular rate of growth is achieved in order to do more to improve social conditions than we are doing at the moment.

kind. Cash benefits include family allowances, pensions, National Insurance benefits, national assistance grants, etc., but not scholarships and educational grants. Benefits in kind include the National Health Service, State education, school health services, school meals, milk and welfare foods and scholarships and education grants. The method of allocating the benefits from State education is to impute to each child the average cost per child of education in the particular category of school he or she is attending. Benefits of the National Health Services are allocated in a similar manner, it being assumed that the total value of all the services (except maternity services, which are separately allocated) is the same for all persons in each of six different categories of the population.

The benefits derived from government expenditure on administration, defence, museums, libraries, parks, roads and so on are not allocated. By their nature, allocation of benefits to individuals of these services would be a haphazard affair.[4]

When looking at these statistics, it is important to bear in mind that results are not shown for pensioner households, so defined if at least three-quarters of the income is derived from Old Age or National Insurance pensions and National Assistance. Results are not given for households with an income of less than £260 a year, and the highest income range given is £2,566-£3,104. Mixed households—that is, households where there are more than two adults (here defined as a person over sixteen years)—are not shown because of the limited number in the sample.

Where the number of households in each 'cell' fell below ten, the information was not published, as it was thought to be too unreliable. With a small sample, too much reliance should not be placed on each individual figure. The Central Statistical Office state that from 1967 onwards the sample of households will be doubled. This should make the estimates more reliable, and it would also greatly assist in the interpretation of the results if the figures were presented with estimates of standard deviation (i.e. estimates of variation found in each figure).

What emerges from this sample? Table 1 presents information for the year 1966. Reading down the left-hand margin, we have information on family grouping, first for one adult then for two adults with nought, one, two, or three children. Across the page information on income range is presented. Beneath each family grouping appear lines

[4] It is interesting to note that, as with all Budget surveys, the amount that people say they spend on alcohol and tobacco is underestimated (by half on alcohol and a quarter on tobacco) and the figures have to be grossed up to allow for this.

numbered, 1, 2, 3 and 4. The first line presents the average gross income (termed original income) found in each income range, while the second line gives this income after taxes have been deducted and benefits added (this will be termed 'effective income'). Line 3 gives the difference between original income and effective income, while line 4 expresses this difference as a percentage of original income. Line 4 thus gives an approximate measure of the progressiveness of the system of taxes and benefits for households of each size; it expresses the net benefits received or net taxes paid.

A recapitulation is in order before commenting on these figures. The estimates gather up the diverse strands present in the British system of taxation and government spending. We have noted that indirect taxes (as currently administered) and flat-rate Insurance and Health contributions are regressive, while income and surtax rates are progressive. On the expenditure side benefits will normally be progressive—that is, forming a larger percentage of lower incomes than of higher incomes, with the important exception of benefits via tax allowances.

The picture that emerges is that within the income range considered (£260-3,104) the overall impact of taxing and government spending in each family category (1 adult, 2 adults, etc.), is progressive to some extent. Higher incomes in general pay a bigger proportion than lower incomes, and some lower incomes benefit to a greater extent than they pay out. However, the progression quickly flattens out for two categories: single adults with average income between £816 and £1,752 pay roughly 30%; and two adults with average income between £1,196 and £2,122 also pay about 30%. It is to be hoped that information will soon be collected on higher income ranges, so that the progression at higher incomes can be ascertained.

The table also shows the degree of progressiveness between categories. For example, comparing the original income range £676-816 per annum, an average of about £14 a week, with an income that is a little more than double this, i.e. an income in the range £1,448-1,752 per annum, an average of £31 a week, we find:

	Income £14 per Week, Taken Net in Tax Per Annum		*Income £31 per Week,* Taken Net in Tax Per Annum	
	£	%	£	%
1 adult	182	24·5	507	32·3
2 adults	90	12·0	488	30·5
2 adults, 1 child	85	11·3	378	23·7
2 adults, 2 children	+70	+9·1	266	16·7
2 adults, 3 children	Not available		96	5·9

Should we be complacent about these results? Do they accord with current ideas about equity? It may be questioned, for example, whether it is the general wish to impose on a family with one child earning £14 a week a net tax of over 11% of their rather meagre income. This is a sum that is only £5 less than that paid by a couple without children in the same income range, whereas the difference between these categories in the £31 a week range is £110.

While increasing income from £14 a week to £31 a week means that a single person pays about 2·8 times more in tax (from £182 to £507), the other categories go up more steeply. Two adults pay 5·4 times more (from £90 to £488), a couple with one child 4·4 times more, while a couple with two children move from the position of benefiting from an addition to income of £70 to one where they pay £266. Once again it can be questioned whether these results are intended.

Conclusions

The evidence is overwhelming that our system of taxes and benefits, in spite of a considerable amount of effort, is neither equitable, nor is it succeeding very well in achieving its declared object of relieving poverty. No method is likely to achieve these objects by 100%, but there is no doubt that, given the desire, considerable improvements could be made.

Each writer has his own suggestions for reform, and groups from each of the main political parties have suggested changes. Reformers can be categorized into those who want to patch up the grossest deficiencies and those who believe more fundamental changes are needed. The author belongs to this second category. The mistake should not be made of thinking that the former solution is necessarily the simpler to execute and administer. The structure is already complex because of patching up in the past. One of the advantages to follow from more sweeping proposals is the simplification which this makes possible.

The accretion principle has been used as a yardstick. This may be thought of as a guide-line by which various taxes can be judged, or as a practical system to which we should make our system adhere as far as possible. Proposals to impose a progressive tax on inheritances, gifts and capital gains, and to cumulate these receipts over a person's lifetime fall into the former category. The proposals to tax these receipts as income falls into the latter category. The latter solution has been favoured in this book, but either alternative would be preferable to the present inadequate system. There are advantages in administration in subjecting all receipts to one tax, and no sound arguments have been found for separate treatment of inheritance, gifts or capital gains. Redistribution of wealth, if this is desired by the community, can continue by a modified form of estate duty, in addition to taxing bequests as income in the hands of the recipient.

Proposed reforms

The prime reform therefore that is suggested is a reversal of the process which has been going on for so many years, whereby income that is subject to income tax is more and more narrowly drawn. In particular, capital gains, gains on the sale of land, gifts and inheritance should be taxed at the same rate as other income. Some form of averaging of income will be needed, as it is needed under the present system, to achieve equity.

Averaging was considered in Chapter 11, and the conclusion was reached that, as well as being desirable, averaging is feasible: it is possible to avoid the heavy burden of recalculating tax due for past years of the averaging period. As a provisional step, the Royal Commission suggestion could be implemented, that where a drop in earned income of 50% or more over the previous years' income occurs, the taxpayer should have his tax recalculated over the proceeding year. This could be supplemented by provision for forward spreading of receipts, such as a gift, legacy or exceptional earnings in one year, when this has the effect of increasing income by 50% or more over the previous year. Income in these cases could be spread in equal amounts over the year of receipt and the next two or three years.

Tax could still be collected for the majority of taxpayers, as at present, under P.A.Y.E. The taxpayer could have the option of having his tax coding, which is notified to his employer, increased if he has income from other sources than his employment. If he wished to keep this information from his employer, arrangements could be made to pay the tax due on his non-employment income, directly to the Inland Revenue, similarly to the arrangements which exist at present under Schedule D tax.

Against the initial upheaval likely to be caused by these changes can be set some substantial benefits. The incentive for tax-avoidance by shuffling assets around would be greatly reduced. The existing bias against earned income and the alleged disadvantages that follow from this would be alleviated. A benefit that cannot be documented, but one that in the author's opinion is likely to bring substantial benefits, would be achieved just because an attempt was being made to achieve equity.

If the tax base is enlarged, tax rates can be looked at afresh.

The present system of a flat rate of tax at 8*s*. 3*d*. in the £1 over a wide range of income and progressive rates of surtax starting at £5,000 needs re-examination in any case.

A criterion for equity

A criterion for equity could be set up in terms of effective income. The first step in this direction would be to extend the survey made by the Central Statistical Office to cover high-income individuals and families. Information on low-income households was made available for the first time in *Economic Trends*, No. 177 (July, 1968). With this information to hand, the difference between original income and effective income (that is, after allowing for tax and benefits) is known, i.e. this figure gives the value of the *net* benefits received or the *net* taxes paid. Policy on taxation and benefits might with advantage take the form of an attempt to formulate and then to attain an equitable-percentage relationship between net benefits received or net taxes paid (as the case may be) and original income for incomes of various levels. In terms of Table 1, this would be to ensure the right degree of progression in line 4. Ideally, a smoothly decreasing amount of net benefit as income increases, leading to a smoothly progressive amount of net taxation as income increases still further. No attempt is made here to judge the break-even point for each class of taxpayer (that is, the level of income at which tax and benefit should cancel each other out), nor to determine the right degree of steepness of the progression.

The criterion just outlined takes into account that a person's standard of living consists of his income (defined on total-accretion lines), less taxation paid, plus the addition of the value of benefits that can be allocated to him. This criterion for assessing equity goes a long way to ensuring that taxpayers in equal positions are treated equally. It does not achieve complete equity, because both the taxes paid and benefits received are averages found from a sample of the population. Those with consumption patterns or in receipt of benefits markedly different from the average will be treated differently. For example, it is generally assumed that under any tax system alcohol and tobacco will continue to bear a high tax for social reasons. If this is to be the case, a person who smokes or drinks more than the average will pay more tax than a person in a similar position who does not smoke or drink. In a like manner, a person who is unfortunate enough to require prolonged medical treatment will 'benefit' more than the average from Health expenditure. It was stated at the end of Chapter 11 that principles in tax are set up as guides, not as inflexible rules. The presumption is that exceptions of the kind noted above to the rule that taxpayers in equal positions are treated equally would be generally accepted as desirable by the majority of people.

This criterion could be used to judge tax and benefit changes. Do they bring the system nearer to the agreed equity position?

Reform of tax allowances and other benefits and poverty

Widening the tax base on total-accretion lines and setting up a criterion for equity would mean that a radical reappraisal of the whole system of tax allowances and other benefits would be possible. For example, the abolition of tax allowances for children would make no difference to low-income earners who do not benefit at present and would worsen the position of those who pay tax and do benefit. There is likely to be some combination of change in tax rates and grants, in lieu of tax allowances, that will bring the system nearer to the agreed equity position. Over time a simplification of the fiscal system can be looked for. In particular, the pretence of high tax rates, which nevertheless have their impact greatly softened by tax allowances, can be overhauled. Benefits paid to those who need them rather than to everybody would mean that the great game whereby the rich apparently have large sums taken away from them in tax, and also apparently large sums given to them by tax allowances, need no longer be played.

The simplest tax reform would be the replacement of tax allowances by tax credits. This would not help the poor person who does not receive enough income to pay tax. This group cannot be assisted by income tax concessions, but it would ensure equal benefits to taxpayers. The effect of a tax allowance varies with the marginal rate of tax paid by the individual. This is so because an individual deducts any allowances due to him before tax is calculated. He will therefore either not reach so high a rate of tax or he will have less income to be taxed at his top rate. The benefits can be substantial to a high-rate surtax payer. For example, if we compare two individuals who have earned income only, where A has an income of £5,000 per annum and B an income of £25,000 that takes him into the top rate of surtax of 10*s.* in the £1. The cost to A of borrowing £3,000 for house-purchase at 7% is £210 per annum. Allowing for the two-ninths earned income relief, A is taxed at 6*s.* 5*d.* in the £1, so he obtains tax relief of £67 7*s.* 6*d.* His net cost is £142 12*s.* 6*d.* For the same net cost, the top-rate surtax payer can borrow about £23,000.

A tax credit, on the other hand, is a sum which is deductible from a person's tax bill. If all allowances were replaced by tax credits, each taxpayer would calculate his tax from his gross income level. Deductions on an agreed scale would then be made from the tax due, according to the circumstances of the taxpayer. If the allowance for a child was £50, then a taxpayer with two children would reduce his tax due by £100, whatever the size of his tax bill. No longer would the benefit mean most to those with highest incomes. The tax revenue gained could be used partly to reduce taxes and partly to provide benefits to those with low incomes.

The standard of equity set up envisaged judging a person's standard of living by taking his income on total-accretion lines, less taxes paid, plus the value of benefits received. Inevitably some persons' and families' effective incomes will fall below that deemed necessary to maintain an adequate standard of living. For these persons additional supplementation is needed. To this problem we now turn.

Supplementation of low incomes

A fairly simple procedure administratively would be to pay a supplement based on the previous year's effective income, with allowance for any known adjustments for the current year—for example, due to a wage-change or due to changes in benefits. The supplement could be paid weekly on the lines of the current pension book. Allocating a Post Office Giro account to all citizens would greatly facilitate the transfer of money to and from the government (suggested by Williams, B. R. (1967)). In time a simplification could be carried out. In place of a host of allowances, paid by a multiplicity of public authorities (e.g. child allowance, cheap milk and school meals, rate rebates, pensions and so on), a single payment could be made. Flexibility would be necessary to meet sudden calamities, so that money could be paid out immediately in respect of illness and unemployment.

A social objection is sometimes made to subsuming benefits into a weekly cash payment. This is, that benefits in kind, such as milk tokens and subsidized school meals ensure, as far as this is possible, that the benefits go to the intended recipient in the form in which they were intended, whereas, to put it in its worst light, cash payments may go straight to the betting-shop or on alcohol or tobacco, and the recipient's family be no better off. If this objection is thought to be sufficiently strong to warrant directed assistance, it still leaves a number of cash payments which can economically be paid out in one sum. The payment of this sum to the woman, in the case of married couples is likely to ensure that in the majority of cases it would be the family that benefited. Provision for payment to the husband, rather than the wife, could be made in exceptional circumstances.

The arguments that such a scheme would sap initiative, encourage idleness, subsidize employers who paid poor wages and the other objections, emotive or real, which are raised against any extension of welfare provisions must be weighed against the undoubted hardship and misery which exists at present.

It should be stressed that society at present makes the choice to assist its members not in any very rational manner, but as the end result of a series of tax imposts, tax concessions and other benefits. The scheme outlined sets out to ensure that no person or family falls below some minimum standard of living. It does so largely within the current system, but envisages this being greatly simplified over time. It suffers, if the past is any guide to the future, from the difficulties of defining what is the minimum standard to be aimed at and, perhaps of more practical importance, the lag that occurs in adjusting the standard to changes in the cost of living. There will probably always be disagreement on the first point, but making the standard and the amount of supplementation to be paid subject to the annual review of Parliament, on the lines of farming subsidies, should go a long way to ensuring that, in a society which is in aggregate becoming richer, all sectors of the population will participate in the increase to some extent. An annual review would also be likely to draw Parliament's attention more forcibly to alternative ways of relieving poverty; for example, raising the skill and wages of lower-paid workers.

The above proposals are rather different to suggestions that are put forward from time to time for a negative income tax (Friedman, M. (1962), 190-5, and Lees, D. (October, 1967)). These schemes envisage income tax being extended down the income scale so that poorer persons would receive payment. Let us take the position of a married man with two children under eleven earning an income of £522 per annum. Considering only the personal, child and earned-income allowances he was entitled in 1968 to the following tax relief:

	£
Earned-income relief, two-ninths of £522	116
Married person's allowance	340
Children's allowance (twice £115)	230
Total	686

There is a discrepancy of £164 between his income and allowances. Such a person under a negative income tax (i.e. a subsidy) would be entitled to receive payment of this sum. Proposals on these lines may be coupled with the suggestion that less than the full 100% negative tax, or subsidy, be introduced. For example, if the negative tax were introduced at the rate of 50% the person in the above example would be entitled to half of the sum of £164, i.e. £82. The reason given for having a negative tax on these lines at less than 100% is to lessen the effect on incentive to work. In the above example, under a full negative tax, for every £1 earned above his wage of £522 the person loses £1 of relief. At a rate of 50% the person loses 10*s*., and it is argued that his incentive to work is therefore greater.

There are a number of objections to a scheme on these lines. The first is that under any system of progressive taxation, tax concessions, benefit the most wealthy. The drawbacks of seeming to impose high tax and giving large concessions has been emphasized sufficiently in this book. The corresponding injustice at the other end of the scale, under a negative income tax, is that the smaller a person's ability to earn the smaller is the grant to which he is entitled because of the two-ninths earned-income relief. This is so whether the smaller earnings are due to laziness, ill-health, permanent disability or unavailability of work. In the example previously given, and asssuming a 100% tax, if the person was made redundant from his job and was unable to find alternative employment, his income would drop from £686 (£522 earnings and £164 benefit) to £507 in benefit. This is so because he loses earned-income relief, which was formerly worth £116. The author believes that the disincentive-to-work argument against giving benefits is greatly overrated, and does not warrant the hardship that it imposes on other categories of person who are genuinely unable to work, or the alternative, which would involve administrative complications in sorting out the idle from other categories of poor persons. In its desire to prevent a minority of work-shy people from benefiting, this scheme continues the current system of public vindictiveness to the majority who are poor through ill-health, disability or inability to get work. Again, to achieve a greater degree of equity, all income-tax concessions, and not just the three mentioned in the example, should be extended to all, although this would greatly add to the administrative complexity. Finally, and perhaps most importantly, tying benefits to tax concessions will arbitrarily alter benefits with every change in those concessions and any change in earned income relief.

The alternative proposals outlined in this section differ from the negative income tax scheme just outlined in envisaging a joint reduction in tax allowances and in tax rates, with supplementation paid to those with low effective incomes, to ensure, as far as this is possible, that no person or family falls below some minimum standard. The payment of this supplement could be termed a 'negative income tax', but it is not linked to existing concessions given by way of tax allowances.

On indirect taxes the conclusion was reached earlier that the value added tax is to be preferred to the existing purchase-tax system and selective employment tax. One of the advantages to be gained by adopting the foregoing standard of equity is that the proportion of revenue raised by indirect taxes, as opposed to income tax, need no longer be subject to the constraint that indirect taxes weighs more heavily on poorer persons. If more tax is to be raised from indirect taxes, equity can still be achieved. Equity was set up in terms of the net benefits received, or net taxes paid, expressed as a percentage of original income. Heavy indirect taxes would fall more heavily on low incomes, so that minimum 'effective incomes' will need to be revised upward and supplementation increased accordingly to those who fall below those levels.

Vindictiveness of the current system

It is not the purpose of this book to pick out all the defects in the system of benefits. However, the charge of vindictiveness which was made above against the current system, which is nevertheless real if unintended, can be illustrated from two recent reports, motivated, it should be said, by public concern.

The wage stop is a rule that ensures an unemployed man does not receive greater social security benefits when he is out of work than he would receive as a wage when he is working. We are told:

> The purpose of the wage stop is not to provide an incentive to a man to get work. The wage stop does not require a man to get less when receiving Supplementary Benefit than he would get when working. What it does is to ensure that an unemployed man's income is *no greater* than it would be if he were in full-time employment.
>
> *Administration of the Wage Stop* (1967), (para. 4).

It emerges from the Ministry of Social Security investigation into the *Circumstances of Families* (1967), which investigated families with two or more children, that in the summer of 1966 there were about 7 million families with children. About half a million of these families, containing 1¼ million children, had incomes from earnings, contributory benefits, family allowances or other sources (but excluding National Assistance) amounting to less than would be paid to a family which qualified for Supplementary Benefit. About 145,000 of these families were fatherless, 160,000 were sick or unemployed, 140,000 men were in full-time work, the remaining 55,000 covered a variety of cases—for example, where there was no mother or where the father worked away from home. Our interest is in the group of families, estimated to be about 160,000 with half a million children in them, whose fathers were disqualified because of the wage stop from receiving full benefits: 140,000 of these fathers were in work, 20,000 unemployed. It is presumably the fear that this 140,000 would leave the labour force to take advantage of higher benefits that is the reason for the wage-stop rule. Of this group of 160,000, it was estimated, from a sample of 2,500, that more than one in five had ill-health in the father or mother. Of the ill fathers 14% thought their ill-health limited their earning capacity.

The wage-stop enquiry investigated a (regrettably) small number of families, fifty-two in all in five different areas, who were unemployed and living on wage-stopped Supplementary Benefit. It was found that most had three or more children, and two-thirds were not in good health: of these 36% were registered disabled persons.

This evidence, in both cases, was confined to asking persons about their physical health, not investigating the group clinically, and mental health was not taken into account. Limited as the evidence is, it points to the fact that disability and ill-health play a considerable part in many of these families' poverty. In some of these cases the circle of poverty is complete: a man receives a low wage because of disability or ill-health and the benefit system cannot raise him above this level.

Raising the wages of the lowest-paid workers is desirable, but would not solve the problem for many of these half-million families whose income is below Supplementary Benefit level—for example, the fatherless families and where disability and ill-health impair earning ability. The hard core of the problem is likely to remain, given a system whereby many benefits are channelled by way of tax relief: inability to reach a high enough level of income means these benefits are never received, and loss of earnings by those who do earn enough to benefit means also the loss of these benefits. To take benefits out of the tax system, on the lines suggested in this chapter, is one way of assisting both the working people and the unemployed: it would remove many of these half-million families from the need to seek assistance.

Administration

The provision of benefits which have been referred to results in an enormous amount of duplication of government administration, and also of form-filling that has to be carried out by the citizen. Different means tests are applied for rent rebates, rate rebates, school meals, welfare foods, educational allowances, child help and so on. Details will be found in *Social Services for All* (1968), No. 382. Where tests are locally administered, great variation is found in assistance given to families in similar circumstances. With such diversity, it is perhaps inevitable that many who are eligible to benefit do not do so; this may be due to a natural pride and the fear of being stigmatized as 'on Assistance', or due to ignorance as to their rights, or to the difficulty in establishing whether they are eligible for benefit.

Computerized records are being set up by a number of ministries. A single computerized service could bring large economies in time, money and manpower. Sewill (1966) gives a brief outline. The simplification of benefits which has been advocated would assist these economies. It seems clear that parallel to a study of benefits should be undertaken a study of administration. The United States Commission set up by Congress to study automation was already reporting along these lines in 1966. The Belgian government has announced that by 1970 administrative details of every inhabitant will be centrally recorded and used by every government department and agency. Compared to the known technical possibilities, we are still in the quill-pen stage: we pay for this in terms of frustration, waste and hardship. Those that object on the grounds that they will be 'just a number' seem to overlook the fact that they already have a National Health Service number and a different National Insurance number, as well as a wide variety of codes used in most of their dealings with central or local government agencies.

Improvements and administrative savings could also be made if services were unified under one authority instead of being fragmented over many authorities and departments as at present. Proposals have already been made on these lines. The Ministry of Health issued a Green Paper, *Administrative Structure of the Medical and Related Services in England and Wales* (1968), in which they put forward for discussion the idea of a 'unified administration of the medical and related services in an area by one authority, in place of the multiplicity of authorities concerned in the present arrangements'. The *Report of the Committee on Local Authority and Allied Personal Social Services* (1968), known as the *Seebohm Report*, likewise comes up with similar proposals. They suggest the establishment of one central social welfare department in each local authority to be responsible for the whole welfare structure administered by local authorities.

The individual *vis-à-vis* the company

An individual as we have seen may be at a serious tax disadvantage compared to a company, whether the company is incorporated or unincorporated in form. Put the other way, an individual may be able to reap substantial tax advantages by forming a company, and a shareholder may reap tax advantages. This is so because companies are allowed to deduct for the using up of capital before arriving at a figure of taxable profit, whereas individuals do not have this right. Also a company is in a more advantageous position in being able to claim for expenses. In recent years expense claims have been tightened up, but important differences still remain.

The adoption of the accretion principle would, we have seen, go a long way to achieving equity. Dividends would be taxed as income, retained profits, if they enhanced the value of the business, would also be taxed as income when the gains were realized.

Difficult questions remain on the extent of company taxation. A change to a V.A.T. in place of the S.E.T. might, it has been argued, be beneficial, and is necessary if Britain is to align herself with Europe. Though a V.A.T. is mainly borne by consumers, the regressive nature of the impost can be taken care of on the lines previously indicated in this chapter.

A V.A.T. at 10% would bring in far more revenue than the S.E.T. and purchase tax, which, it is assumed, would be abolished. Important questions are raised as to which taxes should be reduced or abolished if a V.A.T. is introduced. The time is ripe for a Royal Commission to investigate these alternatives and the differences in treatment for tax of persons and companies in the light of the many changes which have occurred since 1955. It will be argued in the final chapter of this book that such a Commission should have wide terms of reference to look at taxes and benefits as a whole. The V.A.T. and treatment of companies would then form part of its brief.

Summary

After listing the major faults found in the current system, incidence of tax in the traditional sense is discussed. This is rejected in favour of looking at the impact, in so far as costs and benefits can sensibly be allocated to individuals, of government spending and revenue as a whole. The advantage of this approach is that the importance of a particular tax or benefit in relation to the whole can be judged. In time, alternative assumptions about the incidence of various taxes and benefits can be made in order to see how great a difference this makes to the 'burden'.

The conclusions reached, from the limited statistical evidence available, is that the present system, in spite of considerable effort, is not equitable. Nor, as we have seen, is it succeeding very well in relieving poverty.

Further patching up of the system would not seem to be the answer. The present very complicated tax and benefit arrangements are a result of past piecemeal tackling of problems.

It is possible to see improvement taking place from the side of taxation and from the side of benefits. These are inseparably interlinked and cannot sensibly be discussed in isolation from one another, in spite of many past attempts to do so. Discussion of tax benefits must take place against some criterion of equity. One possibility outlined is to take the difference between original income and income after allowing for taxes paid and benefits received, termed 'effective income'. This difference gives the figure of *net* benefits received or *net* taxes paid, as the case may be, and can be related to original income to build up a standard of equity. Ways of supplementing those people with effective income below that judged adequate by society were discussed.

While this chapter necessarily concentrates on types of benefit, complementary to it is a study of administration. Because of the very fragmented administrative set-up, a great deal of waste, frustration and hardship occurs at present. Improvement could be expected; by integration of services under one authority, by simplification and by using known technical possibilities of computers.

Part III
Policy

19
Introduction to policy considerations

Policy to deal with inflation is a subject on which a great deal has been written and argued by eminent authorities without adding substantially to knowledge, and in some cases subtracting from it.

JOHNSON, H. G. (1967), *Essays in Monetary Economics.*

In Part I the monetary system was examined, and in Part II government expenditure, revenue and debt. It is now time to attempt to draw these threads together and examine their effects on the economy.

Much has been written about the effects that are likely to flow from different monetary and fiscal changes. The analysis is frequently conducted at great length with an impressive array of geometric and mathematical expertise. Within the assumptions adopted by the author, the conclusions can seldom be faulted. As exercises in logic, this work probably has value, but as a guide to the best policy to adopt at any one time they unfortunately yield few results. It is seldom that the conclusions can be shown to hold once the restrictive assumptions have been removed.

An added difficulty is the lack of general agreement on a theory explaining the variables usually selected as important for study. The usual variables on which it is desired to see the effects of monetary or fiscal changes are: consumption and saving, investment, prices and output, and work effort.

Since the theories explaining these variables are in dispute, it is not surprising that an explanation of the effect of this or that Budgetary change is, at best, imprecise and subject to doubt.

This chapter looks briefly at each of these variables. It attempts no precise answers to the question: what would happen to each of these if, say, a particular tax was changed? In our present state of knowledge, such a precise answer is impossible. Neither does it attempt a detailed assessment of the use of monetary and fiscal methods in the post-war period. A number of recent full-scale assessments have been made, to which the interested reader can refer: Brittan, S. (1964), Dow, J. C. R. (1964) and Caves, R. E. (1968). Rather, it looks at some of the problems involved in getting even approximate estimates.

Personal consumption and saving

We have seen in the post-war period direct measures, such as rationing and price-control, influencing consumption and saving. What of the influence of fiscal and monetary policy?

To get somewhere, it is necessary to have a theory to work with, even if it is no stronger than the feeling that 'consumption and saving can be changed by altering income'. Keynes, J. M. (1936), 96, said:

> The fundamental psychological law upon which we are entitled to rely with great confidence both *a priori* from our knowledge of human nature and from detailed facts of experience, is that men are disposed as a rule and on the average to increase their consumption as their income increases, but not by as much as the increase in income.

Since this was written over thirty years ago, this 'law' has been the subject of much debate and investigation. Attempts have been made to modify the law to take account of the structure of wealth as well as of income (see Appendix to this chapter). It has been suggested that past levels of income need to be taken into account as well as current levels, that it is 'permanent' or normal income which is the relevant concept, or that it is the flow of income over the life-cycle of the individual that matters. Many of these alternative statements are concerned with the long-run trend in consumption and the influences, economic and social, which bear on this. Management of the economy, as we are concerned with it, is largely a matter of year-to-year control, and here we are on safe ground in asserting that a change in income will be of major importance and will change consumption and saving in the same direction as the change in income. An advanced study of the determinants of consumer expenditure is given by Suits, D. B. (1963), 1-57.

The size of the change will depend on many factors. One of the most important is likely to be the way the income change is distributed over different income groups. Budget studies inform us that, as we move up the income scale, out of each addition to income more is likely to be saved: in economic terms, the marginal propensity to save increases with income. It follows that £1 paid in tax by a person with a high income will tend to reduce saving more than £1 paid by a taxpayer with a small income. Thus a progressive income tax is likely to reduce saving more than a flat-rate tax. Put the other way, taxes which fall mainly on the poor are likely to have more impact on consumption than taxes which fall mainly on the rich.

These generalizations are frequently invoked by advocates of tax changes—for example, those who advocate reducing the rates of income tax in order to increase savings.

Unfortunately, there is no clear empirical evidence on the magnitude of the difference on savings or consumption. If the difference is small, then arguments for tax changes on these grounds can be ignored.[1] If they are large, it is necessary to take them into account. American studies (Musgrave, R. A. (1959), 269-70) suggest that although taxes that affect high-income earners are likely to effect saving more than consumption, the result is easily overstated. Dow, J. C. R. (1964), 270-5, lists British investigations which in general give more weight to the effect on savings. In view of the uncertain nature of the data and the assumptions that have to be made, authoritative statements on the relationships of changes in tax and effects on consumption and saving must await further investigation.

Let us consider a fully-employed economy where the need is to increase saving (that is, reduce consumption expenditure) in order that resources may be released from the consumption to the investment sector. Even if the argument is accepted that the effect of taxing high incomes is to affect savings to a significant extent, it does not necessarily follow that flat-rate taxes are to be preferred. There is an obvious clash between the objective of control over the economy and of redistribution of income and wealth. Political judgments here come to the fore. From the point of view of controlling the economy, it does not matter whether the savings are undertaken by individuals or the government. If a decision has been made about the degree of progression of the tax system that is desired, and if it is desired to reduce consumption, then tax rates can be changed. The change can be made so as to leave the degree of progression of the system unchanged. If this results in less private saving or a slower increase in private saving, this affect can be allowed for in the new rates. This results in the desired level of saving being obtained through a government surplus or reduced deficit.

It is possible (but not perhaps very likely) that this increase in savings of the government sector would result in a shortage of funds for private investment. Numerous ways are available whereby

[1] Differences may be small in two senses. The first, that the change makes no perceptible difference to behaviour. The second, that although the change makes a large difference, the numbers affected by the change are so small, or the amount of money involved is so small, as to make no significant change in overall saving, e.g. if only 1,000 people are affected by a change, then even though it is assumed they save the whole of the amount involved, this will have an insignificant effect on total savings. Any reactions of those who are not directly affected by the change must also be considered.

these funds can be channelled back to private investment. The decision is once more primarily a political judgment. The government could undertake direct investment in firms, or the resources of the Finance Corporation for Industry or the Industrial and Commercial Finance Corporation and kindred organizations could be supplemented. Alternatively, taxes on companies could be reduced or investment grants increased.

One further illustration will be given. At first sight, a change in estate duties is a clear-cut case of a change in taxation that will affect saving more than consumption. However, it has already been pointed out that one way of avoiding estate duties is to give away one's wealth at least seven years before death. To the extent that wealth is given away to younger persons sooner than it would otherwise be given, the consumption of these younger persons is likely to increase.

A consideration therefore of the impact of monetary and fiscal changes on consumption and saving should take account of the impact on different income-groups, because they are likely to have different propensities to consume. Ideally, the effects of different amounts of wealth should also be taken into account and allowance made for shifts of money and assets to different age-groups who are likely to have different spending habits. Dow, J. C. R. (1964), 275, has suggested that an important category to separate out is the self-employed, whose propensity to consume is lower than that of comparable income groups because of higher saving to provide investment for their own business.

The above brief discussion shows some of the more important difficulties that have to be faced if 'hunches' about the effects of tax or monetary changes are to be turned into objective facts. In Britain the matter is further bedevilled by a lack of adequate statistical data—in particular, in relation to figures of savings. The figures of savings that appear in the *National Income and Expenditure* tables (the so-called Blue Book) are completely unreliable. This is so because no attempt is made to arrive at independent estimates of saving. The figure is arrived at by taking estimates of income and deducting estimates of consumption. The resulting residual figure is called 'saving'. Since income and consumption are big magnitudes, even small errors in these estimates can make a large difference in the residual figure. Independent estimates of savings are beginning to be built up, but these have yet to be incorporated in the Blue Book. For details of the figures of savings compared year by year refer to 'More Light on Personal Saving' (April, 1965). Uncertainty is therefore present concerning the amount of savings in the community and who undertakes it. There is a need for better statistics of what is actually taking place and for more consideration of the motives for savings, and how these motives change in response to different economic and social pressures.

Public expenditure can affect consumption and saving as well as changes in tax or monetary policy. The most important part in this respect is likely to be the extent of transfer payments. These, as we saw in Chapter 8, have increased in recent years to a greater extent than other forms of government expenditure. The greater provision of social security payments by the government, in the form of pensions, children's allowances and the like, reduces the need for private provision for these needs, although the extent to which the private sector would voluntarily save to provide for these contingencies is uncertain. Similar considerations apply to so-called 'free services', such as medical care, but the effect is weaker in that much would be spent directly on these services by individuals in the absence of schemes financed out of taxation.

Save as you earn scheme

The Budget in 1969 announced a contractual savings scheme whereby a person over sixteen years can invest up to a maximum of £10 a month in National Savings for five years and obtain a tax-free bonus at the end of the period of £12 for each £60 saved. If the savings are retained for a further two years, without making further contributions the bonus is doubled to £24 for each £60 saved. This bonus is equivalent after five years to a tax-free rate of interest of about 7% a year or in gross terms 12% for a standard-rate taxpayer. The seven-year rate is equivalent to a tax-free rate of interest of about 11% or gross rate around 19%. It is possible to cash the accumulated savings after one year in which case a tax-free rate of interest of only 2½% is paid. A feature of the scheme is that payment can be deducted from income by the employer. A similar scheme is being set up for contractual savings through a building society. Because the bonuses on these savings are paid free of all tax the effective yield to a top-rate surtax payer is around 80%. If, as seems likely, high-rate taxpayers avail themselves of the maximum permitted savings this is an expensive way for the government to induce contractual savings, but inevitable so long as blanket tax-free bonuses are given.

The extent to which this scheme will shift the savings schedule of the community, that is result in more savings at the same level of National Income, and the extent to which it will merely change the type of security savers take up, remains to be seen.

Investment

The post-war period has seen a variety of methods used to influence investment, from direct controls, such as licensing and planning permission, to various monetary and fiscal policies. Even if there was agreement about a theory of investment (which there is not), the presence of so many variables makes it very difficult to pin down the effect of any one of them. Investment has been the subject of a good part of recent economic writing. For an advanced study see Eisner, R. and Strotz, R. H. (1963), 61-337, with a selected bibliography of 666 items!

The 'acceleration principle' makes investment a function of changes in demand. The truth in this principle, that a permanent change in demand calls for a different stock of investment goods, should not blind us to the obvious defects of the principle as a guide to short-term investment decisions. An increase in demand can often be met from previous resources that were idle or not working to capacity. The length of time required to adjust the capital stock, up or down, may run into years, and so on. Much investment needs to be planned for a number of years ahead. For example, once a decision has been made in principle to go ahead with a new factory, a suitable site has to be found, planning permission obtained, contractors engaged before work can commence, and the construction itself may take one, two or more years. Under these circumstances, it might be thought that investment of this type would be insensitive to temporary changes in demand, brought about by a government that was pledged to full employment not intending permanently to alter demand patterns.

Present evidence is far from conclusive, but from surveys of British industry it seems that investment plans do fluctuate considerably according to the current condition of the economy, whether, that is, the period is one of expansion or contraction: stop or go. There are several possible explanations for this. The most unfavourable interpretation to British industry would be that not many firms plan very far ahead or calculate their intended investments in a very rational manner. The White Paper on *Investment Incentives* (1966) quoting an enquiry carried out by the Confederation of British Industry among their members, gave some support to these pessimistic conclusions. However, other factors must also play a part. Some forms of investment have a short time to come to fruition, and it is then more realistic to expect fluctuations in investment according to fluctuations in demand. Again, the cut-back during times of low demand may be due to difficulties in obtaining finance rather than deliberate intentions to cut investment. There is also business confidence to take into account, which may be unduly pessimistic about investment prospects at a time of contraction of demand, and unduly optimistic at a time of buoyant demand.

To the extent that investment does fluctuate with demand, the conclusions for getting growth in the economy are perverse. The stated intention in cutting consumer demand during times of full employment is to release resources for the investment sector. If the effect is also to cut investment, the required growth will not be forthcoming and employment will fall. If deliberate manipulation of consumer demand in one or more particular sectors can be engineered without too large an overspill to other sectors of the economy, then the non-suppressed sectors of the economy will be able and willing to proceed with their investments.

Other explanations of investment lay more stress on the availability of particular types of saving, e.g. ploughed-back profits or the buoyancy of the stock market. British policy, by its frequent discrimination against distributed profits, changes in tax allowances and experiments with initial allowances, investment allowances and now investment grants, has developed policy actively in this field. It has been argued in Chapter 13 that the most dubious part of this policy, and also, it would appear, the least successful, has been the discrimination against dividends. Initial and investment allowances suffered from several drawbacks, as we saw, which it is hoped the new system of grants will overcome.

A third theory of investment makes it a function of rate of return on investment compared to the rate of interest. If the return from real investment is above the cost of borrowing (or above the best return that can be obtained from putting surplus funds into financial assets), then the inducement to invest is strong and vice versa. The impact of the rate of interest will be considered in Chapter 21. It is argued there that one way that the rate of interest can be important is via the stock-market and its influence on the willingness and ability of firms to raise fresh capital and on the flow of new money into the market.

Econometric studies approach the problem of investment by trying to unravel the interconnections between industries. That, for example, it is estimated that every £100 of final output in 1963 in the metal manufacturing trades requires a net input of £1·8 from coal, £0·7 from other mining, £3 from chemicals, £44·5 from metal, £4·7 from engineering, and so on (figures given in *National Income and Expenditure*, Table 21 (1968). For details of a model of the British economy see Stone, R. and others (1962).) If therefore decisions are made this year as to how the economy should grow next year, the details can be fed into the model and the requirements on the economy can be calculated. If details of investment for the next year are known, the shortfall or over-expansion of investment can then be seen and attempts made to get firms to alter their plans accordingly. If industrialists can be convinced of the soundness of the calculations, they have a firmer base on which to plan their own investments. The firm is well aware intuitively that the success or otherwise of its own plans depends to a large extent on what is happening in the rest of the economy: the more facts can replace guesswork, the more steady is investment likely to become. Too much should not be expected from what are admittedly crude models of the interactions in the economy. The hope is that more data will be forthcoming, improvements in method made and the predictions made more reliable.

These theories of what determines investment concentrate attention on differing variables that enter into the decision whether or not to invest. They are not independent variables, but interact with each other, and their respective importance is likely to change over time. Bearing these facts in mind, it is not surprising that evidence of the effect of government measures on investment is hard to pin down.

Prices and output

The adjustments in prices and output that businesses make in response to government policy changes are at least as difficult to sort out as any that have so far been considered.

It is clear that if a manufacturer passes on to his customers the whole of an increase in cost (whether this is due to an increase in purchase tax, in company tax or higher interest charges), the demand for his product may be affected. He may be forced therefore to reconsider his price and so in effect bear part of the increase, at least in the short run.[2] In the long run adjustments can be made to the size of the plant. The industry itself can also expand or contract by the movement of firms into and out of the industry.

Nor are the changes that occur in one sector of the economy likely to be confined to that sector. An increase in the price of, for example, fruit may lead to some *substitution* for fruit of other goods that are unchanged in price, i.e. now relatively cheaper. Likewise, a decrease in the price of fruit may lead to the substitution of fruit for other goods. As well as this substitution effect as the relative prices of commodities change, an *income* effect is apparent.

[2] The response of demand to a change in price is measured by the concept of 'elasticity': the percentage change in quantity divided by the percentage change in price. But elasticity is a measure of response: it merely says that for a particular change in price in the commodity being considered, demand changes by this or that amount. There is still a need to explain in each case the reasons for the particular degree of responsiveness.

INCOME AND SUBSTITUTION EFFECT

A simple example will be given to illustrate the distinction between the substitution and the income effect. Consider an individual's choice between fruit and other commodities and what happens when a tax on fruit is reduced. It is assumed that the individual spends all his income on these items.

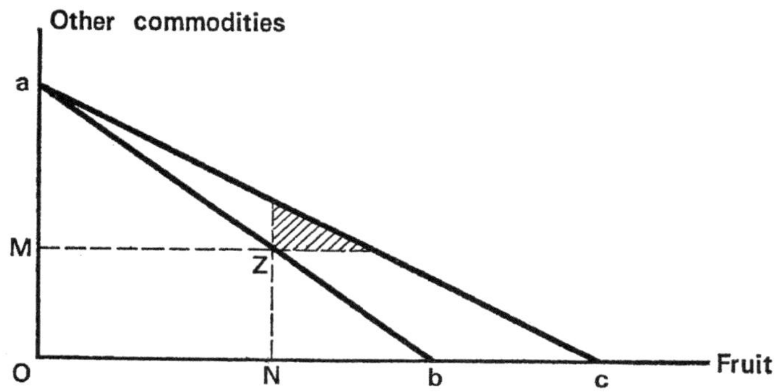

The amount of fruit is plotted along the horizontal axis, the other commodities along the vertical axis. Point *a* represents the amount of commodities other than fruit that could be purchased if the individual spent the whole of his income on these. Likewise, point *b* represents the amount of fruit that could be purchased if the individual spent the whole of his income on fruit. The straight line, joining *a* and *b* indicates the various combinations of each that the individual can purchase with his given income. Let us assume that the individual chooses point Z, which gives him a quantity of OM of other commodities and ON of fruit. Into this picture we now introduce a tax-reduction on fruit; therefore more fruit can be purchased with the same money income as before. Hence we draw the new line, *a, c,* to indicate the position after the tax change. Within the shaded area on the diagram the consumer can now, with his same income, have more of both goods—that is, the effect of a price change enables the consumer to have an increase in consumption. The price change has in effect given the consumer an increase in income, hence the name '*income* effect'. Whereabouts on the new budget line *a, c* the individual will settle cannot be determined. The price change has altered the relative prices, making fruit cheaper, and *substitution* may well take place—that is, more fruit may be purchased because it is now relatively cheaper. The position taken up by the individual on the budget line *a, c,* will depend on the combined results of the income and substitution effects. The strengths of these effects will differ in different cases.

In the simple case considered, a change in the price of fruit, other prices remaining the same, it was concluded that it was not possible as a general rule to pinpoint the exact position that a consumer would take up. The substitution effect would normally be expected to operate to increase demand for the relatively cheaper good, but the income effect is less easy to predict.

AGGREGATE CHANGES IN PRICE AND OUTPUT

The above reasoning deals with the response of an individual manufacturer to a change. In trying to account for aggregate movements in prices and output a number of other considerations need to be borne in mind.

The time element has so far been ignored for exposition purposes. Its presence adds considerable practical difficulties in sorting out the effects of a change. For example, after each recent increase in the tax on tobacco, the consumption of tobacco has fallen for a few weeks or months, only to come back to higher levels. One of the difficulties in sorting out the effects of a change is that the market for tobacco, as for many products, has been an expanding one for many years. Most noticeably, population changes and the spread of smoking among women have increased the market. To say that the consumption of tobacco surpasses its old level is not to say that, in the absence of a tax change, consumption might not be higher than its present level. It is very difficult to separate out statistically the underlying trend in consumption and the change due to the tax measure.

The impact of a change will depend in part on the state of the economy. In conditions of full employment the manufacturer is more likely to pass on increases, reasoning that competitors will follow suit. So relative market shares between himself and competitors in the same industry and also the market share of his industry *vis-à-vis* other industries will be affected slightly or not at all: an increase in price in one sector may lead, that is, to a broad movement in prices over a wide range of goods.

Many countries have experienced a general rise in prices, or inflation, in the post-war period. A number of theories have been developed to try to explain this phenomenon (see Johnson, H. G. (1967), and Bronfenbrenner, M. and Holzman, F. D. (September, 1963), 593-661. Two theories have contended for pride of place: *demand* inflation, which concentrates on the pull which demand can exercise on prices; and *cost* inflation, which lays emphasis on increases in cost forcing up prices. The major emphasis with cost inflation has been put on increases occurring in wages and salaries coming from union pressures. Employers may, however, bid up wages in their demand for labour which tends to blur the distinction between these two theories for practical purposes.

The role assigned to fiscal policy in controlling prices is given different emphasis by these two theories, but both have in common the fact that little emphasis is placed on monetary policy. A reaction against this can be discerned in Johnson, H. G. (1967), and Bronfenbrenner, M. and Holzman, F. D. (September, 1963).

In general, government policy in the post-war period, has been seen as aiding, or hindering, other forces which are moulding prices. British government policy came out of this sheltered position in 1966, when in place of exhortation, control over prices and wages was directly attempted?![3]

Work effort with full employment

The adjustment in the work effort of a community to a fiscal change has been mentioned on several previous occasions.

In order to get a determinate answer, we need to know a great deal. It is worth putting this down, if only to evaluate the exaggerated claims that are sometimes made of the effects on work that will follow from a particular change.

1. It is necessary to know how the change affects each group in the community. A group must be defined in some way to make it economically meaningful, perhaps by occupation or income.
2. The numbers in each group must be determined.
3. The average reactions of each group have to be determined.
4. The weighting to be assigned to each group must be determined, e.g. how should five hours less worked by an accountant be judged in relation to five hours more worked by a dustman?

A determinate answer can only be given if data is available and assumptions are made at the relevant points. Clearly, different assumptions about reactions of each group (e.g. that they will work less hard because they have less income because of the tax change, or that they will work harder to make up for the tax change) will yield different answers. In this context, groups have to take account, not only of the working labour force, but the potential labour force.

[3] A chess-player will recognize the significance of '?!'. In chess notation a '?' is placed after a doubtful move, a '!' after an excellent move. Both signs placed after a move denote a risky move that has the chance of winning or losing the game according to the play of the opponent: signs that could be adopted, with advantage, in economics.

For example, it is frequently asserted that high taxation acts as a disincentive to work, or affects the quality of work, of particular groups. On the other hand, high taxation has been one of the factors leading to married women joining the labour force in order to help out the family income, although in the case where a married couple's joint income brings them into the surtax bracket, tax may be a disincentive to the wife to work (Hockley (May-June, 1967)).

Appendix One of the Royal Commission on the Taxation of Profits and Income (1954) presents the results of an investigation, from a sample of nearly 1,500 persons, of tax on work incentives of industrial workers. It concluded that there was no significant effect on productivity. A bibliography of studies that has been made in the tax-incentive field will be found in Musgrave, R. A. and Shoup, C. S. (1959). Break, G. F. (September, 1957), gives an empirical study amongst solicitors and accountants. Merritt, A. J. and Monk, D. A. G. (1967), and Merritt, A. J. (1968), look at executive remuneration. Titmus, R. M. (1963) (particularly Chapter 11) takes a very broad look at current trends in the economy, and deals *inter alia* with taxation. *The Banker*, March, 1968, contains two articles: one by Cyriax, G., sets out the orthodox case that taxes reduce work incentives; the other, by Daniel, W. W. D., examines evidence against this view. Eisenstein, L. (1961), wittily discusses the art of obtaining a tax system in the interest of particular groups. (Chapter 5 deals with incentive arguments.) Although this book deals with American conditions, the reader should have little difficulty in substituting examples from his own country's institutions and groups.

The difficulties in coming to conclusions in this field can be illustrated from the latest study by Merritt, A. J. (1968). This book gives a valuable look at the remuneration of executives and corporate efficiency.

Merritt argues, among other things, that advantages would follow from higher before-tax executive remuneration, and also advantages would follow from higher net-of-tax benefits. Giving executives, or some of them, the right to stock options on the American pattern is given as one way of increasing net-of-tax benefits.

Higher before-tax remuneration is seen as a way of forcing companies to be more efficient if profitability is not to suffer. However, this is an argument that can be used to justify giving an increase to any category of worker or imposing a swingeing increase in the selective employment tax! Higher after-tax remuneration is recommended on the grounds that it would enable firms to impose stricter work criteria on executives who proved inadequate, since they would have been enabled to provide adequately for this contingency out of their higher net earnings. Again, this argument, if accepted as valid, can be used to justify lower tax on any category of worker. It seems equally plausible to argue that higher remuneration for executives would make it harder for firms to turn out inefficient executives, since it would be known that they would suffer a larger cut in living standards and larger 'golden handshakes' would be needed.

Even if it could be established conclusively that giving stock options would improve the quality and quantity of executives' work, this does not prove that the change is desirable. Before a change can be recommended on these grounds, it is necessary to establish that the reactions of non-executives to this tax privilege would not result in a greater detriment. The change could lead to greater industrial strife by those workers who do not benefit, which would more than outweigh the gain in executive efficiency. This increase in strife could occur through a general feeling that the gulf between 'them' and 'us' had widened, and general antipathy on the part of the ordinary worker to productivity changes which would put more into the pocket of the executive than into his own. It could also occur because the trade unions used this as a lever to be more militant on behalf of their members. The correctness or otherwise of these reactions, whether they are motivated by feelings of vindictiveness or of social justice, is not important in this context. What matters is the strength of the reaction which needs to be measured against the favourable response expected from the change.

Summary

Before it is possible to analyse the effect of a change in government policy, it is necessary to have a theory about how the economy operates.

> When we have no theory about economic affairs, no state of those affairs and no temporal succession of states seems inconceivable. A theory restricts the conceivable states and succession of states to those in which the relations between quantifiable things in the economy conform to some specified rules. Theories differ from each other in the list of quantifiable (not necessarily measurable) things to be considered, and in the precise character of the rules about their interrelation (Shackle, G. L. S. (June, 1961), 200).

In this chapter consumption and saving, investment, prices and output, and work effort have been examined and treated in isolation from each other. In practice they are closely interrelated. A change in government policy may cause significant changes in two or more of them. It is the overall effect that is important. Sometimes changes in different variables will operate in the same direction, e.g. cause a reduction in investment and in work effort, and sometimes changes will tend to cancel each other out.

In judging the implications of economic policy, it has been shown that there is no generally agreed theory to work with. Thus, unfortunately, an analysis even for an observer who is trying to be impartial depends a great deal on which theory is selected and on the weight given to each of the variables. More unfortunately still, it leaves the door wide open for those with special interests to defend to select those theories that serve their cause best. This pessimistic conclusion is not intended as an apologia for inaction. Given the size of the government sector, it is not possible for the government to be neutral. It is an indication of the need for care in accepting the claims put forward for this or that particular measure.

Appendix: wealth effect

In spite of increased attention paid to wealth in recent years, it is still one of the neglected areas in economics. A variety of names have been coined to emphasize one particular aspect of wealth or another, e.g. wealth effect, real balance effect, Pigou effect, Roosa effect. The single term 'wealth effect' will be used here.

It is fairly obvious that, if two persons both have an income of £10,000 after tax, but one person has wealth of £500,000 while the other has wealth of £50,000, then the consumption patterns of the two persons is likely to be very different and the proportions each saves is likely to be different.[4] Unfortunately, we have very little idea how a person's wealth position affects his behaviour. A transfer of income from the wealthy to the less wealthy will have repercussions, but we cannot as yet add in quantitative data.

One aspect of the wealth effect has been looked at, when the idea was examined that a change in the rate of interest may affect capital values, particularly of fixed-interest securities. It is possible that this will deter the holders from selling, but the evidence to date is that this effect is weak. A similarly weak effect may be caused by a general change in the value of money. Supposing there is a deflation, then some assets, e.g. money and government securities, will increase in real value. This may induce some extra spending on behalf of the holders. Once again this effect is likely, in aggregate, to be weak.

[4] The composition of assets in which wealth is held may also be important. Two persons who each have wealth of £100,000, one whose wealth primarily consists of land, the other whose wealth primarily consists of a portfolio of shares, are also likely to have different patterns of consumption and saving.

The extent to which a change in the value of money affects behaviour depends, in part, on the extent *money illusion* is, or is not, present in a community.

In a simple form, money illusion is thinking that one is better off when one's remuneration is increased, although the increase only covers the general increase in prices, or, conversely, thinking that one is worse off because prices are up and ignoring increases in money remuneration.

The problem of money illusion is encountered whenever the price-level changes, whether this is due to changes in indirect taxes or other causes, and likewise is encountered when incomes alter, whether this is due to changes in direct taxes or other causes.

The extent to which consumption alters in response to a price or income change will thus depend on the extent to which money illusion is present in the community. The usual assumption made is to assume that money illusion is absent, or that different people's reactions largely cancel out in the aggregate, but exceptional circumstances may falsify this expectation.

Because economics has in the past built on simple relationships relating consumption and saving to income, largely ignoring the dimension of wealth, it follows that action by the government to regulate the economy based on this simplification can be misleading. It is likely that changes in wealth will proceed fairly gradually over time, and to this extent can be ignored in the short run, but in exceptional circumstances they may be important. For example, most predictions made on how much consumers would spend after the Second World War were too low by a fairly large amount, due to underestimating the build-up of liquid capital during the war. Predictions based on pre-war data were wrong almost certainly because sufficient attention had not been given to the changes in the total and composition of wealth and to changes in its ownership.

20
Policy (continued)

The state of balance of the conventional budget, judged by the eternal knife-edge precepts of Mr Micawber, is the badge of fiscal success or failure. From the economist's point of view, the focus of attention on the size and state of balance of the conventional budget is quite misplaced. Its size does not measure the government's draft on the productive resources of the economy. Its balance does not measure the effect of the government's transactions with the public on the overall economic balance between supply and demand.

TOBIN, J. (1963), 'An Essay on Principles of Debt Management'.

Introduction

Ideally we set out to ask: if a given change is put into effect, what will be the resulting changes and adjustments in the economy? Or, alternatively, what must be changed in order to achieve some desired objective? The change can be in monetary policy, in government spending, revenue and debt, or in direct types of controls, such as hire-purchase regulations. Our ideal has been called 'a state of bliss' and, like most states of bliss, it is difficult to obtain. The complexity, as the previous chapter indicated, nearly defeats us. There is so much to take into account; so little agreed theory and empirical knowledge to work with.

A recognition of this complexity is in itself an important point. The criticism that, given a group of ten economists, there will be *at least* ten different opinions is not so damaging a remark as it at first appears. Given an objective—say, to increase productive investment —there are usually countless ways of achieving this. There is first of all the decision, a political one, whether it is public or private investment, or both, which shall be increased. If some measure of encouragement of private investment is required, consumer spending could be encouraged, which in turn would be expected to feed back a demand for investment, or investment could be encouraged directly. In either case there are numerous combinations of tax changes, monetary changes, or changes in regulations which can bring this about. No two combinations are likely to have exactly the same repercussions on other parts of the economy. Under these circumstances, it would be surprising if a unique 'best' method could be agreed on. A search for a unique solution is likely to be misleading in other ways. For example it is unlikely that a solution which yields a satisfactory result, given full employment of labour, will be satisfactory, given a large measure of unemployment.

One approach to this problem has been indicated previously: the construction of a model of the economy, which can be put in mathematical terms and programmed on to a computer. Alternatives—for example, different tax changes—can then be fed into the model and results compared. Economic models of this type offer exciting possibilities for the future, but their usefulness is at present limited.

Our approach to this problem is necessarily less ambitious. In this chapter an attempt is made to provide a useful analytical framework. Within this framework regulation of the economy is looked at. This leads to a complete rejection of the idea of a 'balanced Budget'. Finally, problems of control and the effects of control are taken up. Monetary and debt policy is left to the next chapter.

Framework

A basically Keynesian framework will be adopted. The national income or national product account will be used. These terms are synonymous, and merely refer to the fact that it is possible to arrive at the same total estimate of a country's activity either by adding up total expenditure in a year or by adding up the incomes received from producing those goods and services.

Looking at it from the expenditure side, the aggregate sought comprises expenditure on consumption goods and expenditure on investment goods. In both cases there is a mixture of private expenditure and of government expenditure. To complete the picture, allowance must be made for the export and import of goods and services and flows of money into and out of the country. The picture in greater detail for the year 1967 is given in Table 1.

From Table 1 we see that out of gross domestic[1] expenditure of £34,320 million, 61% was accounted for by private expenditure, 18% by public expenditure and the remaining 21% went to investment. Of this investment companies and individuals invested about

[1] 'Domestic' refers to the fact that exports, imports and net flows of money into the economy have not been taken into account. When these magnitudes are incorporated the term 'national' is used.

half, the balance being accounted for chiefly by public corporations and local government. In the second part of the table it can be seen that in 1967 rather more goods were imported and property income paid abroad than was exported and received as income from property held abroad.

The word 'gross' in the table refers to the fact that investment relates to the total undertaken in the year, regardless of the fact that some of it was to replace old equipment. If to the sums of private and public expenditures at the top of the table had been added the amount of indirect taxes paid, less subsidies, a figure of £5,211 million, the aggregates would be at market prices instead of factor prices.

Table 1

Gross National Product 1967

			£m	%
Private expenditure on goods and services[2]			21,039	61
Public expenditure on goods and services[2]			6,136	18
	£m	%		
Gross investment:				
Persons	986	(3)		
Companies	2,519	(7)		
Public corporations	1,661	(5)		
Central government	392	(1)		
Local government	1,587	(5)	7,145	21
Total gross domestic expenditure at factor cost			34,320	100
Add: Exports and property income from abroad	8,736			
Deduct: imports and property income paid abroad	8,894		—158	
Add in: value of stock adjustment			130	
Gross national product at factor cost			34,292	

Source: *National Income and Expenditure*, 1968, Tables, 1, 6, 29.

[2] Prices at factor cost, i.e. with indirect taxes subtracted and subsidies added back. In all, taxes less subsidies amounted to £5,211.

Regulation of the economy: the concept of compensatory finance

The figures just given were all in money terms. The government, in its role of regulating the economy, is concerned with the impact of these money flows on the real resources of the economy. It is usual in these days to consider that labour provides the upper limit to the amount of goods and services that can be obtained from the economy, but in other circumstances the limit may be provided by other factors of production. For example, for several years after 1945 the supply of goods and services was chiefly limited by the amount of coal and electricity that could be produced. The aim of the government will be therefore to keep the economy near the level of full employment, with a large enough proportion of the working population producing investment goods to maintain the appropriate ratio of physical capital to output.

If the spending estimates of the various sectors for the next period when added together amount to more goods and services than can be produced after allowance has been made for a certain level of imports and exports, then the authorities will attempt to cut back these plans. Similarly, a shortfall is an indication that in the absence of action to stimulate the economy there will be unemployment and the economy will be producing less than it could. Failure to reduce over-ambitious plans results in inflationary pressure as each group tries to carry out its plans; moreover, there is a spill-over effect into imports and consequently pressure on the balance of payments. A shortfall in spending results in unemployment and deflationary pressure as producers find that some of the goods and services produced remain unsold.

Let us suppose Budget plans for the next year indicate an inflationary gap (plans exceed, at current prices, the output that is possible, allowing for a certain level of imports and exports). The following alternatives are open:

1. (a) Increase income tax to reduce disposable incomes and thereby reduce consumption expenditure.
   (b) Achieve the same result as in (a) by raising indirect taxes or cutting subsidies.

Both of these may be upset by successful attempts to increase incomes.

   (c) An increase in company tax, hoping to reduce dividends or investment or both, or a cut in investment grants.
2. (a) The gap may be closed by cutting the demands of the public sector for goods and services, either on current or capital account.
   (b) By cutting transfer payments.
3. The use of monetary policy by itself or in conjunction with any

of these measures to try to reduce private consumption or private investment.

In every case the impact on the balance of payments must be taken into account, and assumptions made as to whether or not persons and companies are able to compensate for the change.

In the absence of compensating changes, raising income tax does not alter the price-level. The impact falls on income-tax-payers. Indirect taxes raise the price-level to the extent that the tax is passed on in higher prices to those who buy the taxed goods (with the same money incomes, a reduction in real incomes results). To the extent that prices are not increased, this will result in a reduction in profits. In practice, post-war policy has largely failed to prevent compensatory increases either of wages or of profits.

It is necessary to note that the amount needed to be raised under alternative types of taxes is not the same, because the taxes are likely to affect taxpayers with different marginal propensities to consume. The substitution effect of indirect taxes also has to be taken into account, e.g. some demand may spill over to untaxed commodities. Also, the timing of the measures has to be allowed for.

Using the data of Table 1, we will suppose the inflationary gap for 1967 was estimated in 1966 to be £500 million. A cut of this magnitude on consumers' expenditure of £21,039 million is a cut of 2·4%. The same reduction on public expenditure of £6,136 is a cut of 8·1%. Likewise, if private investment is to bear the whole adjustment this amounts to a cut of 14·3%. Correspondingly, if the public sector investment is to bear the whole of the cut, this would amount to a reduction of 13·7%. This simple illustration goes a long way to explain why adjustments are in the main usually carried out on private expenditure: because it is by far the largest component of the national product, a cut of a given magnitude is a smaller proportion of the total, and hence is likely to have a less disturbing effect. There are other reasons for attempting to regulate private expenditure rather than the other components of national income. One is the speed at which measures can be put into effect: investment must be planned for some time ahead and cutting back can prove a very costly process. Another is the argument we have met before that can be summed up by the phrase, 'public squalor, private affluence'. Public spending, whether on current or capital account is often held to be of an essential nature. There is no need to take this statement at its face value: government spending needs examining in the same way as other magnitudes, but also the germ of truth in this statement is obvious. Finally, since the investment is likely to increase the national product in the future, a cut in current consumption is usually preferred to a cut in investment.

When we come to examine the ways in which adjustments can be imposed, it will be found the problem is much more complicated than the above would imply. Whatever measures are used to reduce consumers' expenditure, these are likely to have differential effects on different commodities. Thus to talk of a cut of £500 million on consumers' expenditure only amounting to a reduction of 2·4% is misleading. The impact on particular products and services may be very severe. Also, of course, there are likely to be repercussions on the other components of the national product.

Political factors must also realistically be taken into account. At times this may weigh against cutting private consumption. A cut in private consumption is obvious and may be actively resented. A cut in public expenditure may be less obvious. A cut in investment (private or public) is followed by consequences that are both remote and not easily related to the original cut.

The balanced budget

The idea that a government is virtuous if it matches expenditure with revenue is still a popular one, and one that receives support from a few economists. It will be clear from this chapter so far that this view is rejected. Our starting-point is that the government has a role to play in regulating the economy. The size of the government sector today is such that a neutral policy is in any case not possible. Seen in this context, there may be strong economic reasons for having either a surplus or a deficit on any particular Budget.

Political reasons appear to underly many objections to departing from a balanced Budget. It is argued that government expenditure is too large already, and anything which induces caution in government spending is to be welcomed. Give the government power to spend more than it raises in taxes, so it is argued, and any discipline over its spending is forfeited

Some time has already been spent on looking at government expenditure in detail. The inadequacy of talking of government expenditure as a total, without considering the components of that total, has already been argued. Useful service may be performed by attacking this or that component of government spending as being too high or too low, judging the grounds of the attack on their merits. To argue that there is some fixed percentage of government spending above which inflation or some other evil or evils set in, as well as being a dubious statistical exercise, is not necessarily an argument for cutting government expenditure, any more than it is an argument for cutting private consumption. What matters, for stabilization purposes, is the total demands on the economy in relation to the real resources of the economy; if the former is above the latter, it is an indication that the demands from all sectors should be looked at anew. The decision that it is best to cut expenditure in one sector or the other does not emerge from the statistics.

It is argued that unbalanced Budgets can lead to currency depreciation. The argument is undoubtedly true: there are many examples of governments, unable or unwilling to tax adequately, resorting to the printing press. To argue that a certain consequence *can* happen is not to argue that it *must* happen. If it is feared that the increase in the level of demand causes inflationary pressure, this only points to the fact that offsetting action is required. If it is feared that deficits over a number of years will so add to the money supply as to be inflationary, a similar reply can be made. This is a pointer to the need for offsetting action—for example, to tighten control of the monetary sector, to fund, or to take action to reduce the deficit, which can be done either by increased taxation or by reducing government expenditure. The latter solution of reducing the deficit does not automatically emerge as the best solution.

A further assertion is that deficits are less painful than current taxes in the sense that people take account of current taxes and discount future taxes to service debt. It is argued that this leads to over-expansion of government services. A counter-assertion is also put forward, that traditional concepts of Budgeting have hindered the provision of much-needed services and that failure to separate the debt of the nationalized industries and local authorities (which debt will normally result in the creation of real assets) accentuates this trend to under-provision. While either of these assertions may be true for a particular historical time period, they become increasingly hard to demonstrate in a modern Budgetary setting. Parliamentary procedures are the same whether the source of finance is loans or taxes, and with the growth of Keynesian ideas, whether a government has a deficit or surplus is likely to be dictated by the claims of all sectors on the real resources of the economy.

The argument is sometimes presented in the form of under- or over-pricing in the public sector leading to a misuse of resources. The 'price' of public services is, as indicated earlier, of real economic and social significance: but its connection with the overall Budget surplus or deficit is remote.

The concept of the balanced Budget has an intuitive appeal to the individual because of the analogy with the economy of the private household. But it has no validity in the accounts of a nation. It is dangerous because it conceals the real issues. In the trite phrase the real issue is 'the best use of the nation's resources'. The injection of the dogma, 'Balance the Budget', merely helps to cloud these real issues.

BRITISH OFFICIAL OPINION ON A BALANCED BUDGET

Official British opinion as expressed in White Papers has shifted a great deal. First is a quotation from a paper on *Employment Policy* published in 1944.

> The Government accepts as one of their primary aims and responsibilities the maintenance of a high and stable level of employment after the war . . . to the extent that the policies proposed in this Paper affect the balancing of the Budget in a particular year, they certainly do not contemplate any departure from the principle that the Budget must be balanced over a longer period (foreword and para. 77).

The second quotation is from the *Reform of the Exchequer Accounts*, published in 1963:

> The Chancellor's Budget judgment, as embodied in his tax proposals, takes into account, not only the Government's own direct expenditure on current goods and services and on capital formation, but also the level of demand in other sectors of the economy and the balance of payments. These will be influenced by the Government's own activities—by withdrawal of spending power through taxation and by additions to spending power through grants and other forms of assistance. If the prospective growth of productive resources in the period ahead and the growth of demand upon them at the existing level of taxation are in balance, then the Budget will be a neutral one, with either no changes in taxation or offsetting increases and reductions. If the forecasts show demand to be insufficient, then the object of the Budget will normally be to stimulate demand by reducing taxes. If the demand is expected to be excessive the Budget will normally set out to restrict it by increases in taxation. Although forecasts of the developments of the economy and calculations of the effect of particular tax changes are inevitably imprecise, a judgment has still to be made to decide the general direction of the Budget. The judgment will determine the Government's net borrowing or 'financing' requirements, which then has to be considered in itself from the point of view of debt management and monetary policy.
>
> The proper level of the Government's capital expenditure depends on quite separate considerations (e.g. the building programmes of the social services); and therefore it cannot be linked to the Government's borrowing without artificiality (paras. 33-4).

The contrast between these statements is quite clear. From the first it seems that while the unbalanced Budget could be used for war, it could not be used to fight unemployment, poverty and for the social good. Fortunately, nobody seems to have taken a great deal of notice. The second statement omits all reference to a balanced Budget. The balance that matters in the economy is that between real resources and demands on those real resources. The Budget has a part to play because it influences demands on those resources and also influences the amount of real investment that will be undertaken.

Problems of control

In trying to regulate the economy, the fundamental problem is to *diagnose* the trends in the economy. Has employment, private investment, consumer buying or some other economic magnitude changed? Once a change has been spotted, its importance to the economy must be assessed, and a judgment made on whether the change is a temporary one or if it is likely to continue for some time. In the latter event an assessment is needed on whether the change in question —say, a decrease in employment—will increase in intensity or gradually correct itself.

On the factual side of obtaining information about changes in the economy, much has been done to improve the position, although it remains true that a great deal more can and should be done to improve it still further. The question involves not only obtaining information, but of obtaining it in time for it to be economically useful. The deficiencies in information make it difficult to evaluate government measures since the war. It is not easy to decide whether the correct measures were applied in the wrong situation because of faulty information, or whether other elements in the picture were wrong.

After the prognostication, if action is thought to be necessary, the type of action to be taken must be decided on. Enough has been said to indicate that in most cases a number of alternatives are open which will effect a remedy. The choice of which course of action offers the 'best' solution involves both political and economic judgment. In both cases differences of opinion can legitimately occur. Of particular importance in assessing alternative measures is the *time* scale needed to put the measures into effect, and once put into effect the *time* for them to affect the economy. The position today is better than it used to be. The Chancellor has power to vary purchase tax by 10% between Budgets, company tax has been put on a current-year basis and, so on. Another important consideration is how *flexible* the proposed action is. If the prognostication is wrong because it has either underestimated the effects or overestimated the effects, can the action be changed so as to allow for these revised estimates?

Consideration of the pitfalls of economic management has led a number of people to reject altogether the idea that management of the economy should be attempted. They point to mistakes in the past which have had the effect of the remedy making the situation worse. Since the record of the economy when it was 'unregulated' was one of slumps and booms, with long periods of high unemployment, the attempt at management seems likely to be more fruitful in the long run. As improvement takes place both in our knowledge of what is occurring in the economy and of our understanding of its working, we can hope for better results in the future. The moral to be drawn is not that control of the economy is wrong in principle, but that too much should not be expected from what at present are relatively crude methods. The attempt is worth making because improvements can be expected in the future as we learn from past mistakes.

A different attitude is taken by some persons who do not argue against attempts at regulation as such, but wish to see the building up of new, and the strengthening of existing, 'automatic stabilizers'. An example of an automatic stabilizer is provided by a progressive tax on income. A reduction in aggregate wages paid in a period (due to some of the labour force being unemployed) will result in an automatic reduction in tax from income. Whereas, of course, indirect taxes are paid whether the person buying the goods is employed or unemployed. National Insurance contributions, which are not payable when the person is unemployed, and unemployment benefit, which is paid when a person is out of work, both act as automatic stabilizers. A few writers have suggested that the amount of currency in the economy should be automatically regulated and increased by a small regular percentage each year.

The idea behind the concept of automatic stabilizers is an attractive one. However, in the present state of knowledge of the economy, we cannot hope to dispense with deliberate action to aid the economy. Whether, and under what circumstances, it would be possible to make our economy run smoothly by such automatic stabilizers is beyond the scope of this book.

To summarize this section, a flow diagram is useful. The steps outlined above involve:

Identification of change

↓

Assessment of the likely trends in the changes

↓

Assessment of change and trends on the economy

↙ ↘

No action required | Action required, and need to assess what kind of action should be undertaken

The arrows point out the steps involved in the decision, starting from the top. The third step 'Assessment of change and trends on the economy', leads either to no action being required or to an assessment of what kind of action should be put into effect.

Effect of changes on the economy

In trying to assess the relative merits of alternative policies, it has been shown that it is useful to ask a number of questions—namely, how long before the measure can be put into effect; how long before it then makes its impact on the economy; and: is it flexible?

Management of the economy, however, is only one aim of government, labelled *stabilization* in Chapter 9. Policies need also to be judged in relation to their effects on the *allocation* and *distribution* of resources.

Different policies will almost certainly affect the allocation of resources between private and public goods, between investment and consumption goods, and between types of good in each category. A tax on labour—for example, the selective employment tax—is likely to lead to the substitution of capital for labour in the service sector: indeed, this was one of the reasons for introducing it. Tracing the effects of different policies is likely to be difficult because not only is the stock—that is, the amount already in existence—likely to be affected, but also the flow—that is, the additional amount demanded or supplied over time. Thus, as we have seen, one of the effects of the selective employment tax in its original form was to reduce the demand for part-time workers. Again, a change in tax rates may cause the existing labour force to work less hard or more hard, and may also encourage or discourage married women into the labour force.

Different policies will also almost certainly affect the distribution of resources and move the economy towards, or away from, whatever degree of equity is considered desirable. For example, consumers' expenditure could be regulated by much greater use of purchase tax or the adoption of a value-added tax, but unless compensating action is taken considerable hardship is likely to poorer persons.

When the aims of government are considered as a whole, this limits the extent to which any one measure can be used. Favourable effects in one direction tend to be counterbalanced by unfavourable effects in other directions.

The steps outlined can be continued on a flow diagram:

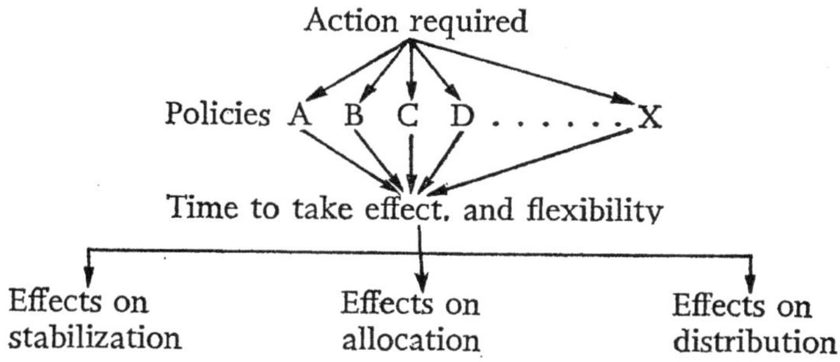

Once it has been decided that action is required, this leads to a consideration of alternative policies indicated by A, B, C, D, ... X. For each policy it is necessary to weigh the time and flexibility elements and their effects on stabilization, allocation and distribution.

Summary

Using the national income figures for 1967, the problem was posed: what alternatives were open to the government if expenditure plans for the following year, of the private and public sectors taken together, exceeded expected output?

The alternatives imply different amounts to be raised by different taxes, different use of resources between public and private goods and different use of resources between consumption and investment goods. The alternatives have only two things in common: they involve unpleasant choices and they require estimates as to whether or not persons and companies are able to compensate for the changes and so nullify the action taken. In practice post-war policy has largely failed to prevent compensatory changes against the increased taxes of either profits or of incomes.

Ideas about a balanced Budget were examined. These ideas have an intuitive appeal to the individual because of the false analogy often made between the economy of the State and of the private household. As is often the case, a number of important issues underlie the discussion about a balanced Budget, and are worth discussing in their own right. To discuss them in the dogmatic context of 'Balance the Budget' obscures rather than illuminates the real issues.

Finally, practical difficulties in establishing just what is happening in the economy, and what measures should be taken if something needs correcting, were outlined and summarized.

21
Monetary and debt policy

. . . economists have had little difficulty in verifying that monetary policy can influence interest rates and credit conditions, and great difficulty in detecting the influences of the latter, or of the quantity of money itself, on economic activity. Nevertheless, very few economists would be prepared to assert, and certainly none has ever attempted to prove, that monetary policy has no influence whatever on the economy.

JOHNSON, H. G. (1967), *Essays in Monetary Economics*.

Introduction

Monetary and debt policy aims at influencing the economic activity of the community by acting on the quantity and composition of money and assets. Indissolubly linked with this is the policy on interest rates. Initially this chapter will be concerned with internal aspects; balance of payments considerations will then be taken up. The last ten years has seen much work in this field at both the empirical and theoretical level. This book attempts no more than to state some of the main issues, many of which have still to be resolved.

Monetary and debt policy

The definition of money as comprising coin, notes and bank deposits was adopted in Part 1. There it was stressed that it must be borne in mind that money has close substitutes in liquid assets, such as Treasury bills. Questions on the quantity of money fall into those dealing with how this quantity can be controlled, and if control can be achieved, is it successful, or does the presence of liquid assets nullify in whole or in part the attempt at control? From a different standpoint, questions were posed on the relation of the quantity of money to prices. Once the simple, but incorrect, idea that there is a direct relation between the two is rejected, it is necessary to look at the reasons for holding money and the effect of other assets on money holdings.

The importance of the composition of assets has been commented on several times. The monetary authorities for much of the post-war period were concerned to reduce the liquidity of the banks for fear that they would use this as a base for extending loans. Also they aimed to reduce the liquidity of the public in general so as to reduce the potential spending power in the economy. The quantity of assets—that is, whether the total is increasing or decreasing—will have repercussions on liquidity, and make it easier or harder for the authorities to maintain the level of liquidity and structure of rates they require.

Monetary policy therefore involves a study of money, assets and interest rates. It is not possible, without drastic simplification, to separate out one of these components for separate study independently of the other components. Indeed, by trying to do so we may obscure the effects we are trying to trace. Monetary and debt analysis thus becomes an attempt to trace the impact on the economy of money, assets and interest rates. An important part of this impact is the action of each of these components on the other.

Money

Working with the definition of money as coin, notes and bank deposits, the conclusion was reached in Part I that the quantity of coin and notes in the British system is not an important policy variable. Control of bank deposits is open to the authorities by a variety of means; the limitations of each measure was dealt with in Chapter 4. These methods were:

1. Open-market operations. } Have direct effects on other
2. Changing Bank Rate. } rates of interest.
3. Use of directives or requests.
4. Special deposits.

1. Open-market sales to the public will tend to depress prices and so drive up the yields on existing securities; conversely, open-market buying will lower yields. Also the issue of new securities will have to take account of the change in yield on old securities. Open-market operations are concerned with government fixed-interest securities and will not thus automatically affect company finance. However, if the change in yield on government securities is expected to be one that will last for some time, it is usual to expect sympathetic changes in other rates, otherwise money will tend to flow to that sector which now offers better terms. As with most relationships, this can be a two-way affair. The yield on existing securities may be used as a

guide by the authorities as to the interest rates to be charged on new government debt. In the words of the *Radcliffe Report*, 'Over much of the period (1945-59), the authorities were therefore entirely passive, indeed fatalistic, in their attitude to the movement of long-term interest rates' (para. 552).

The dilemma is clear: the authorities can set out to control the rates of interest by being willing to buy and sell on the market as required, in which case they cannot have control over the quantity of assets. Or they can control the quantity of assets, in which case they have to forgo control over the rate of interest and let this find the level at which the quantity of assets they have decided on will be held.

2. Changing Bank Rate operates initially on the short end of the market. Given a change in Bank Rate that is expected to continue for some time, it is likely that the long end of the market will be influenced to some extent.

Neither of these two measures as outlined operates directly to change the *quantity* or *supply* of money, as opposed to the *cost* of borrowing. However, it may be the case that open-market operations are undertaken in an attempt to reduce bank deposits and enforce a contraction on banks. By selling securities to the public, the authorities cause the public to exchange some of their bank deposits for government securities—a leakage as far as the banking system is concerned if the authorities do not return the money to the system. The success of this policy depends, as shown earlier, on the willingness of the public to take up new government issues, how they finance these purchases, and on the ease with which the banks can recoup themselves.

Changing interest rates may influence the amount of money people are willing to hold, i.e. the *demand* for money. The higher the rates of interest the more is forgone by keeping a balance in a current banking account. This effect is not thought generally to be very strong. This is the same conclusion that was reached earlier, when the influence of the rate of interest on decision to spend on consumption or investment goods was discussed.

Items 3 and 4. The use of requests and of special deposits do not directly act on interest rates: they are an attempt to restrict the supply of credit that the banks can extend. In Britain it is clear that sufficient pressure can be brought on the banks to make a credit squeeze on the banks effective. The critical question is whether this means an effective squeeze or whether other institutions take up the running.

The conclusion reached earlier was that the presence of other financial institutions with quasi-money assets does to some extent nullify the attempt to limit credit; the expansion that can take place in trade credit and economizing on money balances also helps to limit the effectiveness of a squeeze. However, this is not to say that a squeeze on the banks can be completely counteracted. In particular, certain sectors of the economy—those that traditionally rely on bank credit—are likely to be more seriously affected and to find it more difficult to find substitute finance. In general, small firms and private individuals will be squeezed more than large firms—for example, house purchase, where bridging loans from a bank play an important role, will be affected. Monetary policy has in the past been recommended because its effects were thought to be impersonal, compared to, say, changing indirect taxes, where a decision has to be made as to which articles shall bear the tax. This is seen to be false. A monetary squeeze no less than other measures has directional effects which may be desired or not desired, but cannot be avoided. It remains true, however, that monetary policy has widespread effects on the economy; these are hard to quantify and depend on a number of circumstances—for example, how long the credit squeeze is expected to last.

Monetary assets and rates of interest

We have seen that the monetary authorities are concerned with both the quantity of monetary assets and the composition of them. They are concerned because of the effect on their ability to control the banks and the financial sector, rates of interest, and consumption and investment generally.

The line marked 1 in the diagram below represents the so-called

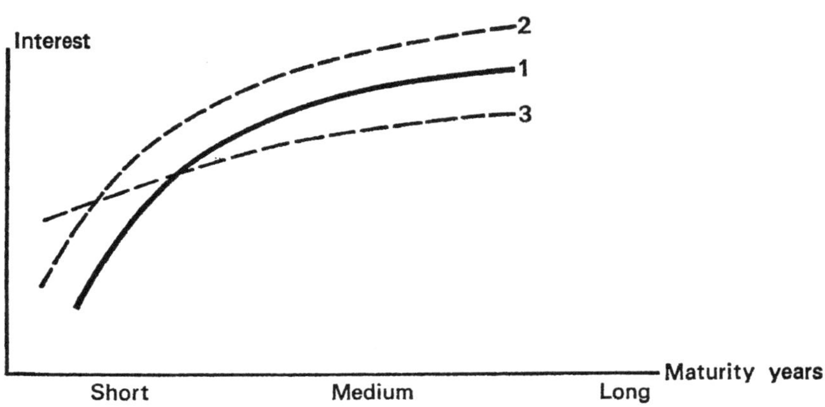

normal-yield curve. It shows the relationship that is usually found between yields and issues of securities of varying maturity, with a similar coupon rate and similar risk in respect of default, e.g. it represents the normal relationship of yield on 6% government securities of varying maturity: other fixed-interest securities will again, as a rule, stand in some stable relationship to yield on government securities.

The yield curve moves sharply up at the short end and then tends to flatten out. The nearer the security is to maturity the more certain is the capital value of the security, the higher yield on longer securities reflects the greater uncertainty as to capital value. An increase in interest rates from say 4% to 6% is not going to make all that difference to the value of a Treasury bill that in any case will be worth its face value in three months. It will make a substantial difference to the market price of a security that is not redeemable for a number of years. Nobody is going to purchase an old security at £100 that yields 4% when a new security that gives 6% can be purchased for £100. The market value of the old security will fall so as to bring its yield into line.

It has already been shown that the monetary authorities can influence the rates of interest in various ways. Here we are talking of a *shift* in the yield curve—say, from curve 1 to curve 2 in the diagram. They can confine their attention to the short end of the market by changing Bank Rate, letting their influence work its way to the longer end of the market. They can conduct open-market operations in longer-term securities and so influence the longer-term direct. Thus selling long-term securities will tend to depress the price and raise the yield; if this is accompanied by an increase in Bank Rate, the yield curve will shift in the direction of curve 2 in the diagram. Selling short-term debt and buying long-term debt will tend to increase the yield on short-term and decrease it on long-term in the manner indicated by curve 3.

One reason why it is necessary to say 'tend to' in any account of influences affecting interest rates is the impossibility of knowing in advance the affect of the influence on expectations and confidence. If a change in Bank Rate, for example, is expected to be reversed in the near future, it is likely to have different results than if it is expected to remain at its new level for some time, and different results again if it is expected to be changed soon in the same direction as the original move.

Other fixed-interest securities, e.g. company debentures, will normally have a slightly higher yield than government securities in order to provide a premium for the risk of default. Again, the action of the market can be expected to keep the yield on government securities and other fixed-interest securities more or less moving together.

When we move to ordinary equity shares of companies, it may be felt intuitively that there should be some connection between yields on fixed-interest securities and yields on equities; but so many other factors play their part in determining the market price of equities that a simple stable relationship is unlikely. In general, we should expect a change in long-term rates on government securities that is expected to last for some time to be reflected in the market for equities by the channelling of some new money, and the channelling of some of the proceeds from the sale of existing securities towards the fixed-interest sector of the market rather than towards the equity market. If such a movement does take place, we have lower prices (i.e. greater yields) in the equity market and the opposite movement in the fixed-interest market. Because risk of default and hopes of gain in the form of dividends paid out by the company and capital value of the equity shares vary so much between companies, and because these hopes and fears need not be linked to (although they may at times be related to) changes in fixed-interest rates, the relationship between equity prices and other security prices is not a direct one. This should not be taken as saying that prices in the two markets are independent of each other. The long-term trend in fixed-interest yields and equity yields will be in the same direction for the reasons indicated: this does not preclude perverse short-term movements in the two kinds of rates.

Influence of interest rates

It has been established so far that the monetary authorities can influence the structure of interest rates in the economy. They do this primarily by Bank Rate and by market operations in their own debt. These effects are fed back by the market and move other fixed-interest rates and perhaps equity rates in the same direction as the movement in government security rates.

It has now to be decided what influence the level of interest rates has on the economy. Here we enter controversial territory. At one extreme we have the view that interest rates are unimportant.

'It seems likely that the interest rates, or the system of rates, will continue to receive from theoreticians the homage due to a ceremonial monarch, without in fact counting for more than such a monarch in the real affairs of western nations' (Shackle, G. L. S. (1961), 252).

Those that hold that interest rates are important have to demonstrate not only a connection between various interest rates (on the lines of the previous section), but a connection between interest rates and real variables in the economy, i.e. between consumption and/or investment.

At several points we have discussed the influence of interest rates, only to conclude that these effects are, at best, very weak ones. Thus both consumption and investment seem relatively insensitive to changes in interest rates. Consumers are affected by changes in down-payment of hire-purchase agreements, but little change is noticed if the interest element of the agreement changes. Many factors are present in a decision whether or not to undertake real investment, and because many investments are required to pay for themselves over a period of a few years a change in interest rates is not likely to change many investment plans. Changes in interest rates are also softened because some fixed-interest charges such as debenture interest and bank overdraft charges, can be offset against tax. If other factors that influence the investment decision change adversely, in addition to an increase in interest rates, an investment project may well be abandoned. For example, if the cost of the investment goes up due to an increase in prices and the expected returns from the investment decrease due to a change in demand for the particular end product of the investment concerned, then these adverse factors will be weighed with the increase in interest rates. In these circumstances it appears to be stretching the use of language and logic to ascribe the investment decision as depending on the rate of interest. As the projected life of the investment goes up the rate of interest plays an increasingly important part: the weight given to this factor has to be increased, but still a variety of factors play their part in the final decision whether to go ahead or not with the investment. Attempts to link changes in the rate of interest with changes in the supply of money via the liquidity effect were also discounted.

Thus far, with the important exception of investments involving long-lived capital installations, we do appear to be dealing with a 'ceremonial monarch' with little real power to influence real variables in the economy. Let us approach this question from a different angle. The stock of financial assets in the economy is very large, and is very large in relation to the flow of new financial assets coming on to the market in any financial period—say, a year. Now the stock of assets must be held by somebody or some institution. Securities can only be sold if somebody else is willing to purchase them. The prices of existing securities will affect the price at which new securities will find willing holders.

It is submitted that, because the amount of existing securities is very large in relation to new issues in a year, the causation runs from the yield on existing securities determining the conditions under which a new issue can be successful rather than from new issues influencing to any great extent the yield on old securities. It is now possible to distinguish two important ways that current yields can influence investment.

Firstly, if current holders of existing securities are content with low yields (i.e. prices of securities are 'high'), firms find the stock market buoyant, and issues of new securities are easier and more profitable. Easier because the market is buoyant, and more profitable because the securities can be issued at a higher price (lower yield). The reverse situation also holds: a depressed market makes it harder and more costly to raise new money by the issue of securities. Thus investment which has to be financed by the issue of securities can be influenced if the stock market can be influenced.[1] It has been argued in the previous section that a change in interest rates on government securities which compete on the market with company issues can have this effect.[2] As an example, the case of an increase in Bank Rate will be taken. Two strands of influence can be picked out: (1) The relative effect: that, because rates on government securities have increased, rates on company securities will have to adjust in the same direction; and (2) effects on confidence. If raising Bank Rate is taken as a sign that a period of restriction is on hand (and particularly if it is accompanied by other measures which depress the

[1] The crucial assumption in this sentence is 'investment which has to be financed by the issue of securities'. Little evidence is available on the extent to which investment, intended to be financed by an issue of securities, is deferred or abandoned, when the stock market becomes unfavourable. The alternative is to go ahead with the investment, if temporary finance is available, with the intention of repaying this when an issue can be made on more favourable terms. Temporary finance is usually costly and is likely to deter the use of this method.

[2] The oral evidence of the representatives of the Issuing Houses Association to the Radcliffe Committee, Minutes of Evidence, Questions 4001-167, is germane. Three strands can be distinguished. Did a change in interest rates affect new issues (1) by freezing the market for technical reasons, i.e. because of interruption of the mechanism for making new issues, (2) by affecting the supply of capital, or (3) by affecting the demand for capital? The effects under (1) and (2) were generally discounted, but the third heading raised some interesting replies: 'The whole terms of an issue depend on the Bank Rate and gilt-edged prices, and if we thought there were likely to be very wide or large fluctuations in the Bank Rate we should just have to be more careful' (Question 4039).

'Presumably it is part of the job of the issuing house, advising their clients, to consider that economic climate, and they would be considering their assessment, in the light of that and of the possibility of a movement in the Bank Rate' (Question 4044).

'But, generally speaking, I would think that the actual mechanical fact of raising the Bank Rate merely means a mechanical adjustment of rates. It might in certain cases make borrowing too expensive; and some people might say that they would not go ahead' (Question 4045).

economy or particular sectors of it), then (1) and (2), taken together, may operate to have a sizeable affect on Stock Exchange prices as a whole or of the particular sectors concerned. In addition, the authorities can influence the market in other ways, e.g. by asking for dividend restraint or altering company tax or allowances.

Secondly, if the return which a firm is receiving from its existing real investment is below the average yield on financial assets, incentive to undertake further real investment will be low. The prudent firm will hold any funds it has in financial assets which will give it a greater return than putting it into real assets. Also it will not attempt to raise money on the market at a cost which exceeds the expected return. This reasoning will not hold in every individual case: it is not difficult, for example, to imagine circumstances where a firm can find profitable real investment outlets even though the yield from its existing real capital is low. However, as an explanation of aggregate behaviour of the real investment market, this influence is likely to be a powerful one.

It may be questioned whether the above reasoning is sufficient to reinstate the influence of interest rates as an important force in the economy. Because it is not possible to point to immediate and direct effects of changes in rates, it is not necessarily correct to assume either that influences are absent or, if present, that they must be weak. Empirical investigations yield as yet no conclusive results. Trying to measure the influence of the rate of interest has much in common with trying to measure the influence of love. We may be quite certain in our minds that both exercise a powerful influence on human affairs, but it is beyond our capacity to demonstrate this conclusively to the sceptic.

External considerations

Monetary and debt policy has major implications for the balance of payments. This is particularly true of a country like Great Britain, which is one of the world's financial centres. One effect follows from the fact that part of the national debt is held by other than British residents. Servicing this part of the debt therefore results in a flow of payments overseas and pressure on the balance of payments. There is thus a possibility that rates of interest considered desirable for internal purposes clash with rates considered desirable for external reasons. The effect on the balance of payments of the external debt depends on a number of considerations. In particular, it depends on whether the overseas holder is prepared (for a time) to hold sterling balances—that is, in effect, to reinvest in sterling securities—or whether these holders convert into gold or foreign currencies. The only official estimate of the effect was given in the *Radcliffe Report* (para. 438). They estimated that a 1% increase in Bank Rate, on the assumption that other short-term rates rise by the same amount, affects the balance of payments adversely to the extent of £15 million a year. This figure can vary a great deal, depending on the amount and type of debt held abroad, the reactions of these holders, and the extent to which transactions are covered in the forward exchange market.

A relative change in interest rates between countries, or changes in confidence, may cause flows of money between financial centres. So-called 'hot' money is money invested short-term for speculative reasons and in order to take advantage of differentials in interest rates. A change in confidence or in interest differentials will reverse the flow. The danger of these flows of short-term money is that they may cause (taking Great Britain as an example) a 'run on the £1'. Since there is nothing to distinguish 'hot' money from other sterling balances (although some idea of the magnitudes involved may be built up from a knowledge of the lenders), an adverse balance of payments caused by the outflow of these volatile funds may so unsettle other foreign holders that they too seek to convert their sterling holdings into gold or foreign currencies, and a run on the £1 is under way. The primary fear is that a devaluation of sterling will take place, which would reduce the value of sterling balances in terms of gold and other currencies. We have therefore an added reason why rates of interest in one country need to take account of rates ruling in other financial centres.

Flows of money between countries depend on much more than differential interest rates; these other influences are usually summed up by the word 'confidence'. In the post-war period Bank Rate has usually been changed only as part of a 'package deal'. That is to say, other things are altered at the same time. For example, an increase in Bank Rate may be accompanied by all, or some, of the following measures: restrictions on the banks; hire purchase made less attractive by increasing the down-payment and decreasing the period over which payments can be spread; restrictions on currency movements; and tax increases. In these circumstances the 'package deal' of which Bank Rate forms a part may restore confidence that sterling is not going to be devalued and result in a substantial improvement in the reserve position—that is, foreign holders are willing to retain their sterling holdings and many of those who caused the adverse outflow by exchanging sterling for gold or other currencies are induced to return to sterling.

This section has confined itself to looking at the main implications of monetary and debt policy on the balance of payments. The subject of the balance of payments is complex: students interested in pursuing it should refer to the literature on the subject. In particular, this book assumes throughout that the present system of fixed exchange rates will be maintained, and policy is looked at in the light of this constraint. There are a few economists who advocate flexible exchange rates and many more who have indicated the need for improvements in the system of international payments. These are important issues which lie outside the scope of this book. From a policy point of view, it is clear that if a satisfactory balance of payments could be achieved by internal means or by international co-operation this would leave more scope for monetary and debt policy to be used to influence the home economy.

Conclusion

The monetary authorities, because of the size and importance of their operations, are not in a position to adopt a 'neutral' policy, where they can leave market forces to determine interest rates and the size and composition of money and assets.

Although policy changes in this field have effects on the internal economy, these effects are not precise, nor can their magnitude be predicted very accurately. Reasons for this stressed the part played by expectations and the effects on confidence. Thus rates of interest above traditional levels may yet stimulate, rather than depress, economic activity, if it is generally thought that rates will shortly go higher and remain higher for some time. Similarly, rates of interest below traditional levels may depress rather than stimulate activity if it is thought rates will shortly go lower and remain lower for some time.

External effects of changes in policy are, unlike internal effects, often very quick to take effect, but they share with internal effects the difficulty of predicting the magnitude of the change. Maintaining confidence that the currency will not be devalued is the most important external role of monetary and debt policy, but monetary and debt policy is only one (although an important one) of the factors affecting confidence.

The conclusions that emerge from consideration of the internal and external effects of monetary and debt policy are contradictory. Internal considerations point to its use as a long-term rather than a short-term instrument of control. External considerations point to its usefulness, particularly in the short-term. This clash goes some way to explain the contradictions that are found in post-war policy.

Given this contradiction, it is possible for purposes of exposition to extract three alternative policies:

At one extreme, policy in this field could concentrate on internal effects. Monetary and debt policies would be pursued with long-term internal economic considerations in mind. Of necessity, this would leave fiscal and other policies to take care of short-term fluctuations and the balance of payments. The chief difficulties are presented by the latter. Control in the short-term was dealt with at length in the previous chapter. Control of the balance of payments is only briefly looked at in this volume. Short-term control by means of capital movements and exchange restrictions are subject to international agreement. More fundamental long-term improvements to the balance of payments by improving Britain's export performance have largely been sought in vain. Fundamental changes in the world's system of international payments require international co-operation and agreement of a kind which has been most conspicuous by its absence.

At the other extreme, policy could concentrate on the external repercussions of monetary and debt policy, leaving internal regulation to be largely carried out by other means. This policy leaves a wide variety of methods open for the achievement of this aim. Thus firms could be at least partially isolated from the effects of high interest rates (set for external reasons) by appropriate tax measures or cheap lending policies. If the structure of the debt judged right for external reasons differed from the structure judged right for purposes of internal control over the monetary system, the banks and other financial institutions could likewise be partially screened by appropriate reserve requirements and other measures.

The third policy makes no attempt to separate the domestic economy from the international economy, considering each as part of an indivisible whole. Monetary and debt policy, where internal and external considerations differ, would compromise, and fiscal and other methods would be used to reinforce the policy where it fell short.

It is not the purpose of this volume to canvass one of these policies over the others. It should be clear from the previous analysis that what is the best policy in one set of circumstances may not be so in another set of circumstances. In economics there is no golden rule that can be applied that allows escape from the long and exhausting examination and evaluation of current and expected conditions.

Summary

This chapter started with a résumé of how effectively the monetary authorities can control the supply of money and credit. The authorities are in the dilemma of being able to influence *either* rates of interest *or* the quantity of assets. Their main influence on rates of interest is by changing Bank Rate and by open-market operations.

The influence of interest rates on the economy is important because it will attract or repel funds from abroad, and is likely to have some effect on long-lived capital investment. Other effects on the economy are harder to pinpoint, although if the stock market can be influenced this is likely to affect companies thinking of raising new money by a stock or share issue. The impact of a change in interest rates is difficult to measure because it depends so much on whether the change affects, and in what direction it affects, confidence and business expectations.

This section of the book set out with the limited aim of showing just how difficult management of the economy is, whether this is attempted by fiscal or monetary means. It is not just that our theories about how the economy operates are imperfect and our knowledge of the facts imprecise: given perfection in both cases, there would still be disagreement because value judgments enter as to which way should be selected out of numerous possible ways to achieve any particular object. This has important policy implications which are developed in the next and final chapter.

22
Conclusions

There are times when some aspects of our economic situation have what is almost a Biblical quality: 'And life becomes harder in those times, and the people refused to co-operate one with another. Citizen was pitched against citizen, and there was disarray in that country's market-place. Few were content with their lot, and none could determine how the fruits of the land should be shared. Whereupon there came unto the midst of the people, a prophet who told them: "There is much waste in the land because the people are divided." And the queen of that country did summon the prophet to the palace, and did charge him to bring peace and prosperity unto the land.'

WILLIAM KEEGAN, *Financial Times*, October 9th, 1967.
Commenting on the Prices and Incomes Board.

Part III of this book sets out to analyse the problems of managing the economy via fiscal and monetary policies. The conclusions are pessimistic: that within the existing state of knowledge effects of policy are frequently uncertain and always difficult to quantify. The need for better data, collected more quickly, seems self-evident. To the author these facts lead to an important positive result: that the first priority of a fiscal system should be equity. Inevitably objectives that include equity, full employment, stability of the value of money, a satisfactory balance of payments, and emphasis on growth will show conflicts. Without equity, the achievement of these other objectives are likely to be harmed. The morale of taxpayers is at a low ebb, as has been brought out at numerous points of this book. The fact is that large numbers of citizens *feel* the current system to be unjust. The most frequent complaints are made about high marginal rates of tax at one extreme, and at the other extreme the existence of large pockets of poverty, particularly amongst the old, the young, and the disabled.

This book has attempted to show that both of these criticisms are largely justified and they follow inevitably from the structure of tax and benefits that has been adopted. Piecemeal adaptation of the system has been ruled out as a solution, since this has resulted in the past in yet more anomalies and complexities in the system. The solution has been envisaged basically in terms of recasting the tax base.

It is clear that a solution on these lines needs to be backed by a full-scale study, with detailed facts and figures; it is equally clear that such a study is beyond the scope of this book and of a single person. One country has recently undertaken such an investigation in depth, and a brief summary of the main recommendations and results follow. It is not suggested that the tax conditions in the two countries are identical, but they do have a lot in common. In particular, there are common problems of high marginal rates of tax that are easily avoided, harsh treatment of low-income families and disincentives that follow from the existing tax structure.

The Report of the Royal Commission on Taxation of Canada, produced in 1966, is a lengthy, complex report in six volumes. The Commission was appointed in 1962 and the inquiry cost nearly $3,500,000: Its major proposals were:

The ability-to-pay principle would be reflected in a new 'comprehensive tax base' that would include, for tax purposes, all net gains in purchasing power, including capital gains and windfalls and many other forms of real income that now are tax-exempt.

Rates of personal income tax would be greatly reduced from the present top rate of 80% to 50%.

New tax-paying units would be created and a different rate schedule would apply to each: families (parents and children under twenty-one, or twenty-five if receiving education) and individuals. Families must aggregate income. Gifts within the family would not count for tax purposes until a child was eligible for tax treatment on his own, when tax adjustments would be made.

Anyone with large fluctuations in income would be permitted to average that income over a five-year period, provided the tax saving amounted to more than $50 (to avoid numerous claims), and provided that income in the lowest year of the average period is less than 75% of income of the highest year. Special averaging rate schedules would be available, so that only one computation of tax needs to be made, instead of a new computation for each year averaged.

Corporations would be taxed at 50%, but the shareholder would receive credit for this. The shareholder, that is, would be liable at his personal rate for gross dividends and capital gains on his shares, but would be credited with the 50% tax paid by corporations.

Studies indicated that as a result of their recommendations and assuming the same amount of revenue raised, 46% of the country's

7 million taxpayers would get income cuts of more than 15%.

The Commission emphasized that their proposals should be considered as part of a 'package deal' and that to select some of their proposals and reject others would probably wreck the intentions of their proposals.

The Commission paid much attention to other objectives besides equity; particularly to the effects on growth. They said that the principal objective was to design a tax system that would be fair, but one that would not erode future sources of income simply in order to redistribute current income. They believe that this goal has been achieved while providing for more Canadian ownership of Canadian industry without discriminating against foreign investors, and also achieving an improved allocation of savings.

> We hope Canadians will accept the challenge implicit in our recommendations. And there can be no doubt that our recommendations constitute a great challenge. Preconceived opinions about taxation are deeply and firmly held. Many will find it difficult to take a new look at old questions. Because some facts cannot be readily ascertained, honest differences of opinion are inevitable. There is a danger that the debate about these minor factual questions will divert attention from the major issues (Vol. I, 2).

There is therefore evidence, backed by detailed investigations, from a country with a tax system not so very different from Britain's and faced with similar problems and inequities, that a tax system can be devised that would overcome many of these problems. The author feels that the time is now overdue for a full-scale investigation on comprehensive lines in this country. The proposed entry to the Common Market already dictates, because they have adopted a system of value-added tax, that this area of taxation be investigated. But yet another Commission with limited terms of reference is not the answer; nothing short of a comprehensive look at the whole field of tax and benefits is likely to be able to come to grips with the problems that have been outlined.

The difficulties of controlling the economy have been stressed. If equity was achieved in the tax and benefit structure, these problems would still remain, but equity could be achieved without harmful effects on other objectives.

Income tax changes would probably still remain the chief method of affecting consumption expenditures. Management would be easier with a wider tax base with a smoother progression and lower marginal rates of tax. Britain has developed over the years a new fiscal weapon in the form of investment allowances and grants to industry, which, despite their drawbacks, can be used to influence investment. If investment grants and allowances are used in this way, the taxation of companies on the lines indicated in Chapter 13 would go a long way to ensuring more equitable treatment between individuals and companies. The shareholder pays income tax both on his gross dividends and any capital gains on the sale of his shares, and can be credited with tax paid by the company. The public at large gain if the investment results in a better or cheaper product. Finally, an indispensable prerequisite for the control of inflation by means of a prices and incomes policy is, it has been argued, a fiscal system that tries to achieve equity.

Society in Britain is fortunate in having reached a stage where it can afford to think, not only in terms of growth, but also in terms of the quality of life of its citizens. The means are available if we have the will.

Works cited

ABEL-SMITH, B. and TOWNSEND, P. (1965), *The Poor and the Poorest*, Bell.

'Administration of the Wage Stop' (1967), Ministry of Social Security.

'Administrative Structure of the Medical and Related Services in England and Wales' (1968), Ministry of Health.

'Annual Report of the Ministry of Health' (1967), H.M.S.O.

'Annual Report of the Ministry of Social Security' (1967), H.M.S.O.

ARTIS, M. J. (1965), *Foundations of British Monetary Policy*, Blackwell.

'Bank Charges' (1967), Report No. 34, National Board for Prices and Incomes.

'Bank Liquidity in the United Kingdom' (December, 1962), *Bank of England Quarterly Bulletin.*

BEVERIDGE, W. H. (1944), *Full Employment in a Free Society*, George Allen & Unwin.

BREAK, G. F. (September, 1957), 'Income Taxes and Incentives to Work', *American Economic Review*, XLVII.

BRITTAN, S. (1964), *The Treasury under the Tories, 1951-1964*, Pelican.

BRONFENBRENNER, M. and HOLZMAN, F. D. (September, 1963), 'Survey of Inflation Theory', *American Economic Review*, LIII, No. 4.

CAVES, R. E. (1968), ed. for the Brookings Institute of Washington, *Britain's Economic Prospects*, George Allen & Unwin.

'Circumstances of Families' (1967), Ministry of Social Security.

COLE, D. and UTTING, J. (1962), *The Economic Circumstances of Old People*, Codicote Press.

'Commentary' (March, 1966), *Bank of England Quarterly Bulletin.*

'Committee on the Working of the Monetary System' (1959), Cmnd. 827.

'Committee on Turnover Tax' (1964), Cmnd. 2300.

'Conditions Favourable to Faster Growth' (1963), National Economic Development Council.

'Control of Bank Lending: the Cash Deposits Scheme' (June, 1968), *Bank of England Quarterly Bulletin.*

'Corporation Tax' (1965), Cmnd. 2646.

CRAMP, A. B. (February, 1963), 'Banks and Their Competitors', *The Banker.*

—— (June, 1966), 'Control of the Money Supply', *Economic Journal.*

—— (October, 1967), 'The Control of Bank Deposits', *Lloyds Bank Review.*

CROUCH, R. L. (December, 1964), 'The Inadequacy of "New Orthodox" Methods of Monetary Control', *Economic Journal.*

—— (August, 1965), 'The Genesis of Bank Deposits, New English Version', *Bulletin of the Oxford Institute of Statistics.*

CYRIAX, G. (March, 1968), 'Tax Incentives—A New Urgency', *The Banker.*

DALTON, H. (1959), *The Inequality of Incomes,* Routledge & Kegan Paul.

DANIEL, W. W. D. (March, 1968), 'Personal Taxation and Occupational Incentives', *The Banker.*

DENMAN, D. R. (1958), *Origins of Ownership,* George Allen & Unwin.

'Development Areas Regional Employment Premium' (1967), Cmnd. 3310.

'Distribution of the National Debt' (March, 1967), *Bank of England Quarterly Bulletin.*

DOW, J. C. R. (1964), *The Management of the British Economy, 1945-60,* C.U.P.

DREES, W., JR. (1967), 'Efficiency in Government Spending', *Public Finance,* XXII, Nos. 1-2/1967.

EISENSTEIN, L. (1961). *The Ideologies of Taxation,* New York: The Ronald Press.

EISNER, R. and STROTZ, R. H. (1963), 'Determinants of Business Investment', contained in *Impacts of Monetary Policy,* Prentice-Hall.

'Employment Policy' (1944), Cmnd. 6527.

'Expert Committee on Compensation and Betterment' (1942), Cmnd. 6386.

FELDSTEIN, M. S. (December, 1967), 'The Effectiveness of the British Differential Profits Tax', *Economic Journal.*

FERGUSON, J. M., ed. (1964), *Public Debt and Future Generations,* University of North Carolina Press.

Financial Accounts of the U.K. H.M.S.O.

'Financial Institutions' (June, 1965), *Bank of England Quarterly Bulletin.*

Financial Statistics (Monthly publication), Central Statistical Office.

FRIEDMAN, M. (1962), *Capitalism and Freedom,* University of Chicago Press.

GRUNDY, J. M. (1956), *Tax Problems of the Family Company,* Sweet & Maxwell.

HARBURY, C. D. (December, 1962), 'Inheritance in the Distribution of Personal Wealth', *Economic Journal.*

HARCOURT, G. C. and WHITTINGTON, G. (June, 1965), 'A Comment on the Irrelevancy of the British Differential Profits Tax', *Economic Journal.*

HEMMING, M. F. W. (August, 1965), 'Social Security in Britain and Certain Other Countries', *National Institute Economic Review,* No. 33.

—— and DUFFY, H. (August, 1964), 'The Price of Accommodation', *National Institute Economic Review,* No. 29.

HOCKLEY, G. C. (May/June, 1967), 'Taxation and the Employment of Married Women', *British Tax Review.*

—— (January/February, 1968), 'Capital Gains and Inflation' and a 'Rejoinder', *British Tax Review.*

—— (March, 1968), 'Incentives under a Value-added Tax', *The Banker.*

'How the Banks Compete for Deposits' (July, 1967), *The Banker.*

'Incidence of Taxes and Social Service Benefits' (February, 1968 and July, 1968), *Economic Trends,* Nos. 172 and 177.

'Inflows and Outflows of Foreign Funds' (June, 1962), *Bank of England Quarterly Bulletin.*

'Investment Incentives' (1966), Cmnd. 2874.
JOHNSON, H. G. (1967), *Essays in Monetary Economics*, George Allen & Unwin.
KALDOR, N. (1955), *An Expenditure Tax*, George Allen & Unwin.
KEYNES, J. M. (1936), *The General Theory of Employment, Interest and Money*, Macmillan.
—— (1940), *How to Pay for the War*, Macmillan.
'Land Commission' (1965), Cmnd. 2771.
LEES, D. (October, 1967), 'Families and Fiscal Reform', *Lloyds Bank Review*.
'London Money Market' (May, 1966), *Midland Bank Review*.
'Management of Money Day by Day' (March, 1963), *Bank of England Quarterly Bulletin*.
MEADE, J. E. (1964), *Efficiency, Equality and the Ownership of Property*, George Allen & Unwin.
MERRITT, A. J. (1968), *Executive Remuneration in the* U.K., Longmans.
—— and MONK, D. A. G. (1967), *Inflation Taxation and Executive Remuneration*, Hallam Press.
MISHAN, E. J. (1967), *The Costs of Economic Growth*, Staples Press.
'More Light on Personal Saving' (April, 1965), *Economic Trends*.
MUSGRAVE, R. A. (1959), *The Theory of Public Finance*, McGraw-Hill.
—— and SHOUP, C. S., eds. (1959), *Readings in the Economics of Taxation*, George Allen & Unwin.
MYRDAL, G. (1960), *Beyond the Welfare State*, Duckworth.
'National Income and Expenditure' (1968), Central Statistical Office.
'Nationalized Industries: A Review of Economic and Financial Objectives', (November, 1967), Cmnd. 3437.
'National Superannuation & Social Insurance Proposals for Earnings-Related Social Security' (1969), Cmnd. 3883.
NEWLYN, W. T. (June, 1964), 'The Supply of Money and Its Control', *Economic Journal*.
'Note Circulation' (March, 1965), *Bank of England Quarterly Bulletin*.
'Official Transactions in the Gilt-edged Market' (June, 1966), *Bank of England Quarterly Bulletin*.
'Overseas and Foreign Banks in London' (September, 1961 and June, 1968), *Bank of England Quarterly Bulletin*.
PEACOCK, A. T. and SHANNON, R. (August, 1968) 'The Welfare State and the Redistribution of Income', *Westminster Bank Review*.
PEACOCK, A. T. (January, 1964), 'Problems of Government Budgetary Reform', *Lloyds Bank Review*.
—— and WISEMAN, J. (1961), *The Growth of Public Expenditure in the United Kingdom*, O.U.P.
'Post Office Giro' (1965), Cmnd. 2751.
PREST, A. R. (1968), 'The Budget and Interpersonal Distribution', *Public Finance*, XXIII, Nos. 1-2/1968.
'Radcliffe Report'. Refer to 'Committee on the Working of the Monetary System' (1959).
'Railway Policy' (November, 1967), Cmnd. 3439.
'Reform of the Exchequer Accounts' (1963), Cmnd. 2014.

'Report of the Canadian Royal Commission on Taxation' (1966). Queen's Printer, Ottawa, Canada.

'Report on the U.S. Commission on Money and Credit (1961), Prentice-Hall.

'Report of the Committee on Local Authority and Allied Personal Social Services' (1968), Cmnd. 3703.

'Report of the Committee on the Taxation of Trading Profits' (1951), Cmnd. 8189.

REVELL, J. R. S. and HOCKLEY, G. C. (July and December, 1960), 'A Survey of the Holders of Local Authority Debt', *Local Government Finance.*

ROBINSON, J. (1962), *Economic Philosophy*, Pelican.

'Royal Commission on the Taxation of Profits and Income' (1954), Second Report, Cmnd. 9105, and (1955) Final Report, Cmnd. 9474.

RUBNER, A. (June, 1964), 'The Irrelevancy of the British Differential Profits Tax', *Economic Journal.*

SANDFORD, C. T. (1965), 'Taxing Inheritance and Capital Gains', Hobart Paper, No. 32.

—— (April, 1967), 'The Swedes can do It, why can't We?' *The Banker.*

'Selective Employment Tax' (1966), Cmnd. 2986.

SEWILL, H. (November, 1966), 'Automatic Unit for National Taxation and Insurance,' Conservative New Techniques, No. 6.

SHACKLE, G. L. S. (June, 1961), 'Recent Theories concerning the Nature and Role of Interest', *Economic Journal.*

SHULTZ, W. J. and HARRISS, C. L. (1965), *American Public Finance*, 8th edition, Prentice-Hall.

SIMONS, H. (1938), *Personal Income Taxation*, Chicago.

'Social Insurance and Allied Services' (1942), Cmnd. 6404.

'Social Services for All?' (1968), various authors, Fabian Society Tracts, Nos. 382-5.

Statistical Abstracts of the U.K., H.M.S.O.

STONE, R. and others (1962), *A Computable Model of Economic Growth*, Chapman & Hall.

SUITS, D. B. (1963), 'The Determinants of Consumer Expenditure: a Review of Present Knowledge', contained in *Impacts of Monetary Policy*, 1-57, Prentice-Hall.

'Taxation of Trading Profits' (1951), Cmnd. 8189.

TEW, B. and HENDERSON, R. F. (1959), eds., *Company Income and Finance, 1949-53*, C.U.P.

TITMUS, R. M. (1962), *Income Distribution and Social Change*, Unwin University Books.

—— (1963), *Essays on 'the Welfare State'*, Unwin University Books.

TOBIN, J. (1963), 'An Essay on Principles of Debt Management', contained in *Fiscal and Debt Management Policies*, Prentice-Hall.

VICKRAY, W. (1947), *Agenda for Progressive Taxation*, New York: The Ronald Press.

WHEATCROFT, G. S. A. (January/February, 1968), 'A Reply to "Capital Gains and Inflation"', *British Tax Review.*

WILLIAMS, B. R. (1967), 'The New Social Contract', Conservative Political Centre.

Further reading

The following is intended as an introduction to books for further reading. The list is far from exhaustive: more specialized references can be obtained from the list of 'Works Cited' in this volume.

THE MONETARY SYSTEM

Committee on the Working of the Monetary System (1959), Cmd. 827.

Day, A. C. L., *The Economics of Money*, 2nd edition 1968, O.U.P.

Sayers, R. S., *Modern Banking*, 7th edition 1967, O.U.P.

PUBLIC FINANCE Texts with U.K. emphasis

Hicks, U. K., *Public Finance*, 3rd edition 1968, C.U.P.

Prest, A. R., *Public Finance*, 3rd edition 1967, Weidenfeld & Nicolson.

OTHER

Musgrave, R. A., *The Theory of Public Finance*, 1959, McGraw-Hill. An advanced theoretical text.

Musgrave, R. A. & Peacock, A. T., *Classics in the Theory of Public Finance*, 1958, New York: The Macmillan Company.

Readings in the Economics of Taxation, 1959, Allen & Unwin.

POLICY

Brittan, S., *The Treasury under the Tories 1951-1964*, 1964, Pelican.

Caves, R. E., ed., *Britain's Economic Prospects*, 1968, Allen & Unwin.

Dow, J. C. R., *The Management of the British Economy 1945-60*, 1964, C.U.P.

Index

For Product Safety Concerns and Information please contact our EU representative GPSR@taylorandfrancis.com
Taylor & Francis Verlag GmbH, Kaufingerstraße 24, 80331 München, Germany

www.ingramcontent.com/pod-product-compliance
Ingram Content Group UK Ltd.
Pitfield, Milton Keynes, MK11 3LW, UK
UKHW022217190926
475702UK00003B/401

9781138704794